SI Conversion Factors for Values in Clinical Chemistry

Component	Present Reference Intervals (Examples)	Present Unit	Conversion Factor	SI Reference Intervals	SI Unit Symbol	Suggested Minimum Increment
acetone (B,S)	0	mg/dL	172.2	0	μmol/L	10 μmol/L
acid phosphatase (S)	0–5.5	U/L	16.67	0–90	nkat/L	2 nkat/L
adrenocorticotropin (ACTH) (P)	20–100	pg/mL	0.2202	4–22	pmol/L	1 pmol/L
alanine aminotransferase (ALT) (S)	0–35	U/L	0.01667	0–0.58	μkat/L	0.02μkat/L
albumin (S)	4.0–6.0	g/dL	10.0	40–60	g/L	1 g/L
aldolase (S)	0–6	U/L	16.67	0–100	nkat/L	20 nkat/L
aldosterone (S)						
normal salt diet	8.1–15.5	ng/dL	27.74	220–430	pmol/L	10 pmol/L
alkaline phosphatase (S)	30–20	U/L	0.01667	0.5–2.0	μkat/L	0.1 μkat/L
$alpha_1$-antitrypsin (S)	150–350	mg/dL	0.01	1.5–3.5	g/L	0.1 g/L
alpha-fetoprotein (S)	0–20	ng/mL	1.00	0–20	μg/L	1 μg/L
ammonia (vP)						
as ammonia (NH_3)	10–80	μg/dL	0.5872	5–50	μmol/L	5 μmol/L
amylase (S)	0–130	U/L	0.01667	0–2.17	μkat/L	0.01 μkat/L
aspartate aminotransferase (AST) (S)	0–35	U/L	0.01667	0–0.58	μkat/L	0.01 μkat/L
bilirubin, total (S)	0.1–1.0	mg/dL	17.10	2–18	μmol/L	2 μmol/L
bilirubin, conjugated (S)	0–0.2	mg/dL	17.10	0–4	μmol/L	2 μmol/L
calcium (S)						
male	8.8–10.3	mg/dL	0.2495	2.20–2.58	mmol/L	0.02 mmol/L
female <50y	8.8–10.0	mg/dL	0.2495	2.20–2.50	mmol/L	0.02 mmol/L
female ≥50y	8.8–10.2	mg/dL	0.2495	2.20–2.56	mmol/L	0.02 mmol/L
	4.4–5.1	mEq/L	0.500	2.20–2.56	mmol/L	0.02 mmol/L
calcium ion (S)	2.00–2.30	mEq/L	0.500	1.00–1.15	mmol/L	0.01 mmol/L
calcium (U), normal diet	<250	mg/24 h	0.02495	<6.2	mmol/d	0.01 mmol/d
carbon dioxide content (B,P,S) (bicarbonate + CO_2)	22–28	mEq/L	1.00	22–28	mmol/L	1 mmol/L
chloride (S)	95–105	mEq/L	1.00	95–105	mmol/L	1 mmol/L
cholesterol (P)						
<29 years	<200	mg/dL	0.02586	<5.20	mmol/L	0.05 mmol/L
complement, C3 (S)	70–160	mg/dL	0.01	0.7–1.6	g/L	0.1 g/L
complement, C4 (S)	20–40	mg/dL	0.01	0.2–0.4	g/L	0.1 g/L
cortisol (S)						
0800 h	4–19	μg/dL	27.59	110–520	nmol/L	10 nmol/L
creatine kinase isoenzymes (S)	0–130	U/L	0.01667	0–2.16	μkat/L	0.01 μkat/L
MB fraction	>5	%	0.01	>0.05	1	0.01
creatinine (S)	0.6–1.2	mg/dL	88.40	50–110	μmol/L	10 μmol/L

(see reverse side)

SI Conversion Factors for Values in Clinical Chemistry

Component	Present Reference Intervals (Examples)	Present Unit	Conversion Factor	SI Reference Intervals	SI Unit Symbol	Suggested Minimum Increment
desipramine (P)						
therapeutic	50–200	ng/mL	3.754	170–700	nmol/L	10 nmol/L
digoxin (P)						
therapeutic	0.5–2.2	ng/mL	1.281	0.6–2.8	nmol/L	0.1 nmol/L
	0.5–2.2	μg/L	1.281	0.6–2.8	nmol/L	0.1 nmol/L
electrophoresis, protein (S)						
albumin	60–65	%	0.01	0.60–0.65	1	0.01
alpha$_1$-globulin	1.7–5.0	%	0.01	0.02–0.05	1	0.01
alpha$_2$-globulin	6.7–12.5	%	0.01	0.07–0.13	1	0.01
beta-globulin	8.3–16.3	%	0.01	0.08–0.16	1	0.01
gamma-globulin	10.7–20.0	%	0.01	0.11–0.20	1	0
estrogens (S) (as estradiol)						
female	20–300	pg/mL	3.671	70–1100	pmol/L	10 pmol/L
ethanol (P)						
legal limit (driving)	<80	mg/dL	0.2171	<17	mmol/L	1 mmol/L
toxic	>100	mg/dL	0.2171	>22	mmol/L	1 mmol
ferritin (S)	18–300	ng/mL	1.00	18–300	μg/L	10 μg/L
fibrinogen (P)	200–400	mg/dL	0.01	2.0–4.0	g/L	0.1 g/L
folate (Erc)	140–960	ng/mL	2.266	550–2200	nmol/L	10 nmol/L
follicle-stimulating hormone (FSH) (P)						
female	2.0–15.0	mIU/mL	1.00	2–15	IU/L	1 IU/L
peak production	20–50	mIU/ml	1.00	20–50	IU/L	1 IU/L
male	1.0–10.0	mIU/ml	1.00	1–10	IU/L	1 IU/L
galactose (P) (children)	<20	mg/dL	0.05551	<1.1	mmol/L	0.1 mmol/L
gases (aB)						
P_{O_2}	75–105	mm Hg (= Torr)	0.01333	10.0–14.0	kPa	0.1 kPa
P_{CO_2}	33–44	mm Hg (= Torr)	0.01333	4.4–5.9	kPa	0.1 kPa
gamma-glutamyltransferase (GGT) (S)	0–30	U/L	0.01667	0–0.50	μkat/L	0.01 μkat/L
glucose (P)-fasting	70–110	mg/dL	0.05551	3.9–6.1	mmol/L	0.1 mmol/L
growth hormone (P,S)						
male (fasting)	0.0–5.0	ng/mL	1.00	0.0–5.0	μg/L	0.5 μg/L
female (fasting)	0.0–10.0	ng/mL	1.00	0.0–10.0	μg/L	0.5 μg/L
haptoglobin (S)	50–220	mg/dL	0.01	0.50–2.20	g/L	0.01 g/L
hemoglobin (B)						
male	14.0–18.0	g/dL	10.0	140–180	g/L	1 g/L
female	11.5–15.5	g/dL	10.0	115–155	g/L	1 g/L

(continued on last two pages)

4th edition

LABORATORY TESTS & DIAGNOSTIC PROCEDURES with NURSING DIAGNOSES

Jane Vincent Corbett, RN, EdD
Professor and Chair, Adult Health Department
School of Nursing
University of San Francisco
San Francisco, California

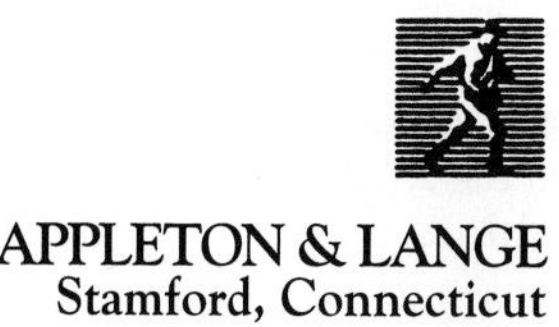

APPLETON & LANGE
Stamford, Connecticut

Notice: The author and the publisher of this volume have taken care to make certain that the doses of drugs and schedules of treatment are correct and compatible with the standards generally accepted at the time of publication. Nevertheless, as new information becomes available, changes in treatment and in the use of drugs become necessary. The reader is advised to carefully consult the instruction and information material included in the package insert of each drug or therapeutic agent before administration. This advise is especially important when using new or infrequently used drugs. The publisher disclaims any liability, loss, injury, or damage incurred as a consequence, directly or indirectly, or the use and application of any of the contents of the volume.

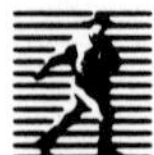

96 97 98 99 00 / 10 9 8 7 6 5 4 3 2 1

Prentice Hall International (UK) Limited, *London*
Prentice Hall of Australia Pty. Limited, *Sydney*
Prentice Hall Canada, Inc., *Toronto*
Prentice Hall Hispanoamericana, S.A., *Mexico*
Prentice Hall of India Private Limited, *New Delhi*
Prentice Hall of Japan, Inc., *Tokyo*
Simon & Schuster Asia Pte. Ltd., *Singapore*
Editora Prentice Hall do Brasil Ltda., *Rio de Janeiro*
Prentice Hall, Upper Saddle River, *New Jersey*

Corbett, Jane Vincent.
Laboratory tests and diagnostic procedures with nursing diagnoses / Jane Vincent Corbett. — 4th ed.
p. cm.
Includes bibliographical references and index.
ISBN 0-8385-5595-0 (pbk. : alk. paper)
1. Diagnosis, Laboratory. 2. Diagnosis. 3. Nursing diagnosis.
I. Title
[DNLM: 1. Diagnosis, Laboratory—nurses' instruction.
2. Diagnostic Tests, Routine—nurses' instruction. QY 4 C789La 1996]
RT48.5.C67 1996
616.07′5—dc20
DNLM/DLC
for Library of Congress 95-36448

ISBN 0-8385-5595-0

9 780838 555590 90000

Acquisitions Editor: David P. Carroll
Production Editor: Karen W. Davis
Designer: Libby Schmitz

PRINTED IN THE UNITED STATES OF AMERICA

To Rod and Rhonda Jane, who gave me the space and time to make this book a reality and whose contributions were invaluable.

CONTENTS

PREFACE

For this fourth edition, outdated tests and procedures have been deleted and many new ones included. As before, examples used include all age groups (newborn to the aged) from a variety of practice settings. The extensive reference list for each chapter has been updated with an even stronger focus on current nursing literature that emphasizes research.

Related tests or procedures are grouped so that common nursing diagnoses can be highlighted. The nursing diagnoses presented in this book are not meant to be used in cookbook form. The nurse can read about the test and *possible* nursing diagnoses but then must evaluate the actual clinical situation and apply what seems appropriate. The purpose of this book is to make nurses think more, not less. The case studies in Part II give the reader an opportunity to practice interpreting lab data to formulate nursing diagnoses.

As health care becomes more and more technical, the multitude of diagnostic procedures and laboratory tests continues to grow. Nurses can become dazzled by the technical details and discouraged about keeping pace with these advances. This book is based on the belief that the nurse's role in relation to diagnostic testing should continue to focus on the human element. Professional nurses are involved in health teaching, client preparation, and assessment for adverse reactions to diagnostic procedures. Thus, from a nursing point of view, detailed technical information on diagnostic procedures, using a disease or systems model, may not be the most helpful. Witness the difference in nursing care needed for a client who undergoes a liver biopsy compared with a client who undergoes a liver scan. Although both tests are used to diagnose potential disease in the same organ, there is no similarity in the nursing care. Yet, for some tests the disease state is an important focus. The pathophysiologic conditions that cause altered laboratory values are explained in an easy-to-understand format. Medical diagnoses and medical interventions are discussed when that information is pertinent to the nurse who may be assisting with treatment. A discussion of usual medical intervention for a particular set of circumstances is included to show how nursing use is related to and yet different from medical use of laboratory data (Corbett and LaBorde, 1994). The independent role of the nurse is emphasized throughout.

Each chapter of this book is organized as an independent study unit complete with objectives, an organizing theme with background information (called an expository organizer), and test questions. The organization and content of the chapters is based on research conducted by the author (Corbett, 1985). This book, meant to be both scholarly and practical, is intended for use in both the academic and the clinical setting. For example:

1. Undergraduate and graduate nursing students can use the book as a textbook in theory classes that integrate laboratory data as one aspect of nursing care.
2. Practicing nurses can use the book to update themselves in specific areas. The content in this book has been used extensively for continuing education courses for RNs.
3. Nurses in clinical settings can use the book as a quick reference. By consulting the index or the listing for each chapter, the nurse can retrieve information about one specific test.

It is intellectually challenging to broaden one's knowledge in a field, and in nursing we often have the added benefit of seeing that our increased knowledge is of direct benefit to the client. My enthusiasm and sense of purpose in writing this book stem from my belief that students and practicing nurses will be able to use the practical information in the book to improve the care of many clients. I hope the reader finds the book informative, interesting, and useful in the practice of nursing.

I welcome written comments, which can be sent to me at the following address:

Dr. Jane Vincent Corbett
University of San Francisco
Ignatian Heights
San Francisco, CA 94117

or via Internet:
corbett@usfca.edu

Corbett, J.V. (1985). *The effects of two types of preinstructional strategies on two levels of cognitive learning from a written study unit.* Dissertation for School of Education, University of San Francisco. Reprints available from University Microfilms International, Ann Arbor, MI.

Corbett, J.V. and LaBorde, A. (1994). Nurses' perceptions of usefulness of laboratory data for nursing practice. *Journal of Continuing Education in Nursing 25* (4), 175–180.

ACKNOWLEDGMENTS

The writing of this fourth edition was done while I was on sabbatical from the University of San Francisco. My thanks to all my colleagues who have always been willing to share their expertise with me.

The students at the University of San Francisco have given me many helpful suggestions for the fourth edition.

The format for this book was based on work completed for my doctoral dissertation. I am grateful to S. Alan Cohen, EdD, Joan Hyman, EdD, and William Schwarz, EdD, who helped me gain an in-depth knowledge about how written strategies such as behavioral objectives and expository organizers can influence cognitive learning from study units. Eleanor Hein, RN, EdD, Jean Nicholson, RN, MS, Mae Timmons, RN, EdD, and Ginny Jones, RN, BS, also helped a great deal with their careful critiques of Chapter 13, which was used as the prototype chapter.

A large number of nurses from various clinical settings have participated in my continuing education classes. I am particularly indebted to them for the discussion on the case studies included in this edition.

Also, many practicing nurses have participated in my surveys about laboratory tests. The data from the surveys were useful for updating and refining the content for this fourth edition.

Carol Bailey, RN, MS, Kaiser Hospital, San Francisco, has been most helpful in obtaining information for this edition. Other people at Kaiser, such as Sunny Holland, RN, Cardiac Catheterization Lab, and Elaine Vaughn, Director of Diagnostic Imaging Services, have also been helpful in answering many of my questions and allowing me to observe numerous types of diagnostic procedures. The University of California at San Francisco (UCSF) provided me with excellent library resources and the opportunity to observe clinical tests and consult with various experts.

4th edition

LABORATORY TESTS & DIAGNOSTIC PROCEDURES with NURSING DIAGNOSES

LABORATORY TESTS

USING LABORATORY DATA

- Laboratory Reports and the Nursing Process
- Nursing Functions in Laboratory Testing, Including Point-of-care Testing
- "Normal" Reference Values and the Variability of Test Results
- False-positive Tests and False-negative Tests
- New Technology for Diagnostic Testing
- Establishing the "Normal" Value
- Measurements in Laboratory Reports
- Screening Tests for Asymptomatic Adult Populations
- Laboratory Personnel

OBJECTIVES

1. Describe how laboratory data can be used in the framework of the nursing process and how nursing use differs from medical use of data.
2. Describe the traditional functions of nurses in relation to laboratory tests, including peripheral testing.
3. Identify the two nondisease factors that cause the greatest variations in normal reference values for laboratory tests.
4. Compare the meanings of the terms *specificity* and *sensitivity* in relation to diagnostic tests.
5. Explain in general terms how the normal curve and percentiles are used to establish normal reference ranges for laboratory tests.
6. Explain the meaning of the measurement symbols in the conventional laboratory system and in the SI system.

7. Describe the purpose of each of the basic diagnostic screening tests recommended for asymptomatic adult populations.
8. Define how nurses can foster smooth working relationships with personnel in the laboratory department.

In discussing several issues that are pertinent to the nurse's utilization of laboratory data, this chapter touches briefly on the nursing process, on the differences between nursing care and medical care, and on the traditional roles of the nurse in relation to diagnostic tests. Emphasis is given to the many factors that influence test results, such as physiology, drug interference, and the statistical methods used to determine "normal" ranges. A comparison of conventional measurements and SI units is included, and the purpose of screening tests is explored. The last section in the chapter discusses ways that the nurse can effectively work with personnel in other departments.

LABORATORY REPORTS AND THE NURSING PROCESS

Up to the early 1970s, problem solving was emphasized as a way of thinking about the needs of clients. About that time, most nursing educators started turning to the nursing process, which is an elaboration of the problem-solving technique used by all disciplines. In essence, the *nursing process* is a way of systematically identifying the needs of patients or clients and then logically planning the appropriate nursing actions to meet those needs. (The term *client* is used in this book, but *patient* may be substituted if one wishes.) Most practicing nurses use the nursing process even though they may be unsure about how to describe it step-by-step in writing. However, nursing students learn to develop care plans based on the nursing process in a very systematic manner. Yet, whether written or not, the nursing process, as a way of thinking, helps the nurse provide nursing care that is based on more than guesswork or generalizations about clients. This process is a deliberate way of using data to make the assessments and to identify the problems that are under the jurisdiction of the nurse. The evaluation and the modification of care are also essential components of the nursing process. The format for a written nursing care plan is shown in Table 1–1.

Collection of Data (Assessment)

Nurses use a variety of ways to collect data, including physical assessment and interviewing; laboratory data constitute only one small part of the entire clinical situation. Consequently one can never use the laboratory data apart from other clinical data. For example, although an increased specific gravity is one objective sign of dehydration or a fluid volume deficit, the nurse must collect other data that may be relevant to this client's situation. If the client has just undergone diagnostic tests with radiopaque dye (Chapter 20), the specific gravity is not a meaningful contribution to data collection.

TABLE 1–1. USE OF LABORATORY DATA IN NURSING PROCESS

Collection of Data (Assessment)	Nursing Diagnosis or Statement of Problems (Analysis)	Client/Nurse Goals (Planning)	Interventions (Nurse-to-Nurse Orders Implementation)	Evaluation and Modification Needed (Evaluation)
Cannot use left arm to hold glass; mouth is dry; skin turgor poor; I&O for last 24 hours I = 800 O = 600 s.g. = 1.036 hct 50% BUN 35 mg	Fluid volume deficit related to inability to feed self	Client remains hydrated with a s.g. no higher than 1.020 *Short-term:* Client drinks at least 1,000 mL on the day shift and 600 mL on the evening shift	Give mouth care at least once a shift Ask client what type of fluids are wanted—does not like *water* Assist client to drink out of glass—likes straw In addition to meals, offer 250 mL of fluids at: 10 AM 2 PM 4 PM 8 PM	Intake for 2–10: 7–3 PM 1,000 mL 3–11 PM 650 mL Client's s.g. now 1.015 on 2–11 2–11: continue with plan

Note: Although a nursing diagnosis may arise from the use of one or two laboratory tests, more often many tests and much clinical data are needed to fashion an individualized care plan. This text helps the reader by suggesting *potential* nursing diagnoses related to specific abnormal test results. The nurse must then gather relevant clinical data to validate the use of those diagnoses in a given situation.
I, intake; O, output; s.g., specific gravity; hct, hematocrit; BUN, blood urea nitrogen.

Nursing Diagnosis (Analysis)

Taking all the collected data, nurses must then formulate a *nursing diagnosis*, which is a problem within the scope of nursing practice. In a national conference held in 1972, nurses identified a list of nursing diagnoses that were generally agreed to be under the control of the nurse. Since then the list has been periodically updated by national meetings of nurses called the North American Nursing Diagnosis Association (NANDA). NANDA is also involved in activities to include nursing diagnoses in the International Classification of Diseases (ICD) structure (Fitzpatrick and Zanotti, 1995). Although many nurses use this official and quite specific list of nursing diagnoses, others may prefer to use their own words to describe client problems. The important point is that nurses must make sure the diagnosis or problem is truly within the scope of nursing and that other health care workers understand the terminology. Carnevali (1984) noted that one requirement for the complete establishment of the process and products of nursing diagnosis in the health care field is that nursing textbooks take a nursing perspective. As noted in Brandon and Hill (1994) almost all books on laboratory tests now have a definite nursing perspective, and some emphasize nursing diagnoses.

A nursing diagnosis is not the same as a medical diagnosis. Although medicine is focused on the diagnosis and treatment of disease, nursing focuses on the care, comfort, and support of people whose patterns of daily life are in some way threatened. Nursing focuses on restorative support, nurturance, comfort measures, and health teaching. Over the years, nursing diagnosis has moved from a basic concept about the nature of nursing toward theory-based diagnostic categories that can be tested in clinical practice (Gordon, 1979, 1990).

Many client problems can be identified by means of the nursing process. For example, through assessment, the nurse may discover that Mr. Smith's urine has become concentrated because he cannot feed himself and no one has been offering him any fluids between meals. Thus the nursing diagnosis would be a fluid volume deficit caused by an inability to obtain fluids. However, dehydration, or a fluid volume deficit, may be caused by a serious medical problem such as ketoacidosis. The second case warrants medical interventions such as insulin administration and intravenous fluids (Chapter 8). Other examples are as follows:

1. An elevated direct bilirubin often causes itching in clients. What *comfort* measures by the nurse may be effective? (Alteration in comfort)
2. A client has a low serum potassium level. What *health teaching* does the client need about foods rich in potassium? (Knowledge deficit)
3. A woman is to undergo a hystosalpingogram as part of an infertility work-up. The nurse observes that the client is very anxious. What can the nurse do to prepare the woman and to give her *nurturance*? (Moderate anxiety)
4. A young child has a low hemoglobin reading. What can the nurse teach the parents that would be *restorative support*? (Alteration in nutritional requirements)

The nursing process is effective if one knows the answers to go with the questions raised above. Hence the subsequent chapters provide the information necessary for planning individualized client care. Only potential nursing diagnoses are listed for each test. The nurse must decide if the diagnosis is really appropriate for a particular client. Students, clinicians, and researchers must continue to be flexible and creative in the use and validation of nursing diagnoses (Avant, 1990).

Writing Goals for Client Outcomes

With the nursing diagnosis, the nurse can write client/nurse goals in behavioral terms. The goal should be acceptable to the client and compatible with medical goals. For example, in Mr. Smith's case, an immediate short-term goal is to have him drink so many milliliters of fluid during each shift. The long-term goal is that he not show any signs of dehydration (i.e., his specific gravity remains in a normal range).

Nursing Interventions (Implementation)

The nurse then plans the nursing actions or interventions needed to reach the goals. She or he may consult with the client about how to best achieve a mutually acceptable goal. Maybe Mr. Smith needs to be fed completely. Maybe he could feed himself and drink fluids if he were properly positioned. Maybe the client would drink juice better than water. Collaboration with the physician and with other health team members (such as the dietitian) is often necessary.

Nurses write goals and interventions in various ways. These interventions, called *nurse-to-nurse orders*, need to be written in the card file. The important point is to differentiate between actions that depend on physicians' orders and those that are independent nursing actions. Too often nurses communicate their own orders only by word of mouth. While nursing as a profession becomes more assured of its uniqueness, one hopes that nurse-to-nurse orders will become a more common practice. Another way to define the collective expertise of nurses has been the nursing interventions classification system (NIC), which lists and defines 336 nursing interventions. The NIC, published in 1992, is designed to make the contributions of nurses visible in health information systems. Research continues on the use of NIC in various settings (Bulechek et al., 1994; McClosky and Bulechek, 1995).

Evaluation of Goals or Expected Outcomes

Evaluation is necessary to see if the goals or expected outcomes were met. If goals are not achieved, what needs to be modified? For example, a specific gravity measurement can be considered evidence that the client has regained a normal fluid balance. *Responsibility* and *accountability* in nursing mean that nurses take responsibility for the quality of client care and that they are accountable if the care does not meet certain standards. Hence evaluation is an integral part of accountability.

NURSING FUNCTIONS IN LABORATORY TESTING, INCLUDING POINT-OF-CARE TESTING

Integrating Laboratory Data into Nursing Practice

As health care has become more complex and technological, nurses have been increasingly expected to integrate laboratory data into their practice (Cushing, 1985; Northrop, 1986; Kee and Hayes, 1990; Calfee, 1991). Although nurses are expected to use laboratory data in their nursing practice, not all nurses may feel comfortable with this role. A nursing research study identified a lack of knowledge about clinical importance and time constraints as the two most common barriers to the use of laboratory data (Corbett and LaBorde, 1994). In addition to using laboratory data to formulate nursing diagnoses, nurses must determine if the results of a test need to be reported immediately to a physician or if the report is not urgent. The nurse may also need to alert other health care workers or the client and family about symptoms to watch for or precautions to take. Although abnormal results may require immediate attention, normal results may also have great diagnostic importance in ruling out certain diseases. The importance of both normal and abnormal results is emphasized for each of the tests in the following chapters.

Gathering Information from Charts

In collecting data from a chart, nurses should always look at the latest laboratory data first to see the current status of the client and to note trends in the data. One of the hardest things for novices to figure out is the meaning of the abbreviations used for many of the laboratory tests and diagnostic procedures. *ANA* on a chart, for example, has nothing to do with the American Nurses Association! It stands for *antinuclear antibody test*, which is a test performed for systemic lupus erythematosus (SLE). The standard abbreviations used to denote laboratory tests are listed in Appendix E and those for diagnostic procedures in Appendix F. Learning these abbreviations makes reading charts and collecting data much easier.

Transcribing Orders and Ordering Laboratory Tests

Generally, because the procedures for transcribing orders and filling out laboratory requisitions vary from institution to institution, this skill is best learned by in-service or on-the-job training. In this book, the essential points to include on the laboratory requisitions are discussed in relation to each test. Ordering laboratory tests is a skill usually reserved for experienced nurse clinicians in special situations. In some clinical settings, however, nurses may order certain laboratory tests in accordance with the hospital's standardized orders. For example, the regulations for nursing practice in California note that ordering routine laboratory tests, such as urinalysis, occult blood tests, or wound cultures, may be part of basic health care given by the nurse (Chow, 1986).

Testing by Nurses

Several simple tests require only a drop or two of blood or urine and no special equipment. Some of these tests include the dipsticks for urine chemistry, slide tests for occult blood, and simple procedures such as specific gravity reading by refractometers. In special care units, such as intensive care units or emergency departments, nurses may also operate automated equipment that measures blood gases or hematocrits.

Nurses must be aware of the potential problems with administering such tests. For instance, the diagnostic test kits are reliable only if the nurses follow the instructions. Another problem is that test materials may not be properly cared for. Bottles are left open, materials get wet or hot, and the issue date of the test is unknown. Aides, inexperienced nurses, or interns may not perform the test accurately, or the technician may be color-blind. (All laboratory workers are tested for color blindness as a requirement for their job.)

If nurses are not comfortable with the procedures used for testing, they should request in-service training. Many of the manufacturers of diagnostic kits provide in-service education free-of-charge to nurses and other health care workers. Also, many teaching aids about products may be obtained by writing directly to the manufacturer or by talking to the local sales representatives.

Point-of-Care Testing

The availability of sophisticated wet and dry chemistry systems (automatic analyzers) that can be used outside the traditional centralized laboratory has made it possible to perform many tests in the physician's office or in small clinics. Handheld portable analyzers that require only a few drops of blood can simultaneously perform many measurements such as electrolyte, glucose, blood urea nitrogen (BUN), and hematocrit values within 2 minutes. These portable analyzers have proved useful in settings such as emergency departments (Woo et al., 1993). This "point-of-care testing," as it is called in the medical and nursing literature, has come about not only because of the technological advances but also because of changes in reimbursement practices (Pysher and Daly, 1989). Nurses or other health care providers who are nontechnical in relation to laboratory procedures may be responsible for performing some of these tests. Nanji et al. (1988) found that reliable results are more likely to be obtained by nontechnical personnel if diluting or pipetting steps are not required. Not having to send specimens to a laboratory does mean faster results usually at a lower cost. Issues about quality control continue to be a concern. Proficiency testing for quality control in laboratories had been voluntary for many years. However, with the passage of the Clinical Laboratory Improvement Act of 1988 (CLIA), effective in 1992, proficiency testing became mandatory for all laboratories doing laboratory tests categorized as "moderately complex" or "highly complex." All tests are categorized as "waived," moderately complex, or highly complex. The level of test is determined by assessing the relative difficulty of doing the test and the relative risk to the client if the test is performed incorrectly (Flynn, 1994). Blomberg (1993) reported that an estimated 13% of physician office laboratories would discontinue office laboratory testing and others would reduce the scope of their testing rather than face the regulatory risks of CLIA. Issues remain about the best way to ensure implementation of these regulations, about which tests should be waived, and about benefits versus costs of mandatory federal regulation (Noble, 1993; Kaplan et al., 1995). The reader is encouraged to find out the latest federal regulations as well as specific state laws that determine which tests can be performed by other than trained laboratory personnel. For example, what laboratory tests can be performed in a clinic run by a nurse practitioner? What tests can be done in a free clinic that relies on mostly volunteer help?

Preparation of the Client for a Laboratory Test

The nurse's role includes preparing the client physically and psychologically. As a client advocate, the nurse can make sure that the client has adequate knowledge of what is to be performed. As information giver or health teacher, the nurse can also seek additional input from other members of the health team so that the client gives informed consent. The responsibilities of nurses in implementing a doctrine of informed consent are related to their role within the health team, the facility at which health care is given, and current law. In the past few years, there has been more emphasis on clients' rights as states have enacted laws to enforce the doctrine of informed consent.

Collection and Transportation of Specimens

Venous Samples

Experienced nurses often draw venous blood for blood work. When they do, they must avoid the following possible causes of hemolysis, which invalidates tests such as potassium or lactic dehydrogenase (LDH) determination:

1. Skin too wet with antiseptic
2. Moisture in the syringe or collection tube
3. Prolonged use of a tourniquet or clenching of fist
4. Use of a small-gauge needle to withdraw a large volume of blood
5. Use of suction on the syringe
6. Vigorous shaking of the blood specimen
7. Not removing the needle from the syringe before expelling the blood into the collection tube
8. Vigorous expulsion of blood from the syringe into the collection tube

Other precautions are not drawing blood from an arm in which there is an intravenous catheter because the values are changed by the solution being infused. Intracatheter or scalp vein needles used for blood samples should be inserted 30 min before fasting samples, which could be affected by stress, are obtained (Tallman, 1982). Reker and Webb (1986) emphasized the usefulness of a serial sampling technique to avoid multiple vein punctures. McAffee et al. (1990) illustrated how to draw blood safely from a vascular access device. The meanings of the various colors for tubes are explained in Table 1–2. For example, a red top on a tube means *no additives*. Most venous blood samples for chemistry are collected without additives or in the red and black tube that separates the serum; the tubes are noted as serum separator tubes (SST). These tubes are often referred to as "tiger tops" or "speckled reds" (Flynn, 1994). Chapter 13 describes techniques for arterial blood samples.

Finger, Earlobe, and Heel Sticks

For many tests performed with a portable analyzer, capillary blood obtained with a finger stick is used, rather than blood obtained by means of venipuncture. The earlobe may occasionally be used for tests such as hematocrits. The usual procedure is to cleanse with 70% alcohol, dry with a gauze sponge, and puncture with a sterile blade deep enough to get a free flow of blood. The first drop of blood is discarded, and enough blood is collected to fill a capillary tube supplied by the laboratory. Or a drop of blood may be put onto special filter paper. It is important not to squeeze to obtain capillary blood because the squeezing causes tissue fluids to dilute the sample. Warming the site a few minutes before the puncture greatly increases blood flow, as does selecting a lancet with the needed puncture depth. In infants, heel sticks are used to obtain capillary blood. The lateral aspects of the heel are used to avoid the plantar artery. If several different collection tubes are needed, they should

TABLE 1–2. MEANING OF COLOR CODE FOR BLOOD SPECIMENS

Color of Tube Top	Contents	Use
Red	No additives No separator	Most chemistry, serology, and blood banking
Red and black	Silicone gel to separate serum from cells[a]	Most chemistry and serology
Green	Heparin	Special tests such as ammonia levels, blood gases
Lavender	EDTA	Hematology, some chemistry and blood banking
Blue	Sodium citrate	PT, PTT, and other coagulation tests
Gray	Glycolytic inhibitor such as oxalate and fluoride	Glucose

[a] The use of the silicone gel, which separates the cells from the plasma, makes it easier for the laboratory worker to obtain the serum. The gel is more expensive, however. Tubes should be rotated if additive is present so it will mix with the specimen.
EDTA, ethylenediaminetetraacetate; PT, prothrombin time; PTT, partial thromboplastin time.

be collected in the following order: blood gases, slides and smears, EDTA tubes, other additive tubes, and plain serum tubes.

The AIDS epidemic has led to much concern about the safety of health workers who handle needles, because needle injuries continue to occur (Jagger et al., 1988). All workers who must handle needles and blood samples must be aware of how to protect themselves and others. The cost and benefits of universal precautions continue to be studied, and practices may not always follow the latest guidelines from the Centers for Disease Control (Doebbeling and Wenzel, 1990). Nurses must make sure that they are knowledgeable about how to handle safely all types of specimens.

Urine and Other Specimens

The procedure for urine collection, including 24-hr testing, is detailed in Chapter 3. Chapter 16 gives explicit details on all the types of specimens collected for cultures.

After a specimen is collected, the way it is stored and transported to the laboratory can affect the test values. For example, blood gases or anaerobic cultures must not be exposed to the air. The nurse must check with the laboratory to determine if there are any special requirements about the transportation of specimens.

Seeing That Stat Tests Are Stat

The word *stat* means "at once." Because a stat request interrupts the normal laboratory routine, a test should be marked *stat* only when the results really do need to be known as soon as possible. In most stat situations, someone should hand-carry the specimen to the laboratory. The nurse should be familiar with the preparation needed and with the expected results of stat tests because these tests are done in emergency situations when there is little time to review. Table 1–3 lists 22 tests done stat by at least 90% of the hospitals in one survey.

TABLE 1–3. TESTS MOST COMMONLY DONE AS STAT PROCEDURES

Name of Test	Discussed In
Complete blood count (CBC)	Chap. 2
Urinalysis (UA)	Chap. 3
Blood urea nitrogen (BUN)	Chap. 4
Electrolytes (Na, K, Cl, bicarb)	Chap. 5
Blood gases	Chap. 6
Calcium	Chap. 7
Glucose	Chap. 8
Acetone (serum)	Chap. 8
Bilirubin	Chap. 11
Amylase	Chap. 12
Prothrombin time (PT)	Chap. 13
Partial thromboplastin time (PTT)	Chap. 13
Platelet count	Chap. 13
Fibrinogen	Chap. 13
Type and cross match	Chap. 14
Direct Coombs	Chap. 14
Transfusion reaction investigation	Chap. 14
Inoculate media for cultures	Chap. 16
Gram stains	Chap. 16
Alcohol	Chap. 17
Salicylates	Chap. 17
Cerebrospinal fluid (CSF)	Chaps. 16 & 25

Based on studies reported in the work by Barnett et al. (1978).
See Ravel (1995) for more information on cost of stat procedures.

Educating Consumers About the Use of Home Test Kits

Advanced technology has made it possible for several tests to be approved by the United States Food and Drug Administration (FDA) for use by consumers. The first such home tests, in 1977, were for pregnancy (Chapter 18). Now a variety of home test kits are available for screening, such as the one for serum cholesterol. Munroe (1994) discussed the important role of the pharmacist in helping consumers understand that they are self-testing not self-diagnosing. Nurses also need to be knowledgeable about the home test kits available and how clients may use them for self-monitoring.

"NORMAL" REFERENCE VALUES AND THE VARIABILITY OF TEST RESULTS

Laboratory values in the medical literature are referred to as *normal reference values* or *reference values* and not as *normal values*, because each laboratory must determine what is "normal" for a test performed in a specific laboratory. *The use of any of the reference values in this book may be hazardous to the well-being of clients unless values are verified by the local laboratory. No book can be the authority on what is normal for a specific laboratory.*

For the most part, the reference values used throughout this book are those periodically published in the *New England Journal of Medicine.* (See Appendix A for the address to write to obtain reprints of all the printed values.) These values, based on the ones used at Massachusetts General Hospital, have been published periodically since 1946 (Jordan et al., 1992). Reference values for some tests were gained from Young (1987) and from various hospitals in San Francisco, California. Other sources for reference values are listed in each chapter and with the tables in the appendices.

Variables That Affect Test Results

Besides the obvious differences in technique and method, many other variables can influence laboratory reference values. Age and sex are the chief physiologic factors that change the "norms." Pregnancy alters the normal reference values. (See the tables in Appendices A, B, C, and D for examples of changes in values in different populations.) Reference values for adults are often better documented than those for children.

Other physiologic factors, such as diet, time of day, activity level, and stress, may alter what is "normal" for a test. For example, hormones (Chapter 15) have a diurnal variation, so the time of day must be recorded when the specimen is drawn. Geographic location, altitude, temperature, and humidity may also affect results. Racial or ethnic variation can also cause different reference values for different groups, but usually ethnic or racial differences are not of much importance for most tests. How much a drug alters a laboratory value may depend on the dosage, timing, physiology of the client, and other variables such as the mixture of drugs. The reader must consult pharmacology references or other more specialized texts than this book for details on drug interactions, both from the physiologic effects and the chemical effects on laboratory results. Only the more common drug interferences are included in this text.

FALSE-POSITIVE TESTS AND FALSE-NEGATIVE TESTS

Specificity

If a test is 100% *specific,* it reacts positively only when the client actually has the condition being tested. No laboratory test is 100% specific because there is always a factor, such as drugs, that can effect a false-positive reaction. For example, the radioimmunoassay (RIA) test for pregnancy is very specific because almost all women who have a positive test are indeed pregnant. However, the VDRL (Venereal Disease Research Laboratory) test for syphilis is not highly specific (i.e., a large number of people can have a positive VDRL even though they do not have syphilis). The danger of false-positives is that the client may receive additional tests and treatments that are unnecessary.

Sensitivity

The *sensitivity* of a test is the degree to which a test detects disease without yielding a false-negative diagnosis. No test is 100% sensitive, because there is always some possibility that the test will not reveal the abnormality even though it is present. For example, the direct agglutination technique of detecting pregnancy is not as sensitive as the RIA method (Chapter 18). So with the direct agglutination method, there are more false-negatives than with the RIA method (i.e., the client is pregnant, but the agglutination method does not reveal it).

In disease states, false-negative tests mean that clients are misclassified as not needing treatment or care when actually they *do* need treatment. As another example, the electrocardiogram (ECG) is not a sensitive test for coronary disease before a myocardial infarction. In other words, coronary disease is not detected by this particular test. Thus a person may have a "normal" ECG one day and a myocardial infarction the next. Larson (1986) described several quantitative methods used to evaluate the validity of screening tests in nursing research.

NEW TECHNOLOGY FOR DIAGNOSTIC TESTING

Specificity and sensitivity are important criteria when a new test is introduced into practice. Balint (1978, p. 291) suggested five questions to decide whether a new test or a diagnostic procedure is worthwhile:

1. Does the new procedure provide a greater specificity and sensitivity than current methods?
2. Is the new information valuable in client management?
3. Is the new approach as effective in routine clinical practice as it is in selected populations of a university center?
4. Does the test provide answers not provided by clinical findings and established diagnostic procedures?
5. In light of the other four factors, is the test cost effective?

The past few years have seen an amazing array of new technology for diagnostic testing. Many of these techniques have improved the sensitivity and specificity of testing by labeling specific antigens and antibodies so that very small amounts of a hormone, a drug or other substance can be identified. The technique for labeling first used radioisotopes and was thus called radioimmunoassay (RIA). Rosalyn Yalow received a share of the 1977 Nobel prize for the development of this technique. Alternative labels to radioisotopes, which are less expensive and do not have the problems associated with radioactive materials, have been developed. These newer techniques include enzyme immunoassay (EIA), fluorescence immunoassay

(FIA), enzyme-linked immunosorbent assay (ELISA), and others (Kaplan et al., 1995). These initials may be used with the test to let the clinician know the type of testing used.

The polymerase chain reaction (PCR) is a technique used to make copies of a sequence of DNA. Amplification makes it possible to study very small amounts of biologic material, even dried blood spots. RNA can also be used, provided it is first converted to DNA with a reverse transcriptase step. For example, PCR is very useful to assay the RNA in the hepatitis C virus (Silva et al., 1994). PCR, introduced in 1985 and first used in a court case in 1986, is also used in the clinical setting to identify sample mix-ups of blood and even urine (Weedn, 1993). To make a match of DNA, a nucleic probe is needed. A nucleic acid probe is a replica or construct of the DNA or RNA of the cell or organism to be detected. The probe is labeled with a radioisotope or other tag. Commercial kits that rely on nucleic acid probes with PCR (NA-PCR) have been available since 1990. For commercial kits, the amplified sample of DNA fragments are probed by a complementary fragment of DNA bound to membrane strips. Testing for organisms (Chapter 16) and for genetic diseases (Chapter 28) are examples of the use of techniques that may be called DNA probes, PCR tests, or just DNA testing (Kaplan et al., 1995; Ravel, 1995).

Chapter 21 describes the many types of scans now available. In many other chapters, the impact of technology on the development of new tests or on improvement of the sensitivity and specificity of older tests is evident.

ESTABLISHING THE "NORMAL" VALUE

It should be increasingly apparent that "blind faith" in the validity of laboratory tests is simply not realistic. In addition to the problems already discussed, even the so-called normal value can be misleading. The normal ranges are determined by testing a large sample of healthy people and then analyzing the results by statistical methods.

The Normal Curve

One such method is the *normal curve* or *Gaussian distribution.* In this method a cutoff point, which usually consists of two standard deviations from the mean or average, is determined for each side of the curve. In other words, the lowest 2.5% and the highest 2.5% are outside the normal range. Even without a statistical background, the reader should be able to appreciate that any system with cutoff points automatically means that some *healthy* people in the sample do not fall within the normal range. Also, if the distribution is not normal, the curve is skewed. (Most students who have been exposed to grading by the bell curve know the situation in which students who do exceptionally well are called "curve wreckers" by those on the other end of the curve.) Most physiologic parameters do not fall in normal distributions, and so it is usually incorrect to speak of averages and normal curves in relation to laboratory data (Ravel, 1995).

The Percentile Ranking System

The percentile ranking system is usually a better method than the curve because data that do not have a normal distribution can still be ranked. *All* the values are ranked, and a percentage is given for each value in relation to the other values. The value in the middle (the median) is at the 50th percentile. This means 50% of the scores are higher and 50% are lower. When laboratory data are ranked by percentiles, a cutoff point must be established to indicate an abnormality. For example, values above the 95th percentile are usually considered beyond the normal reference values. Thus 5% of *healthy* people are *unhealthy* according to this statistical determination of "normalcy."

Nurses do not have to determine normal ranges or even understand the underlying statistics. They do, however, need to realize that a margin of error arises from the arbitrary setting of limits. In effect, with each laboratory test, the results *may* be outside the normal range entirely because of mathematical probability. It should be stated again, if a laboratory test is considered normal up to the 95th percentile, then five times out of 100 a test will show an abnormality *even though the client is not ill.* If the client undergoes two tests, the probability that both will be within the normal range is 0.95 times 0.95 or 90.25%. With three tests, the probability is 0.95 times 0.95 times 0.95 or 85.7375%. The point is that if a client has a battery of tests, such as the SMA discussed at the end of this chapter, the possibility is great that some of the tests will be abnormal purely because of chance (Sox, 1986).

MEASUREMENTS IN LABORATORY REPORTS

Conventional Measurements

Probably most of the measurements used in laboratory reports, such as *mL* (milliliter) or *mg* (milligram), are already very familiar. A list of the common abbreviations used for metric measurements is included in Table 1–4, and a more complete list is included as Appendix G. Note that *mg/dL* means so many milligrams in a deciliter, which is 1/10 of a liter, or 100 mL. In other words, a blood sugar report of 90 mg/dL is the same as 90 mg/100 mL.

The terms *picogram* (pg) and *nanogram* (ng) are also commonly used, now that it is possible to detect trace amounts of substances such as hormones or drugs.

The measurement used for electrolytes is *milliequivalent* (mEq). The exact meaning of this term, as well as how milligram can be converted to milliequivalent, is explained in Chapter 5. *Milliosmoles* (mOsm) is used to express the concentration of body fluids. (See Chapter 3 for a definition of milliosmoles in relation to urinary osmolality.) Note that *mOsm* is different from *mmol*, which is discussed next.

SI Measurement System

SI units are based on a comprehensive form of the metric system called *Le Système Internationale d'Unités* (hence SI). The rationale for the adoption of this international

TABLE 1–4. METRIC MEASUREMENTS USED IN LABORATORY REPORTS[a]

	Nonmetric Equivalent
Length	
Meter (m) →	39.37 in
Centimeter (cm) = 1/100 m →	2.5 cm = 1 in
Millimeter (mm) = 1/1,000 m	
Weight	
Kilogram (kg) →	2.2 lb
Gram (g) →	453 g = 1 lb
Milligram (mg) = 1/1,000 of a g	
Microgram (μg) = 1/1,000 of a mg	
Nanogram (ng) = 1/1,000 of a μg	
Picogram (pg) = 1/1,000 of a ng	
Femtogram (fg) = 1/1,000 of a pg	
Volume	
Liter (L) = 1,000 mL (or 1,000 cc[b]) →	1.05 qt
Deciliter (dL) = 100 mL or 1/10 of a L	
Milliliter (mL) = 1 mL or 1/1,000 of a L	

[a] See Appendix G for an expanded list of measurement terms used in laboratory reports.
[b] Note that "mL" and "cc" are interchangeable.

system is to provide a common language for all the various disciplines all over the world (Young, 1974, 1987). Used not only for the biologic sciences but also for all sciences, SI uses *moles* as the basic unit for the amount of a substance and *kilograms* for its mass. Length is still by *meter.*

The most profound change in laboratory reports effected by SI is that concentration is expressed as an amount per volume (moles or millimoles per liter) rather than as a mass per volume (grams or milligrams per 100 mL or dL). For some laboratory tests, the numbers stay the same even though the unit is new. For example, the normal range for potassium (K) in the conventional system is 3.5 to 5.0 *mEQ/L,* and it is 3.5 to 5.0 *mmol/L* in SI. Some of the other tests involve a radical change in numbers, so health workers must totally relearn the reference values. For example, the conventional reference value for glucose of *70 to 100 mg/dL* becomes *3.9 to 5.6 mmol/L* in SI.

Because of the drastic change in many laboratory reports, the conversion is taking place slowly in the United States. Plans are underway for a change to the new system, which seems to be more evident in the literature than in clinical practice (Corbett, 1989; Walter and Keen, 1990; Weeth, 1990; Campion, 1992). At present, many laboratories report results in both conventional and SI units. Appendix A gives the reference values in both conventional and SI units. Also, the work by Young (1987) is an excellent source for conversion tables for SI units. Excerpts are duplicated on the inside covers of this book.

SCREENING TESTS FOR ASYMPTOMATIC ADULT POPULATIONS

Biochemical profiles (BCPs) consist of a battery of tests, usually six or 12, in which the client's individual results are compared against the normal reference values. BCP tests are provided by automatic analyzers from a number of manufacturers. The battery of tests is often called *SMA* because this was the first brand name commonly used: SMAC, for *sequential multiple analysis computer* by Technicon Corporation. More correctly, the test should be called a BCP.

Almost two decades ago, Blue Cross and Blue Shield (1979) recommended the phasing out of *routine* admission test panels. BCPs were to be performed only on the order of the physician. The introduction of diagnostic-related grouping (DRG) led to more curtailing. The emphasis is now that laboratory tests and other diagnostic procedures should be determined by the nature of the client's problem, which must be detected by means of careful history taking and physical examination. Blue Cross and Blue Shield commissioned a series of articles to help physicians become more aware of appropriate diagnostic testing (Sox, 1986), and education programs to reduce orders for unnecessary tests have been tried at some institutions (Dowling et al., 1989).

The cost of testing compared with its usefulness is an issue that perplexes health care today. Kaplan et al. (1985) noted that in the absence of specific indications, routine preoperative tests contributed little to client care decisions. In their study, only 1–2% of the tests were abnormal. In summary, the use of a test does not always mean better client care, but it does mean increased cost. However, Showstack et al. (1985) found that laboratory tests were not a major factor of rising costs.

In the past few years, several expert panels have identified screening tests that are recommended for all asymptomatic adults. The most agreement is for routine blood pressure measurements, serum cholesterol levels every 5 years (Chapter 9), mammograms yearly for women after age 50 (Chapter 20), and Pap smears every 1–3 years for women starting at the age of first intercourse (Chapter 25). Less agreement exists for routine mammograms for women younger than 50 years (Chapter 20), occult blood testing (Chapter 13) and sigmoidoscopy (Chapter 27) as routine screens for colonic cancer, and use of the prostate-specific antigen (PSA) (Chapter 14) to screen all men older than 50 years for prostatic cancer (Goldbloom et al., 1993; Sox, 1994). Nurses need to be aware of the recommended screening tests so they can educate clients about practical and cost-effective primary care.

LABORATORY PERSONNEL

Who Works in a Clinical Laboratory?

The Pathologist

The laboratory is directed by a physician with a specialty in pathology, which focuses on the use and interpretation of laboratory tests in the diagnosis and treatment of disease. Because they often interpret the results of laboratory tests to the attending physician, pathologists are often called the "doctor's doctors." In addition to helping with clinical decision making, the pathologist plays an important role in the accreditation and inspection of the laboratory (Blomberg, 1993).

Medical Technologist

The actual management of the laboratory is carried out by a medical technologist who has had additional training in management and administration. Usually the director of the laboratory establishes the policies and procedures that affect nursing. In most states, medical technologists have a bachelor's degree in a biologic science, which includes a year or more of study in a school of medical technology. States have their own medical technology examination, but a national examination is also available for certification.

Medical technologists typically become specialists in different areas, such as serology, hematology, or bacteriology. Nurses should understand how the laboratory is organized well enough that they do not call the chemistry section, for example, for the results of a culture and sensitivity test.

Laboratory Assistants

The meaning of the commonly used term *lab technician* is not precise. Medical technologists want to be known as medical technologists because any lab assistant may be called a lab technician. Laboratory assistants have a high school diploma and on-the-job experience or training in certain laboratory techniques. Laboratory assistants draw blood, process specimens, and assist in performing some of the more routine tests in the laboratory.

Cooperating with Laboratory Personnel

Too often nursing and laboratory personnel conflict with each other rather than cooperate for the good of the client. Laboratory personnel complain that specimens are not marked correctly—that they are lost or otherwise ineptly handled by the nursing staff. Clients are not always correctly prepared for examinations, or the laboratory personnel are not informed of changes in orders. On the other hand, nurses complain that the laboratory personnel are insensitive to the individual needs of the client, late with stat requests, curt and demanding with nurses, and so forth. Unfortunately, both departments often have legitimate reasons for complaining, but poor communication between the departments often allows small problems to become large frustrations (Stocker, 1985; Flynn, 1994).

For their part in this ongoing feud, nurses need to perform their functions as accurately as possible. The information in the rest of this book should enable nurses to function better in preparing the client for laboratory testing, as well as make them sensitive to what the laboratory personnel needs to know about any special problems with clients. For example, if the nurse knows a client is disoriented and potentially combative, the laboratory personnel should be warned about this attitude before they draw blood or perform other procedures. Nurses forget that they are often the only health professionals who see the client for more than 15 min at a time.

Nurses in hospitals also have to face a fact of hospital life: Although they often complain that they must always plan their care around visits from physicians, laboratory personnel, radiology personnel—who drop in for brief contacts with the client—these people must have access to the client. Whereas the emphasis in nursing is on caring and nurturing to meet not only the physical needs but also the psychosocial needs of the client, such is not always the emphasis of health workers who are trained to do more technical jobs. Nurses can foster smooth relationships with other health care workers by making the client available whenever possible. At the same time, because they spend more time with the client than the others, nurses can often be advocates for the sick client who must deal with a host of other people in a fragmented way.

In general, nurses need to work in a spirit of cooperation with other health care personnel so that each can function well. If they have specific problems with the laboratory—stats not stat, lost reports—nurses should collect written data about the problem and present the report to the nursing supervisor so that changes can be made. Complaining to other nurses during a coffee break accomplishes little if no other action is taken.

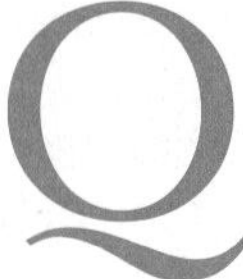

1. Mrs. Rhoades has a urine specific gravity of 1.030 and other clinical signs of a fluid volume deficit. In using the nursing process, the nurse should use this information about specific gravity not only to make an assessment of the problem but also to
   - **a.** Diagnose the pathophysiology or underlying disease
   - **b.** Initiate treatment of the disease
   - **c.** Evaluate the effectiveness of nursing interventions
   - **d.** Determine the rate of intravenous infusion of fluids
2. The traditional functions of the nurse in relation to laboratory tests has never included
   - **a.** Transcribing physicians' orders and writing requisitions for the laboratory
   - **b.** Collecting and transporting specimens to the laboratory
   - **c.** Conducting simple testing on the unit
   - **d.** Scheduling the times when tests are performed by laboratory personnel on the unit
3. Which of these two factors are generally the most common reasons for variations in normal reference values for laboratory tests?
   - **a.** Genetic factors and drugs
   - **b.** Sex and age
   - **c.** Activity levels and stress
   - **d.** Geographic location and diet

4. If a test yields too many false-positives, the test is described as

   a. Not very sensitive
   b. Too sensitive
   c. Not specific
   d. Highly specific

5. If the normal curve is used to establish normal references for laboratory values, the results for a large sample of healthy people are compiled, and the normal range is usually designated as

   a. 37.5% above and 37.5% below the average (75% of all scores)
   b. The lower half of the sample (50% of all scores)
   c. Any value within the range (100% of all scores)
   d. Two standard deviations above and below the average (95% of all scores)

6. In conventional laboratory reports, the smallest amount of a substance would be measured by weight as a

   a. ng
   b. pg
   c. mcg
   d. mg

7. Laboratory results measured in SI units are reported as amount per volume as expressed by

   a. Milliequivalents (mEq)
   b. Milliosmoles (mOsm)
   c. Millimoles (mmol)
   d. Milligrams (mg)

8. Which of the following tests is of questionable value as a basic screening test for asymptomatic adult populations 50–65 years of age?

   a. Annual blood pressure checks
   b. Complete blood count (CBC) and urinalysis every 2–3 years
   c. Annual mammograms for women
   d. Serum cholesterol levels every 5 years

9. Cindy Barrows is a new nurse manager who wants to help her staff develop a good relationship with the laboratory personnel. Which one of the following actions by the nursing staff would be counterproductive to achieving this goal?

   a. Calling the laboratory to seek information about client preparation for an unfamiliar test
   b. Seeing that stat specimens are hand-delivered to the laboratory and that only real emergencies are marked *stat*
   c. Making sure that special needs of the client are conveyed to personnel from other departments who must interact with the client
   d. Complaining only to other nurses about the mistakes made by the laboratory personnel

▼ REFERENCES

Avant, K. (1990). The art and science in nursing diagnosis development. *Nursing Diagnosis, 1* (2), 51–56.

Balint, J. (1978). When is a new test a valid test. *American Journal of Digestive Diseases, 23,* 291–292.

Barnett, R., et al. (1978). Medical usefulness of STAT tests. *American Journal of Clinical Pathology, 69,* 520–523.

Blomberg, D.J. (1993). The clinical pathologists of tomorrow. *American Journal of Pathology, 100 Suppl 1* (4), S22–S23.

Blue Cross/Blue Shield. (1979). Limits of admission test payments. *American Journal of Nursing, 79* (4), 572.

Brandon, A., and Hill, D. (1994). Selected list of nursing books and journals. *Nursing Outlook, 42,* 71–82.

Bulechek, G.M., McCloskey, J.C., Titler, M.G., et al. (1994). Report on the NIC Project: Nursing interventions used in practice. *American Journal of Nursing, 94* (10), 59–66.

Calfee, B. (1991). Protecting yourself from allegations of nursing negligence. *Nursing 91, 21* (12), 34–39.

Campion, E.W. (1992). A retreat from SI units (Editorial). *New England Journal of Medicine, 327* (1), 49.

Carnevali, D. (1984). Nursing diagnosis: An evolutionary view. *Topics in Clinical Nursing, 5* (4), 10–20.

Chow, M. (1986). *Regulation of nursing practice in California*. San Francisco: California Nurses Association.

Corbett, J.V. (1989). Conversion to SI units (Letter to the editor). *Nursing Research, 38* (3), 61.

Corbett, J.V., and LaBorde, A. (1994). Nurses' perceptions of usefulness of laboratory data for nursing practice. *Journal of Continuing Education, 25* (4), 175–180.

Cushing, M. (1985). Lessons from history: The picket-guard nurse. *AJN, 85* (10), 1073–1076.

Doebbeling, B., and Wenzel, R. (1990). The direct costs of universal precautions in a teaching hospital. *JAMA, 264* (16), 2083–2087.

Dowling, P., et al. (1989). An education program to reduce unnecessary laboratory tests by residents. *Academic Medicine, 64* (7), 410–412.

Fitzpatrick, J.J., and Zanotti, R. (1995). Where are we now? Nursing diagnosis internationally. *Nursing Diagnosis, 6* (1), 42–47.

Flynn, J.C. (1994). *Proceedings in phlebotomy*. Philadelphia: W.B. Saunders.

Gordon, M. (1979). The concept of nursing diagnosis. *Nursing Clinics of North America, 14,* 487–495.

Gordon, M. (1990). Toward theory-based diagnostic categories. *Nursing Diagnosis, 1* (1), 5–11.

Goldbloom, R., Oboler, S.K., and Sox, H.C. (1993). Periodic health evaluation: What to include in the evaluation. *Patient Care, Feb 28,* 14–28.

Jagger, J., Hunt, E.L., Brand-Elnaggar, E., et al. (1988). Rates of needle-stick injury caused by various devices in a university hospital. *New England Journal of Medicine, 319,* 284–288.

Jordan, C.D., Flood, J.G., Laposata, M., et al. (1992). Normal reference laboratory values. *New England Journal of Medicine, 327* (10), 718–724.

Kaplan, E., et al. (1985). The usefulness of preoperative laboratory screening. *JAMA, 253* (24), 3576–3581.

Kaplan, A., Jack, R., Opheim, K.E., et al. (1995). *Clinical chemistry. Interpretation and techniques*. (4th ed.). Baltimore: Williams & Wilkins.

Kee, J.L., and Hayes, E.R. (1990). Assessment of patient laboratory data in the acutely ill. *Nursing Clinics of North America, 25*, 751–759.

Larson, E. (1986). Evaluating validity of screening tests. *Nursing Research, 35* (3), 186–188.

McAfee, T., Garland, L.R., and McNabb, T.S. (1990). How to safely draw blood from a vascular access device. *Nursing 90, 20* (11), 42–43.

McCloskey, J., and Bulechek, G. (1995). Validation and coding of the NIC taxonomy structure. *Image, 27* (1), 43–49.

Munroe, W.P. (1994). Home diagnostic kits. *American Pharmacy, NS 34* (2), 50–58.

Nanji, A., et al. (1988). Near patient testing: Quality of laboratory test results obtained by non-technical personnel in a decentralized setting. *American Journal of Clinical Pathology, 84* (6), 797–800.

Noble, D. (1993). Controversies in the clinical chemistry laboratory. *Analytical Chemistry, 65* (11), 547A–551A.

Northrop, C. (1986). Lessons from the law: Look and look again. *Nursing 86, 16* (1), 43.

Pysher, T., and Daly, J. (1989). The pediatric office laboratory: A look at recent trends. *Pediatric Clinics of North America, 36*, 1–25.

Ravel, R. (1995). *Clinical laboratory medicine: Clinical application of laboratory data*. (6th ed.). St. Louis: Mosby–Year Book.

Reker, D., and Webb, E. (1986). Multiple blood samples without multiple blood sticks. *RN, 49* (4), 39–41.

Showstack, J., et al. (1985). The role of changing clinical practice in the rising costs of hospital care. *New England Journal of Medicine, 313* (19), 1201–1206.

Silva, A.E., Hosein, B., Boyle, R.W., et al. (1994). Diagnosis of chronic hepatitis C: Comparison of immunoassays and the polymerase chain reaction. *American Journal of Gastroenterology, 89* (4), 493–496.

Sox, H.C. (1986). Probability theory in the use of diagnostic tests. *Annals of Internal Medicine, 104* (1), 60–65.

Sox, H.C. (1994). Preventive health services in adults. *New England Journal of Medicine, 330* (22), 1589–1595.

Stocker, S. (1985). No more Dracula jokes, please. *Nursing 85, 15* (4), 104.

Tallman, V. (1982). Effect of venipuncture on glucose, insulin and free fatty acid levels. *Western Journal of Nursing Research, 4* (1), 21–34.

Walter, R., and Keen, C. (1990). SI Units: A whole hearted effort is needed (Letter to the editor). *JAMA, 264* (8), 974.

Weedn, V.W. (1993). Where did this come from? Identification of sample mix-ups by DNA testing (Editorial). *American Journal of Clinical Pathology, 100* (6), 592–593.

Weeth, J. (1990). SI Units: What do internists think? (Letter to the editor). *Archives of Internal Medicine, 150* (1), 221.

Woo, J., McCabe, J.B., Chauncey, D., et al. (1993). The evaluation of a portable clinical analyzer in the emergency department. *American Journal of Clinical Pathology, 100* (6), 599–605.

Young, D. (1974). Standardized report of laboratory data: The desirability of using SI units. *New England Journal of Medicine, 290*, 368–373.

Young, D. (1987). Implementation of SI units for clinical laboratory data. *Annals of Internal Medicine, 106*, 114–129.

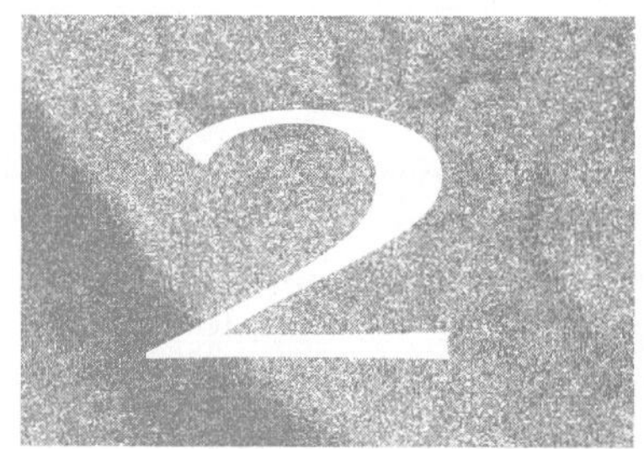

HEMATOLOGY TESTS

- Red Blood Cell Count
- Hematocrit
- Hemoglobin
- Erythrocyte Indices: Mean Corpuscular Volume, Mean Corpuscular Hemoglobin, and Mean Corpuscular Hemoglobin Concentration
- Red Blood Cell Distribution Width
- Serum Folic Acid and Vitamin B_{12}
- Serum Iron Levels, Total Iron-Binding Capacity, Transferrin Saturation, Serum Ferritin Levels, and Free Erythrocyte Protoporphyrin
- Glucose-6-Phosphate-Dehydrogenase
- Reticulocyte Count
- Erythropoietin Assay
- Peripheral Blood Smear
- Erythrocyte Sedimentation Rate
- Total White Blood Cell Count and Differential

OBJECTIVES

1. Describe the purpose for each of the different tests done by hematology analyzers.
2. Identify appropriate nursing diagnoses for clients with increased and decreased hemoglobin (hgb) and red blood cell count (RBC) levels.
3. Anticipate how a change in the hydration status of a client affects hematocrit (hct) results.

4. Describe how acute and chronic blood loss, iron deficiency anemia, and pernicious anemia change the erythrocyte indices.
5. Prepare teaching plans, which include specific information on drugs and diet, for clients with abnormal serum folic acid, B_{12}, iron, or glucose-6-phosphate-dehydrogenase (G-6-PD) levels.
6. Give examples of clinical situations in which an elevated reticulocyte count is an expected physiologic response.
7. Plan appropriate nursing interventions for a client who has an increasing erythrocyte sedimentation rate (sed rate or ESR).
8. Compare and contrast reference values for the differential (diff) white blood cell (WBC) count in children, in adults, and in pregnancy.
9. Define the meaning of the phrase "shift to the left" with regard to the diff WBC count.
10. Identify appropriate nursing diagnoses for clients with increased and decreased levels of the different types of leukocytes.

Routine hematology tests can be performed by automatic counters, so the results are more reliable than the older method of counting under a microscope. Table 2–1 lists the tests routinely completed with a hematology analyzer, a standard instrument in all laboratories. If the WBC count is abnormal, it is necessary to know which of the five types of WBCs is increased or decreased. The test of the five WBC types is called a *differential.*

Sometimes only one component of the complete blood count (CBC) is needed. For example, if the primary concern is assessing blood loss, a hct performed a few hours after the bleeding gives an index of the severity of the blood loss. With undiagnosed anemia, it would be important to have RBC, hgb, and hct readings. These three different measurements of the erythrocytes (red blood cells) are the figures used to compute the erythrocyte indices: (1) mean corpuscular volume (MCV), (2) mean corpuscular hemoglobin (MCH), and (3) mean corpuscular hemoglobin concentration (MCHC).

TABLE 2–1. USUAL TESTS DONE AUTOMATICALLY BY CELL COUNTERS[a]

Hct	Hematocrit
Hgb	Hemoglobin
WBC	Leukocyte or white blood cells (differential requires separate test)
RBC	Erythrocyte or red blood cells
MCV	Mean corpuscular volume (RBC distributed width can also be calculated)
MCH	Mean corpuscular hemoglobin
MCHC	Mean corpuscular hemoglobin concentration

Platelet counts may also be performed with some counters.

[a]Can perform all tests on 1 mL of blood. Blood is collected in a vacuum tube with EDTA as anticoagulant (lavender top).

A reticulocyte count gives an indication of the rate of production of RBCs. One test that involves erythrocytes and that is discussed in this chapter is the sed rate, or ESR, but it really has nothing to do with erythrocyte production or function. The sed rate or ESR is a test for inflammatory reactions. A peripheral smear of blood is prepared to look for abnormal blood cells. This chapter mentions some of the common terms used on laboratory reports of peripheral smears. Related hematology tests (e.g., serum iron levels, folic acid, B_{12} levels, and G-6-PD) are also mentioned because they may be needed to assess a persistent and unexplained anemic state. Although platelets are formed by the bone marrow, these fragments of tissue are not really blood cells in the true sense of the words. Platelets are covered with tests of clotting factors in Chapter 13.

▼ RED BLOOD CELL COUNT

The RBC count is a count of the number of RBCs per cubic millimeter (mm^3) of blood. In addition to other less understood mechanisms, a hormone named *erythropoietin*, secreted mainly by the kidney, stimulates the production of RBCs by the red bone marrow. Tissue hypoxia causes an increased secretion of erythropoietin.

Preparation of Client and Collection of Sample

There is no special preparation of the client for this test, which requires 1 mL of venous blood. EDTA is used as the anticoagulant (lavender top vacuum tube).

REFERENCE VALUES FOR RBC COUNT	
Adult: Men	4.6–5.9 million (or 10^6)/mm^3
Women	4.2–5.4 million/mm^3
Pregnancy	Slightly lower
Newborn	5.5–6, gradually decreases
Children	4.6–4.8, varies with age

Values increase at high altitudes. See Tikly et al. (1987) for ethnic variations.

Increased RBC (Polycythemia or Erythrocytosis)

Clinical Significance. Physiologic increases in RBC counts occur with a move to high altitude or after increased physical training. In both instances, the underlying reason is a response to an increased need for oxygen. At high altitude there is less oxygen in the atmosphere, so the bone marrow increases the production of RBCs. In the event of prolonged physical training, the increased muscle mass requires more oxygen.

The RBC count may be elevated for many pathologic reasons. One is a disease of unknown origin called *polycythemia vera,* the name of which implies that it is a true (vera) increase in RBC count. The increase in this case is not caused by an oxygen need, as it is in all other cases of polycythemia, which are termed *secondary polycythemia* or *erythrocytosis.* No general agreement has been reached regarding using the term *polycythemia* to indicate an increase in RBC count as well as other cells and *erythrocytosis* to designate an increase in RBC count alone. Two common clinical examples of secondary polycythemia, or more specifically erythrocytosis, are clients with chronic lung diseases and children with congenital heart defects who display cyanosis. The increased RBC count is an attempt to compensate for the chronic hypoxia brought on by the disease state.

In care for a client with an elevated RBC count, the nurse must differentiate primary from secondary polycythemia. In the event of primary polycythemia, medical treatment is geared to slowing the overactive bone marrow. Radioactive phosphorus has been used for more than 40 years (Herring et al., 1986). If the polycythemia or erythrocytosis is secondary to a state of chronic hypoxia, therapeutic measures are geared toward correcting the cause of the hypoxia. For example, the child with a congenital heart defect may undergo surgical treatment. For a client with chronic lung disease, hypoxia may not be treatable (see Chapter 6 on hypoxia).

▼ POSSIBLE NURSING DIAGNOSIS RELATED TO ELEVATED RBC COUNT

Risk for Injury Related to Possible Formation of Venous Thrombi

One of the basic problems that occurs with polycythemia, regardless of the cause, is that the blood becomes more viscous, and this increased viscosity makes the client more susceptible to the formation of venous thrombi. A key goal for the client with polycythemia is to maintain adequate hydration. In some cases, it may be desirable to increase fluids to a set level, such as a minimum of 2,000 mL a day for an adult. Before assuming that fluids need to be increased, assess the overall status of the client, particularly the cardiovascular status. Both children with congenital heart defects and adults with chronic lung disease may often be on the verge of congestive heart failure. Confer with the physician to determine the optimal hydration state for individual clients. It is important that any client with polycythemia or erythrocytosis not become dehydrated. For example, it may be harmful for the client to avoid taking anything by mouth for an extended time before tests.

Encouraging Activity. The client with polycythemia needs as much activity as possible so that venous stasis does not contribute to the risk for venous thrombosis.

Decreased RBC

Clinical Significance. A low RBC can result from

1. Abnormal loss of erythrocytes
2. Abnormal destruction of erythrocytes
3. Lack of needed elements or hormones for erythrocyte production
4. Bone marrow suppression

The term *anemia* is a nonspecific term that can mean a decrease in the total number of RBCs, in the hgb level of RBCs, or in both the number and the hgb content of RBCs. Thus, if the RBC count is low, looking at hgb levels is also important to classify the type of anemia. The classification of different types of anemia is covered in the section on erythrocyte indices.

It is not necessary for a RBC count to be used routinely to check for bleeding because the hct can be performed more quickly. Refer to the section on hct to see the nursing implications when the low RBC count is due to blood loss.

If the low RBC count is caused by a condition other than blood loss, then hgb levels and a peripheral smear that identifies the shape and size of erythrocytes may be necessary to identify the type of anemia. Erythropoietin assay (EPO) may be done. Refer to the sections on hgb and on erythrocyte indices for related nursing diagnoses in different types of anemias.

▼ HEMATOCRIT

The hematocrit (hct, PCV, or Crit) is a fast way to determine the percentage of RBCs in the plasma. When the serum is centrifuged, the WBCs and platelets rise to the top in what is called the *buffy coat.* Because the heavier RBCs are packed in the bottom, the hct is sometimes also called the *packed cell volume* (PCV). The hct is reported as a percentage because it is the proportion of RBCs to the plasma. Note that the results are based on the assumption that the plasma volume is normal. A hct is useful as a measurement of RBCs *only if the hydration of the client is normal.*

Preparation of Client and Collection of Sample

Because the hct can be performed on capillary blood, a client may undergo a finger stick (or heel stick for infants) rather than a venipuncture (see Chapter 1 for the procedure for heel and finger sticks). The first drop of blood is discarded. Enough blood is collected to fill a capillary tube supplied by the laboratory, and a small adhesive strip can be placed over the site. The stick method should be noted on the laboratory requisition because capillary values may be 5–10% higher than values by venipuncture. Do *not* squeeze the tissue to get capillary blood, because doing so adds tissue fluids, which dilute the sample.

REFERENCE VALUES FOR HCT

Adult: Men	42–52%
Women	37–48%
Pregnancy	Decreases, particularly in last trimester as serum volume increases
Newborn	Up to 60%
Children	Varies with age

Capillary blood may be 5–10% higher. Values are increased in high altitudes.

Relation to Hemoglobin Levels

If the RBC count and hgb are both normal, the hct is about three times the hgb. So a client whose hct is 45% would be expected to have a hgb level of about 15 g.

Increased Hematocrit

Clinical Significance. Because the hct is a proportion (or percentage) of RBCs to volume, any decrease in the volume of plasma causes an increase in hct, even though the RBC count has not increased. For example, in a client with a burn, plasma can be lost in large amounts through damaged capillaries in the burned area. The loss of fluid from the vascular space makes the blood very concentrated, and hence the hct may be as high as 60 or 65%.

If the client's hydration status is normal, an elevated hct signifies a true increase in RBC count. Reasons for an increased RBC count (polycythemia) are discussed in the section on RBC count.

▼ POSSIBLE NURSING DIAGNOSIS RELATED TO ELEVATED HCT

Fluid Volume Deficit

When caring for a client with an increased hct, it is essential to find out if this is a reflection of (1) decreased plasma volume or (2) a true increase in RBC count. If all clinical assessments point to lack of volume, measures to increase the plasma volume are needed. For example, parenteral fluid replacement is an essential part of the treatment for a client with severe burns. In other, less severe situations, it may be sufficient to increase oral ingestion of fluids to overcome dehydration.

If the elevated hct reflects an increased number of RBCs, additional fluids may be appropriate to decrease blood viscosity. The precautions for overhydrating a client with polycythemia are discussed in the section on increased RBC count, as was a nursing diagnosis related to the risk for the development of venous thrombi.

Decreased Hematocrit

Clinical Significance. A decreased hct can be due to either (1) an overhydration of the client, which increases the plasma volume, or (2) a true decrease in the number of RBCs. The second reason for the low hct is much more common. (See the section on RBC count for the causes of decreased numbers of RBCs.)

One of the important uses for the hct is assessing the magnitude of blood loss. It is important for nurses to realize that a blood specimen for a hct drawn immediately after a massive blood loss will probably be normal because both plasma and RBCs have been lost in equal proportions. Within a few hours after a bleeding episode, assuming the client has adequate fluid balance, the plasma volume returns to normal by a shift of some interstitial fluid into the plasma. The RBCs, however, cannot be replaced so quickly. The bone marrow takes about 7 days to make new cells, and those cells need another 4 days to mature. So a few hours after the bleeding episode, the plasma volume is back to normal and the hct becomes low because the RBCs that were lost in the hemorrhage are still missing. *A hct must always be interpreted in relation to the time the sample is drawn and to the probable hydration status of the client at the time.*

▼ POSSIBLE NURSING DIAGNOSES RELATED TO DECREASED HCT

Risk for Fluid Volume Excess

In the rare situation in which a low hct reflects an increased plasma volume, the client may show other signs and symptoms of excess fluid. Therapeutic measures may include a decrease in fluid intake. However, hct is not a key assessment tool for volume expansion. (See the discussion on low serum sodium levels, Chapter 5, as a test for overhydration; see also Chapter 4 on osmolality.)

Risk for Activity Intolerance Related to Loss of Blood

Paleness of the skin and the conjunctiva is a clue that there has been considerable blood loss. Checking for pallor of the conjunctiva is particularly helpful for assessing black clients. Because the plasma volume is usually replaced within a few hours after a bleeding episode, clients with low hct may have normal blood pressures. If there is not enough fluid to shift in the vascular space to make up the loss, the blood pressure falls and the client shows signs of shock. However, if the blood loss is not severe enough to produce shock, the pulse may still give a clue to the magnitude of blood loss: The pulse increases when the client sits up—the "tilt" test. The pulse may become even more elevated if much exercise is attempted because the oxygen-carrying capacity of the blood is diminished. When the hct is as low as 28%, the cardiac rate may be increased, even at rest. Monitoring the pulse before and after activity helps one assess the effect of the low hct on the individual client.

(continued)

▼ POSSIBLE NURSING DIAGNOSES RELATED TO DECREASED HCT (*continued*)

Weakness and fatigue on exertion should be taken into account when planning activities. It may be better not to bathe the client, change the bed linens, and mobilize the patient all at the same time. If a low hct continues to drop, a key nursing implication is to assess for signs of continued bleeding. A detailed description of nursing assessments for occult (hidden) bleeding is covered in Chapter 13 on clotting factors.

Differences Between Acute and Chronically Low Hematocrits. The effect of the low hct on the client depends not only on how low the hct is but also on whether the loss is acute or chronic. If the hct is low because of a sudden blood loss, signs of shock may quickly develop. A client with a chronically low hct may have only a few symptoms because the body has had time to adjust to the low number of RBCs. For example, clients undergoing renal dialysis often tolerate a hct as low as 18%. (The low hct in renal failure is partially due to a lack of the hormone erythropoietin, which is normally produced by the kidney.) A client with sickle cell anemia is another example of a client who may have a few symptoms related to a hct as low as 18–20%. (In sickle cell anemia, the RBCs have an abnormal type of hgb, which decreases the life of the cells.) The essential point to remember about interpreting the low hct is to understand not only the reason for the low hct but also whether the drop is acute or chronic.

Alteration in Nutritional Requirements for Iron and Protein

A client with a low hct needs adequate iron and protein in the diet so that the bone marrow can manufacture additional RBCs. A client who has a lack of protein may produce less protein hormones such as erythropoietin. If oral intake is possible, the nurse may help the client choose foods that are high in protein and iron. Foods rich in iron are liver, egg yolk, lean beef, and prune juice (Cerrato, 1985). Iron derived from animal products, called *heme iron,* is readily available for absorption. Iron from all other sources, called *nonheme iron,* is often not absorbed well because of dietary inhibitors. Food fortification to increase the consumption of bioavailable nonheme dietary iron has been effective in reducing the prevalence of iron deficiency anemia, particularly in young women and children. There is no evidence that iron fortification at currently recommended levels is harmful, but research continues in this area (Lynch, 1994). A dietitian can be useful to help plan optimal nutrition for clients with demonstrated deficiencies in iron or protein intake.

Knowledge Deficit Related to Iron Supplements

Once a client is deficient in iron, as happens with a chronic blood loss, it may be difficult to increase iron intake by diet alone. Sometimes iron supplements are prescribed. Clients need to be aware that iron supplements cause the feces to become dark greenish-black and that iron can be constipating. Iron is better absorbed in an acidic stomach, but some iron combinations are better tolerated with food. The client should not take antacids and iron together, because the iron is much less soluble in an alkaline medium. Other drugs, such as tetracycline and cholesterol-lowering drugs, also reduce iron absorption. The usual therapeutic plan is to continue iron supplements for about 3 months after the hct is back to normal because the body takes this long to build up a reserve of iron. Clients are usually quite interested in knowing the change in hct reading, and their inquiry can be a good occasion to explain why iron supplements are needed. Nurses need to also reinforce the message that iron products are the leading cause of accidental poisoning in children (Corbett, 1995).

Risk for Infection

Anemia with an accompanying iron deficiency may lessen the immunologic defenses of the client. Iron deficiency is often associated with other nutritional deficiencies that predispose the person to infections (Lyle, 1992). Thus measures to protect an anemic client from infection are warranted. (See Chapter 16 on infection control in clients at high risk.)

Alteration in Comfort

In addition to the fatigue and weakness discussed earlier, clients with anemia also are easily chilled. Extra blankets and warm clothing should be provided.

Risk for Alteration in Breathing Pattern

Dyspnea usually does not develop unless the hct is quite low. When the hct is low, the amount of oxygen to the tissue is reduced, but arterial blood gases are normal. Simply increasing the percentage of oxygen in the inspired air (FIO_2) does not solve the problem. For example, an anemic client with dyspnea would probably benefit more from a transfusion of RBCs than from O_2 administration. (See Chapter 6 on oxygen therapy, which may be needed for symptomatic relief.)

Risk for Alteration in Thought Processes

Some investigators believe that iron deficiency in children is accompanied by an impairment of intellectual performance and behavioral changes. Decreased work performance may occur in adults depending on the degree of the deficiency (Lyle, 1992). Nurses should be aware of clients who are at high risk for chronic anemia and malnutrition because of the possible socioeconomic consequences of being unable to perform optimally at school or in the workplace.

Risk for Injury Related to Use of Blood Transfusions

If the hct is less than 25–30%, a physician may order blood, usually in the form of packed cells, to replace the erythrocytes. Packed cells are used when the

(*continued*)

▼ POSSIBLE NURSING DIAGNOSES RELATED TO DECREASED HCT (*continued*)

client needs the RBCs but not additional plasma. No set figure means the client needs blood. As discussed earlier, some clients have a chronically low hct with few symptoms. Depending on the symptoms and on the individual circumstances, blood may be given before clients have a hct as low as 25 or 30%. For example, if a client is going to surgery, it is important that the hct not be too low—"too low" usually meaning less than 30%. Because blood transfusions can cause additional problems, such as allergic reactions or transmission of viruses, the physician may choose to let the body replenish erythrocytes normally whenever this is feasible. (See Chapter 14 for a discussion on transfusion reactions and nursing actions to prevent injury.) As a rough guideline, a unit of whole blood or packed cells raises the hct about 3% in an adult.

▼ HEMOGLOBIN

Hemoglobin is composed of a pigment (*heme*), which contains iron, and a protein (*globin*). If each erythrocyte has the normal amount of hgb, the hct is roughly three times the hgb level. A hct of 45% would indicate about 15 g of hgb. It is not necessary to perform both tests to assess for bleeding. As already discussed, the hct is a simpler test to monitor blood loss. If RBCs are abnormal in size or shape, or if hgb is not being produced normally, the hgb level cannot be estimated from the hct. Hgb levels are necessary as part of the assessment for various types of anemia. (See the erythrocyte indices for an explanation of how the hgb level is used with hct and RBC tests to provide clear information about erythrocyte abnormalities.)

Preparation of Client and Collection of Sample

Venous blood is used for the test. EDTA (lavender top vacuum tube) is used as the anticoagulant in the collection tube. Hgb can also be assessed on blood collected with a finger stick. This rapid measurement gives results comparable to those of standard laboratory techniques (Cohen and Seidl-Friedman, 1988).

REFERENCE VALUES FOR HGB

Adult: Men	13.0–18.0 g/100 mL
Women	12–16 g/100 mL
Pregnancy	11–12 g/100 mL

Newborn	17–19 g/100 mL average % of fetal hemoglobin 1 day 77% 3 wk 70% 4 mo 23%
Children	14–17 g/100 mL, depending on age

Values increase in high altitudes. To convert to SI units, 1.6 g = 1 mmol.

Increased Hemoglobin Level

Clinical Significance. Because a normal RBC already contains the optimum amount of hgb, any increase in hgb level must be evaluated in relation to the number and size of the erythrocytes. (See the discussion on erythrocyte indices for an explanation of how the hgb level is used with the hct and RBC count to determine if the erythrocyte is hypochromic [less color], normochromic, or [very rarely] hyperchromic.)

Decreased Hemoglobin

Clinical Significance. Because hgb is a component of the RBC, all the conditions that cause a low RBC count also result in a low hgb level. Some of the common conditions for a low RBC count are blood loss, hemolytic anemia, and any type of bone marrow suppression.

Hgb levels are low in clients who have abnormal types of hgb, or hemoglobinopathies. RBCs with abnormal types of hgb tend to be fragile and easily destroyed in the vascular system. The normal hgb in adults is almost all adult hgb (hgbA) with only a very small amount (0–2%) of fetal hgb (hgbF). A process called *hemoglobin electrophoresis* can identify the specific type of abnormal hgb that is present. More than 200 hgbs can be identified, but only a few cause symptoms.

In thalassemia major, the client has an unusual amount of hgbF and abnormalities in the synthesis of hgb. In sickle cell anemia, the client has an abnormal hgb called *sickle hemoglobin* (hgbS). (See Chapter 18 for screening tests for sickle cell anemia and for thalassemia, which are both genetically determined.)

It is possible to have a normal RBC count with a low hgb level. For example, with iron deficiency anemia, the count may be near normal but each cell has less hgb than normal. This is called *hypochromic* (less than normal color) anemia. The cells also tend to be *microcytic* (smaller than normal). Women in general need more iron than men because of the loss of iron in the menstrual flow, and women who have heavy flow may be prone to low hgb levels. The demand for iron is increased in pregnancy. If a woman begins pregnancy with low iron reserves, she may become severely anemic as the pregnancy progresses. It is recommended that a pregnant woman be tested for hgb levels at the beginning of pregnancy, about midpregnancy, and during the month before delivery. Because there is a normal drop in hgb levels in the last trimester, due to the expanded plasma volume, some lowering in hgb levels is "normal." This lowering is sometimes called the *physiologic anemia of pregnancy*. If the mother does not have enough stored iron to meet the demands of the fetus, iron supplements may be needed.

▼ POSSIBLE NURSING DIAGNOSES RELATED TO DECREASED HEMOGLOBIN

Most of the nursing diagnoses for a client with a low hgb level are covered in the section on low hct. Additional insights about the clinical significance of low hgb levels are covered in the section on erythrocyte indices. (See the section on MCH and MCHC for nursing implications for hypochromic and normochromic anemias.)

▼ ERYTHROCYTE INDICES

To make the nonspecific term *anemia* more meaningful, it is necessary to see whether the individual RBCs are of normal size and whether they have the normal amount of hgb. One can make the determinations by comparing the results of the hgb, hct, and RBC count. In laboratories that use automated counters—and all of them do now—the indices are automatically figured as part of the CBC. Nurses never need to calculate the indices, but the formula for each is given, because the formulas make it easy to explain the meaning of the results. In the examples used, the client has a hct of 40%, a hgb level of 13.5 g, and a RBC count of 4.5 million/mm^3. Note that with these figures, all the indices would, of course, be normal.

Preparation of Client and Collection of Sample

There is no need to draw additional blood because the indices are derived from the hct, hgb level, and RBC count.

Mean Corpuscular Volume

The MCV describes the mean or average size of the individual RBC in cubic micrometers (μm^3). The hct percentage is multiplied by 10 and is divided by the RBC count to provide the MCV.

REFERENCE VALUES AND EXAMPLE FOR MCV

Reference values	MCV = 86–98 μm³
Formula	$MCV = \frac{\text{hct (\%)} \times 10}{\text{RBC (millions/mm}^3\text{)}}$
Client example	$\frac{40 \times 10}{4.5} = 89\ \mu m^3$

Newborns and infants have higher values.

Change in the MCV

Clinical Significance. The MCV is an indicator of the size of the RBCs. If the MCV is lower than 86 μm³, the erythrocytes are *microcytic*, or smaller than normal. RBCs are microcytic in some types of anemia, such as iron deficiency anemia and lead poisoning. Thalassemia minor and thalassemia major (Cooley's anemia), which are genetic diseases, also cause microcytosis. (See Chapter 18 on screening tests for the thalassemias.) If the MCV is higher than 98 μm³, the erythrocytes are *macrocytic*, or larger than normal. Macrocytic RBCs are characteristic of pernicious anemia and folic acid deficiencies. Macrocytosis is common in liver disease and is sometimes used as a marker of recent alcohol intake. MCV also has been described as predictor of mortality in clients with advanced cirrhosis (Abad-Lacruz, et al., 1993). If the MCV is within normal reference range, the erythrocytes are *normocytic*, or of normal size. Anemia due to acute blood loss results in normocytic anemia.

The size of the RBCs is not enough to diagnose the reason for the anemia, but with other indices (MCH and MCHC), the anemia can be classified by size and color. Other tests, such as the peripheral blood smear, can identify the characteristic cell shapes of various pathologic conditions.

Mean Corpuscular Hemoglobin

MCH is the amount of hgb present in one cell. The result is reported by weight in picograms (pg). The weight of hgb in the average cell is obtained by multiplying the hgb level by 10 and dividing the result by the RBC count.

REFERENCE VALUES AND EXAMPLE FOR MCH

Reference values	MCH = 28–33 pg
Formula	$MCH = \frac{\text{hgb (g/100 mL)} \times 10}{\text{RBC (in millions/mm}^3\text{)}}$
Client example	$\frac{13.5\ g \times 10}{4.5} = 30\ pg$

Mean Corpuscular Hemoglobin Concentration

The MCHC is the proportion of each cell occupied by hgb. Because this is a proportion, the results are reported in percentages. To get the percentage, the hgb is divided by the hct and multiplied by 100.

REFERENCE VALUES AND EXAMPLE FOR MCHC

Reference values	MCHC = 32–36%
Formula	$\text{MCHC} = \frac{\text{hgb (g/100 mL)}}{\text{hct}} \times 100$
Client example	$\frac{13.5}{40} \times 100 = 33.8\%$

Changes in MCH and MCHC

Clinical Significance. These two parts of the erythrocyte indices are discussed together because both are ways to determine whether the erythrocytes are *normochromic* (normal color), *hypochromic* (less than normal color), or *hyperchromic* (more than normal color). Some institutions only obtain the MCH. A MCHC less than 32% (or a MCH < 28 pg) indicates that the erythrocytes have a decrease in hgb concentration (hypochromic). Iron deficiency anemia is the most common type of hypochromic anemia. Chronic conditions that cause anemia may show some hypochromia, but they are usually not as marked as when there is a true deficiency of iron. Certain genetically caused anemias such as thalassemia (Cooley's anemia) cause hypochromia. With many types of anemia, the remaining cells have the normal amount of hgb and hence are called normochromic. Hyperchromia (an abnormally high MCHC) is not seen except for a few rare conditions. As a rule, normal RBCs can hold only so much hgb, so the cells cannot be hyperchromic.

▼ RED BLOOD CELL DISTRIBUTION WIDTH

The RBC cell distribution width (RDW) is calculated from the MCV and the RBC. The variation of the width of the cell may help assess types of anemia. Reference values are usually 11.5–14.5%. The RDW may become abnormal before anemia occurs (Ravel, 1995).

▼ POSSIBLE NURSING IMPLICATIONS RELATED TO DIFFERENT TYPES OF ANEMIA

It is important for the nurse to understand that abnormal erythrocyte indices are useful in classifying types of anemia, but they are not enough to establish a definite medical diagnosis. The history of the client, physical assessment

TABLE 2–2. CLASSIFICATION OF ANEMIAS BY ERYTHROCYTE INDICES

Laboratory Results	Classification	Example of Common Pathologic Condition
MCV, MCH, and MCHC all normal	Normocytic, normochromic anemias	Acute blood loss
Decreased MCV, decreased MCH, and decreased MCHC	Microcytic, hypochromic anemias	Iron deficiency
Increased MCV, variable MCH and MCHC	Macrocytic anemia	Vitamin B_{12} deficiency, folic acid deficiency

findings, and other tests are needed to determine the cause of the anemia. Some general nursing diagnoses for clients with anemia are discussed under the sections on RBC, hgb, and hct. Other general nursing implications can be classified under the three categories of anemia. Table 2–2 lists the three categories and common pathologic conditions that could cause each type.

Microcytic, Hypochromic Anemias. Most likely this type of anemia is due to an iron deficiency if other causes such as thalassemia minor are ruled out. The serum iron level can be measured, as can the iron-binding capacity and ferritin and transferrin levels discussed later. As discussed earlier, in the section on hgb, it is difficult to correct an iron deficiency with diet alone. (See the section on hgb for what to teach a client about iron therapy.)

Normocytic, Normochromic Anemias. The cause could range from acute blood loss to a chronic genetic problem such as sickle cell disease. With a normocytic anemia, iron supplements may not be needed, but the nurse should make sure that the client has adequate protein and iron in the diet because of the continuing need for an increased production of RBCs. If the anemia is of genetic origin, the nurse's role centers on helping the client and the family adjust to a chronic disease. (See Chapter 18 on genetic screening.) Anemia is but one sign of a larger pathologic problem.

Macrocytic Anemias. This type of anemia may be hypochromic, normochromic, or very rarely hyperchromic. The two most common reasons for macrocytic anemias are vitamin B_{12} deficiency and folic acid deficiency. These two anemias are also called *megaloblastic anemias. Megaloblastic* refers to the appearance of a certain type of RBC precursor in the bone marrow and often in the bloodstream. (See the next section for two possible nursing diagnoses related to vitamin B_{12} and folic acid deficiencies.)

▼ SERUM FOLIC ACID AND VITAMIN B_{12}

Both vitamin B_{12} and folate can be measured in the serum when the initial laboratory results show macrocytosis (elevated MCV), a low reticulocyte count (discussed later), and hypersegmented neutrophils. These tests are used to help in diagnosing a macrocytic anemia that may be due to dietary deficiency or malabsorption.

Preparation of Client and Collection of Sample

Check with the laboratory about food or drug interference. The test for folic acid requires 1 mL of serum. The test for vitamin B_{12} requires 12 mL of serum.

REFERENCE VALUES FOR FOLIC ACID AND VITAMIN B_{12}

Folic acid	Greater than 3.3 ng/mL (Borderline 2.5–3.2 ng/mL) (Aged may have lower values)
Vitamin B_{12}	205–876 pg/mL (Borderline 140–204 pg/mL) (Aged may have lower values)

Some laboratories may measure the folic acid in red cells rather than in serum. Red cell values should be greater than 160 ng/mL (Gottfried, 1994).

▼ POSSIBLE NURSING DIAGNOSIS RELATED TO VITAMIN B_{12} DEFICIENCY

Knowledge Deficit Related to Need for Vitamin B_{12} Injections

Because vitamin B_{12} is present in all animal protein, a diet deficiency is rare. Pernicious anemia (a type of macrocytic anemia) refers to a pathologic inability of the body to absorb vitamin B_{12} because of the lack of the intrinsic factor in the stomach. (The Schilling test is a test for B_{12} absorption; see Chapter 22.) Nurses can help clients understand that not all types of "tired blood" can be treated with over-the-counter vitamin and iron mixtures. Clients often do not understand that anemia is only a symptom. The underlying pathologic reason for the anemia must be determined to ensure its successful treatment. For example, if the macrocytic anemia turns out to be caused by pernicious anemia, the client needs vitamin B_{12} shots for the rest of his or her life. So the nurse will probably be involved in helping the client and a member of the family learn to give injections. The importance of lifelong therapy must be emphasized to prevent relapses. Savage and Lindenbaum (1983) found it took about 5 years for pernicious anemia to develop when clients stopped taking their vitamin B_{12} injections.

▼ POSSIBLE NURSING DIAGNOSIS RELATED TO FOLIC ACID DEFICIENCY

Increased Nutritional Requirements for Folic Acid

Vitamin B_{12} is present in all animal protein, so rarely do people in the United States develop a true deficiency. However, unless vegetables are fresh, folic acid deficiency can develop because most of the folic acid is destroyed by heat.

Pregnancy and the use of oral contraceptives are situations in which a macrocytic anemia may occur because of an increased need for folic acid in the diet. Recent studies have shown that an adequate intake of folic acid in childbearing women reduces the risk of neural tube defects. Nurses have been instrumental in educational programs to inform all women of childbearing age to consume 0.4 mg of folic acid daily (Romanczuk and Brown, 1994). Folic acid antagonists, such as methotrexate used for cancer treatment, may deplete the client of folic acid, as may inflammatory bowel disease. It may be necessary for some clients to take oral supplemental vitamin preparations that are high in folic acid. Orange juice is a good natural source of folate. Folic acid can also be given subcutaneously if malabsorption is a problem.

Alcohol abuse may contribute to the development of a macrocytic anemia caused not only by folate or B_{12} deficiency but also by other, unknown factors. In such cases, diet teaching is of little avail until other problems are addressed. It is important for the nurse to see abnormal indices in relation to the client's total situation. It is important that the exact cause of the macrocytic anemia be identified because folic acid replacements can reverse the anemia, but folic acid cannot prevent the degeneration in the spinal cord from a persisting vitamin B_{12} deficiency caused by pernicious anemia.

▼ SERUM IRON LEVELS, TOTAL IRON-BINDING CAPACITY, TRANSFERRIN SATURATION, SERUM FERRITIN LEVELS, AND FREE ERYTHROCYTE PROTOPORPHYRIN

Several of the tests discussed in this section are used to assess iron deficiency anemias. These tests are not *routine* for all clients who take iron supplements; the screening tests of hgb, hct, and MCV combined with the medical history often are sufficient. The tests in this section are reserved for further evaluation of clients with microcytic, hypochromic anemia who do not respond to iron therapy. These tests are also used to evaluate iron metabolism and storage in diseases such as hemochromatosis, a genetic disorder that results in excessive iron deposits in organs.

Serum Iron Levels

Serum iron (Fe) levels can be measured directly. Because there is a diurnal variation in serum iron, with lower evening values, blood levels should be drawn in the morning (Pittiglio and Sacher, 1987). The client should not take any iron supplements for at least 24 hr before the test is performed.

Total Iron-Binding Capacity

Iron is transported in the bloodstream by transferrin, a plasma protein. Normally about one-third of the available transferrin transports iron. The total iron-binding capacity (TIBC) is a measurement of the transferrin available to bind more iron. The TIBC is used with the serum iron to calculate transferrin saturation.

Transferrin Saturation

Transferrin saturation is not a direct measurement. It is calculated from the results of the serum iron and the TIBC. The formula is

$$\frac{\text{Serum iron}}{\text{TIBC}} \times 100 = \text{\% of transferrin saturation}$$

Serum Ferritin Levels

Ferritin, the predominant iron storage protein, is directly related to the amount of iron storage in a healthy adult. However, illnesses such as infections, inflammations, and malignant diseases cause increased levels and thus may make ferritin level unreliable as an indicator of iron stores. If there are no chronic illnesses, serum ferritin determination is a very cost-efficient and reliable test for detecting iron deficiency. Malnutrition causes decreases, and thus ferritin levels, along with transferrin levels, are also used to assess protein depletion (see Chapter 10).

Free Erythrocyte Protoporphyrin

Erythrocyte protoporphyrin is used in the final step of heme synthesis. If iron is not present, the protoporphyrin is not incorporated into the hgb. Thus a measurement of free erythrocyte protoporphyrin (FEP) provides one of the most sensitive early detectors of iron deficiency. And because the FEP remains within the RBC for the entire life span of the cell, it can also be used to diagnose iron deficiency anemia even after administration of iron is started (Pittiglio and Sacher, 1987). Hemoglobin disorders such as thalassemia do not cause an increase, so the FEP is widely used to distinguish thalassemia trait from iron deficiency anemia. (The FEP measures porphyrins, of which 95% are the free erythrocyte.)

Preparation of Patient and Collection of Sample

Blood specimens for serum iron and TIBC are collected in *iron-free* tubes. Specimens for serum ferritin and FEP can be placed in either green or lavender top tubes. Check with the laboratory for amounts needed. Only iron must be drawn in the morning.

REFERENCE VALUES FOR IRON, FERRITIN, TIBC, TRANSFERRIN, AND FEP

Serum iron	50–150 μg/dL (higher in men)
Serum ferritin	Normal 20–400 ng/mL Borderline deficient 13–20 ng/mL Deficient 0–12 ng/mL Elderly may have iron deficient erythropoiesis with ferritin levels as high as 75 ng/mL Holyoake, et al., 1993)
Total iron-binding capacity (TIBC)	250–410 μg/dL
Transferrin saturation	20–50%
FEP	<35 μg/dL

Clinical Significance. Iron deficiency anemia results in a low serum iron level, an increased TIBC, and decreased transferrin saturation. In addition, the serum ferritin level is low and the FEP increased. When there is no obvious cause of an iron deficiency, further investigations are necessary to identify the underlying pathologic condition. For example, iron deficiency anemia may be caused by an adenocarcinoma of the gastrointestinal tract, which often causes occult bleeding. (See Chapter 13 on hemoccult testing.)

Elevations of serum iron, serum ferritin, and transferrin saturation with a decrease in the TIBC are characteristic of *hemochromatosis*, a genetic disorder of iron metabolism that causes organ damage from iron deposits. Excessive iron intake, which results in a condition called *hemosiderosis*, also causes elevations of the serum iron, serum ferritin, and transferrin saturation.

▼ POSSIBLE NURSING DIAGNOSIS RELATED TO CHANGES IN IRON REQUIREMENTS

Alteration in Nutritional Needs

Nurses should be aware of the recommended daily requirements of iron for young children (15 mg), men (10 mg), and women of childbearing age (18 mg), as well as the specific needs during pregnancy and for the newborn. Diet teaching may help prevent deficiencies, but iron supplements may be needed as discussed in the section on hgb. Some iron supplements come with ascorbic acid to help absorption of the iron.

For clients with iron storage problems, 1 or 2 pints (0.47 or 0.94 L) of blood may be removed each week until iron stores are normal. Afterward, therapy is continued every 2–4 months. A client with an overload problem should not eat large amounts of iron-containing foods, such as red meat, or take any type of iron supplement. The American Liver Foundation (1-800-223-0179), Cedar Grove, NJ, 07009, has excellent educational material for the client with hemochromatosis.

▼ GLUCOSE-6-PHOSPHATE-DEHYDROGENASE

Glucose-6-phosphate-dehydrogenase is one of many enzymes normally present in the erythrocytes. Some people have a lack of this enzyme because of a genetic defect. Hemolytic anemia may develop if the person is exposed to certain drugs, infections, or an acidotic state. Examples of drugs that cause hemolysis of erythrocytes in susceptible people are the sulfas and aspirin. Several laboratory tests detect a deficiency of this enzyme.

Preparation of Client and Collection of Sample

There is no special preparation of the client. The test requires 9 mL of venous blood collected in a tube with a special anticoagulant (anticoagulant citrate dextrose [ACD]). Various laboratories may perform other types of tests that require only a few milliliters of blood with other anticoagulants. A screening test may be done before the quantitive measurement. An increased reticulocyte count falsely elevates G-6-PD.

REFERENCE VALUES FOR G-6-PD	
All groups	5–15 U/g hgb

G-6-PD Deficiencies

Clinical Significance. The G-6-PD test may be used to determine if a hemolytic anemia is due to a lack of this specific enzyme. Other enzymes, such as pyruvate kinase, may also be deficient in the erythrocytes and cause anemia, but a lack of G-6-PD is more common. The lack of the enzyme is a sex-linked recessive trait carried on the X chromosomes, and mutations produce the variants that are identified (Beutler et al., 1989). The effect is more pronounced in men. (See Chapter 18 for a discussion of genetic diseases.) Unless the person either is exposed to drugs that cause the hemolysis or has a severe infection or an acidotic state, he or she is typically unaware of the defect.

▼ POSSIBLE NURSING DIAGNOSIS RELATED TO DRUGS AND FOODS TO AVOID

Knowledge Deficit

A client who has a lack of G-6-PD must not be given any drugs that can cause hemolysis. Clients need health teaching about exactly which drugs are to be avoided. For example, many over-the-counter drugs contain aspirin. Certain foods, such as fava beans, are not tolerated if the defect is the Mediterranean variant. Different variants may cause different intolerances.

▼ RETICULOCYTE COUNT

Reticulocytes are the less mature type of RBCs in the bloodstream. They are called reticulocytes because they show a fine network (reticulum) when stained. After about 4 days in the bloodstream, the cell loses this reticulum and becomes a mature RBC. The reticulocyte count (retic count) is valuable because it is a measurement of bone marrow function.

Preparation of Client and Collection of Sample

There is no special preparation of the client. The laboratory needs less than 1 mL of blood.

REFERENCE VALUES FOR RETIC COUNT	
Adult	0.5–2.5% of the total RBC count
Pregnancy	Slight increase
Newborn	Increased 3–5% first week

Increased Reticulocyte Count

Clinical Significance. An increase in the percentage of reticulocytes indicates that the release of RBCs into the bloodstream is occurring more rapidly than usual. Because this is a physiologic response to the need for more RBCs, the retic count may be as high as 10% after an acute blood loss. Such an increase is also expected when the appropriate treatment is begun for a specific type of anemia. For example, when a client with iron deficiency anemia is given iron supplements, the retic count may go as high as 32%. An increase in the retic count after therapy for anemia has begun is an encouraging sign that the bone marrow is responding to the treatment. Clients with sickle cell anemia usually have retic counts of 5–10% because of the increased destruction of RBCs.

Decreased Reticulocyte Count

Clinical Significance. In certain macrocytic anemias (see the discussion under erythrocyte indices), cell development is arrested before the reticulocyte stage. For example, in pernicious anemia, the ineffective production of RBCs leads to a low retic count. A decrease in reticulocytes, particularly after a bleeding episode, indicates an abnormal response of the bone marrow. The client needs further medical evaluation to determine the reason for this lack of erythrocyte production.

▼ ERYTHROPOIETIN ASSAY

Erythropoietin (EPO), a hormone produced primarily by the kidney, is the most important regulator of RBC production. Assays of this hormone may use either the RIA or ELISA methods discussed in Chapter 1. With the RIA there may be some cross-reactions with other plasma proteins. The ELISA method is more specific,and the results are known within 24 hr compared with several days for the RIA method. Both tests have problems in measuring subnormal levels (Wognum et al., 1989).

Preparation of Patient and Collection of Sample

There is no special preparation of the patient. Conventional labs require 1 mL of venous blood. Commercial kits are available, and thus the test may also be carried out as decentralized testing. The results are comparable to laboratory results (Hubbard and Wheeler, 1989).

REFERENCE VALUES FOR EPO
Less than 19 m/U/mL

Clinical Significance. An increased EPO, sometimes nearly double the normal value, is found in most types of anemia because the body is trying to increase the production of RBCs. One exception is the anemia of renal disease, because in this type of anemia, the kidneys have lost the ability to produce even normal amounts of EPO. EPO is available as a therapeutic injection (Epoetin alfa), and nurses may be case managers for clients undergoing dialysis who receive this drug (Sasak and Giordano, 1990). An increased EPO is found in polycythemia caused by hypoxia (secondary polycythemia) but is normal for polycythemia vera. Nursing diagnoses related to anemia and polycythemia are discussed earlier in this chapter, and nursing diagnoses for renal failure are presented in Chapter 4.

▼ PERIPHERAL BLOOD SMEAR

The peripheral blood smear is useful for the identification of abnormalities in erythrocytes, leukocytes, and platelets. If necessary, a bone marrow aspiration or biopsy may be performed as a follow-up test for abnormal results (see Chapter 25). Hematology studies include technical details about red cell and white cell morphology. Some of the more common terms that may appear on laboratory reports are as follows:

- Descriptive terms for RBCs
    1. *Anisocytosis* means that the cells vary in size.
    2. *Poikilocytosis* means that the cells are irregular in shape.
    3. *Rouleaux formation* is a laboratory phenomenon in which RBCs stick to one another. (Note that this is the basis for the sed rate.)

4. *Basophilic stipplings* are a characteristic pattern of dark spots caused by some abnormalities of hgb synthesis. This phenomenon is seen in lead poisoning and severe anemias.
5. *Howell Jolly bodies* are small remnants of nuclear material found in certain hemolytic and megoblastic anemias and after a splenectomy.

- Descriptive terms for WBCs

1. *Atypical lymphocytes* (Downey cells) are characteristic of infectious mononucleosis, hepatitis, and other viral and allergic reactions. They are also present with certain malignant neoplasms of the bone marrow.
2. *Myelocytes* and *metamyelocytes* are two stages of immature leukocytes that are normally in the bone marrow, not in the bloodstream. Pathologic conditions in bone marrow production may cause the release of various immature forms into the bloodstream.
3. *Blasts* are primitive cells found in certain malignant neoplasms that involve the bone marrow.
4. *Dohle bodies* are small pear-shaped inclusions in the cytoplasm found in some anemias and malignant neoplasms, and after ingestion of toxic substances.

- Descriptive term for platelets

1. *Thrombocytopathy* means abnormal-looking platelets. (See Chapter 13 for a discussion of platelet counts.)

▼ ERYTHROCYTE SEDIMENTATION RATE

The sed rate, or ESR, measures the speed with which RBCs settle in a tube of anticoagulated blood. The results are expressed as millimeters in an hour (mm/hr). An increase in plasma globulins or fibrinogen causes the cells to stick together (rouleaux formation) and thus to fall faster than normal. If the cells are smaller than normal (microcytic), they also fall faster than normal. And if they are larger than normal (macrocytic), they fall more slowly than normal. The laboratory takes into account any change in the size of the erythrocyte and corrects for this.

Because so many different conditions can cause an increase in globulins, fibrinogen, or other substances that can cause erythrocytes to clump together, the sed rate is a very nonspecific test. (See the discussion on C-reactive protein, Chapter 14, for another test of inflammation.) Both the sed rate and the C-reactive protein indicate a pathologic condition, but they do not identify the source. Sometimes the sed rate is explained as "showing how hot the fire (inflammation) is, but not where it is."

Preparation of Client and Collection of Sample

The test requires a minimum of 5 mL of anticoagulated blood. EDTA is used as the anticoagulant (lavender top vacuum tube).

REFERENCE VALUES FOR SED RATE

Westergren Method	
Adult: Men	1–13 mm/hr
Women	1–20 mm/hr
Pregnancy	44–114 mm/hr
Aged: Men older than 50 years	1–20 mm/hr
Women older than 50 years	1–30 mm/hr
Children	1–13 mm/hr
Wintrobe Method	
Adult: Men	1–9 mm/hr
Women	1–20 mm/hr

Upper limbs are not clearly defined after the age of 60 years.

Increased Sed Rate

Clinical Significance. A marked increase in the sed rate during pregnancy is a normal occurrence because there is an increase in globulins and in the fibrinogen level in pregnancy. A pathologic reason for an increased sed rate is usually an inflammation or tissue injury. For sed rates greater than 100 mm (in the nonpregnant client, of course), the most likely causes are infections, malignant tumors, or collagen vascular diseases. The sed rate is often used to monitor the course of rheumatoid arthritis or pelvic inflammatory disease (PID) or infectious states in clients with acquired immune deficiency syndrome (AIDS). A micro-ESR is an inexpensive, easy bedside screening test for neonatal sepsis. Values increase with postnatal age (day of life plus 3 mm/hr). Up to 15 mm/hr is normal (Gerdes, 1994).

▼ POSSIBLE NURSING DIAGNOSIS RELATED TO ELEVATED SED RATE

Activity Intolerance

If the sed rate is used as a screening device, the results may not be useful in planning nursing care because an abnormal sed rate requires more testing to determine the underlying pathophysiologic condition. If the disease is known, the results of the sed rate are helpful in assessing the acuteness of the inflammatory process. For example, a client with rheumatoid arthritis may exhibit an increasing sed rate, which is one clue that the client may need therapeutic interventions to control the inflammation, as well as limitation of activity to allow inflamed joints to rest.

A decreasing sed rate is indicative of a lessening of the inflammatory response. The change in the sed rate should alert the nurse to confer with the physician about reevaluating limitations placed on a client who has rheumatoid arthritis. As another example, clients who take antibiotics for PID may undergo sed rates to determine if the pelvic inflammation is subsiding and thus if more activity is allowed.

Decreased Sed Rate

Clinical Significance. A low rate is usually not clinically significant. Clients with polycythemia vera, hypoalbuminemia, sickle cell anemia, or a deficiency in blood Factor V have decreased sed rates.

▼ TOTAL WHITE BLOOD CELL COUNT AND DIFFERENTIAL

Two measurements of WBCs are commonly performed. One is the count of the total number of WBCs in a cubic millimeter of blood (WBC count). The other is the determination of the proportion of each of the five types of WBCs in a sample of 100 WBCs (differential). The first measurement, the WBC count, is an absolute number of so many thousand WBCs per cubic millimeter (/mm^3). The second measurement, the differential, is percentages because it is a report of the proportion of each type cell in a sample of 100. The precision of automated counters makes it easy to do an actual or absolute count of the various types of leukocytes. This absolute count is more useful than the differential. For example, if the total WBC count is 10,000/mm^3 with 2% bands (immature neutrophils) and 48% segmented or mature neutrophils, the absolute neutrophil count (ANC) per cubic millimeter is 5,000 (48% + 2% × 10,000). The ANC is useful for monitoring the effect of chemotherapeutic drugs that cause neutropenia.

It is important to understand that the differential is reported in percentages because an increase in the percentage of one type of cell always means a decrease in the percentage of another type even *though* the absolute number for the second type of cell may not decrease. For example, a man has a normal WBC count of 10,000/mm^3, with a neutrophil count of 60% and a lymphocyte count of 30%. One can figure out that the man has 3,000 lymphocytes per cubic millimeter (10,000 total × 30%). If this man gets a severe bacterial infection, his total WBC may rise to 20,000/mm^3. In a severe bacterial infection, almost all the increase in WBC count is due to an increase in neutrophils. The differential count now shows 75% neutrophils and only 15% lymphocytes, but this does not mean the man has fewer lymphocytes. He has 15% of 20,000, or 3,000, lymphocytes per cubic millimeter, just as before. Only the proportions have changed.

REFERENCE VALUES FOR WBC DIFFERENTIAL

Adult: Men and women		
Total WBC count	4,300–10,800/mm³	(Smokers tend to have higher rates)
	%	Absolute Count
Bands or stabs (young neutrophils)	0–4	0–432
Neutrophils or segs	45–74	1,935–7,942
Eosinophils	0–7	0–756
Basophils	0–2	0–216
Lymphocytes	16–45	688–4,860
Monocytes	4–10	172–1,080
Differential adds to 100%[a]		

Pregnancy	The leukocytosis of pregnancy (up to 16,000/mm³) is due mostly to an increase in the neutrophils with only a slight increase in lymphocytes
Newborn	Day of birth 18,000–40,000/mm³. Drops to adult levels within 2 weeks. Reference values for differential have wide ranges depending on time after birth. Neutrophils predominate for first few days, but eventually lymphocyte predominance is seen
Children	Until about age 3 years or later, lymphocytes are more prominent than neutrophils. WBC counts up to 14,500/mm³ may be in normal range depending on age. Consult specific laboratory for relative values for the differential at different ages.
Aged	Some sources suggest total WBC may decrease slightly with age

[a]If the laboratory uses certain automated instruments to count the WBC, some large cells may not take the stain properly. These large unstained cells (LUC) may make up to 3% of the normal specimen. If there are more than 3% unstained cells, the laboratory performs a microscopic examination (peripheral smear) to identify the abnormal cells.

Increase in Neutrophils and Bands (Neutrophilia)

Clinical Significance. Neutrophils, classified as polymorphonuclear leukocytes (PMNs), seem to be the body's first defense against bacterial infection and severe stress. Normally most of the circulating neutrophils are in the mature form, which the laboratory can identify by the way the nucleus of the cell is segmented. Hence some laboratories call mature neutrophils *segs* or segmented neutrophils. In contrast, the nucleus of the less mature neutrophil is not in segments, but still in a band, so the lab calls these immature neutrophils *bands*. Another name for the bands are *stabs*, a name that comes from the German for rod. Notice that there are at least two names for mature neutrophils (segs, segmented neutrophils) and two names for immature neutrophils (bands or stabs).

An increased need for neutrophils causes an increase in both the segs (mature neutrophils) and the bands (immature or young neutrophils).

When a client may have appendicitis, one of the questions is, "Does the client have a shift to the left?" When laboratory reports were written by hand, the bands or stabs were written first on the left-hand side of the page. Hence, a "shift to the left" means that the bands or stabs have increased. Table 2–3 demonstrates what a shift to the left would look like in comparison to a normal differential in *an adult.*

Although with a shift to the left, the lymphocytes appear to have decreased, as explained earlier, the differential is only a percentage. The total number of lymphocytes has not changed, but the neutrophils have increased. In bacterial infections the total WBC does increase, and an examination of the differential enables one to determine that the increase is due to an increase in both immature and mature forms of neutrophils. Although an increased percentage of bands has been the conventional method for determining infection, an increased ANC may be of more value (Hoyer, 1993).

The slang "shift to the right" is rarely if ever used to describe the alteration toward the other side of the neutrophil differential. A *shift to the right* is used to imply that there are abnormal hypersegmented neutrophils, seen in some anemias and in liver disease. Some authors may call an increase in mature neutrophils a shift to the right (McConnell, 1986).

Besides bacterial infections, an increase in neutrophils can be due to various inflammatory processes, physical stress, or tissue necrosis such as that in myocardial infarction or in severe burns. Newborns delivered by cesarean section have higher WBC counts than those delivered vaginally (Hasan, et al., 1993). Neutrophils are increased in granulocytic leukemia and in many other malignant diseases. Emotional stress can also increase the neutrophil count but usually not as dramatically as a physical stress. Blood transfusions have recently been added to the list of possible causes of leukocytosis (Fenwick, et al., 1994).

TABLE 2–3. COMPARISON OF NORMAL DIFFERENTIAL TO A "SHIFT TO THE LEFT" IN AN ADULT WITH AN ACUTE BACTERIAL INFECTION[a]

	Stabs or Bands (%)	**Neutrophils or Segs (%)**	**Eosinophils (%)**	**Basophils (%)**	**Lymphocytes (%)**	**Monocytes (%)**
Normal differential—total WBC 9,400	3	61	4	1	26	5
"Shift to the left"—total WBC 14,300	10 ↑	65	3	1	17	4

[a]In addition to the shift to the left note that the absolute neutrophil count (ANC) has increased from 4,216 to 10,715 as determined by multiplying the total WBC count by the percentages of bands and segs. ↑, or higher.

▼ POSSIBLE NURSING DIAGNOSES RELATED TO ELEVATED NEUTROPHILS

Risk for Infection and Spread to Others

When a client has an elevated neutrophil count, one of the first things to determine is whether the client has an infection. If so, should he or she be isolated to protect others? Although infection is not the only reason for an increased neutrophil count with a shift to the left, it should always be considered along with other factors. (See Chapter 16 for culture collections.) In the absence of any signs of infection, the nurse can assess whether there has been another assault to the body that has caused the bone marrow to increase the number of neutrophils.

Knowledge Deficit Related to Measures to Promote Recovery

The increase in neutrophils is actually a healthy response—a defense mechanism against an insult to bodily integrity. The nurse can help clients maximize their defense against assaults by promoting rest, adequate nutrition, and plenty of fluids. As the body successfully overcomes the assault, bacterial or otherwise, the neutrophil count falls back to normal. This falling neutrophil count is an objective assessment that therapeutic measures have been successful.

Decreased Neutrophil Count (Neutropenia)

Clinical Significance. Although most bacterial infections cause an increase in the neutrophil count, some bacterial infections (e.g., typhoid, tularemia, or brucellosis) cause a decreased neutrophil count (neutropenia). (See Chapter 14 on serologic tests for infectious diseases.) Many viral diseases, such as hepatitis, influenza, measles, mumps, and rubella also cause a decreased neutrophil count. (Most of these viruses cause lymphocytosis.) An overwhelming infection of any type may completely exhaust the bone marrow and cause neutropenia. Newborns, in particular, may deplete their bone marrow storage (Pittiglio and Sacher, 1987). Neutropenia is an indicator of sepsis in the newborn (Gerdes, 1994). (See Chapter 16 on blood cultures.) Some drugs, particularly those used to treat cancer, can cause severe bone marrow depression. Radiation therapy also carries the risk of neutropenia. Antibiotics such as nafcillin, penicillins, and cephalosporins can induce neutropenia, as can psychotropic drugs such as lithium, the phenothiazines, and tricyclic antidepressants. Some adults may have a chronic benign neutropenia that is sometimes called *ethnic neutropenia* because it appears more often in blacks and Yemenite Jews (Russin et al., 1990).

The diagnosis of neutropenia in the pediatric population is fairly common. Most neutropenia observed in children is mild and occurs during viral infections. More severe forms of neutropenia may be hereditary or caused by serious disease such as collagen vascular disease.

▼ POSSIBLE NURSING DIAGNOSES RELATED TO LOW NEUTROPHIL COUNT

High Risk for Infection

Clients with neutropenia (an absolute count of neutrophils less than 2,000) are prone to infections, and those with agranulocytosis (an absolute count less than 500) may have a rapid progression to a fatal sepsis (Russin et al., 1990). Therefore, the nurse should carefully assess the WBC count to see any downward trends, and the client should be closely monitored for any signs of infection such as sore throats, cough, or an occult rectal abscess. Fever may be the only symptom. (See Chapter 16 on tips for collecting cultures.)

Until 1983, reverse isolation was used for patients with neutropenia, but newer protocols based on research and the recommendations of the Centers for Disease Control (CDC) emphasize meticulous handwashing as being the most important factor in protecting neutropenic clients from infection (Russin, et al., 1990; Flyge, 1993). Exposure to any people with colds or other infectious diseases should be curtailed. Scrupulous personal hygiene must be maintained, and the environment must be controlled for bacterial sources such as fresh flowers or stagnant water. In addition, a "neutropenic diet" is served that avoids fresh fruit and raw vegetables. Granulocyte colony-stimulating factor (G-CSF) or filgrastim (Neupogen), made by DNA recombinant technology, may be used to prevent severe neutropenia in clients receiving chemotherapeutic drugs (Groopman, et al., 1989; Conover, 1990; Katzung, 1995). For newborns, who sometimes have depletion of neutrophils, transfusions of neutrophils may be given to increase the storage pool (Etzioni, 1994).

Risk for Injury Related to Drugs That Cause Neutropenia

The nurse has the responsibility of checking the latest WBC count before giving drugs that may cause neutropenia. The nurse must confer with the physician, and the drug must be withheld if the neutrophil count drops below a certain number. The *nadir* is the point at which the WBC count drops to the lowest level after chemotherapy. Because in adults most WBCs are neutrophils, the change in neutrophils most affects the total count. But neutropenia may be present even with a normal number of other types of WBCs.

For clients undergoing chemotherapy for cancer, the WBC count and differential may be ordered daily. Some nurses become "chemotherapy specialists" and, under the supervision of a physician, take over the functions of cancer drug preparation and administration, client education, and monitoring of side effects, including the effects on the hematologic system.

Increased Eosinophil Count (Eosinophilia)

Clinical Significance. The actual function of the eosinophils is not clearly understood, but they are associated with antigen–antibody reactions. The most common reasons for an increase in eosinophils (eosinophilia) are allergic reactions such as asthma, hay fever, or hypersensitivity to a drug. Parasitic infestations, such as round worms, are another reason for an eosinophil increase. Other conditions in which eosinophils increase are certain skin diseases and neoplasms.

▼ POSSIBLE NURSING DIAGNOSES RELATED TO EOSINOPHILIA

Knowledge Deficit Related to Avoidance of Allergens

If an increased eosinophil count has been attributed to a specific allergen, the nurse may be involved in helping the client learn to avoid the allergen. Otherwise, the eosinophil count may just be useful as an indication that the client is likely to have a history of allergies. This fact should then be taken into account in planning diets and assessing for allergic reactions to new drugs.

Risk for Injury Related to Infestation

If the elevated eosinophil count is due to a possible parasitic infestation, the nurse should question whether stool precautions are necessary. (See Chapter 16 for the collection of stool specimens for parasites.)

Decreased Eosinophil Count

Clinical Significance. Increased levels of adrenal steroids decrease the number of circulating eosinophils. For example, a decrease in eosinophils would be expected for a client with an allergy who begins corticosteroid therapy. Before the refinement of tests to measure corticosteroid levels directly, a drop in the eosinophil count after injection of adrenocorticotropic hormone (ACTH) (Thorn test) was an indirect measure of functioning adrenal glands. (See Chapter 15 for cortisol measurements.)

Changes in the Basophil Count

Clinical Significance of Increase in Basophils. The purpose of basophils in the bloodstream is not well understood. Few conditions seem to increase this relatively rare type of WBC. Leukemia and other pathologic alterations in bone marrow production may give rise to an increase in basophils.

Clinical Significance of Decrease in Basophils. Because the normal basophil count is considered to be 0–2%, a decline is not likely to be detected unless absolute counts are completed. Corticosteroids, allergic reactions, and acute infections all may lower the basophil rate.

Increased Lymphocyte Count (Lymphocytosis)

Clinical Significance. Lymphocytes are the principal components of the body's immune system, but only a small proportion of them circulate in the bloodstream. In the bloodstream, most are T lymphocytes (60–95%) rather than B lymphocytes (4–25%) or non-B or non-T lymphocytes (5–10%). The non-B–non-T lymphocytes are now called natural killer (NK) cells (Ravel, 1995). To help assess immune deficiencies, such as AIDS, the laboratory must perform specialized tests of T lymphocytes. In the differential, all lymphocytes are grouped together. In adults, lymphocytes are the second most common type of WBC, after neutrophils. In children up to at least the age of 3 years, the lymphocytes are more numerous than the neutrophils. Even in older children, the percentage of lymphocytes nearly equals or even surpasses the percentage of neutrophils.

Lymphocytes increase in many viral infections, such as mumps or infectious hepatitis; they also increase with pertussis, with infectious mononucleosis, with some tumors, and often with tuberculosis. (See Chapter 14 for serologic tests for infectious mononucleosis.) *Chronic* bacterial infections cause an increase in lymphocytes. A common reason for marked lymphocytosis (80–90%) is lymphocytic leukemia. Ninety percent of all leukemias, both acute and chronic, are lymphocytic. Acute lymphocytic leukemia is much more common in children, whereas chronic lymphocytic leukemia is most common in older adults. Children also have a rather benign disease called *infectious lymphocytosis* in which the lymph count is quite high.

▼ POSSIBLE NURSING DIAGNOSES RELATED TO LYMPHOCYTOSIS

Risk for Alteration in Health Maintenance

If the lymphocyte count is extremely high, the physician orders other tests to establish the possible existence of leukemia. The nurse needs to be aware of the specific type of leukemia diagnosed, because treatment measures and prognosis differ for different subcategories of the disease, and some types are curable (Sullivan et al., 1990). The peripheral blood smear, maybe along with a bone marrow biopsy, is needed to differentiate clearly the type of abnormal white cells (see Chapter 25). Three potentially lethal complications in a leukemic client are (1) infection caused by the lack of normal WBCs, (2) hemorrhage caused by the lack of platelets, and (3) hyperuricemia caused by the increase

(*continued*)

▼ POSSIBLE NURSING DIAGNOSES RELATED TO LYMPHOCYTOSIS (*continued*)

of uric acid from cell destruction. (See Chapter 4 for a discussion about high serum uric acid levels in certain malignant diseases such as leukemia. See Chapter 13 for a discussion on low platelet counts, or thrombocytopenia.)

Risk for Injury Related to Infectious Process

If the lymphocyte count is not due to a malignant disease, the important question is whether the client has an infection that may be transmitted to others. Other measures, discussed under increased neutrophil counts, also apply because the nurse needs to help the person resist the assault that has triggered an immune response. The increased lymphocyte count is needed for a defense against a viral or chronic bacterial infection.

Decreased Lymphocyte Count (Lymphopenia)

Clinical Significance. Since the advent of the human immunodeficiency virus (HIV), a virus that affects T lymphocytes, much research has been done on the various types of T lymphocytes. Lymphocyte phenotyping uses flow cytometry to detect the many different types of lymphocytes. These subsets of lymphocytes are identified by their clusters of differentiation (CD), which react to a cluster of monoclonal antibodies. For example, CD4 are the helper-inducer cells. (See the section on lymphocyte immunophenotyping.) AIDS causes a reduction in the total number of lymphocytes as well as changes in the ratios of the types of T lymphocytes. Adrenal corticosteroids and other immunosuppressive drugs also cause a decrease. Autoimmune diseases such as systemic lupus erythematosus commonly cause leukopenia and lymphopenia. Severe malnutrition also decreases the absolute number. Because increases in neutrophils occur for many reasons, decreased percentages of lymphocytes may often be explained by changes in the neutrophil count. Review the discussion in the beginning of this chapter if it is not clear why a marked increase in the percentage of neutrophils always causes a decrease in the percentage of lymphocytes, even though the absolute number of lymphocytes has not decreased.

▼ POSSIBLE NURSING DIAGNOSIS RELATED TO LYMPHOPENIA

Risk for Infection Related to Lack of Immunologic Protection

A client with a true (or absolute or actual) decrease in the number of lymphocytes is immunodeficient. This client may need extensive protection from sources of infection. Also, if an immunodeficient client does get an infection, there may be few signs or symptoms that this assault is occurring. So the nurse needs to use careful assessment techniques to detect early infections in the absence of the classic signs such as fever. For example, clients undergoing chronic steroid therapy may have lower-than-normal levels of lymphocytes, and so it should not be surprising that these clients sometimes have tuberculosis or other infections. Clients with AIDS are likely to have infections such as cytomegalovirus (CMV) (Chapter 14) or *Pneumocystis carinii* infection. (See Chapter 27 on bronchoscopy.)

Nurses can often help clients with chronic lowered resistance find ways to enhance their health by diet, rest, and all the measures too often overlooked as "simple" health habits. Sometimes the objective sign of a laboratory test can prompt the nurse to evaluate the total health of the client.

Lymphocyte Immunophenotyping

The use of flow cytometry has made it possible to identify many types of lymphocytes. This identification of subsets of lymphocytes is most useful in assessment of the immunologic status of a client. The lymphocytes are identified by their CD, each of which reacts with a cluster of specific antibodies. The CD nomenclature was developed after some types of cells were already identified by other types of reagents, so laboratories may use other descriptions on laboratory reports. However, CD designations have become the most common method for reporting results; many laboratories also include descriptive names (Peddecord, et al., 1993).

Preparation of Client and Collection of Sample

Whole blood is collected. No special preparation of the client is required.

REFERENCE VALUES FOR LYMPHOCYTES

Cell type	Mean (%)	Range (%)	Mean (cells/μL)	Range (cells/μL)
CD3 (Total T cells)	71	55–87	1,586	781–2,391
CD19 (Total B cells)	5	1–9	277	17–537
CD4 (Helpers)	43	24–62	1,098	447–1,750
CD8 (Suppressers)	42	19–65	836	413–1,260
CD4/CD8 Ratio	1.25	0.5–2.0		

Flow cytometric analysis of peripheral blood lymphocyte subsets in children have shown that both the total and some subsets of T lymphocytes are higher in children until the age of 3 years. See Kotylo, et al. (1993) for values from 6 months to 3 years.

Clinical Significance. The reader is encouraged to review the immunology literature to find the most up to date use of lymphocyte phenotyping. Only two examples are given here.

The CD4 T-lymphocyte count has become important in the diagnosis and treatment of clients with HIV-1 infection. A CD4 count less than 200 is a diagnostic case marker for acquired immune deficiency syndrome (AIDS). This test is also used as a criterion for initiating antiviral therapy for clients with HIV infection and for evaluating the response to therapy.

The CD3, the total count of B lymphocytes, is used to assess the efficacy of OKT3 monoclonal antibody therapy in transplant recipients.

Increased Monocyte Count

Clinical Significance. Like basophils and eosinophils, monocytes are but a small percentage of the total WBC count. (Monocytes are present in tissues as macrophages.) Monocytes act as phagocytes in some chronic inflammatory diseases. A clinically significant increase of monocytes, for example, accompanies tuberculosis. Some protozoan infections such as malaria, as well as some rickettsial infections such as Rocky Mountain spotted fever, cause increases in the monocyte count. (See Chapter 14 on tests for rickettsial infections.) Monocytic leukemia, acute or chronic, also causes an increased monocyte count, but monocytic leukemia is far less common than the lymphocytic type. Chronic ulcerative colitis and regional enteritis both cause an increased monocyte count, as do some collagen diseases. As a rule, the condition that causes increased monocytes is more likely to be a chronic condition, but further investigation for a specific pathologic condition is necessary to make the monocytic count useful in the clinical situation.

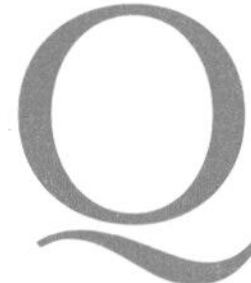

1. Mrs. Landy lost a large amount of blood during a mastectomy. A hematocrit (hct) drawn in the recovery room was 43%. It is now 12 hr after the operation, and the hct just read is 37%. Which action by the nurse is appropriate?

   a. Take the client's blood pressure and call the physician immediately because Mrs. Landy is most likely bleeding again

   b. Slow down the rate of intravenous infusion of fluids until the physician can be notified because Mrs. Landy is probably overhydrated

   c. Consult the physician for further fluid orders because Mrs. Landy is probably slightly dehydrated

   d. Notify the physician of the lab report when rounds are made in a couple of hours because this drop in hct is expected because of a fluid shift from the interstitial space

2. The test that is most frequently done to assess for loss of blood is the

a. RBC count **b.** Hgb
c. Hct **d.** CBC

3. The practice of being n.p.o. for routine tests is likely to be detrimental for an adult female patient who has a

a. Hemoglobin (hgb) of 9 g/100 mL
b. Red blood cell (RBC) count of 7 million/mm^3
c. Hematocrit (hct) of 30%
d. White blood cell (WBC) count of 3,000/mm^3

4. As a rough guide, each unit of packed cells given to an adult raises the hematocrit about

a. 3% **b.** 6%
c. 9% **d.** 12%

5. Assuming that the erythrocyte indices are normal, the estimated hemoglobin level (hgb) for a client whose hct is 30% would be about

a. 6 g **b.** 8 g
c. 10 g **d.** 12 g

6. Mrs. London has a hgb of 11 g because of a continuing blood loss from a heavy menstrual flow. Which of the following nursing actions is the most appropriate?

a. Encourage additional fluids to prevent thrombus formation
b. Explain that increased physical activity stimulates increased production of red blood cells
c. Assess dietary intake of protein and iron
d. Prepare the client for the eventual need for blood transfusions to correct the anemia

7. Anemia caused by a recent blood loss would most likely be

a. Microcytic (↓ MCV), hypochromic (↓ MCHC)
b. Macrocytic (↑ MCV), normochromic (normal MCHC)
c. Normocytic (normal MCV), hypochromic (↓ MCHC)
d. Normocytic (normal MCV), normochromic (normal MCHC)

8. A low reticulocyte count would be expected for which one of the following clients?

a. Mr. Joseph, who has an untreated macrocytic anemia caused by vitamin B_{12} deficiency
b. Mrs. Lars, who has been receiving iron supplements for iron deficiency anemia

c. Timmy Logon, who recently moved to a high altitude
d. Ms. Garfield, who had acute blood loss last week after a miscarriage

9. Mrs. Toby has rheumatoid arthritis that flares up occasionally. Her erythrocyte sedimentation rate (sed rate) is higher than it has been. The home care nurse is planning a visit to evaluate the need for a change in care. In regard to this lab test, the nurse should consult with the physician about teaching Mrs. Toby to

a. Take additional fluids to prevent dehydration
b. Decrease fluid intake to prevent circulatory overload
c. Increase her activity to promote the full range of motion of all joints
d. Decrease her activity to promote the rest of joints, which are actively inflamed at present

10. Mary Smith, a nurse practitioner in a Women's Health Clinic, sees many clients of childbearing age. As part of her health teaching Mary needs to inform the women that the risk of having a child with a neural tube defect is lessened if the woman has an adequate intake of

a. Vitamin B_{12} **b.** Iron
c. Folic acid **d.** Vitamin C

11. Mr. Jelco is receiving chemotherapy for treatment of cancer of the colon. His last white blood cell (WBC) count was 2,500/mm^3. On the basis of this laboratory report, a nursing care plan must include nursing interventions to

a. Protect from infection **b.** Protect from stressful situations
c. Prevent stasis of circulation **d.** Prevent dehydration

12. Mr. Jelco's white blood cell (WBC) count is now 2,000, and the differential showed 40% neutrophils and 2% bands. Therefore the client's absolute neutrophil count (ANC) is

a. 1,640 **b.** 1,260
c. 840 **d.** 660

13. Eosinophil counts are usually elevated when the client

a. Has had an allergic reaction **b.** Is undergoing corticosteroid therapy
c. Has a viral infection **d.** Has a bacterial infection

14. Clyde Easton has been HIV-positive for a little more than 3 years. Which of the following laboratory reports would be the best indicator that his condition has progressed from HIV-positive to acquired immune deficiency syndrome (AIDS)?

a. CD4/CD8 ratio of 1.5 **b.** CD19 count of 100
c. CD3 count of 500 **d.** CD4 count of 200

15. Mary Rogers is undergoing antibiotic therapy because of pelvic inflammatory disease (PID). The nurse checks the WBC count and differential to assess if Mary has a shift to the left. Characteristic of a shift to the left is

a. An increase in stabs or bands (immature neutrophils)
b. A decrease in eosinophils
c. An increase in lymphocytes
d. A decrease in monocytes

▼ REFERENCES

Abad-Lacruz, A., Cabré, E., González-Huix, F., et al. (1993). Routine tests of renal function, alcoholism, and nutrition improve the prognostic accuracy of Child-Pugh score in nonbleeding advanced cirrhotics. *American Journal of Gastroenterology, 88* (3), 382–392.

Beutler, E., Kuhl, W., Vives-Corrons, J., and Prchal, T. (1989). Molecular heterogeneity of glucose-6-phosphate-dehydrogenase. *Blood, 74* (7), 2550–2555.

Cerrato, P. (1985). Hidden malnutrition in geriatric patients. *RN, 48* (7), 60–62.

Cohen, A., and Seidl-Friedman, J. (1988). HemoCue system for hemoglobin measurement: Evaluation in anemic and nonanemic children. *American Journal of Clinical Pathology, 90* (3), 302–305.

Conover, A. (1990). GM-CSF may boost WBC counts. *American Journal of Nursing, 90* (4), 29.

Corbett, J.V. (1995). Accidental poisoning with iron supplements. *MCN American Journal of Maternal Child Nursing, 20* (4), 234.

Etzioni, A. (1994). Neutrophil function in the newborn: A review. *Israel Journal of Medical Science, 30*, 328–330.

Fenwick, J.C., Cameron, M., Nalman, S., et al. (1994). Blood transfusion as a cause of leucocytosis in critically ill patients. *Lancet, 344*, 855–856.

Flyge, H.A. (1993). Meeting the challenge of neutropenia. *Nursing 93, 23*, 61–64.

Gerdes, J.S. (1994). Clinicopathologic approach to the diagnosis of neonatal sepsis. *Israel Journal Medical Science, 30*, 430–441.

Gottfried, E.L. (1994). *Clinical laboratory manual.* San Francisco: San Francisco General Hospital.

Groopman, J., Molina, J., and Scadden, D. (1989). Hematopoietic growth factors. *New England Journal of Medicine, 321* (21), 1449–1456.

Hansan, R., Inque, S., and Banerjee, A. (1993). Higher white blood cell counts and band forms in newborns delivered vaginally compared with those delivered by cesarean section. *American Journal of Clinical Pathology, 100*, 116–118.

Herring, W., et al. (1986). Why is that hematocrit so high? *Patient Care, 20* (1), 46–75.

Holyoake, T.L., Stott, D.J., McKay, P.J., et al. (1993). Use of plasma ferritin concentration to diagnose iron deficiency in elderly patients. *Journal of Clinical Pathology, 46*, 857–860.

Hoyer, J.D. (1993). Laboratory medicine and pathology: Leukocyte differential. *Mayo Clinic Proceedings, 68*, 1027–1028.

Hubbard, J., and Wheeler, D. (1989). Erythropoietin measurement by EIA. *Laboratory Medicine, 20* (12), 849–854.

Katzung, B. (ed.). (1995). *Basic and clinical pharmacology.* (6th ed.). Norwalk: Appleton & Lange.

Kotylo, P.K., Fineberg, N.S., Freeman, K.S., et al. (1993). Reference ranges for lymphocyte subsets in pediatric patients. *American Journal of Clinical Pathology, 100,* 111–115.

Lyle, R.M. (1992). Iron status in active women: Is there reason to be concerned? *Food and Nutrition News, 64* (5), 35–37.

Lynch, S.R. (1994). Overview of the relationship of iron to health. *Contemporary Nutrition, 19* (4), 1–4.

McConnell, D. (1986). Leukocyte studies. *Nursing 86, 16* (3), 42–43.

Peddecord, K.M., Benenson, A.S., Hofherr, L.K., et al., 1993. Variability of reporting and lack of adherence to consensus guidelines in human T-lymphocyte immunophenotyping reports: Results of a case series. *Journal of Acquired Immune Deficiency Syndromes, 6,* 823–830.

Pittiglio, D., and Sacher, R. (1987). *Clinical hematology and fundamentals of hemostasis.* Philadelphia: F.A. Davis.

Ravel, R. (1995). *Clinical laboratory medicine: Clinical application of laboratory data.* (6th ed.). St. Louis: Mosby–Year Book.

Romanczuk, A.N., and Brown, J.P. (1994). Folic acid will reduce risk of neural tube defects. *MCN: American Journal of Maternal Child Nursing, 19* (6), 331–334.

Russin, S., et al. (1990). Neutropenia in adults: What is its clinical significance? *Postgraduate Medicine, 88* (2), 209.

Sasak, C., and Giordano, E. (1990). Case management of the anemic patient: Epoetin alfa—Focus on patient teaching. *American Nephrology Nursing Association Journal, 17* (2), 188–189.

Savage, D., and Lindenbaum, J. (1983). Relapses after interruption of cyanocobalamin therapy in patients with pernicious anemia. *American Journal of Medicine, 74* (5), 765–772.

Sullivan, M., et al. (1990). Clinical and biological heterogeneity of childhood B cell acute lymphocytic leukemia: Implications of clinical trials. *Leukemia, 4* (1), 6–11.

Tikly, M., Blumsohn, D., Solomons, H., et al. (1987). Normal hematological reference values in the adult black population of the Witwatersrand. *South African Medical Journal, 72,* 1355–1356.

Wognum, A., Landsorp, P., Eaves, A., Krystal, G. (1989). An enzyme-linked immunosorbent assay for erythropoietin using monoclonal antibodies, tetrameric immune complexes, and substrate amplification. *Blood, 74* (2), 622–628.

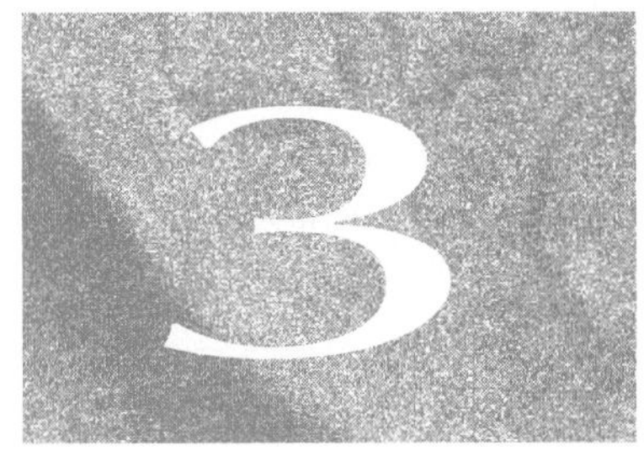

ROUTINE URINALYSIS AND OTHER URINE TESTS

- pH of the Urine
- Specific Gravity of the Urine
- Protein in the Urine (Proteinuria)
- Sugar in the Urine (Glycosuria)
- Ketones in the Urine
- Examination of Urine Sediment
- Addis Count
- Nitrites
- Leukocyte Esterase
- Urinary Porphyrins
- Delta-aminolevulinic Acid
- Urinary 5-Hydroxyindolacetic Acid
- Collection of 24-hour Urine Specimens

OBJECTIVES

1. State three important nursing considerations in obtaining the urine for routine urinalysis and for random testing.
2. Recognize findings on a routine urinalysis report that may have pathologic significance.
3. Summarize important points about the various types of dipsticks and other reagents used by the nurse for urine testing.
4. Explain when periodic tests of urine pH, specific gravity, protein, sugar, and ketones may be useful in planning and modifying nursing goals.

5. Describe what should be taught to a client about any 24-hr urine collection.
6. Give examples of common tests and the types of preservatives used for 24-hr urine specimens.

Because a routine urinalysis is indeed routine for almost every client, the nurse needs to understand fully the meaning of each component of urinalysis. All these tests are screening tests that may indicate the need for a more thorough assessment. Several of the tests can be completed quickly with the use of chemically impregnated paper strips that can be dipped into a urine specimen. In some situations, the nurse may use this "dipstick" method as one part of the assessment. It is important to make sure that the materials for testing are fresh (note the date on the container) and that the directions are followed exactly. Some strips must be read within a certain time limit, and specific directions should always be included with the testing equipment. Because color changes are the basis for the results of the dipstick test, good light is needed, and personnel need to be examined for color blindness. (See Chapter 1 on testing by nurses.)

Specific techniques for each component of the urinalysis are covered in this chapter. Table 3–1 is a summary of reagent strips for urinalysis. Specific tips on the two methods of testing for glucose in the urine are described in regard to the special points to note when nurses are actually performing the tests, although finger sticks for glucose are more useful.

The last part of the chapter presents the correct procedure for collecting 24-hr urine specimens. The final table lists the usual substances tested with 24-hr specimens, whether any preservatives are needed, and where the test is covered in detail in later chapters.

COLLECTION OF URINE SPECIMENS

For a routine urinalysis, the laboratory needs at least 10 mL of urine. The perineal area in women or the end of the penis in men should be cleaned before the urine is collected. For a female client, collecting midstream urine lessens the contamination of the urine from vaginal secretions or menstrual flow; use of a vaginal tampon also helps in this respect. For infants, wiping with a sterile wipe may stimulate voiding or a collection bag can be attached to the genitalia. A cotton ball in a diaper can be used for quick collection of urine for dipstick testing. Urine also can be collected from regular or superabsorbent diapers (Hermansen and Buches, 1988). Stebor (1989) noted that a specific gravity from diaper urine is accurate for at least 4 hr after urination, but times for sugar and protein need further research.

If a *culture and sensitivity* are to be completed in addition to the routine urinalysis, the urine has to be in a sterile container. In that case, collecting a clean-catch urine sample may necessitate the use of an antiseptic solution as well as cleansing of the area. Urine for culture and sensitivity is discussed in Chapter 16.

If the client is instructed to bring in a urine specimen from home, any small clean jar with a tight-fitting nonrusty lid may be used. The first voided specimen in the morning is ideal for routine urinalysis because the urine is concentrated, and any abnormalities will be more pronounced in the screening tests.

TABLE 3–1. REAGENT STRIPS FOR URINALYSIS

Substance Tested and Tips on Interpreting	Further Discussion in Addition to Chapter 3
pH—Colors range from orange through yellow and green to blue to cover entire range of urinary pH. Make sure not to let urine remain on test strip, or the acid reagent from neighboring protein may run over and make pH acid or more acid.	Chap. 6 on respiratory and metabolic alkalosis and acidosis
Protein—Detects as little as 5–20 mg albumin/dL. May be false-positive with alkaline urine. Does not test for Bence-Jones protein.	Chap. 10 on protein electrophoresis
Glucose—Enzyme method specific for glucose only. So need reduction method (Clinitest) for any other types of sugar. May be affected by ascorbic acid. Large quantities of ketone may depress color.	Chap. 8 on tests for galactosemia
Ketone—Provides results as small, moderate, and large. Reacts with acetoacetic acid and acetone but not beta-hydroxybutyric. PKU or L-dopa can cause false-positive.	Chap. 8 for serum ketone tests
Bilirubin—Sensitive to 0.2–0.4 mg bilirubin/dL. Icotest tablets are more sensitive. May be affected by chlorpromazine (Thorazine), phenazopyridine (Pyridium), ethoxazene (Serenium), or ascorbic acid.	Chap. 11 for tests of bilirubin
Occult blood—More sensitive to hemoglobin and myoglobin than intact erythrocytes. Complements the microscopic exam. Affected by ascorbic acid and some infections that produce peroxidase.	Chap. 13 for detecting occult bleeding
Nitrites—Any pink color suggests urinary infection, but a negative result does not provide sufficient proof of no bacteria, because some bacteria do not produce nitrates. Affected by ascorbic acid. High specific gravity may inhibit.	Chap. 16 on urine cultures
Leukocytes—Positive test for leukocyte esterase suggests urinary tract infection. Avoid contamination by vaginal secretions.	Chap. 16 on urine cultures
Urobilinogen—False-positive with porphobilinogen, P-amino-salicylic acid or azo dyes, such as phenazopyridine, found in sulfisoxazole (Azo Gantrisin) or phenazopyridine (Pyridium).	Chap. 11 for more on urobilinogen
Ascorbic acid—If ascorbic acid is as high as 25 mg/dL, the strip turns purple. Alerts that glucose, nitrite, occult blood, and bilirubin may not be accurate because of interference from ascorbic acid.	

Complete information on all testing products is available by contacting companies that make diagnostic kits.

Urine specimens need to be examined within 2 hr. Urine that is left standing too long becomes alkaline because bacteria begin to split urea into ammonia. Visualization of microscopic casts and the test for protein are inaccurate if the urine has undergone a conversion to a high pH (i.e., if it has become alkaline). Urine should be refrigerated if the specimen cannot be sent to the laboratory within 2 hr.

REFERENCE VALUES FOR ROUTINE URINALYSIS

pH	4.3–8 with a mean of about 6 (depends on diet)
Specific gravity	
Adult	Range of 1.001–1.040. Random sample usually about 1.015–1.025

Infant to 2 years	Range of 1.001–1.018
Aged	May have a lower range because of decreasing concentrating ability
Protein	Usually negative; a few healthy people may have orthostatic proteinuria
Sugar	Usually negative; may be trace in normal pregnancy. Lactosuria common in last trimester
Ketone	Should be negative
Nitrites and leukocyte esterase (LE)	Both should be negative
Microscopic sediment[a]	
Crystals	Usually have little clinical significance (see discussion)
Casts	Most are pathologic; a few hyaline casts are considered normal
WBCs	Should be only a few white blood cells in the urine (less than 4–5 per high-power field)
RBCs	Only an occasional red blood cell is expected (less than 2–3 per high-power field)

[a] Performed only if protein, blood, nitrites, or LE are positive.

COLOR OF URINE

Normally the color of the urine, from light yellow to dark amber, depends on its concentration. *Urechrome* is the name of the pigment that gives urine the characteristic yellow color. When the reason for a color abnormality is not known, the laboratory must perform a chemical analysis to determine the cause. Usually the nurse or the client first notices that something is wrong with the urine color. Such changes should always be called to the attention of the physician and recorded in the nurse's notes. Staff of one urology unit developed a urine color wheel to standardize vague and variable descriptions of urine color (Cooper, 1993).

A number of things can cause a change in the color of urine. If the client is known to be taking a medication that causes color changes in the urine, this information should be written on the laboratory slip. It is also important that clients be told about expected color changes in the urine so they do not become unnecessarily concerned. For example, phenazopyridine (Pyridium), a drug used as a urinary tract analgesic, causes the urine to turn orange. Table 3–2 lists 29 other drugs that can color urine. Some foods, such as beets or rhubarb, may cause color changes in the urine, as do some dyes used in food. Purulent matter in the urine gives urine a cloudy appearance. Blood makes the urine dark and "smoky" looking. Pseudomonal infections of the bladder may give the urine a greenish color. Bilirubin turns the urine a dark orange that foams on shaking. (The other reason that urine may foam is the presence of large amounts of protein.)

TABLE 3–2. DRUGS THAT CAN COLOR URINE

Generic Name and Brand Name of Drug	Color Produced in Urine
Acetophenetidin	Pink-red
Amitriptyline (multisource)	Blue-green (rare)
Anisindione (Miradon)	Orange in alkaline urine, pink-red-brown in acid urine
Cascara (multisource)	Red in alkaline urine, red-brown in acid urine
Chloroquine (Aralen)	Rusty yellow or brown
Chlorzoxazone (Paraflex)	Orange or purple-red (rare)
Danthron (multisource)	Pink in alkaline urine
Deferoxamine (Desferal)	Red
Ethoxazene (Serenium)	Orange-red
Furazolidone (Furaxone)	Brown
Iron preparations (multisource)	Dark brown or black on standing
Levodopa (multisource)	Dark brown on standing, red or brown in hypochlorite toilet bleach
Methocarbamol (multisource)	Brown, black, or green on standing
Metronidazole (Flagyl)	Dark brown on standing (rare)
Nitrofurantoin (multisource)	Brown, yellow
Phenazopyridine (Pyridium, also in Azo-Gantrisin)	Orange-red
Phenindione (multisource)	Orange-red in alkaline urine
Phenolphthalein (multisource)	Pink-red in alkaline urine
Phenothiazine (multisource)	Pink-red, red-brown
Phensuximide (Milontin)	Pink, red, red-brown
Phenytoin (Dilantin)	Pink, red, red-brown
Primaquine	Rusty yellow (red or dark brown a sign of inherited hemolytic anemia reaction)
Quinacrine (Atabrine)	Intense yellow, especially in acid urine
Quinine and derivatives	Brown to black
Riboflavin	Intense yellow
Rifampin (multisource)	Red-orange
Sulfasalazine (multisource)	Orange-yellow in alkaline urine
Tolonium	Blue, green
Triamterene (Dyrenium)	Pale blue fluorescence

Compiled from Slawson (1980, p. 4) and Cooper (1993).

ODOR OF URINE

Old urine has the very characteristic smell of ammonia because bacteria split the urea molecules into ammonia. If a freshly voided urine specimen has a foul odor, there may be a urinary tract infection (i.e., bacteria are converting urea to ammonia in the bladder).

A foul odor in freshly voided urine, however, may also be due to drugs or food. Asparagus gives a distinct smell to the urine. The unusual odor should be charted and called to the laboratory's attention for any needed further investigations. Some metabolic abnormalities caused by genetic defects can cause a peculiar odor in the urine of newborns. (See Chapter 18 on tests for genetic defects.)

▼ pH OF THE URINE

Higher pH means toward the alkaline side, and *lower pH* means toward the acid side. Normally the pH of urine tends to be lower, or acidic, largely because of diet. Meat and eggs contribute much of the acid metabolic wastes, whereas most fruits and vegetables, including citrus fruits, contribute to an alkaline urine. Thus a meatless diet would be one reason why the pH of urine may be higher than usual.

Most bacteria that cause urinary tract infections, with the exception of *Escherichia coli*, make urine alkaline because the bacteria split urea into ammonia and other products. The urea-splitting properties of many bacteria also explains why urine left standing at room temperature for more than 2 hours usually turns alkaline from bacterial contamination.

Urine pH varies in different types of acidosis and alkalosis. All forms of acidosis cause a strongly acid urine because the body is trying to compensate for the acidotic state by excreting hydrogen ions. If the acidotic problem is renal in origin, however, the kidneys may not be able to secrete large amounts of hydrogen ions; so the urine is not strongly acid. One might expect that in alkalosis the urine would become alkaline because the body would tend to retain hydrogen ions to compensate for the alkalotic state. Yet the pH of the urine often remains acid even with severe types of alkalosis because the kidneys are obligated to excrete hydrogen ions if potassium ions are not available. The relations among potassium levels, acid–base balance, and urine and blood pH levels are discussed in detail in Chapter 6 on blood gases.

▼ POSSIBLE NURSING DIAGNOSIS RELATED TO pH TESTING

Knowledge Deficit Related to Measures to Control Urine pH

Usually changes in the pH of urine are not very important because the pH fluctuates with food and with the metabolic state of the client. Sometimes, however, it may be necessary to see that the urine remains alkaline or acid. For example, if a client has a tendency to form uric acid or cystine stones, it may be desirable to keep the urine alkaline or at least as high as 6.5. Sometimes medications are given to achieve an alkaline urine. The nurse may need to teach the client to monitor the pH of the urine to see that it remains alkaline. This teaching is made easy by means of the dipstick method.

In other situations it may be desirable that the urine pH remain strongly acid (about 5.5). The two common clinical justifications for not letting the urine ever be alkaline are

1. Alkaline urine promotes the growth of certain organisms in the urine.

2. Alkaline urine promotes the formation of calcium phosphate renal stones in susceptible people. Calcium oxalate stones are not affected by urine pH.

For example, people with quadriplegia are prone to the formation of renal stones because of the higher calcium content in the urine that results from a lack of mobility. Such clients are also prone to urinary tract infections because of urinary stasis caused by loss of bladder control. Increasing the acidity of the urine may help prevent both infections and calcium stones. Often such clients drink cranberry juice several times a day to increase the acidity of their urine (Kinney and Blount, 1979). Milk products may be limited, as may citrus fruits, which leave an alkaline ash. However, vitamin C tablets help acidify the urine. Leiner (1995) noted that multiple studies have not supported the use of cranberry juice or avoiding dehydration as effective measures to prevent urinary tract infections, but these measures are often promoted.

Testing the pH of Vaginal Secretions

Dipsticks may also be used on vaginal secretions. The vaginal secretions are usually acidic, but the presence of amniotic fluid makes an alkaline reaction. The pH is a test to assess if the amniotic "bag of waters" has broken.

Dipsticks for the pH of Gastric Contents

The pH of the gastric contents is strongly acid, whereas the contents below the pylorus are alkaline. A dipstick test of secretions from a long gastrointestinal tube, such as a Cantor, helps assess if the tube has progressed through the pylorus. Metheny et al. (1989) used pH to predict feeding tube placement. The pH of gastric secretions is useful in monitoring the effectiveness of medications, such as cimetidine (Tagamet), given to reduce gastric acidity. (See Chapter 13 on combination pH and occult blood tests for gastric contents.)

▼ SPECIFIC GRAVITY OF THE URINE

The specific gravity is a measure of the density of the urine compared with the density of water, which is 1.000. The higher the number, the more concentrated is the urine unless there are abnormal constituents in the urine. Adults have a wide range from very dilute to very concentrated. In infants, the upper limits for specific gravity are much lower than the adult limits because the immature kidneys are not able to concentrate urine as effectively as mature kidneys. Often nurses may measure specific gravity as part of an assessment of fluid balance, using either a urinometer or a refractometer. Do not use urine contaminated with feces or toilet paper because these solutes elevate the specific gravity (McConnell, 1991).

Two Methods for Testing Specific Gravity

Urinometer

An older method to test specific gravity uses a float called a *urinometer* or *hydrometer*. The float has been calibrated to the 1.000 mark when floating in distilled water at 68–72°F (20.2–22.4°C).

A test tube is filled with 20 mL of urine, and the float is placed into the liquid. The higher the density of the urine, the more the float rises in the urine. The calibrated mark on the float that the urine covers is the specific gravity reading. Reading the marks exactly is sometimes difficult because the numbers are very small and close together. However, a reading of 1.011 or 1.012 is acceptable, because only wide variations are clinically significant.

Refractometer

The refractometer looks like a small telescope. Only a drop of urine is needed. This drop is placed on a slide at the end of the scope, and the refractor is held up to a light. The instrument must be kept level. The density of the particles in the urine determine the direction of the beam of light through the eye of the scope. The refractor is calibrated to translate the refractive index into the standard way of reporting the specific gravity. For example, if the light beam is at the 1.026 mark, this figure is recorded as the specific gravity of the urine.

The refractor has an added advantage of measuring the protein content in the same drop of urine. The protein measurements are on the right side of the scale. Knowledge about the presence of protein in the urine is important in measuring specific gravity because protein in the urine makes specific gravity falsely high.

REFERENCE VALUES FOR SPECIFIC GRAVITY	
Adult	Range of 1.001–1.040 with random samples of about 1.015–1.025
Infant to 2 years	1.001–1.018
Aged	May have a decrease in concentrating power so that upper limits are lowered

Increase in Specific Gravity

Clinical Significance. The specific gravity is falsely high if glucose, protein, or a dye used for diagnostic purposes is in the urine. All these abnormal constituents increase the density of the urine. If they are not present, the high specific gravity means the kidneys are putting out very concentrated urine, for which there are two reasons: (1) the client is lacking in fluids, or (2) there is an increased secretion of antidiuretic hormone (ADH), which causes a decrease in urine volume. Trauma, stress reactions, and many drugs cause increased ADH secretion.

If the urine does not contain protein, glucose, or dyes, a high urine specific gravity most often indicates that the client needs additional fluids. It is much rarer that a high specific gravity would be caused by an increased secretion of ADH.

Nurses should understand, however, the nature of a phenomenon called *surgical diuresis*. In a client who has experienced considerable stress, such as a major surgical procedure, the urine specific gravity is higher than normal because additional fluid is being held in reserve in the vascular system because of the presence of extra ADH and other hormones. As the stress lessens, ADH and other hormones, such as the glucocorticosteroids, return to normal levels, and the fluid that was held in reserve is then excreted. This excretion of extra urine a few days after an operation is sometimes referred to as surgical diuresis. It is important for nurses to understand the nature of this kind of fluid retention so that they do not overload clients with fluids because the specific gravity is a little higher than normal.

▼ POSSIBLE NURSING DIAGNOSIS RELATED TO ELEVATED SPECIFIC GRAVITY

Fluid Volume Deficit

A specific gravity that continues to increase or that remains high when stress is not an overriding factor is a clear indication that the client is not achieving adequate fluid intake. In acutely ill clients, this condition necessitates medical orders for increased intravenous infusion of fluids. In the nursing home setting or for clients with chronic problems, it may be up to the nurse to devise ways to provide the client with oral fluids. A specific gravity that drops back to normal is an objective evaluation that the client is no longer dehydrated. Specific gravity readings are more objective than charting "concentrated" urine.

The nurse also needs to be aware of clients who could be dehydrated because of a shift of fluid into a "third space." The normal two spaces are intracellular fluid and extracellular fluid compartments. A third space is any fluid collection that is physiologically useless, such as edema or ascites. "Third spacing" creates the potential for hypovolemia and decreased renal output.

Decreased Specific Gravity

Clinical Significance. A low specific gravity is indicative of dilute urine. Dilute urine is normal if the client has consumed a considerable amount of fluids. Diuretics cause a large urine output with a low specific gravity. Chapter 4 contains a discussion of tests for serum and urine osmolality. These tests are much more accurate in determining the actual dilution or concentration of the urine as compared with the dilution or concentration of the plasma. Specific gravity readings are only crude indicators of fluid imbalances in serious conditions.

Sometimes a client has a *fixed specific gravity* around 1.010. (This reading is usually pronounced as "ten-ten" because "one-point-zero-one-zero" is much harder to say.) A fixed specific gravity does not change even when the client becomes dehydrated. This continuously low specific gravity indicates that the kidneys have lost the ability to concentrate urine. The fixed specific gravity is always about 1.010 because 1.010 is the density of the plasma.

Another rare reason for a continuously low specific gravity is a deficiency of ADH. If not enough ADH is being secreted by the posterior pituitary gland, the kidneys excrete too much water. This condition is called *diabetes insipidus*.

▼ POSSIBLE NURSING DIAGNOSES RELATED TO LOW SPECIFIC GRAVITY

Risk for Fluid Volume Excess

Often a careful assessment of the client's total fluid intake uncovers the explanation for a low specific gravity. If the intake is larger than normal, it may be necessary to evaluate the possibility that the client is in danger of a fluid overload. For example, clients may be receiving intravenous fluids in addition to oral intake. Intake and output records and daily weights help assess any fluid overload.

Risk for Alterations in Health Maintenance

A persistently low specific gravity when the fluid intake is not high is a serious sign that necessitates medical evaluation. A low specific gravity of a routine early morning specimen indicates the need for a thorough assessment of the renal system and an evaluation of ADH secretion if the physician deems it necessary. People with fixed low specific gravities (1.010) may have difficulty getting medical insurance because they are considered at high risk for future renal problems.

A client who is known to have a fixed specific gravity of 1.010 needs to be kept well-hydrated so that the kidneys can effectively remove waste products. As kidney disease progresses, fluid restrictions and other interventions may be needed. The two common tests for renal function, BUN and creatinine, and the possible nursing diagnoses related to each are covered in Chapter 4.

▼ PROTEIN IN THE URINE (PROTEINURIA)

Qualitative Method

Most often protein in the urine is checked by the dipstick method. This method does not detect the presence of abnormal proteins such as the globulins and the

Bence-Jones protein of myelomas. For most screening purposes, however, the dipstick method is adequate (see Table 3–1 for one type of dipstick). Nurses often use it for testing for albumin in the urine of prenatal clients. People with diabetes are prone to renal disease, so they may undergo yearly checks for microalbumin, which is discussed later in this section. If there is a need to check the urine for protein other than albumin, the laboratory uses other agents such as sulfosalicyclic acid. The dipsticks are designed to be used with acid urine, so there may be a false-positive for protein if the urine is highly alkaline. Time is not critical in reading the results. Note the exact color chart for each particular brand.

REFERENCE VALUES (QUALITATIVE METHOD) FOR PROTEIN IN URINE

Trace	As little as 5–30 mg/dL
1+	30 mg/dL
2+	100 mg/dL
3+	300 mg/dL
4+	More than 2,000 mg/dL

Quantitative Method

The finding on one random sample should be negative. For clients who may have orthostatic or postural proteinuria, a second urine sample should be collected before arising from bed. If random samples are persistently positive for protein, a quantitative (24-hr) sample may be collected. A 24-hr specimen should show less than 150 mg of protein. (See Table 3–6 for the details about collection.) A quantitative assessment of proteinuria can also be performed on a random urine sample if the laboratory measures the protein-osmolality ratio. (See urine osmolality measurements in Chapter 4). A urinary protein-osmolality ratio greater than 2.2 indicates a level of albumin more than 3.0 g per 24 hr (Wilson and Anderson, 1993).

Microalbuminuria

Normally the urine contains less than 15 µg/mL of albumin. However, the dipsticks for albumin only begin showing a trace of albumin at levels of about 250 µg/mL. The range between these two numbers is above normal, but it is not recognized as overt proteinuria. This condition is referred to as *microalbuminuria*. The term means a small amount of albumin, not a small albumin molecule (Kaplan et al., 1995).

This test is most useful for detecting early nephropathy in clients with diabetes. If the test is positive, interventions can be planned to prevent a rapid decrease in renal function. If glucose control is not optimal, the client needs help achieving tight glucose control (see Chapter 8). Other interventions include limitations in dietary protein (see Chapter 10 on normal protein requirements) and drugs, if needed, to maintain a normal blood pressure. Angiotensin-converting enzyme (ACE) inhibitors may be useful in delaying progression of renal disease (Katzung, 1995).

Clinical Significance. Severe stress can cause proteinuria, but this is usually a temporary occurrence. Persistent protein in the urine is a common characteristic of renal dysfunction. Almost all types of kidney disease cause mild (up to 500 mg a day) to moderate (up to 4,000 mg a day) protein leakage into the urine. For children, more than 25 mg/kg a day should be investigated (Bastl et al., 1986). Some people have proteinuria that is called *orthostatic* or *postural* because it occurs only when the person is in the upright position. Usually no renal abnormalities are associated with this apparently benign condition. Preeclampsia and toxemia of pregnancy cause massive loss of protein in the urine. In what is called the *nephrotic syndrome*, which may be the end result of many diseases that cause renal dysfunction, the protein loss is as much as 4,000 mg a day. Albumin is the primary protein lost in all these conditions. Myelomas and certain other malignant tumors cause large protein losses, too, but because these proteins are abnormal, it is necessary for the laboratory to use special quantitative methods to determine the presences of these proteins. (See Chapter 10 on urine protein electrophoresis.)

▼ POSSIBLE NURSING DIAGNOSES RELATED TO PROTEINURIA

Alteration in Health Management

Persistent protein in the urine is an indication for further assessment of the renal system. The nurse may be the one to explain to the client how to collect another specimen before the client gets out of bed. If the proteinuria is due to renal dysfunction, other laboratory tests should be completed to assess the degree of impairment. (See Chapter 4.) A client with diabetes who tests positive for albuminuria may need help in achieving optimal glucose control (see Chapter 8), tight blood pressure control, and restrictions in protein intake (see Chapter 10).

Alteration in Health Management for Pregnant Clients

For a pregnant client, a check for protein in the urine is a routine part of each prenatal visit. If repeated dipsticks with a clean-catch specimen show proteinuria, a quantitative analysis is performed. In pregnancy a 24-hr urine collection for protein should not contain more than 500 mg. In the event that the pregnant client begins to show protein in the urine, it is important to assess carefully for hypertension and edema. Proteinuria, hypertension, and edema are the classic triad for preeclampsia.

▼ SUGAR IN THE URINE (GLYCOSURIA)

There are two different methods of screening for glucose in the urine:

1. Dipsticks change color in the presence of glucose because of the reaction of an enzyme, glucose oxidase.
2. Tablets (Clinitest) use the reducing properties of cupric oxide to cause a color change in the presence of glucose and of other sugars.

Dipstick (Enzymatic) Method

The dipstick or enzymatic method is easy: A tape is dipped into the urine and read for color changes after 1 min. If there is a color change on the darkest area, one should wait an additional minute to make the final comparison with the color chart.

The tapes should not be used if they are outdated. The activity of the tape or tablet can be checked by doing a mock test of a cola drink, because commercial beverages (except for diet ones!) all contain more than 2% glucose. The tapes should not be stored in a hot or humid room (such as the bathroom).

As the enzyme method is specific for glucose *only*, this method should be used if the client is taking any drugs that may make a false-positive with the reducing method. Such drugs are salicylates, penicillin, cephalosporins, ascorbic acid, and probenecid. Table 3–3 is a summary of drug effects using both methods.

Tablets (Reducing) Method

Sometimes it is necessary to check for the presence of sugars other than glucose. The reducing method detects the presence of fructose, galactose, lactose, or the pentoses.

TABLE 3–3. DRUGS THAT CAN AFFECT GLUCOSE TESTING

Reduction method	
False-positive	Ascorbic acid
	Cephalosporins (e.g., Keflin, Ancef)
	Chloramphenicol (Chloromycetin)
	Levo-dopa
	Methyldopa (Aldomet)
	Nalidixic acid (Neg Gram)
	Probenecid (Benemid)
	Penicillin
	Salicylates (high dosages)
	Sulfonomides
	Tetracyclines
	Sugars other than glucose (i.e., lactose, fructose, galactose, and pentoses)
Enzyme methods	
False-positive or negative	Phenazopyridine (Pyridium, Azo-Gantrisin)
False-negative	Ascorbic acid
	Levo-dopa (only Clinistix)
	Methyldopa
	Salicylates (high dosages) (only Clinistix)
	Cancer metabolites

For example, in screening the urine of an infant for potential abnormal sugars in the urine, it would be essential to use Clinitest tablets (Ames Products) and not enzyme tests. (See Chapter 8 on galactosemia and lactose intolerances.)

In what is called the *five-drop method,* five drops of urine and 10 drops of water are added to a test tube. When the Clinitest tablet is added, a boiling action occurs. This chemical reaction makes the bottom of the test tube hot. After the boiling stops, wait 15 sec and then gently shake the tube. Then compare the sample with a chart. Urine that is free of sugar remains blue. There may be a whitish sediment in the urine, but this is not clinically significant. Increasing amounts of glucose turn the urine from green to brown to orange.

As the boiling reaction is taking place, it is important to watch because the color may go very quickly to a dark brown color, which signifies more than 2% sugar. If so, this change is called a *pass-through reaction,* and it should be recorded as more than 2%. Otherwise the dark color that occurs *after* the initial reading at 15 sec should be ignored. Only the color change at 15 sec is compared with the chart.

The *two-drop method* uses the same tablet and amount of water but only two drops of urine. The two-drop method, by making the urine more dilute, avoids the "pass through" effect. Use the specific color chart for each method.

Increased Glucose in the Urine (Glycosuria)

Clinical Significance. Glucose in the urine signifies either (1) hyperglycemia (see Chapter 8 for a detailed discussion of the causes of hyperglycemia) or (2) a decreased renal threshold for glucose.

The *renal threshold* for glucose is usually about 160–190 mg/100 mL of blood; in other words, no sugar is spilled into the urine until the blood sugar rises above this level. Various situations, including diabetes, may cause a blood glucose level higher than 160 mg, and may alter the renal threshold for glucose. For example, in pregnancy the renal threshold for glucose may be lowered so that small amounts of glycosuria may be present and are usually not considered abnormal. Lactosuria is common in the third trimester. Clients receiving hyperalimentation have glycosuria if the intravenous solution (which has very concentrated sugar) is infused faster than the pancreas can produce insulin. Hereditary defects, such as galactose intolerance, cause a positive Clinitest, because a positive result with the reducing method can indicate the presence of sugars other than glucose. But such defects do not effect a positive result with enzyme dipsticks.

▼ POSSIBLE NURSING DIAGNOSES RELATED TO GLYCOSURIA

Knowledge Deficit Related to Urine Testing Techniques

Clients with diabetes need instructions on how to monitor glucose levels. Finger sticks for blood glucose are more accurate (see Chapter 8), but sometimes urine tests are easier. Gray (1985) and Carr (1990) noted that elderly clients may have visual problems, lack of manual dexterity, and some short-term memory loss, so they need careful assessment of their capabilities.

A double-voided specimen for periodic testing of sugar in urine is desirable. The client empties the bladder and then voids again as soon as possible. With this procedure one is sure that the urine reflects the current status, which is a particularly important condition if insulin is ordered, to cover any glycosuria. From a practical point of view, obtaining two specimens from a client may not be possible, so it is always wise to test the first voiding, too. Clients receiving hyperalimentation at home may also need instruction on urine testing for glucose.

Risk for Fluid Volume Deficit

A high concentration of sugar in the blood acts as an osmotic diuretic, so water is excreted as the sugar spills into the urine. The presence of glycosuria, from any cause, alerts the nurse that the client needs additional fluid intake and could undergo severe dehydration if the glycosuria is allowed to continue. (See Chapter 8 for a discussion on hyperglycemic hyperosmolar nonketotic coma [HHNK].) If the glycosuria is due to hyperalimentation therapy, the physician may eliminate the spilling of glucose in two different ways: (1) slow down the rate of the concentrated sugar solution or (2) order insulin to help the body use the large load of glucose.

In a client with diabetes a continued spilling of sugar leads not only to severe dehydration but also to ketonuria and eventually to ketoacidosis as the ketone bodies build up in the serum. The nurse needs to be aware that the presence of a positive acetone with a positive sugar indicates a need for immediate medical intervention. (See the discussion on ketoacidosis in Chapter 8 and on metabolic acidosis in Chapter 6.)

▼ KETONES IN THE URINE

Ketones are metabolic end products of fatty acid metabolism. When the body does not have sufficient glucose to use for energy, the excretion of ketones increases. The three ketone bodies in the urine are acetone, acetoacetic acid, and β-hydroxybutyric acid. Test strips and tablets check only for acetone and acetoacetic acid, but this is sufficient because a change in the small amount of acetone signifies the same degree of change in the other ketones. Acetoacetate and acetone can also be measured in the serum (see Chapter 8).

As in the tests for sugar, acetone can be tested either with a dipstick or with a tablet. Both methods show a deepening purple color when acetone is present. The scale indicates small, moderate, or large amounts of acetone. Symptomatic ketosis occurs at levels of about 50 mg/dL or when the client has moderate acetone in urine testing. Urine containing phenylketones (PKU, Chapter 18) or L-dopa metabolites may give false-positive results.

REFERENCE VALUES FOR KETONES

Normal urine should not contain enough ketones to give a positive reading

Small	20 mg/dL
Moderate	30–40 mg/dL
Large	80 mg/dL or greater

Clinical Significance. The presence of ketones in the urine signifies that the body is using fat as the main source of energy. Fats are used when glucose is unavailable to the cells. Glucose may not be available because it is not being transported to the cells, as in diabetes, or because glucose is lacking in the body because of starvation, vomiting, fasting, or an all-protein diet. The American Diabetes Association recommends that clients test for ketones when their blood sugar level is more than 240 mg/dL (Doeren and Friedman, 1992).

▼ POSSIBLE NURSING DIAGNOSES RELATED TO KETONES IN URINE

Risk for Injury Related to Development of Diabetic Acidosis

If the client is known to have diabetes, ketonuria (a positive acetone by testing) indicates that the insulin and glucose balance is not satisfactory. An abundance of glucose is in the bloodstream, but it is unavailable to the cells. A client with diabetes and a positive acetone has switched to using fats as the primary source of energy because the lack of insulin prohibits the transport of glucose to the cells. As the ketones accumulate, they use up the bicarbonate buffer (see Chapter 6), and ketoacidosis can develop. Extra fluids help the body eliminate excess ketones. (See Chapter 8 for more information about ketoacidosis and the other treatments needed.)

Alteration in Nutritional Needs, Less than Body Requirements of Carbohydrates

If the acetone is positive because of a starvation state, the positive ketone is associated with a negative glucose in the urine and normal blood sugar. A search must be made for other reasons why the cells do not have glucose. Questions to be asked would be

1. Has the client had a reduced amount of food?
2. Has there been a lot of vomiting?
3. Is the client trying to lose weight by being on an all-protein diet?

Depending on the circumstances, the client needs glucose in some form so that fats and proteins do not continue to be the primary source of energy. The client also needs extra fluids so that the ketones can be excreted by the kidneys. Clients on tube feedings that are very high in protein may show ketones in the urine unless they also receive adequate glucose in the feeding, along with plenty of water to rid the bloodstream of the ketones.

▼ EXAMINATION OF URINE SEDIMENT

As part of a urinalysis, the urine sediment is centrifuged and examined microscopically for crystals, casts, red blood cells (RBCs), white blood cells (WBCs), and bacteria or yeast. Table 3–4 contains a brief summary of the meaning of each of these findings. Some laboratories only do a microscopic examination on special request unless the routine urinalysis is positive for protein, blood, nitrites, or WBC esterase. If occult blood is suspected, the microscopic analysis is better for detection than the dipsticks. If urine is collected with a syringe and needle from the port of a Foley catheter, the needle should be removed before the urine is squirted into the specimen cup. Pushing the urine through the needle may damage cells and casts. Red cell casts dissolve within 20 min (Bastl et al., 1986).

TABLE 3–4. SUMMARY OF URINE SEDIMENT FINDINGS

WBCs	Normally there should not be more than a few white blood cells in the urine (4–5 per high-power field). Infections or inflammations anywhere along the urinary tract cause an increase of WBCs in the urine.
RBCs	Normally there should be only an occasional red blood cell in the urine (2–3 per high-power field). An increased number of RBCs in the urine indicates bleeding somewhere in the urinary system, which may be caused by renal disease, trauma, or a bleeding disorder. In women it is important to make sure that the urine was not contaminated by the menstrual flow. Insertion of a tampon and a collection of midstream urine are ways to prevent this contamination.
Crystals	Most crystals have little clinical significance. If the client is taking drugs that may cause crystallization in the urine, such as some of the sulfa drugs, this finding may be clinically important.
Casts	A few hyaline casts are considered normal, but all other casts need to be evaluated by the physician. Unlike crystals, casts are suggestive of kidney disease. Casts are a compacted collection of protein, cells, and debris that are formed in the tubules of the kidneys. Those that form in the distal tubule have a narrow caliber. Those that form in the collecting tubules tend to be very broad. Broad granular casts are sometimes called *renal failure casts* because they indicate renal destruction. The width and composition of the cast is important in the diagnosis of and prognosis for renal disease. (Shuman et al., 1978; Kaplan et al., 1995).
Bacteria or yeast	Often the presence of a few bacteria or yeasts is indicative only of contamination from the perineal area, but a culture and sensitivity may need to be performed if a large number of bacteria are noted on routine screening. Chapter 16 discusses the nursing implications for obtaining a urine specimen for a culture and sensitivity or for a smear. See the tests for nitrites and leukocyte esterase discussed in this chapter.

▼ ADDIS COUNT

The Addis count is a quantitative measurement of the RBCs, leukocytes, and casts in a 12-hr overnight urine specimen. Protein level and specific gravity also may be calculated. Fluids may be restricted before the test so urine will be concentrated. Some laboratories may want a 24-hr specimen with a restriction of 200 mL of fluid for each meal. (See the later discussion on 24-hr urine collection techniques.) The Addis test may be used to evaluate the course of renal disease by comparing results over time.

REFERENCE VALUES FOR 12-HR URINE SPECIMEN FOR ADDIS COUNT	
Red blood cells	Not more than 500,000
White blood cells	Not more than 1 million
Hyaline casts	Not more than 50,000

INDIVIDUAL URINE TESTS

Random urine specimens may be needed for various other tests besides a routine urinalysis; Table 3–5 shows some tests that are performed on a single specimen. Two of these, nitrites and leukocyte esterase, have become part of a routine urinalysis as noted in Table 3–1.

TABLE 3–5. EXAMPLES OF TESTS ON URINE (OTHER THAN ROUTINE URINALYSIS OR 24-HR URINE SPECIMENS)

Test	Reference Value	Specimen	Information About Test
Bence-Jones protein	Negative	First morning specimen	Chap. 10
Human chorionic gonadotropin (HCG)	Negative (unless pregnant)	First morning specimen	Chap. 18
Tests for occult blood Hematest (Ames) Hemastix (Ames) Hemoccult (Smith, Kline, French)	Negative	Random	Chap. 13 on tests to detect bleeding. Note microscopic exam is more sensitive test.
Porphobilinogen	Negative	Freshly voided specimen	This chapter
Bilirubin	Negative	Random	Chap. 11
Urobilinogen	Up to 1.0 Ehrlich units/2 hr	2-hr specimen (1–3 PM)	Chap. 11
Nitrites	No pink color	Clean-catch or midstream specimen	This chapter and Chap. 16
Leukocyte esterase	Negative	Random, clean-catch	This chapter

▼ NITRITES

Most species of bacteria, such as those of the family *Enterobacteriaceae*, if present in the urine, cause the conversion of nitrates, which are derived from dietary metabolites, to nitrites. Thus a dipstick for nitrites is a check for urinary infections. A negative nitrite test or negative culture does not provide proof that the urine is free of all bacteria, particularly if there are clinical symptoms to the contrary. Some bacteria do not produce nitrites. Note that the nitrite test is usually combined with the leukocyte esterase (LE) test discussed next.

Preparation of Client and Collection of Sample

Optimal results are obtained by using a first morning urine sample that has been "incubating" in the bladder for 4 hr or more. The urine should be collected by a clean-catch midstream technique (see Chapter 16 on clean-catch urine specimens), and it should be tested within an hour of voiding. As an alternative to the clean-catch method, the client may wet the strip by holding it in the urinary stream.

REFERENCE VALUES FOR NITRITES

Nitrate reagent	Turns pink if bacteria are present. The pink color is *not* quantitative in relation to the number of bacteria present. Ascorbic acid or a high specific gravity may invalidate the results. Blood or other pigments in the urine can interfere with the color changes.
Cultures	Usually growth of 100,000/mL is considered evidence of a bacterial infection. (See Chapter 16 on culture reports.)

A specialized dipstick for nitrites can also be used for a culture. Immediately after the strip is read, it is put into a transparent bag. The dipstick has two miniaturized culture areas that support both gram-positive and gram-negative bacteria. If the dipstick is to be cultured, it must not be touched. The dipstick in the bag is put into an incubator for a minimum of 18 hr. Results are ready within 18–24 hr. Various companies make diagnostic culture kits (see Chapter 16).

▼ LEUKOCYTE ESTERASE

The LE test identifies enzymes found in granulocytes, histiocytes, and *Trichomonas* species. The test detects 5–15 WBCs per high-power field and thus has an advantage over the microscopic examination because the LE test detects both lysed and intact cells. The combination of LE with the nitrite test (discussed earlier) provides a sensitive screen for predicting urinary tract infections. Lum and Thiemke (1989) found the combination of the two tests had 95% sensitivity and 85% specificity for detecting urinary tract infection in women with dysuria. For pregnant women, the LE test is used to test for infection in the amniotic fluid (Hoskins et al., 1990).

Preparation of Client and Collection of Sample

Dipsticks, such as Leukostix (Ames Products), are used the same way as other reagent strips for urinalysis. Concentrated urine is most satisfactory for testing. The dipstick for Leukostix is read at 2 min by comparing with a color chart and noting trace to +++. Color changes that occur after 2 min have no diagnostic value. Ascorbic acid and some antibiotics may interfere with the test.

REFERENCE VALUES FOR LE

A result matching any color block designated by a + sign indicates the presence of increasing amounts of leukocytes in urine. A "trace" reading should be retested with a fresh urine specimen. Positive results for LE and nitrites may be followed up with a urine culture (see Chapter 16).

▼ URINARY PORPHYRINS

Porphobilinogen, coproporphyrins, and uroporphyrins are intermediaries in the synthesis of heme, which is part of hgb and of several enzymes. Delta-aminolevulinic acid (ΔALA) is an important enzyme for the formation of porphobilinogen. Abnormalities of porphyrin metabolism may be either genetic or caused by drug intoxication, usually lead. Several tests can be completed to demonstrate an abnormality in the metabolism of heme. Because the porphyrins are precursors of the pigment (heme), the urine may be burgundy or pink when exposed to black light.

Preparation of Client and Collection of Sample

Coproporphyrin and uroporphyrin usually require a 24-hr urine specimen with a preservative. Testing for porphobilinogen is performed on a random urine specimen, consisting of 10 mL of freshly voided urine. Specimens should be protected from light.

REFERENCE VALUES FOR PORPHYRINS

Coproporphyrin	50–250 μg per day
Uroporphyrin	0
Porphobilinogen	0

Abnormal Porphyrins

Clinical Significance. Elevations of these tests are indications of one of the porphyrias, which are several different diseases that may be acute or chronic. The disease may be difficult to diagnose because it mimics so many other conditions. At present, treatment is symptomatic. Acute intermittent porphyria, the most common, can be precipitated by barbiturates. Coproporphyrins may document toxicity to lead (see Chapter 17). Because some types of porphyria are genetic diseases, studies should also be performed on relatives of affected clients.

▼ DELTA-AMINOLEVULINIC ACID

ΔALA is an enzyme needed for the proper conversion to porphobilinogen in the metabolic formation of heme. Although ΔALA is not present in the urine of healthy people, it is present in lead intoxication. Also, ΔALA may be elevated in certain kinds of genetic deficiencies of porphyrin metabolism (the porphyrias). This test is commonly performed for lead exposure and poisoning (Ravel, 1995).

Preparation of Client and Collection of Sample

A 24-hr urine sample should be collected (see instructions at the end of this chapter). Specimen should be protected from light. Various methods require different preservatives.

REFERENCE VALUES FOR ΔALA
1–7 mg/day

Clinical Significance. See Chapter 17 for the use of this test in relation to lead poisoning.

▼ URINARY 5-HYDROXYINDOLEACETIC ACID

Glands in the gastrointestinal tract secrete the hormone serotonin. Carried in the platelets, serotonin is a vasoconstrictor that is especially important to small arterioles after tissue injury. It is also a regulator of smooth muscle contraction, such as in peristalsis. The chief metabolite of serotonin, excreted in the urine, is 5-hydroxyindoleacetic acid (5-HIAA). Certain tumors, called *carcinoid tumors*, of the argentaffin cells in the gastrointestinal tract may begin to secrete abnormal amounts of serotonin. Hence a measurement of the amount of 5-HIAA in the urine is a help in diagnosing carcinoid tumors.

Preparation of Client and Collection of Sample

The client must not eat foods such as bananas, tomatoes, plums, avocados, eggplant, or pineapples because all these foods contain a large amount of serotonin. Because many drugs may also affect the test results, the nurse must check with the laboratory about specific drug interactions. The urine is collected in a special container with 10 mL of HCl or boric acid. Follow the procedure for a collection of 24-hr specimen (discussed at the end of this chapter).

REFERENCE VALUES FOR 5-HIAA	
24-hr screening test	Negative
Quantitative test	2–9 mg/day—women lower than men

Clinical Significance. An elevated level of 5-HIAA in the urine is evidence of increased serotonin, which may be caused by carcinoid tumors. These tumors may be either benign or malignant. Note that tumors in other organs may sometimes produce serotonin. (See Chapter 15 on ectopic hormone production by tumors.) The symptoms of serotonin excess may include cyanotic episodes, flushing of the skin, diarrhea, abdominal cramps, and bronchial constriction. The nurse should note and record any type of symptoms that occur during the time the client is undergoing studies for a possible carcinoid tumor. The principal clinical manifestations of the syndrome are due to biologically active agents released by the tumor. In addition to the release of serotonin, bradykinin, histamine, and adrenocorticotropic hormone (ACTH), other substances are released. Treatment involves surgical removal of the tumor. These tumors are usually slow-growing, and drug therapy may be used. Platelet serotonin is the most sensitive and consistently increased marker for long-term monitoring for most types of carcinoid tumors (Kema, et al., 1994).

▼ COLLECTION OF 24-HOUR URINE SPECIMENS

These collections are useful only if *all* the urine is collected for 24 hr. Even if "just one specimen" is discarded, the test is not valid. The nurse must make sure that the client fully understands the importance of saving all the urine. Because of the problem with incomplete urine collections, laboratories sometimes check the creatinine present in the urine to validate that the urine is representative of a full 24 hr. Assuming the client does not have renal problems, a creatinine value below the normal range for age and body weight suggests an incomplete collection.

To begin the 24-hr urine collection, the client voids and *discards* the urine so that the urine from the previous night is not included. Then all the urine for the next 24 hr is saved and put into a large collection bottle. If a client voids and discards the urine at, say, 8:20 AM, the test ends at 8:20 AM the next day. The client should do a final voiding as close to 8:20 AM as possible so that the last urine in the bladder can be included. The urine specimen should be sent to the laboratory as soon as possible. The times for beginning and ending the urine collection should be noted on the requisition.

The laboratory supplies the collection bottle, along with any preservative needed. (See Table 3–6 for common 24-hr urine specimens and the preparations

TABLE 3–6. 24-HOUR URINE SPECIMENS

Substance Tested	Reference Values (d = 24-hr day)	Preservative Needed	Information About Test
Aldosterone	5–19 μg/d	Refrigerate	Chap. 15
Amylase	24–76 U/mL	None	Chap. 12—may do for only 2 hr
Calcium	300 mg/d or less	Need 10 mL of HCl	Chap. 7
Catecholamines			
Epinephrine	<20 μg/d	Need 10 mL of HCl (pH kept 2–3)	Chap. 15
Norepinephrine	<100 μg/d		
Coproporphyrine	50–250 μg/d Children <80 lb; 0–75 μg/d	5 g of Na carbonate	This chapter
Creatinine	15–25 mg/kg body weight	None	Chap. 4
Creatinine clearance	Male: 95–135 mL/min Female: 85–125 mL/min	None	Need serum creatinine (Chap. 4)
Delta-aminolevulinic acid	1–7 mg/d	None	See this chapter and Chap. 17
5-HIAA	2–9 mg/d (women lower than men)	10 mL of HCl	See this chapter
Lead	≤120 μg/d	None	Make sure lead-free container (Chap. 17)
Pregnanetriol	Men: 1–2 mg/d Women: 0.5–2 mg/d Children: <0.5 mg/d	Refrigerate	Chap. 15
Phosphate	1 g/d—varies with intake	10 mL of HCl	Chap. 7
Potassium	25–125 mEq/d	None	Chap. 5
Pregnanediol	Men: <1 mg/d Women: 1–8 mg/d	Refrigerate	Chap. 15
Protein	<150 mg/d	None	See quantitative and qualitative tests in this chapter and notes for pregnancy
Sodium	40–220 mEq/d	None	Chap. 5
17-Ketosteroids	Varies with age and sex	None	Chap. 15
17-Hydroxysteroids	3–8 mg/d (women lower than men)	None	Chap. 15
Urea nitrogen	6–17 g/d	None	Chap. 4
Uroporphyrin	0–30 μg/d	5 g of Na carbonate	See this chapter
Vanillylmandelic acid	Up to 9 mg/d	12 mL of HCl	Chap. 15

Note that most laboratories prefer all 24-hr urine specimens iced. Check with the laboratory for the specific technique used and reference values.

needed.) Clients need to be told if there is a preservative, so that no direct contact occurs with a toxic solution. The laboratory should also notify the nurse or the client if certain drugs or foods invalidate the test. (See the discussions in the various chapters on specific points for each test.) If a preservative is not used, a few specimens, such as those for hormones, must be refrigerated. Usually refrigeration is preferred for most urine tests, but the nurse should validate this requirement with the laboratory. The rationale for refrigeration is to inhibit bacterial growth, which may interfere with some tests.

For toddlers, when a diaper is used at night, a 12-hr specimen may have to suffice. For infants, urine may be collected in disposable paste-on collection bags. Rarely, it may be necessary to insert a Foley catheter to obtain a 24-hr urine collection from a child. The danger of a urinary tract infection is a disadvantage.

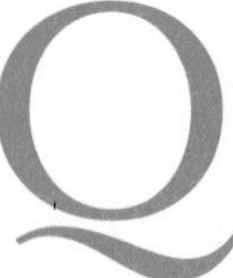

1. A specimen of urine for a routine urinalysis should be

   a. At least 60 mL
   b. Put into a sterile container
   c. An early morning specimen, if possible
   d. Sent to the laboratory as a stat procedure

2. Which of the following tends to make the urine pH higher?

   a. Meat b. Eggs
   c. Cranberry juice d. Citrus juices

3. Marie Cotton has just been taught how to perform blood glucose checks for her newly diagnosed diabetes. She asks the clinic nurse what other tests she should carry out if her blood glucose level is more than 240 mg/dL. The nurse responds by instructing Marie to follow-up an elevated blood glucose level by performing a urine dipstick for

   a. Glucose b. Specific gravity
   c. Protein d. Ketones

4. In interpreting the meaning of specific gravity of a urinalysis for a child younger than 2 years, it is important for the nurse to realize that in a child this young, the maximum specific gravity is

   a. Much lower than for an adult
   b. Higher than for an adult

c. Essentially the same as the adult range
d. Fixed at 1.010

5. Which of the following clients demonstrates the concept of a "fixed" specific gravity?

   a. Mrs. Jung, who has a specific gravity of about 1.025 on three early morning urine specimens
   b. Mr. Louis, who has a specific gravity of 1.010 on a random urine specimen
   c. Mr. Tagelino, whose specific gravity remains about 1.008 while he is taking diuretics
   d. Mrs. Foley, whose specific gravity was 1.010 during a prolonged period of fluid restriction

6. A client is asked to obtain a urine specimen before arising to rule out orthostatic or postural

   a. Glycosuria   b. Ketonuria
   c. Proteinuria   d. Hematuria

7. The nurse in a prenatal clinic has just tested Mrs. Ames' urine and found it to be 0.5% for glucose and 3+ for protein by the dipstick method. There will be a 30- to 40-min delay before the client sees the physician. She says she is "feeling okay" so she wishes to have her appointment rescheduled. Which action by the nurse would be the most appropriate?

   a. Reschedule her appointment for another day because glucose and protein in the urine are not uncommon in the third trimester of pregnancy
   b. Say nothing about the urine test but insist that she wait to see the physician because the clinic schedule is always full
   c. Take a nursing history from the client and tell her the glucose in her urine needs investigation by the physician because she may be diabetic
   d. Take her blood pressure, check her ankles, and explain why it is necessary to make these assessments to help the physician evaluate the seriousness of the proteinuria. Emphasize that it is important for the client to wait to see the physician

8. Jacob Cohen, 55 years of age, has had insulin-dependent diabetes mellitus (IDDM) for more than 5 years. He has had yearly urine dipstick tests for albumin. He asks the nurse why the physician has ordered a new test, a "microalbuminuria." The most accurate reply by the nurse would be: "The microalbuminuria test is

   a. A 24-hour urine test to check for very small particles of albumin."
   b. A more sensitive test than the regular dipstick test. Tiny amounts of albumin can be detected."

c. The same test you have been having each year. The name just denotes a new technique."

d. A procedure that compares the albumin in your urine with the microalbumin in your blood."

9. Marilyn is a 19-year-old college freshman who is quite obese. She has come to the campus health clinic because she feels very tired. A routine CBC and urinalysis are normal except for a trace of acetone. (Urine sugar was negative.) Based on these laboratory findings, which question by the nurse will most likely help detect the reason for the abnormal ketones?

   a. Have you been eating a lot of fats lately?
   b. Have you been under a lot of stress?
   c. Is there a history of diabetes in your family?
   d. Have you been on a strict reducing diet lately?

10. Mrs. Zorba is in the last trimester of her pregnancy. Dipstick tests for nitrites and leukocyte esterase in the urine were positive. Her specific gravity was normal. These positive reactions are evidence of

   a. Preeclampsia
   b. Normal dietary metabolites of protein
   c. Possible urinary tract infection
   d. Possible lack of ascorbic acid in her diet

11. Mr. Leggins is to collect a 24-hr specimen for urine coproporphyrins for possible lead toxicity. He has been given a container with the necessary preservative. Which of the following instructions by the nurse is correct?

   a. Begin the test exactly at 8 AM and collect all urine until 8 AM the next day
   b. Discard the first urine specimen tomorrow morning and then collect all the urine for the next 24 hr
   c. Discarding only one specimen will not create a problem if he can estimate the amount lost
   d. Consume large amounts of fluids so the urine will be dilute

▼ REFERENCES

Bastl, C., et al. (1986). Diagnosing kidney disease early. *Patient Care, 20* (4), 28–52.

Carr, P. (1990). Home blood glucose monitoring: It's not for everyone. *Nursing 90, 20* (10), 50.

Cooper, C. (1993). What color is that urine specimen? *American Journal of Nursing, 93* (8), 37.

Doeren, E., and Freidman, N. (1992). Urine testing still in style. *Diabetes Forecast, 45* (9), 62–64.

Gray, D. (1985). Elderly diabetics and urine testing. *Geriatric Nursing, 6* (6), 332–334.
Hermansen, M., and Buches, M. (1988). Urine output determination from superabsorbent and regular diapers under radiant heat. *Pediatrics, 81*, 428–431.
Hoskins, I., et al. (1990). Leukocyte esterase activity in amniotic fluid: Normal values during pregnancy. *American Journal of Perinatology, 72* (2), 130–132.
Kaplan, A., Jack, R., Opheim, K.E., et al. (1995). *Clinical chemistry: interpretations and techniques*. (4th ed.). Baltimore: Williams & Wilkins.
Katzung, B. (ed.). (1995). *Basic and clinical pharmacology*. (6th ed.). Norwalk: Appleton & Lange.
Kema, I.P., de Vries, E.G., Slooff, M.J., et al. (1994). Serotonin, catecholamines, histamine, and their metabolites in urine, platelets, and tumor tissue of patients with carcinoid tumors. *Clinical Chemistry, 40* (1), 86–95.
Kinney, A., and Blout, M. (1979). Effect of cranberry juice on urinary pH. *Nursing Research, 28* (5), 287–290.
Leiner, S. (1995). Recurrent urinary tract infections in otherwise healthy adult women. *Nurse Practitioner, 20* (2), 48–56.
Lum, G., and Thiemke, W. (1989). Evaluation of a scoring system for leukocyte esterase-nitrite dipstick screening for urine culture. *Laboratory Medicine, 20* (10), 692–695.
McConnell, E. (1991). How to use a urinometer. *Nursing 91, 21* (10), 28.
Metheny, N., et al. (1989). Effectiveness of pH measurements in predicting feeding tube placement. *Nursing Research, 38* (5), 280–285.
Ravel, R. (1995). *Clinical laboratory medicine: Clinical application of laboratory data*. (6th ed.). St. Louis: Mosby–Year Book.
Shuman, B., et al. (1978). An improved technique for examining urinary casts and a review of their significance. *American Journal of Clinical Pathology, 69* (1), 18–23.
Slawson, M. (1980). Thirty-three drugs that discolor urine and/or stools. *RN, 43* (1), 40–41.
Stebor, A.D. (1989). Post urination time and specific gravity in infants' diapers. *Nursing Research, 38* (4), 244–245.
Wilson, D.M., and Anderson, R.L. (1993). Protein-osmolality ratio for the quantitative assessment of proteinuria from a random urinalysis sample. *American Journal of Clinical Pathology, 100*, 419–424.

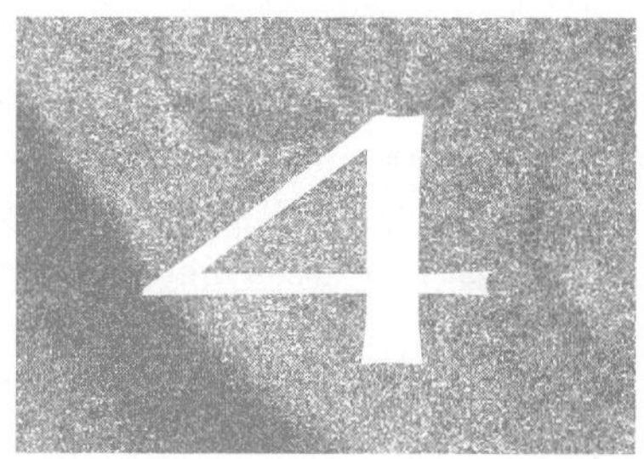

RENAL FUNCTION TESTS

- Blood Urea Nitrogen
- BUN-to-Creatinine Ratio
- Urinary Urea Nitrogen and Nitrogen Balance
- Creatinine Levels in Serum
- Creatinine Clearance Test
- Serum and Urine Osmolality
- Uric Acid (Serum and Urine)

OBJECTIVES

1. Compare and contrast the factors that affect BUN and serum creatinine levels.
2. Explain the rationale for checking BUN or serum creatinine levels before administration of certain antibiotics.
3. Describe the nursing diagnoses that are appropriate when a client has markedly elevated BUN and serum creatinine levels.
4. Given the values for urinary urea nitrogen and the client's intake of protein, calculate the nitrogen balance to determine if dietary adjustments are warranted.
5. Compare the usefulness of urine osmolality to the measurement of urine specific gravity.
6. Given various changes in serum and urine osmolality, plan appropriate nursing interventions.

7. Prepare a teaching plan that helps a client with high serum uric acid levels to decrease the possibility of renal stones.
8. Describe the role of the nurse in preparing clients for creatinine clearance tests.

Some of the tests discussed in this chapter are used only for renal assessment, whereas others have several purposes. For example, serum creatinine levels, urine creatinine levels, and the creatinine clearance tests are all used only to evaluate renal function, and only renal dysfunction changes the result. However, BUN, also used primarily to assess renal function, can be affected by other factors and may be used to assess fluid volume deficit. The urinary urea nitrogen is used to assess nitrogen balance. Tests for serum and urine osmolality are useful not only in assessing renal function but also for assessing fluid requirements and fluid imbalances. The discussions of urine osmolality should be read after one has read about specific gravity measurements in the previous chapter. One test covered in this chapter, uric acid, is not really a test for renal dysfunction, but uric acid is likely to be elevated in severe renal dysfunction. Therefore, the discussion on uric acid fits into a general discussion about renal dysfunction, even though it is not used as an assessment tool for the severity of the dysfunction.

▼ BLOOD UREA NITROGEN

The BUN test measures the amount of urea nitrogen in the blood. Urea, a waste product of protein metabolism, is formed by the liver and carried in the blood to the kidneys for excretion. Because urea is cleared from the bloodstream by the kidneys, the BUN can be used as a test of renal function. However, protein breakdown, dehydration, overhydration, and liver failure all invalidate the BUN as a test for renal dysfunction.

Preparation of Client and Collection of Sample

There is no special preparation of the client. The laboratory needs 1 mL of blood or serum for the test.

REFERENCE VALUES FOR BUN	
Adult	8–25 mg/dL May be slightly higher in men than in women
Pregnancy	Values may decrease about 25%
Newborn	Values tend to be slightly lower than adult ranges
Aged	Values may be slightly increased because of lack of renal concentration

Increased BUN

Clinical Significance. Diseased or damaged kidneys cause an elevated BUN because the kidneys are less able to rid the blood of the waste product urea. Even if the kidneys are not diseased or damaged, conditions in which renal perfusion is decreased result in an increase of urea in the blood. Thus a client in shock or one in congestive heart failure may have higher-than-normal BUN levels caused by poor circulation to the kidneys. A client who is severely dehydrated may also have an elevated BUN level because of the lack of volume to excrete waste products. Because urea is an end product of protein metabolism, a diet high in protein, such as tube feedings, may cause some increase in the BUN level. Bleeding into the gastrointestinal tract also causes an elevated BUN because digested blood is a source of protein. For example, loss of 1,000 mL of blood into the gastrointestinal tract may elevate the BUN to 40 mg/dL.

▼ BUN-TO-CREATININE RATIO

Because creatinine is changed only by renal dysfunction, a comparison of the BUN with the serum creatinine is useful. A client with a BUN of 15 mg might have a serum creatinine level of about 1.0 mg. If the client becomes dehydrated or has increased protein (such as with gastrointestinal bleeding), the BUN increases whereas the creatinine does not; so the ratio of 15:1 would be increased in dehydration or in protein breakdown. However, the ratio of BUN to creatinine would be less than 15:1 in low-protein intake, overhydration, or severe liver failure, which reduces the BUN but not the creatinine level. BUN-to-creatinine ratios may range from 1:6 to 1:20. Ravel (1995) considered 1:10 to be the mean but noted that variability in protein intake and mass of voluntary muscle can cause the ratio to be misleading.

Use of BUN or Creatinine to Monitor Nephrotoxic Drugs

BUN and creatinine levels are also used to monitor clients who are receiving drugs known to be potentially nephrotoxic, such as antibiotics classified as aminoglycosides. Some of the aminoglycosides are gentamicin, tobramycin, and netilmicin. Before administering a drug that is known to be potentially nephrotoxic, nurses should look at the client's BUN and creatinine levels. If either level is higher than the reference range, they should withhold the drug until consulting the physician. Because aminoglycosides tend also to be toxic to the eighth cranial nerve, assessments of auditory and vestibular functions are ways to monitor for neurotoxicity. The impaired hearing or dizziness that may occur is more likely if the drug is continued when there is renal dysfunction. Measurements of the levels of drugs in the serum are completed so that a therapeutic level can be maintained. (See Chapter 17 for a discussion about the measurement of serum levels of aminoglycosides such as gentamicin.) It is important to keep the client well-hydrated when aminoglycosides are used because they are excreted almost unchanged in the urine.

▼ POSSIBLE NURSING DIAGNOSES RELATED TO ELEVATED BUN

Risk for Fluid Volume Deficit

Because an increased BUN may be caused by anything that causes poor renal perfusion or renal dysfunction, it is important to look at the BUN in relation to the pathologic process for the individual client. If the BUN is due to poor renal perfusion, the focus is on increasing renal flow. For example, if the client has dehydration, this must be corrected. However, if the elevated BUN reflects actual renal damage, fluids may have to be restricted or increased, depending on the phase of acute renal failure. The client is most likely to have severe fluid and electrolyte imbalances during the oliguric-anuric phase and the late diuretic phase (Baer, 1990). The nurse must monitor the necessary fluid requirements and keep accurate intake and output (I&O) records. Table 4–1 compares BUN and creatinine in various stages of renal disease. Note that the BUN-to-creatinine ratio may help identify dehydration rather than renal disease. Also see the discussion on serum and urine osmolality for other assessments of a fluid volume deficit.

If the elevated BUN can be traced to a great increase in protein in the diet, a reduction of protein or an increase of fluid intake or both helps the kidneys eliminate the excess urea. For example, increased fluids are needed with high-protein supplements.

Alterations in Nutritional Requirements of the Problem Nutrients: Potassium, Sodium, and Protein

Because urea is not the only substance that increases in the bloodstream as renal dysfunction persists, the nurse must be alert to which medications and foods may be contraindicated. Sodium and potassium are excreted by the kidneys. Sodium may have to be restricted, and supplemental potassium is contraindicated in a client who has progressive renal dysfunction. (See Chapter 5 on hyperkalemia and hypernatremia.) Usually protein in the diet is not restricted for mild renal insufficiency, but one would question a high-protein diet, which would tend to increase the BUN even more. The protein level may have to be adjusted to maintain lean body mass and still not cause a high BUN. Once the client is on dialysis the dietary restrictions may be lessened. Inadequate nutrition, as measured by serum albumin levels (Chapter 10), is associated with higher mortality rates (Owen, et al., 1993). (See Chapter 7 for a discussion of supplemental calcium and the restriction of phosphorus in renal disease.)

Children and adolescents with renal failure present additional nutritional problems because of the needs of their growing bodies. Few infants are given fluid restrictions. Yet as with adults, sodium, potassium, and protein are the problem nutrients. Infants may be experiencing life-threatening hyperkalemia (high potassium level), even though the BUN is not greater than 35 mg/dL.

Impairment of Skin Integrity

Azotemia means an increase of nitrogenous waste products in the serum. *Uremia* is the broader name given to the toxic condition in which the kidneys are not able to excrete urea and other substances such as potassium, creatinine, and organic acids. In the days before the advent of peritoneal and renal dialysis, clients with high levels of BUN would have a condition called *uremic frost,* which consisted of urea crystals that were being excreted through the sweat glands. Fortunately urea levels can be lowered now with dialysis before clients experience toxic uremia. Still, itching is often a problem, and the potential for skin breakdown is always present.

Risk for Injury Related to Weakness and Possible Confusion

Clients with a mild gradual increase in BUN level may not have many symptoms. The level of BUN that causes symptoms in clients varies tremendously. As BUN levels continue to rise, the client is likely to experience fatigue, muscle weakness, and some nausea and vomiting. There may be a decline in mental awareness, drowsiness, or confusion. Nurses need to assess the mental and physical capabilities of any client with an increased BUN level to ensure safe care. Clients who may be slightly confused or unsteady on their feet need careful watching. Hypertension and arrhythmias may limit activity, so blood pressure and pulse must be closely monitored. Hatch (1990) noted that many of the most troublesome symptoms of uremia are really those of anemia, and the use of erythropoietin injections to raise the hct may eliminate fatigue, dyspnea, angina, and depression. (See Chapter 2 on erythropoietin assays.)

Alterations in Health Maintenance Related to Need for Readjustment of Medications

Clients with elevated BUN and creatinine levels may need modifications in their drug regimen. For example, clients with diabetes need less insulin as their renal function decreases. Other common drugs that have a prolonged effect in clients with compromised renal function include digoxin, phenothiazines, meperidine, and several antibiotics. The nurse must be aware of possible overdose and the necessity to explain its possibility to clients so ongoing monitoring is carried out. The creatinine clearance test, discussed later in this chapter, is an objective evaluation of the actual extent of renal damage and helps the physician reevaluate the needed dosage changes of maintenance drugs.

Risk for Infection Related to Alterations in the Immune System and Phagocytosis

Clients undergoing chronic dialysis have an increased risk for infection not only because of the invasive devices used but also because of a decrease in lymphocytes and alterations in the functioning ability of lymphocytes, mono-

(*continued*)

▼ POSSIBLE NURSING DIAGNOSES RELATED TO ELEVATED BUN (*continued*)

cytes, and neutrophils (Lewis, 1990). Nursing interventions to protect the client from infection are a high priority. (See Chapter 2 on lymphocytes, monocytes, and neutrophils and ways to enhance resistance to infection.)

Alteration in Bowel Elimination Related to Constipation

Clients with chronic renal disease often have problems with constipation because of restricted fluid intake and lack of exercise. Increasing fiber in the diet may be limited because many high-fiber foods are high in potassium and phosphorus. Usually, these clients do need stool softeners on a regular basis, and the sodium and calcium in these products are not sufficient to warrant concern (Chambers, 1983). (See Chapter 7 for a discussion on high phosphorus and magnesium levels and the danger of some laxatives for clients with renal failure.)

Risk for Disturbance in Self-esteem and Self-concept

The psychological needs of the client usually decrease if the client has a type of acute renal failure that is reversible. However, many types of renal damage are not reversible. As renal function becomes compromised, many pathologic changes occur (Table 4–1). These changes and the need for alterations in lifestyle can be devastating to the client and significant others. Depression, anxiety, and a feeling of powerlessness may develop as clients consider possible options such as home or hospital hemodialysis, peritoneal dialysis, or an eventual renal transplant. Stark and Hunt (1983) suggested that the nurse find the coping methods previously used by the clients for major life changes and help them use the successful methods for the present crisis. A psychiatric nurse or a social worker may also be used for support.

TABLE 4–1. POSSIBLE CONTINUUM OF CHRONIC RENAL DISEASE

Reduced or diminished renal reserve	BUN may be slightly high or high-normal, but no problems unless stress (infections, surgery, emotional crisis) challenges limited reserve. Creatinine levels within normal range.
Renal insufficiency	BUN mildly elevated. May not tolerate high-protein intake. Impaired urine concentration (see serum osmolality). Mild anemia. Stress easily impairs renal function. Creatinine level beginning to rise (see Table 4–2).
Renal failure	Both creatinine and BUN are elevated. Levels vary with severity and other factors. Other abnormal tests may be hypernatremia, hyperkalemia (Chapter 5), anemia (Chapter 2), hypocalcemia, hyperphosphatemia (Chapter 7).
End-stage renal disease	Serum creatinine greater than 10 mg/dL. BUN rises somewhat proportionately. Other tests mentioned are increasingly abnormal.

See text and Stark (1994) for more details.

Decreased BUN

Clinical Significance. Just as dehydration may cause an elevated BUN, overhydration causes a decreased BUN. An increase in antidiuretic hormone (ADH) is a pathologic reason for dilute plasma. Increases in plasma volume, such as in pregnancy, reduce the BUN level. A marked decrease in protein breakdown also tends to lower the BUN. Usually a BUN that is slightly lower than the reference values has little clinical significance. Because urea is synthesized by the liver, severe liver failure causes a reduction of urea in the serum. Yet, the inability of the liver to form urea results in an increase in other nitrogenous products, such as ammonia, so tests for ammonia levels are much more clinically significant in liver dysfunction than are lowered BUN levels. (See Chapter 10 on ammonia levels.)

▼ POSSIBLE NURSING DIAGNOSIS RELATED TO DECREASED BUN

Risk for Fluid Volume Excess

Because a decreased BUN raises the possibility of expanded plasma fluid volume, some attention should be given to the overall hydration status of the client. Yet the test by itself is not helpful in identifying plasma dilution. (See the section on serum osmolality in this chapter and Chapter 5 on serum sodium as tests for plasma dilution.)

▼ URINARY UREA NITROGEN AND NITROGEN BALANCE

The urinary urea nitrogen can be measured and compared with the amount of protein ingested to determine the nitrogen balance of the client. There is about 1 g of nitrogen in each 6 g of protein, and the loss of nitrogen is about 4 g from stool and insensible loss. Based on these facts the following formula has been devised:

$$\text{N balance} = \frac{\text{Protein intake (g)}}{6.25} - (\text{24-hr urinary urea nitrogen} + 4)$$

A value less than 0 indicates a negative nitrogen balance as shown in the following example:

$$\text{N balance} = 50/6.25 - (6 + 4) = -2$$

A negative nitrogen balance is an indication that the client needs a greater protein intake (see Chapter 10).

Preparation of Client and Collection of Sample

See Chapter 3 on the method for collecting 24-hr urine specimens. No preservation is needed. The dietician usually assesses protein intake. The nurse must accurately record all food intake.

REFERENCE VALUES FOR URINARY UREA
6–17 g of urinary nitrogen in 24 hr

REFERENCE VALUES FOR NITROGEN BALANCE	
0 or greater	(see earlier discussion for formula)

▼ CREATININE LEVELS IN SERUM

Creatinine is the waste product of creatine phosphate, a high-energy compound found in skeletal muscle tissue. The measurement of serum *creatinine* is useful in evaluating any type of renal dysfunction in which a large number of nephrons have been destroyed. Late afternoon values are reported to be about 20–40% higher than morning values. This variation may be related to meals (Ravel, 1995).

Preparation of Client and Collection of Sample

The laboratory needs 1 mL of venous blood. High doses of ascorbic acid or barbiturates may distort the results. Ketone bodies and cephalosporin antibiotics may elevate the results.

REFERENCE VALUES FOR SERUM CREATININE	
Adult: Men	0.6–1.5 mg/dL
Women	0.6–1.1 mg/dL Values tend to be slightly higher for men because of their larger muscle mass
Pregnancy	Values are reduced in pregnancy, presumably because creatinine clearance is markedly increased
Newborn	Lower than children
Children	0.2–1.0 mg/dL. Slight increases with age because values are proportional to body mass

TABLE 4–2. RELATIONSHIP OF CREATININE LEVELS TO ESTIMATED AMOUNT OF NEPHRON LOSS

Creatinine Level	Estimated Loss of Nephron Function
Normal creatinine (0.6–1.5 mg/dL)	Up to 25% loss
Creatinine level >1.5 mg/dL	>50% nephron function loss
Creatinine level of 4.8 mg/dL	As much as 75% nephron function loss
Creatinine level of ~ 10 mg/dL	90% loss of nephron function—end-stage kidney disease

Increased Creatinine Level

Clinical Significance. The only pathologic condition that causes a clinically significant increase in serum creatinine level is damage to a large number of nephrons (Table 4–2). Unlike the BUN, the serum creatinine level is not affected by protein metabolism and is only minimally affected by the hydration state of the client.

As discussed in the section on BUN, a change in the BUN-to-creatinine ratio may be useful in pinpointing the primary factor that needs correction. Because the creatinine is not increased until at least one-fourth of the nephrons are nonfunctioning, it is usually not elevated in diminished renal reserve as is the BUN. Thus clients with an increased creatinine are most likely to have potentially severe renal impairment. Like the BUN, serum creatinine is used to detect potential renal damage when nephrotoxic drugs, such as the aminoglycoside antibiotics, are used. Serum creatinine levels are also routinely measured for all dialysis clients and for clients who have had renal transplants. Some renal transplant units prefer to monitor a rise in the serum concentration of B_2 microglobulin, a serum protein, as the earliest indicator of renal transplant rejection (Kaplan et al., 1995). Because creatinine levels rise and fall more slowly than BUN levels, creatinine levels are often preferred for long-term assessment of renal function.

▼ POSSIBLE NURSING DIAGNOSES RELATED TO ELEVATED CREATININE

See section on BUN.

Decreased Creatinine Level

Clinical Significance. A decreased serum creatinine level may indicate atrophy of muscle tissue. However, if skeletal muscle problems are suspected, the serum creatine is used. Note also that the creatine kinase (CK) is an important enzyme test for muscular disease. (See Chapter 12 on CPK or CK.)

▼ CREATININE CLEARANCE TEST

The creatinine clearance test is used as an indication of the glomerular filtration rate (GFR). The test compares the serum creatinine level with the amount of creatinine excreted in a volume of urine for a specified time. The time may be 2, 12, or 24 hr. Kaplan et al. (1995) noted that a 24-hr collection is not more accurate and is inconvenient. At the beginning of the test, the client empties his or her bladder, and this urine is discarded. Thereafter, all the urine voided during the specified time period is collected. (See Chapter 3 on 24-hr urine collections. No preservative is needed.)

Sometime during the test period, a blood sample is drawn to determine the serum creatinine level. The rate of creatinine clearance is thus determined by the following formula:

$$\frac{\text{Urine creatinine} \times \text{Urine volume}}{\text{Creatinine in serum}} = \text{Creatinine clearance rate}$$

expressed in millimeters per minute per 1.72 m^2 of body surface.

REFERENCE VALUES FOR CREATININE CLEARANCE

Adult: Men	95–135 mL/min Varies with the amount of lean body mass, so muscular men are usually in the upper limits of the range
Women	85–125 mL/min
Pregnancy	May be as high as 150–200 mL/min
Premature and newborn infants	35–65 mL/min
Children (older than 1.5 years)	55–85 mL/min
Aged	Values diminish with age even if no renal disease exists. Glomerular filtration rate declines about 10% per decade after 50 years of age

Decreased Creatinine Clearance

Clinical Significance. A decreased creatinine clearance rate is an indication of decreased glomerular function. In preeclampsia, the creatinine clearance drops as it does with renal impairment. However, the lesions on the kidney for preeclampsia are reversible, so there are no long-term problems (Groër and Shekleton, 1989). Creatinine clearance rate is a more sensitive indication of renal dysfunction than serum creatinine alone because the serum creatinine may remain normal until the creatinine clearance is less than half than normal. Creatinine clearance is also used to evaluate the progression of renal disease. A minimum creatinine clearance of about 10 mL/min is necessary to maintain life without the use of renal or peritoneal dialysis.

The results of the creatinine clearance test, together with other assessments of renal dysfunction, help determine the long-term plans for the client. Clients may have repeated creatinine clearance tests because changes in the results may be more clinically significant when compared over a period of time.

▼ SERUM AND URINE OSMOLALITY

The osmolality of serum, urine, or any other fluid depends on the number of active ions or molecules in a solution. The osmolality of a solution reflects the total *number* of osmotically active particles in the solution, without regard to the size or weight of the particles. In laboratory reports, osmolality is expressed in milliosmoles per kilogram of water (mOsm/kg water).

Although nurses do not need to know how to calculate milliosmoles, they may find it helpful to understand conceptually the meaning of a milliosmole (mOsm). A milliosmole is 1/1,000 of an osmole. *Osmoles* are a standard of measurement based on the freezing point of a solution: As the number of osmotically active particles in a solution increases, the freezing point decreases. For example, a lower temperature is needed to freeze a salt solution than to freeze plain water. As a standard of measurement, one osmole is the amount of a particular solute that lowers the freezing point of 1 kg of water 1.86°C. With a standard measurement of osmoles and of milliosmoles for clinical studies, the precise concentration of active solutes in the serum and urine can be calculated. Although sodium is the principal constituent of serum osmolality, urea nitrogen is also one of the major factors in urine osmolality.

Serum Osmolality

Sodium, BUN, and blood glucose levels are important factors in determining serum osmolality. In severe dehydration serum osmolality increases. Chapter 5 discusses hypernatremia as a type of hyperosmolar dehydration, and Chapter 8 discusses hyperglycemic hyperosmolar nonketotic (HHNK) dehydration. An estimate of serum osmolality may be obtained from the laboratory values of sodium, potassium, BUN, and blood glucose, as shown in Table 4–3. The osmolality calculated from labora-

TABLE 4–3. ESTIMATION OF SERUM OSMOLALITY FROM LABORATORY VALUES FORMULA

2(Na) + BUN/2.8 + Blood glucose/18
Example of normal reference values
2(135) + 12/2.8 + 110/18
270 + 4.29 + 6.11 = 280 mOsm[a]

[a] *Osmolal gap.* This gap is the difference between the estimated (calculated) and the measured serum osmolality. A gap of more than 10 mOsm provides a clue to unusual solutes (Ravel, 1995).

tory values may be as much as 9 mOsm less than the measured one. This difference between the measured and the estimate is called the *osmolal* or *osmole gap*. Unmeasured substances such as methanol or ethanol increase this gap even greater, because each 0.10 mg/dL of ethanol raises the serum osmolality about 22 mOsm (Ravel, 1995). Thus a serum osmolality may be useful for screening for alcohol ingestion. Chapter 17 discusses the direct measurement of blood alcohol levels.

Urine Osmolality

Urine osmolality, like specific gravity, is a measurement of the concentration of the urine. (See Chapter 3 on the specific gravity of urine.) Urine osmolality reflects the total number of osmotically active particles in the urine, without regard to the *size* or *weight* of the particles. As a result, high sugar concentrations, proteins, or dyes do not disproportionately raise urine osmolality as they do the specific gravity of the urine. The urine osmolality test has at least three other advantages over the specific gravity:

1. The temperature variable is controlled with the osmolality determination, so the results are more accurate.
2. Because the osmolality test is a more sensitive measurement, a small change in the amount of solutes is evident with the osmolality test, but not with the specific gravity.
3. The urine osmolality can be compared with the serum osmolality to provide a more definitive idea of the fluid balance or imbalance.

The disadvantages of the osmolality test are that it cannot be completed immediately by the nurse as can the specific gravity and it is more expensive.

Preparation of Client and Collection of Sample

There is no special preparation of the client for the test. Depending on the type of machine used, the laboratory can perform an osmolality on as little as 2–5 mL of serum or urine.

REFERENCE VALUES FOR SERUM AND URINE OSMOLALITY

Serum osmolality	Range 280–296 mOsm/kg water. Usually about 285 (290 mOsm = 1.010 specific gravity)
Urine osmolality	Extreme range of 50–1400 mOsm/kg water, but average is about 500–800 mOsm (800 mOsm = 1.022 specific gravity). Newborns have low urine osmolality
	After an overnight fast (14 hr), the urine osmolality should be at least three times the serum osmolality (Basil et al., 1986)

TABLE 4–4. CLINICAL IMPLICATIONS OF CHANGES IN OSMOLALITY

Serum Osmolality (280–296 mOsm)	Urine Osmolality (500–800 mOsm)	Clinical Significance
Normal or increased	Increased	Fluid volume deficit
Decreased	Decreased	Fluid volume excess
Normal	Decreased	1. Increased fluid intake or 2. Diuretic use
Increased or normal	Decreased (with no increase in fluid intake)	1. Kidneys unable to concentrate urine or 2. Lack of ADH (diabetes insipidus)
Decreased	Increased	Syndrome of inappropriate secretion of ADH (SIADH) can be caused by stress, trauma, drugs, or malignant tumor

Note: See discussion in text under high and lower urine osmolality for more details on clinical significance and possible nursing diagnoses. Note that alcohol can increase serum osmolality. See Table 4–3 for note on osmolal gap.

Increased or High Urine Osmolality

Clinical Significance. A high urine osmolality, when the serum osmolality is normal or increased, indicates that the kidneys are conserving water (Table 4–4). As the serum osmolality rises, because of the presence of abnormal solutes or to hemoconcentration, the urine osmolality should also rise: the higher the number of milliosmoles in the urine, the more concentrated is the urine. This is the expected physiologic response to a lack of fluids for metabolic needs.

A less-than-normal serum osmolality and a high urine osmolality do not constitute a normal physiologic response. For some reason the plasma remains dilute. An increased level of the ADH causes a dilution of the plasma and a more concentrated urine. This syndrome is called syndrome of inappropriate ADH secretion (SIADH). SIADH can be difficult to detect and may be life-threatening in acutely ill children (McElroy and Davis, 1986). Some drugs, trauma, or stress reactions may cause an increased production of ADH, but this reaction is usually transitory. Advanced age may increase susceptibility to an increased secretion of ADH (Goldstein et al., 1983).

▼ POSSIBLE NURSING DIAGNOSES RELATED TO INCREASED URINE OSMOLALITY

Risk for Fluid Volume Deficit

A very high urine osmolality means that the client is dehydrated. A moderately high urine osmolality is probably also due to a lack of fluids, as long as it is not due to fluid retention resulting from an increased ADH level. The urine osmo-

(*continued*)

▼ POSSIBLE NURSING DIAGNOSES RELATED TO INCREASED URINE OSMOLALITY (*continued*)

lality should be used as only one part of the data base about the fluid balance of the client. Other factors, such as clinical signs of dehydration, total intake and output, weight gain or loss, and the pathologic state of the client, must all be taken into account. The serum osmolality, if available, helps to determine the amount of dehydration present. The type and method of fluid replacement depend on the cause and severity of fluid loss.

Risk for Fluid Volume Excess

If the client's retention of fluids is possibly due to an increased level of ADH, extra fluids may not be warranted even though the urine osmolality is high. For example, in a client who is recovering from an operation, concentrated urine may be normal for 2 or 3 days after the operation, because ADH is holding some extra fluid in the plasma. As the stress level decreases, hormone levels return to normal, and the extra fluid is released. This is sometimes called *surgical diuresis*. A similar diuresis occurs after other kinds of stress such as extensive burns. A comparison of serum and urine osmolality may be helpful in differentiating a slightly increased urine osmolality due to fluid retention from one that continues to increase because of a basic lack of fluids. It isimportant neither to overload clients with fluids nor to let them become dehydrated. Nurses can use the serum osmolality as one objective measurement.

Low Urine Osmolality

Clinical Significance. Urine osmolality should always be higher than serum osmolality unless there is a known reason for the excretion of dilute urine, such as increased fluid intake or the use of diuretics (Table 4–4). In the case of either, the serum osmolality is expected to be within normal range as the excess fluid is excreted. What is not expected is a continuing low urine osmolality when the serum osmolality begins to increase. With the client in a dehydrated state, the urine osmolality should be quite high. If the serum osmolality is normal and the urine osmolality remains about 280 mOsm/kg water, this set of conditions indicates an inability to concentrate urine, which may be an early sign of renal damage. Or it may be caused by a lack of secretion of ADH, which causes the client to have very dilute urine all the time. This pathologic lack of ADH is called *diabetes insipidus*.

▼ POSSIBLE NURSING DIAGNOSES RELATED TO LOW URINE OSMOLALITY

Risk for Fluid Volume Imbalances

Because dilute urine is expected in clients undergoing diuretic therapy, the main nursing concern is to monitor fluid balance so that not too much fluid is lost. A low urine osmolality is also expected if the goal is to increase fluids to make the urine dilute. Urine osmolality can be an objective evaluation that an increased fluid intake is having the desired results. (Recall that a client who is not getting enough fluids has a consistently high urine osmolality.)

Risk for Alteration in Urinary Elimination

Eventually with renal dysfunction, the urine osmolality may remain the same as the plasma level, which is about 290 mOsm/kg water. Chapter 3 explained that a "fixed" urine specific gravity is always about 1.010, because this is the specific gravity of the plasma. The comparison of urine and plasma osmolalities is a more sensitive measurement of this same concept. Nursing implications for clients with an inability to concentrate urine include a careful assessment of the amount of fluids they need to excrete waste products. Dehydration must be avoided.

Knowledge Deficit Related to Replacement of ADH

Much more rarely, a decreased urine osmolality may be related to a lack of ADH, in which case nurses would observe that the client is excreting huge amounts of urine. ADH levels can be measured with an immunoassay. Medical treatment includes the prescribing of ADH replacement either parenterally or by nasal spray (Katzung, 1995). Nurses may be responsible for teaching the client how to take the drug and how to observe for any side effects or complications.

▼ URIC ACID (SERUM AND URINE)

Uric acid is the end product of purine metabolism. Purines, which are in the nucleoproteins of all cells, are obtained from both dietary sources and from the breakdown of body proteins. The kidneys excrete uric acid as a waste product.

The exact level of uric acid that is considered pathologic is controversial. In recent years it has been generally recognized that the so-called normal ranges of uric acid are quite wide. In light of this ambiguity and because uric acid levels show day-to-day and seasonal variations in the same person, clinicians usually order several uric acid levels over a period of time. Urine uric acid levels may also be used to evaluate gout or determine overexcretion of uric acid.

TABLE 4–5. EXAMPLES OF FOODS HIGH IN PURINES

Liver	Lentils
Sardines	Mushrooms
Anchovies	Spinach
Kidneys	Asparagus
Sweetbreads	

Preparation of Client and Collection of Sample

An overnight fast is needed. To perform the test, the laboratory needs 1 mL of serum, which has to be sent immediately to the laboratory. It may be useful to ask about a dietary history of intake of purine-rich foods. For urine specimens the laboratory may require use of an alkaline preservative in the 24-hr bottle. (See Chapter 3 on client instructions for 24-hr collections.)

REFERENCE VALUES FOR SERUM URIC ACID

Adults: Men	3.6–8.5 mg/dL
Women	2.3–6.6 mg/dL
Pregnancy	In early pregnancy, the levels fall about one-third but rise to nonpregnant levels by term
Children (10–18 yr): Boys	2.0–5.5 mg/dL
Girls	2.0–4 mg/dL
	Striking rise in boys 12–14 yr coincides with puberty. Rise in girls may occur 12 yr (Harlan et al., 1979)
Aged: Men older than 40 yr	2–8.5 mg/dL
Women older than 40 yr	2–8.0 mg/dL
	Rise in women is related to menopause

Uric acid levels tend to vary from day to day and from laboratory to laboratory.

REFERENCE VALUES FOR URINE URIC ACID

250–750 mg/24-hr specimen	Influenced by purine content in diet (Table 4–5)

Increased Uric Acid Level (Hyperuricemia)

Clinical Significance. Although gout, a disease much more common in men than women, is the specific disease associated with consistently high serum uric acid levels, several other conditions commonly cause hyperuricemia:

1. The most common is renal impairment because the kidneys normally excrete uric acid. However, because the level of the uric acid increase does not correlate with the severity of the renal disease, serum uric acid is not used as a test of renal function. (The BUN and creatinine tests are the two basic blood tests for renal function.)
2. A variety of drugs, such as thiazides and some other diuretics, can cause an abnormal elevation of serum uric acid by impairing uric acid clearance by the kidneys.
3. In preeclampsia and particularly in eclampsia, serum uric acid levels are quite high, partially because of the reduced GFR.
4. Another common reason is abnormal cell destruction, such as that associated with neoplasms. In neoplastic disease, chemotherapy or radiation therapy may further elevate serum uric acid levels because of the accelerated destruction of cells. Allopurinol, which prevents uric acid elevation, is sometimes started 24 hr before chemotherapy.
5. With prolonged fasting or chronic malnutrition, uric acid levels are higher than normal, because of the breakdown of cells.

▼ POSSIBLE NURSING DIAGNOSES RELATED TO ELEVATED URIC ACID LEVELS

Alteration in Comfort Related to Joint Pain

Because some clients have asymptomatic hyperuricemia, the basic nursing assessments for pain are not always a clue that there is a problem with uric acid. The symptoms of gout are caused by deposits of urate crystals in the joint. For clients with gout, the warning symptom may be discomfort from the bedspread resting on a toe or swelling and pain in one joint. Usually the pain becomes intense and requires frequent pain medication until the gout is brought under control.

Alteration in Fluid Requirements

Whatever the reason for the high uric acid level, the danger is that uric acid, in the form of urates, crystallizes in an acid urine and forms renal stones. In the absence of a contraindication, clients with high levels of serum uric acid need a liberal intake of fluids to prevent renal stones. "Liberal intake of fluids" should be put into specific terms, such as enough fluid to maintain a urine output of 2,000 mL/day. The specific gravity test (Chapter 3) is useful to evaluate whether the urine is dilute enough.

Knowledge Deficit Related to Any Dietary Modification

Dietary restrictions are usually not emphasized because drugs are used to reduce persistently high levels of serum uric acid. However, foods that are high

(continued)

▼ POSSIBLE NURSING DIAGNOSES RELATED TO ELEVATED URIC ACID LEVELS (*continued*)

in purines (such as sardines, anchovies, and organ meats) should probably be completely eliminated from the diet (Table 4–5); the nurse can also find out whether other meats, poultry, or fish should be restricted in their total amounts (Shellenbarger and Krouse, 1994). Alcohol is to be avoided because it inhibits urate excretion. It is important that clients with high levels of serum uric acid have adequate nutrition, because fasting or starvation diets cause more of an increase in serum acid levels. Any needed weight reduction must be accomplished gradually. Maintaining adequate nutrition for a client undergoing chemotherapy may be very difficult; failure to do so may compound the serum uric acid problem.

Knowledge Deficit Related to Medications

Depending on the level of the serum uric acid and the underlying pathophysiologic condition, the physician may order

- For acute attacks
    1. Colchicine, which does not seem to affect uric acid metabolism but does decrease urate crystal deposition
    2. A nonsteroidal anti-inflammatory drug (NSAID), as an alternative to colchicine
- For maintenance therapy
    1. Uricosuric agents, which promote the elimination of urate salts, such as probenecid (Benemid) or sulfinpyrazone (Anturane)
    2. Drugs that interfere with the production of uric acid levels, such as allopurinol (Zyloprim)

Clients need to be taught the specifics about the drug ordered for them because maintenance therapy will probably be continued for years or even for life (Katzung, 1995).

In addition to hydration and medications, a third factor may be helpful in decreasing the possibility of renal stones from hyperuricemia: an alkaline urine. Normal urine has an acid pH because cheese, eggs, bread, meat, fish, poultry, and some fruits and vegetables contribute to acid waste products. An acidic urine, pH as low as 5.5, may contribute to urate crystallization (Metheny, 1982). Because one cannot routinely achieve alkalinization of the urine without severe dietary restrictions, medication such as sodium bicarbonate or potassium citrate may be used to make the urine pH higher or closer to the alkaline side.

The effectiveness of either dietary modifications or drug treatments should be periodically evaluated by testing the pH of the urine. This is easily performed by using the dipstick method described in Chapter 3. Nurses should teach clients to test their own urine.

Decreased Serum Uric Acid Level

Clinical Significance. Decreased levels usually reflect an increase in plasma volume such as with SIADH or the effect of drugs. Renal tubular defects and liver disease also can decrease serum uric acid levels. Idiopathic hypouricemia commonly is transient. There are no specific clinical symptoms with low uric acid levels.

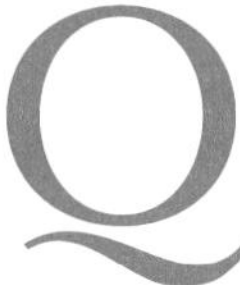

1. Mrs. Balboa, a client with congestive heart failure, has a slightly elevated BUN. What is the most likely explanation for the abnormal BUN?
   a. Plasma dilution caused by aldosterone increase
   b. Increased protein breakdown caused by stress
   c. Poor renal perfusion
   d. Impaired liver function

2. Because some antibiotics may be nephrotoxic, BUN and creatinine levels should be checked before the administration of antibiotics classified as which of the following?
   a. Aminoglycosides, such as gentamicin
   b. Cephalosporins, such as cephapirin
   c. Penicillins, such as penicillin G
   d. Tetracyclines, such as doxycycline

3. Mr. Tod's latest laboratory reports show a BUN of 75 mg and a creatinine level of 6.0 mg. (Reference values for the hospital are BUN 8–25 mg/dL and creatinine 0.6–1.5 mg/dL.) Which nursing action would be appropriate based on the laboratory information?
   a. Take vital signs every 2 hr
   b. Question whether potassium should be continued in the intravenous solution
   c. Encourage the intake of protein foods in the diet
   d. Encourage more active ambulation

4. Mr. Bobbins is to have a 4-hr creatinine clearance test begun this morning. He had just emptied his bladder. For this test, what should he be instructed to do?

   a. Save a urine sample each time he urinates so this can be compared with serum creatinine levels drawn every 30 min
   b. Save all the urine voided in the next 4 hr after he is given a dose of creatinine intravenously
   c. Continue to take nothing by mouth while the urine is being collected as a 4-hr specimen
   d. Save all urine for 4 hr and expect to have blood drawn once for a serum creatinine level

5. For testing for renal function and fluid balance, urine osmolality is a superior test to urine specific gravity because urine osmolality

   a. Can be performed faster on the clinical unit
   b. Detects the presence of specific electrolytes
   c. Is not changed much by sugar, protein, or radiographic dyes
   d. Requires less urine

6. When SIADH occurs in response to severe stress, which of the following are the laboratory reports for serum and urine osmolality most likely to reflect?

   a. A slight increase in serum and urine osmolality
   b. A slight decrease in serum osmolality and an increase in urine osmolality
   c. A slight decrease in serum and urine osmolality
   d. A slight increase in serum osmolality and a decrease in urine osmolality

7. Mrs. Regola has a serum osmolality of 290 mOsm/kg and a urine osmolality of 1,400 mOsm/kg. On the basis of this information, the nurse should assess this client for effects of which of the following?

   a. Fluid overload
   b. Fluid volume deficit
   c. Lack of antidiuretic hormone
   d. Renal dysfunction

8. A urine osmolality of 300 mOsm/kg or a specific gravity of 1.010 on a first voided morning urine specimen is an indication that the client needs to be further assessed for which of the following?

   a. Fluid volume deficit
   b. Circulatory overload
   c. Renal dysfunction
   d. Nothing (this is a normal finding)

9. Higher-than-normal serum uric acid levels are likely for which one of the following?

   a. Jackie, age 8, who is undergoing chemotherapy for leukemia
   b. Mrs. Dillon, age 63, who has rheumatoid arthritis

c. Jennifer, age 21, who has pelvic inflammatory disease
d. Mrs. Benidito, age 34, who is 2 months pregnant

10. Which of the following foods are highest in purine content?

a. Dairy products b. Organ meats
c. Grains d. Citrus fruits

11. What are the two measures, other than drug therapy, that help reduce the possibility of the formation of uric acid renal stones?

a. Forcing fluids and keeping urine alkaline
b. Exercise and consuming liberal amounts of fluids
c. Exercise and keeping urine acid
d. Forcing fluids and keeping urine acid

▼ REFERENCES

Baer, C. (1990). Acute renal failure. *Nursing 90, 20* (6), 34–39.

Basil, C., et al. (1986). Diagnosing kidney disease early. *Patient Care, 20* (4), 28–52.

Chambers, J. (1983). Bowel management in dialysis patients. *American Journal of Nursing, 83* (7), 1051–1052.

Goldstein, C., Braunstein, S., and Goldfarb, S. (1983). Idiopathic syndrome possibly related to age. *Annals of Internal Medicine, 99,* 185–188.

Groër, M., and Shekleton, M. (1989). Basic pathophysiology: A holistic approach. St. Louis: Mosby.

Harlan, W., et al. (1979). Physiological determinants of serum urate levels in adolescence. *Pediatrics, 63* (4), 564–567.

Hatch, F. (1990). Reversing the anemia of renal failure. *Hospital Practice, 25,* 25–34.

Kaplan, A., Jack, R., Opheim, K.E., et al. (1995). *Clinical chemistry interpretations and techniques.* (4th ed.). Baltimore: Williams & Wilkins.

Katzung, B. (1995). *Basic and clinical pharmacology.* (6th ed.). Norwalk: Appleton & Lange.

Lewis, S. (1990). Alteration of host defense mechanisms in chronic dialysis patients. *American Nephrology Nursing Association, 17* (2), 170–180.

McElroy, D., and Davis, G. (1986). SIADH and the acutely ill child. *MCN: American Journal of Maternal Child Nursing, 11* (3), 193–196.

Metheny, N. (1982). Renal stones and urinary pH. *American Journal of Nursing, 82* (9), 1372–1375.

Owen, W.F., Lew, N.L., Liu, Y., et al. (1993). The urea reduction ratio and serum albumin concentration as predictors of mortality in patients undergoing hemodialysis. *New England Journal of Medicine, 329,* 1001–1006.

Ravel, R. (1995). *Clinical laboratory medicine: Clinical application of laboratory data.* (6th ed.). St. Louis: Mosby–Year Book.

Shellenbarger, T., and Krouse, A. (1994). Treating and preventing kidney stones. *MEDSURG Nursing, 3* (5), 389–394.

Stark, J.L. (1994). Interpreting BUN/creatinine levels. *Nursing 94, 24* (9), 58–61.

Stark, J.L., and Hunt, V. (1983). Helping your patient with chronic renal failure. *Nursing 83, 13* (9), 59–63.

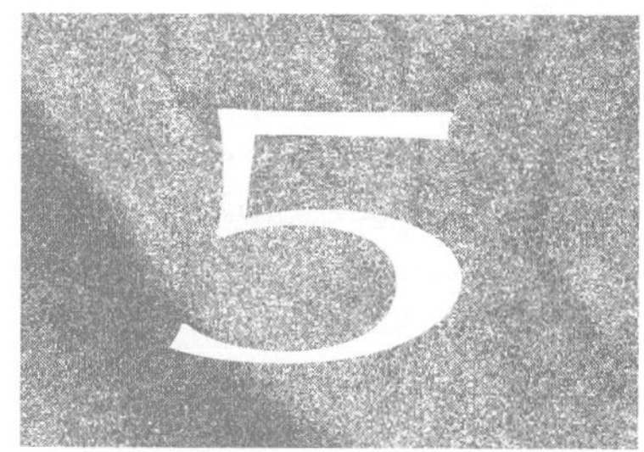

FOUR COMMONLY MEASURED ELECTROLYTES

- Anion Gap
- Serum Sodium
- Urine Sodium
- Serum Potassium
- Urine Potassium
- Serum and Urine Chloride
- Serum Bicarbonate or Carbon Dioxide

OBJECTIVES

1. State which of the four commonly measured electrolytes show wide variation in different age groups and in pregnancy.
2. Differentiate between milligrams (mg) and milliequivalents (mEq) in relation to measurements of electrolytes in the serum and in replacement therapy.
3. Give examples of how the serum cations and anions are kept in electrical neutrality by the kidney and by shifts into and out of cells.
4. Explain the effect of water deficit and water overload on serum sodium levels.
5. Describe nursing assessments that might help identify clients with increased and decreased serum sodium levels.
6. Identify possible nursing diagnoses for clients with hypernatremia and hyponatremia.
7. Explain why serum potassium levels may not accurately reflect total body potassium levels.

8. Describe the nursing assessments that might help identify clients with increased or decreased serum potassium levels.
9. Identify possible nursing diagnoses for clients with hyperkalemia and hypokalemia.
10. Explain the clinical significance of the relationship of serum chloride to serum bicarbonate.

Although many electrolytes are in the blood, when electrolytes (or "lytes") are ordered as a laboratory test, the test is for the four common ones discussed in this chapter. A shorthand method of reporting lytes on a client's chart is

140	4
103	27

Sodium and potassium are the two values on top, and chloride and bicarbonate are on the bottom. Laboratory evaluations of these four basic electrolytes are critical in the assessment of fluid and electrolyte balance as well as acid–base balance.

This chapter focuses primarily on the serum levels of the first three and on the urine levels of sodium and potassium. Because the reference values for these three electrolytes are essentially the same for all populations after the newborn period, it is expedient for nurses to memorize them. Only bicarbonate is substantially changed according to age and pregnancy.

Bicarbonate is discussed in the next chapter in relation to acid–base balance and arterial blood gases. The discussion explains why some laboratories may report serum bicarbonate levels with a test called the "CO_2 content."

The three less commonly measured electrolytes—calcium (Ca^{2+}), magnesium (Mg^{2+}), and phosphate (PO_4^-)—are covered in Chapter 7.

INTERPRETING SERUM ELECTROLYTE REPORTS

When interpreting the reports of serum electrolytes, one must always keep in mind that the laboratory report reflects only *serum* levels. It may not be an accurate reflection of the body's total electrolyte level. Generally, the level of electrolytes in the serum is very close to the electrolyte levels in the interstitial fluid with one exception. Interstitial fluid does not have the plasma proteins found in serum. Because the electrolytes can shift readily from plasma to interstitial fluid, or vice versa, the extracellular fluid remains similar in substances other than the plasma proteins.

But the electrolytic compositions of extracellular (serum and interstitial) fluid and intracellular (cell) fluid are strikingly different. Sodium (Na^+) and chloride (Cl^-) are the two principal electrolytes in the extracellular fluid, whereas potassium (K^+), magnesium, and phosphate are the principal intracellular ions (Table 5–1). Shifts of electrolytes do occur between the cells and the extracellular fluid but not in large amounts. So the measurement of only serum levels cannot always accurately reflect the status of the electrolytes in the individual cells. For example, during a pathologic state, such as acidosis, more potassium may shift out of the cells because more

TABLE 5–1. COMPOSITION OF ELECTROLYTES IN SERUM, INTERSTITIAL FLUIDS, AND CELLS

Fluid	Principal Electrolytes	
■ **EXTRACELLULAR**		
Serum	Na^+	Sodium
	Cl^-	Chloride
	HCO_3^-	Bicarbonate
Interstitial	Almost the same as plasma (note no plasma proteins)	
■ **INTRACELLULAR**		
Cellular	K^+	Potassium
	Mg^{2+}	Magnesium
	PO_4^-	Phosphate

hydrogen (H^+) ions are moving into the cell. Thus the serum level may seem normal or even high, yet the cells are becoming deficient in their main electrolyte, potassium.

Serum sodium and chloride levels rarely reflect the total sodium or chloride content in the body because a change in these levels causes a corresponding change in the volume of the plasma. Sodium and chloride are responsible for most of the osmotic pressure in extracellular fluids. So if the sodium and chloride ions increase in the plasma, they retain more water in the plasma. Hence the concentration of sodium is still reported as 135–145 mEq and the chloride as 100–106 mEq, both *per liter of fluid*. More sodium and chloride (i.e., more salt) in the plasma holds more water in the vascular system and eventually in the interstitial spaces (edema).

MEASUREMENT BY MILLIEQUIVALENTS

Electrolytes are reported in milliequivalents (mEq) rather than in milligrams (mg). The reason is that milligrams measure only the weight of the chemical element, and equal weights do not mean equal chemical activity. For example, it takes 39 mg of potassium to equal 23 mg of sodium in a measurement of chemical activity based on a common standard (Table 5–2). The standard of equivalents is based on how

TABLE 5–2. CONVERSION OF MILLIGRAMS TO MILLIEQUIVALENTS

Measurement of Weight	Measurement of Chemical Activity
23 mg of sodium (Na^+)	1 mEq
39 mg of potassium (K^+)	1 mEq
36 mg of chloride (Cl^-)	1 mEq
30 mg of bicarbonate (HCO_3^-)	1 mEq
■ **PROBLEM 1**	
1,000 mg of sodium = mEq	
Solution: 1,000 ÷ 23 = 43 mEq	
■ **PROBLEM 2**	
40 mEq of potassium = mg	
Solution: 40 × 39 = 1,560 mg	

many grams of an element or compound liberate or combine with 1 g of hydrogen. Because it takes 23 g of sodium to liberate 1 g of hydrogen, the equivalent weight of sodium is 23 g. A *milliequivalent*, the term used in laboratory reports, is one one-thousandth (1/1,000) of an equivalent. If it takes 23 g to make 1 equivalent, 23 *mg* equals 1 mEq.

The important point to remember about the standard of equivalents and milliequivalents is that 1 mEq of one element always has the same chemical activity as 1 mEq of another element. If milligrams or grams are used to measure the amount of electrolytes in diets or medications, the amount of electrolyte milliequivalents must be converted to discuss the physiologic effect of the drugs or diet. For example, a diet of 1,000 mg of sodium (not sodium chloride) would provide about 43 mEq of sodium. This figure is derived from the fact that it takes 23 mg of sodium to make 1 mEq: 1,000 mg divided by 23 mg equals 43 mEq. A more detailed discussion about sodium and salt is covered in the section on sodium. Usually sodium is measured in milligrams.

Potassium is the other electrolyte that may sometimes be measured in milligrams in medication or diet prescriptions. A diet that contains 1,560 mg of potassium supplies 40 mEq of potassium (it takes 39 mg of potassium to equal 1 mEq: 1,560 mg divided by 39 equals 40 mEq). Medications, such as potassium chloride, may be marked in both milligrams and milliequivalents. It is much easier to understand the physiologic effect of electrolytes when the dosage is noted in milliequivalents as well as in milligrams or volume. Although medications list the electrolyte composition clearly, physicians sometimes order—and nurses sometimes record—only that the client took a teaspoon of a potassium supplement and not how many milliequivalents are contained in the teaspoon.

CHEMICAL ELECTRICAL NEUTRALITY

All electrolytes in the serum carry either negative charges (*anions*) or positive charges (*cations*). These negative and positive charges must always be in perfect balance so that the serum remains neutral. The electrical neutrality of the serum is essential in understanding why certain electrolytes may be lost or retained in the serum, even though this upsets acid–base balance.

One way for the body to always maintain an equal number of positive and negative ions in the serum is shifting of electrolytes from the cells or vice versa. For example, when bicarbonate (HCO_3^-) levels are reduced in the serum, other negative ions must replace the missing negative bicarbonate ions. To keep the electrical balance in the serum neutral, chloride can shift out of the erythrocytes. This *chloride shift* occurs in the transport of carbon dioxide. Another example involves the relationship of the positive ions potassium and hydrogen. When the level of serum potassium falls, there is an increased shift of potassium out of the cells to keep the serum potassium normal. As potassium comes out of the cell, hydrogen diffuses into the cell to replace the loss of positive ions intracellularly. This shifting of electrolytes from plasma to cells and vice versa is actually a more complex situation, because the kidneys are also working to remove any excess ions from the bloodstream.

Because sodium, hydrogen, and potassium are all positive ions, a change in one means change in the others. In the distal tubules of the kidney, sodium is usually reabsorbed in exchange for either potassium or hydrogen ions. If there is an abundance of hydrogen ions to excrete, the kidney does not excrete many potassium ions. However, if the potassium level in the serum is low, the kidneys have to continue to excrete hydrogen ions even when the hydrogen is needed to maintain the acid–base balance of the serum. The relation of increased potassium levels to acidosis, as well as that of decreased potassium levels to alkalosis, is discussed in the section on potassium.

When the sodium ion is reabsorbed by the kidney, a negative ion of either chloride or bicarbonate must be reabsorbed also. If one of these two negative ions is low in the serum, more of the other must be absorbed to maintain the proper amount of anions (negative ions). This inverse relation between chloride and bicarbonate is an important consideration in some types of metabolic acid–base imbalances.

▼ ANION GAP

Table 5–3 shows the amount of the positive ions (Na^+ and K^+) compared with the amount of negative ions (Cl^+ and HCO_3^-). For the two cations (positive ions) and two anions (negative ions) that are measured in the serum, there seem to be more positive ions than negative ions, because some of the anions are not measured. This difference between the number of cations and the number of measured anions is called the *anion gap*. Actually, this gap (of 14 mEq in Table 5–3) is made up of unmeasured anions such as sulfates, phosphates, and organic acids. Usually these unmeasured anions are about 8–16 mEq, depending on the particular references used by a laboratory. The anion gap is extensively used for quality control in the laboratory as a check that there is no error in the measurement of electrolytes.

The clinical importance of the anion gap is that it is increased in the types of metabolic acidosis in which organic or inorganic acids are increased in the bloodstream. This increase in the anion gap is helpful in identifying the type of acidosis present. If there is no change in the unmeasured anions in metabolic acidosis, the decreased bicarbonate level (a negative ion) is replaced by an increased serum chloride level (another negative ion). Other much rarer situations may cause changes in the anion gap, but for general purposes, nurses use only the concept of the anion gap in caring for clients with metabolic acidosis.

TABLE 5–3. CATIONS AND ANIONS IN SERUM

Positive Ions (Cations)		**Negative Ions (Anions)**		**Unmeasured Anions**
Sodium	140 mEq	Chloride	103 mEq	Phosphates
Potassium	4 mEq	Bicarbonate	27 mEq	Sulfates
				Organic acids
Total	144 mEq	Total	130 mEq	(gap of 14 mEq)
		144 − 130 = gap of 14 mEq[a]		

[a]Note: If laboratories do not use potassium in the equation, the anion gap is usually 8–12 mEq rather than 8–16 mEq.

By this point the reader may be a little bewildered by so many references to acid–base balance when this chapter is supposed to be on electrolytes. Electrolyte disturbances and acid–base imbalances are so intimately connected that it is hard to learn about one and not the other. Following the summary of acid–base balances in the next chapter, Table 6–6 provides general guidelines of how each electrolyte is changed in the four different types of acid–base imbalance. The concept of the anion gap is also explored in Chapter 6, in the discussion on the three types of metabolic acidosis.

Preparation of Client and Collection of Sample

Usually, all four electrolyte tests are routinely carried out, but sometimes only one is ordered, particularly the potassium. Potassium is, after glucose, the most requested stat test in the hospital (Lutomski and Bower, 1994). It is especially important that the blood sample not be traumatized because hemolysis of cells makes the potassium report inaccurate. (Recall that potassium is an intracellular ion.) A 0.5-mL sample is obtained by means of venipuncture and collected in a tube without additives. The client does not need to be fasting. Portable analyzers that use capillary blood are also available for point-of-care testing.

REFERENCE VALUES FOR COMMON ELECTROLYTES

Sodium (Na^+)	135–145 mEq/L
Potassium (K^+)	3.5–5.0 mEq/L (slightly more in newborns)
Chloride (Cl^-)	100–108 mEq/L
Bicarbonate (HCO_3^-) (measured as CO_2 content)	
Adult	24–30 mEq/L
Pregnancy	19–20 mEq/L (see P_{CO_2} levels in Chapter 6 for explanation of reason for lower bicarbonate levels in pregnancy). During the puerperium, the serum bicarbonate again increases and the chloride decreases slightly (DeCherney and Pernoll, 1994).
Infant	20–26 mEq/L
Children	Slightly lower than references for adults

All four electrolytes may be reported in moles per liter (mmol/L) rather than mEq if the SI is adopted by a laboratory. There is no change in basic numbers for these four electrolytes (see Chapter 1 on SI units).

▼ SERUM SODIUM

Sodium has the highest concentration of all the electrolytes measured in the serum, and yet changes in its level are not commonly seen, because its concentration is always correlated with fluid balance. Because sodium is the primary factor in maintaining osmotic pressure in the extracellular fluid, changes in sodium are hidden because "water goes where salt is." So one must always interpret a change in serum sodium levels in relation to possible fluid overload or dehydration. A rough estimate of plasma osmolality (discussed in Chapter 4) can be calculated from the sodium level by multiplying the sodium level by 2. A normal serum sodium of 140 mEq/L times 2 would equal a normal plasma osmolality of about 280 mOsm/kg water.

The serum level of sodium is not totally dependent on diet because the kidneys can conserve sodium when necessary. The hormone aldosterone causes a conservation of sodium and chloride and an excretion of more potassium. The daily requirement of sodium for an adult is about 2,000 mg. In children, the usual requirement is about 250–500 mg and for infants, 50 mg/kg a day (Hay et al., 1995). Many American diets contain much more than these daily minimums. Some authorities estimate that the average diet may contain as much as 4–8 g of sodium. The American Heart Association suggests a maximum intake of 2 g of sodium or 5 g of sodium chloride per day.

It is necessary to measure sodium, not just sodium chloride, in the diet because sodium is present in forms other than salt. For example, monosodium glutamate is added to many foods in the American diet. Most American diets can be substantially reduced in sodium by avoiding very salty foods and not adding extra salt to foods at the table. One gram of sodium chloride is about 0.6 g chloride and about 0.4 g, or 17 mEq, of sodium (400 mg divided by 23 equals 17 mEq). Table 5–4 lists the amount of sodium in different proportions of salt and food substances. Table 5–5 describes the meaning of sodium labels for food.

REFERENCE VALUES FOR SODIUM

Adult	135–145 mEq/L

The same reference values are used for all age groups. The hemodilution that occurs with pregnancy may cause a drop of 2–3 mEq within general values.

TABLE 5–4. RELATIVE SODIUM CONTENT OF FOODS

Foods with about 500 mg sodium (22 mEq)	1/4 scant tsp salt (40% of salt is sodium)
	3/4 tsp monosodium glutamate
	1/2 boullion cube
	1 cup (240 mL) tomato juice
	average serving of cooked cereal
	1 hotdog
	1 1/2 oz (42 g) ham
Foods with about 250 mg sodium (11 mEq)	1 oz (28 g) canned tuna
	2/3 cup (158 mL) buttermilk
	5 salted crackers
Foods with about 200 mg sodium (9 mEq)	1 slice bread
	2 slices bacon
	3 oz (84 g) shrimp
	1/2 oz (14 g) cheese
	1 tbsp (15 mL) catsup

The American Heart Association has a wealth of literature on low-sodium diets.

TABLE 5–5. MEANING OF SODIUM LABELS FOR FOOD

"Sodium free"	Less than 5 mg of Na^+ per serving
Very low sodium	35 mg or less of Na^+
Low sodium	140 mg or less of Na^+
Reduced sodium	Processed to reduce usual level of Na^+ by 75%
Unsalted	Processed without salt

Note: Also teach clients to note the actual sodium content for specific foods (Table 5–4).

Increased Serum Sodium Level (Hypernatremia)

Clinical Significance. An increase in the serum sodium level becomes apparent only when there is not sufficient water in the body to balance the increasing sodium level. Because sodium has an osmotic action, an increase in serum sodium pulls water into the vascular system from the interstitial spaces and the cells. When the laboratory test for *serum* sodium level is elevated, the client is depleted in water, not only in the extracellular compartment but also in the cells (Table 5–6). Thus many cases of an increase in *total body* sodium do not cause an increased *serum* sodium level. For example, clients with congestive heart failure have sodium retention caused by the action of the hormone aldosterone. However, the retention of sodium means an equal retention of water, so the serum sodium level remains about 140 mEq per *liter* of fluid.

For the serum sodium level to be increased on a laboratory report, it is necessary that either (1) there is a large increase in sodium *without* a proportional increase in water or (2) there has been a loss of a large amount of water *without* a proportional loss of salt. Under most circumstances, increasing sodium intake without increasing water intake is not likely because an increased sodium intake makes a person very thirsty. If the client is receiving intravenous fluid, such as normal saline solution, it may be possible to overload with sodium. Intravenous solutions of normal saline contain 0.9% sodium chloride, that is, 0.9 g of salt in 100 mL or 9 g in 1,000 mL. This percentage is 154 mEq of sodium and 154 mEq of chloride per liter. Infants who receive exchange transfusions with stored bank blood may become

TABLE 5–6. CLINICAL SITUATIONS COMMONLY ASSOCIATED WITH SERUM SODIUM ABNORMALITIES

- **HYPERNATREMIA**—serum Na increased (↑) 145 mEq/L
  Dehydration is the most frequent cause
  Overuse of intravenous saline solutions
  Exchange transfusion with stored blood
  Impaired renal function
- **HYPONATREMIA**—serum Na decreased (↓) 135 mEq/L
  Excessive water—"dilutional" hyponatremia
  Loss of sodium by vomiting, diarrhea, gastrointestinal suctioning, or sweating
  Use of diuretics, diabetic acidosis, Addison's disease, or renal disease, which all cause increased loss of sodium via urine

See text for explanation of why fluid volume changes are usually the underlying cause for changes in serum sodium levels.

hypernatremic because stored blood has high sodium levels. An intravenous infusion of dextrose 5% in water is given to prevent overload of sodium.

The much more common reason for an increased serum sodium level is a loss of a large amount of water without a proportional loss of sodium. For example, diarrhea or vomiting may cause a severe decrease in total body water, particularly in infants. Not all dehydration results in an increased sodium level, however, because just as much sodium may be lost as water; this loss of equal amounts of sodium and water is called *isotonic dehydration*, and is the type that occurs in most infants hospitalized for a fluid volume deficit caused by vomiting or diarrhea. In dehydration caused by a loss of water or a lack of water intake, the sodium loss is not proportional, and hence the dehydration is *hypertonic*. Even in the early stages of hypertonic dehydration, the serum sodium level is not elevated because water is pulled from the interstitial spaces to keep the sodium at a normal dilution in the serum.

A serum sodium level that begins to rise above normal is a sign of a serious deficit of water that has extended to the cellular level. Another term for this type of dehydration is *hyperosmolar dehydration*. The serum is increased in osmolality, not because of a total sodium increase, but because of a total body water deficit.

▼ POSSIBLE NURSING DIAGNOSES RELATED TO HYPERNATREMIA

Fluid Volume Deficit

The initial symptom of hypernatremia is likely to be thirst, which, if the person is unconscious, confused, or very young, is a subjective symptom that is not communicated to the nurse. Other clinical assessments that correlate with a high serum sodium level include elevated temperature, dry, sticky mucous membranes, and little or no urine output. The specific gravity of the urine is high if the kidneys are still able to concentrate urine. The hematocrit (hct) is increased when the water deficit is severe. In infants, a high-pitched cry and depressed fontanels are other signs of severe water deficit. Hyperactive reflexes and irritability may lead to seizures in infants with high sodium levels.

In adults, each 3 mEq of serum sodium above the usual reference range represents a deficit of about 1 L of fluid. Thus a serum sodium level of 157 mEq would be about 12 mEq above the reference of 135–145 mEq. This excess indicates a deficit of about 4 L of fluid. Because 1 L of water weighs 1 kg (2.2 lb), a loss of 4 L means a weight loss of nearly 9 lb (4 kg). In a small child, the loss of even a liter of fluid would constitute severe dehydration because a loss of 2.2 lb may be 10% of the total weight of the child. The most accurate measurement of the amount of water deficit is the client's loss of weight. Daily weights should be part of the nursing assessment for any clients experiencing fluid losses.

(*continued*)

▼ POSSIBLE NURSING DIAGNOSES RELATED TO HYPERNATREMIA (*continued*)

Assisting with Treatments. For hypernatremia caused by a water deficit, the therapeutic interventions focus on replacing the lost water. If oral intake is not possible, physicians order intravenous fluids to hydrate the client. Fluid deficits need to be corrected gradually, particularly in infants. A decrease in serum sodium more than 0.5–1.0 mEq/L an hour may cause cerebral edema, seizures, and severe injury to the central nervous system (CNS) (Hay et al., 1995). Fluid orders may have to be changed every few hours depending on the response of the client and the results of serial sodium levels. If the dehydration was caused by gastrointestinal problems, food is gradually added back to the diet. The BRAT diet (bananas, rice cereal, applesauce, and tea or toast) is easy on the gastrointestinal tract.

Preventing Sodium Overload. Often the nurse may be able to prevent hypernatremia caused by water deficit by careful observation of clients at risk. For instance, clients who are not taking enough oral fluids may become water-deficient. Those who are receiving normal saline solutions (0.9% NaCl) should be checked for any signs of hypernatremia. Intravenous solutions for maintenance are usually only one-half normal saline (0.45% NaCl) or even one-fourth normal saline (0.25% NaCl). Normal saline solutions (0.9% NaCl) are not used for maintenance solutions unless the client has hyponatremia. Infants who receive blood exchange usually have a peripheral line for infusion of dextrose 5% in water (D_5W), because the stored blood is high in sodium.

Fluid Volume Excess Related to Excess Sodium

When both sodium and water are retained in excessive amounts, the symptoms are different from when sodium is in excess. The signs and symptoms of increased total body sodium levels are weight gain, elevated blood pressure, dyspnea, and pitting edema (the common signs of fluid retention). In adults, edema becomes apparent only after about 3 L of water are retained; this amount of water retention would mean 3 kg or 6.6 lb of weight gain before the edema shows. Thus weight gain is the most sensitive detector of early fluid retention.

Knowledge Deficit Related to Need for Sodium Restriction

A client with both sodium and water retention is often prescribed diuretics or a low-sodium diet. Also, clients with hypertension usually eat low-sodium diets. About 30% of clients with hypertension can benefit from a 500-mg sodium diet, but because compliance is difficult, a more moderate goal is usually set (Cerrato, 1985). A diet of 500 mg is very restrictive. It allows only 22 mEq of sodium a day (500 mg divided by 23 mg equals 22 mEq). A teaspoon of salt has 2,000 mg of sodium or 87 mEq. (See Table 5–5 on the meanings of sodium labels.)

The effectiveness of sodium restriction is determined by the absence of fluid retention or a reduction in blood pressure and *not by the serum sodium level.* Nurses may need to go over this point several times with clients. It may be difficult for clients to see a need to restrict sodium and salt intake when the laboratory report is "normal" for sodium. The American Heart Association has excellent teaching material about low-sodium diets. Chloride titrate strips have been used to test the urine to assess a large sodium intake (Luft et al., 1984).

Decreased Serum Sodium Level (Hyponatremia)

Clinical Significance. Like serum sodium increases, serum sodium decreases are not accurate reflections of total body sodium levels because sodium is usually lost with water. The more common reason for a low serum sodium is an excess of water in the body. The water excess can be caused by giving salt-free intravenous fluids. Also, in stress and severe illness, there may be an increased production of antidiuretic hormone (ADH), which causes an increase in total body water. The syndrome of inappropriate ADH secretion (SIADH) can also be caused by various drugs such as antidepressants and psychotropics (Sandifer, 1983). Compulsive water drinking by mentally ill clients can cause hyponatremia or water intoxication (Stanley-Tilt, 1989). Most cases of water excess are usually terminated by an increased urine output, which restores the sodium and water balance. (See Chapter 4 on serum and urine osmolality.)

Although a real water excess is the more common reason for a low serum sodium level, actual sodium depletion can also be a cause of a low serum sodium level. Ordinarily, the hormone aldosterone conserves sodium, but a continual loss of sodium with only water replacement and no sodium replacement eventually leads to true sodium depletion. For example, a client who is taking diuretics and consuming a restricted sodium diet may experience massive sodium depletion from the body. Excessive sodium loss also occurs in

1. Some types of renal failure, in which there is "salt wasting"
2. Diabetic acidosis, in which polyuria contributes to a great loss of sodium
3. Vomiting and diarrhea, particularly in young children, if gastrointestinal losses are replaced only with water
4. Vigorous exercise, in which perspiration can deplete sodium
5. Deficiency of adrenal corticosteroids (Addison's disease). The severe hypotension of an Addisonian crisis occurs because the total body sodium is not enough to keep fluid in the vascular system. (See Chapter 15 on cortisone tests.)

▼ POSSIBLE NURSING DIAGNOSES RELATED TO LOW SERUM SODIUM LEVELS

Fluid Volume Excess Related to Water Intoxication

Although this discussion differentiates the symptoms of hyponatremia (low sodium level) caused by fluid excess from those caused by a true sodium deficit, the clinical signs and symptoms usually are not so clear-cut.

When the low serum sodium level is due to just an excess of body water, the client has a weight gain equal to the amount of excess liters retained. For example, a client undergoing routine maintenance administration of intravenous fluids should not be gaining weight because the caloric intake is minimal. (A bottle of 1,000 mL of dextrose 5% contains only 50 g of dextrose.) In fact, an adult client who is undergoing maintenance use of intravenous fluids of dextrose 5% usually loses about half a pound a day. If the client is gaining weight at all, this weight has to be water. A gain of a pound means the retention of more than 500 mL of fluid. (Every nurse should memorize the fact that a liter of water weighs 1 kg (2.2. lb), or a pound for every pint.)

The other symptom of water excess is an increased urine output. If the water excess continues and if the kidneys cannot eliminate the excess water, the water diffuses into the interstitial spaces and eventually into the cells. The edema that develops is generalized; it is not contained in dependent areas such as the feet. So, for example, the face may look a little puffy. Edema of brain cells causes nausea and vomiting and eventually convulsions when the serum sodium is as low as 120 mEq. Many cases of compulsive water drinking in mentally ill clients are not detected until a seizure occurs (Rinard, 1989). This condition is a hyposmolar imbalance.

Careful nursing assessment of the intake and output records, as well as of weight gains, for clients who are susceptible to fluid overload can do much to prevent severe water intoxication. For example, elderly clients may have an increase in ADH that makes them more susceptible to hyponatremia (Goldstein et al., 1983).

Intravenous fluids for all ages must contain the appropriate amount of sodium. Malpractice suits have occurred because nurses did not realize that salt-free fluids were not appropriate after complex operations (Regan, 1981).

Assisting with Treatment. The primary treatment of water excess is to restrict fluid intake for a while. Diuretics may be used for both adults and children if the water excess is severe (McElroy and Davis, 1986). To evaluate objectively that the fluid balance is returning to normal, one must keep accurate records of intake, output, and weight loss.

Altered Nutrition Related to Sodium Depletion

Nurses need to be aware of clients who may be experiencing true depletion of sodium, because this type of low serum sodium level can often be prevented if early symptoms of sodium depletion are noticed. For example, clients undergoing nasogastric suctioning can lose large amounts of sodium if very large amounts of water rather than normal saline solution are used to irrigate the nasogastric tube. Repeated tap water enemas in the elderly may also cause hyponatremia, as can large doses of diuretics. With mild to moderate depletions of sodium, the serum sodium level remains within the normal reference range while the urine sodium becomes low. (See the next section on urine sodium levels.) As the total sodium becomes low, the client has anorexia, apathy, and sometimes a sense of impending doom. Confusion may occur, particularly in elderly clients. Muscle cramps, weakness, and diarrhea reflect the lack of sodium for normal muscle contractions. Eventually the low serum sodium leads to hypotension and shock because there is a loss of osmotic pressure in the vascular system. Infants, although they may be lethargic, may not have symptoms until the sodium level is low enough to cause edema and seizures.

Assisting with Sodium Replacement. The therapeutic measures for true sodium depletion are geared toward replacing both sodium and lost fluid. Usually the intravenous solution used for replacement is normal saline solution (0.9% NaCl), although in extreme cases, a hypertonic (3% NaCl) saline solution may be used. Nurses must carefully monitor clients who are receiving hypertonic intravenous fluids, because too rapid an infusion of a hypertonic solution is very dangerous. The hypertonic solution not only can cause hemolysis of red blood cells but also can pull a large amount of fluid into the vascular space, leading to circulatory overload (Culpepper et al., 1986). The hypertonic solutions of salt are rarely used now (Metheny, 1990; Hay et al., 1995). Either normal saline solution (0.9% NaCl) or Ringer's lactate (another isotonic solution) can supply enough sodium to safely make up the deficiency.

Knowledge Deficit Related to Specific Need for Replenishing Sodium

Because the body can conserve sodium, it is not necessary to instruct clients to eat high-sodium foods over a long period. Yet clients who may become sodium-depleted because of vomiting, diarrhea, or vigorous exercise should drink salty replacement fluids such as broths instead of water alone. For infants, special formulas of electrolytes are used to replace gastrointestinal losses. Athletes who perform vigorous exercises know to replace lost fluids with special oral electrolyte preparations that are commercially available. In the past, salt tablets were often used by people who engaged in intense physical

(*continued*)

▼ POSSIBLE NURSING DIAGNOSES RELATED TO LOW SERUM SODIUM LEVELS (*continued*)

activity; it is now generally recommended to replace salt more gradually by dietary increases or salty fluids. One cup (240 mL) of tomato juice has 486 mg of sodium (see Table 5–8).

As mentioned, the United States diet usually contains more than enough sodium. But sometimes clients may follow too restricted a sodium diet. For example, nurses may need to assess the dietary habits of elderly clients to make sure that their sodium restrictions are not too severe, particularly if they begin taking diuretics. Children with cystic fibrosis lose extra sodium in their sweat. (See Chapter 18 on the sweat test for CF.) Clients who take lithium must also have plenty of sodium in the diet. (See Chapter 17 on lithium toxicity.)

▼ URINE SODIUM

Normally the amount of sodium excreted in the urine varies with sodium intake. Increased amounts of aldosterone in the serum cause a decreased secretion of urine sodium. (See Chapter 15 on serum and urine aldosterone levels, which may also be ordered.) Conversely, a decreased level of aldosterone activity causes an increased loss of sodium in the urine. Diabetic acidosis and diuretics also cause an increased loss of sodium. Various types of renal failure may cause either increased losses or retention of sodium. Poor perfusion to the kidney (prerenal azotemia) may lead to a low urine sodium, whereas acute tubular necrosis may cause a high urine sodium level (Bongard and Sue, 1994). The values of urine sodium must be interpreted in view of the total clinical situation and can be quite complicated to interpret (Ravel, 1995).

Preparation of Client and Collection of Sample

See Chapter 3 on 24-hr urine collections. No special preservative is needed. The diet of the client should be noted as to the amount of sodium intake.

REFERENCE VALUES FOR URINE SODIUM
40–220 mEq/24 hr or 30 mEq/L (diet-dependent)
Full-term infants have sodium clearance of about 20% of adult values

▼ SERUM POTASSIUM

Potassium is primarily an intracellular ion, but the small amount in the serum is essential for normal neuromuscular and cardiac function. Small changes in serum potassium level can have profound effects on cardiac muscle. In a normal state of health, adequate potassium is easily obtained by eating a variety of foods. Potassium, 40–80 mEq/day for an adult, should be consumed every day because potassium, unlike sodium, is not conserved well by the body. The kidneys continue to excrete 40–80 mEq/day even when there is no intake.

Although potassium can also be lost in gastrointestinal drainage, the kidneys excrete almost all the potassium. The renal mechanism for potassium ion excretion is shared with another positive ion, hydrogen. Either a potassium or hydrogen ion is excreted when a sodium ion is reabsorbed by the kidney. This relationship partially explains why potassium levels are increased in acidosis and decreased in alkalosis. The shifting of potassium and hydrogen ions into and out of the cells in acid-base imbalances also contributes to marked changes in potassium levels. (See Chapter 6 on acid–base balances.)

Pseudohyperkalemia can be caused by fist clenching during phlebotomy, so the client should not clench the fist when blood is drawn (Don et al., 1990). Thrombocytosis falsely elevates potassium levels, so an elevated platelet count should be recorded (Lutomski and Bower, 1994).

REFERENCE VALUES FOR SERUM POTASSIUM

3.5–5.0 mEq/L

In pregnancy there may be a fall of about 0.2–0.3 mEq caused by increased volume

Newborns 4.0–6.0 mEq/L

Increased Serum Potassium Level (Hyperkalemia)

Clinical Significance. The most important cause of an increased serum potassium level (hyperkalemia) is inadequate renal output (Table 5–7). Thus hyperkalemia is always a problem in the oliguric phase of renal failure unless potassium intake is limited. (See Chapter 4 for the distinction between renal insufficiency and renal failure.)

TABLE 5–7. CLINICAL SITUATIONS COMMONLY ASSOCIATED WITH SERUM POTASSIUM ABNORMALITIES

- **HYPERKALEMIA**—serum K^+ increased (↑) 5 mEq/L (or above 6.5 in newborns)
  Renal failure
  Too rapid intravenous infusion of K^+ replacement
  Initial reaction to massive tissue damage
  Associated with metabolic acidosis (see Chapter 6)
- **HYPOKALEMIA**—serum K^+ decreased (↓) 3.5 mEq/L
  Diuretics, particularly thiazides
  Inadequate intake when n.p.o., vomiting, or receiving K^+-free IV feedings
  Large doses of corticosteroids
  Aftermath of tissue destruction or high stress
  Associated with metabolic alkalosis (see Chapter 6)

See text and references at end of chapter for further details.

The intake of too much potassium in medications can also cause an increased serum potassium level. An overdose from oral supplements of potassium is unlikely, but the danger is real with intravenous use of potassium in high concentrations (Schwartz, 1987). Other medications, such as penicillin K, which contains potassium ions, can cause hyperkalemia if renal output is not adequate. (See Chapter 4 on BUN and creatinine levels as assessments of renal function.)

Because potassium is primarily an intracellular ion, anything that causes massive cell destruction increases the serum potassium level. Thus massive tissue injury or a burn causes the release of potassium from damaged cells. Although the serum potassium level may increase after cellular damage, the actual total body potassium is decreased. Thus the hyperkalemia that occurs with a burn or an injury is followed by hypokalemia.

Because aldosterone and other steroids cause a retention of sodium and an increased excretion of potassium, conditions in which hormones are decreased may cause an increased serum potassium level. For example, in Addison's disease, malfunctioning of the adrenal cortex reduces the corticosteroid level. Serum sodium levels are decreased, and serum potassium levels may be increased. (See Chapter 15 on laboratory tests for cortisone.)

Although almost all diuretics cause an increased loss of potassium, there are three exceptions. Spironolactone (Aldactone) is an aldosterone antagonist and thus causes increased retention of potassium. Triamterene (Dyrenium) does not affect aldosterone, but it, too, is a diuretic that may cause hyperkalemia. Triamterene acts directly on the distal tubules to cause excretion of serum sodium and retention of serum potassium as does amiloride (Midamor). These agents can cause severe, even fatal, hyperkalemia in susceptible clients such as those with liver or renal disease (Katzung, 1995). Hyperkalemia may also occur with the angiotensin-converting enzyme (ACE) inhibitors.

Hyperkalemia is often associated with metabolic acidotic states. In acidosis, the kidney must excrete more hydrogen ions, which means less secretion of potassium ions by the renal selection mechanism. In addition, an abundance of hydrogen ions in the serum means that some of these ions go into the cells, which drives potassium out of the cells. Thus, in acidotic states, the total body potassium is not increased, but more potassium ions are present in the serum. Serum potassium rises about 0.6 mEq/L for every 0.1 decrease in blood pH. If the acidotic state is due to diabetic ketoacidosis, the lack of insulin compounds the problem of hyperkalemia because potassium needs insulin, as does glucose, to be transported into the cell. (See Chapter 8 on ketoacidosis.)

▼ POSSIBLE NURSING DIAGNOSES RELATED TO ELEVATED POTASSIUM LEVELS

Risk for Injury Related to Effect of Hyperkalemia on Heart and Other Muscles

Probably the most important thing to remember about checking for symptoms of increasing serum potassium levels is that many of the symptoms are nonspecific. Potassium is important to nerve and muscle function, but so are most of the other electrolytes. Early symptoms of hyperkalemia may be irritability, nausea, diarrhea, and abdominal cramping. Later symptoms may include skeletal muscle weakness. The muscle weakness can progress to a flaccid-type paralysis with difficulty in speaking and breathing.

Hyperkalemia is usually an emergency situation because a high serum potassium level can cause cardiac arrhythmias that can lead to cardiac arrest: The heart stops in diastole. Because the clinical signs of hyperkalemia can be confused with other conditions (hypokalemia can also cause paralysis), the level of serum potassium must be assessed by the laboratory report, not by physical symptoms alone. Remember that the serum laboratory test may not reflect the total body potassium. The electrocardiogram (ECG) is a very sensitive indicator of intracellular potassium, even when the serum potassium still seems normal. Nurses need to be able to identify hyperkalemia on an ECG strip (Raimer, 1994). High-peaked T waves and a prolonged QRS interval are typical findings for hyperkalemia.

Assisting with Medical Interventions. Although there is no *specific* antidote for hyperkalemia, several different medications may be used to treat a high serum potassium level:

1. Sometimes calcium gluconate is given intravenously to lessen cardiac toxicity. Calcium may be particularly useful if the calcium levels were initially low or borderline. Calcium is not used if the client is taking digitalis, because digitalis and calcium have a synergistic effect on the heart.
2. Sodium bicarbonate may be given intravenously if acidosis is present. As the pH of the blood returns to normal, potassium shifts back into the cells. Also, when the pH is normal, the kidney can secrete more potassium ions because there is not a demand to excrete so many hydrogen ions.
3. Intravenous solutions with glucose and insulin help promote the reentry of potassium into the cells, even for clients who do not have diabetes.
4. Sodium polystyrene sulfonate (Kayexalate), given orally or by enemas, is a sodium–potassium exchange resin.
5. For a client with chronically high potassium levels caused by renal failure treatment includes peritoneal dialysis or hemodialysis.

Knowledge Deficit Related to Sources of Potassium

The nurse needs to find out whether the hyperkalemia is likely to be a chronic or recurring situation. If so, the client needs to be taught to read the labels on foods and medications to determine whether they are high in potassium.

(*continued*)

▼ POSSIBLE NURSING DIAGNOSES RELATED TO ELEVATED POTASSIUM LEVELS (*continued*)

For example, most salt substitutes are composed of large amounts of potassium. Instant coffee and other prepared foods may have potassium as one of the ingredients.

Teaching about eliminating potassium from the diet may also have to be carried out. To reinforce client behavior, a contract may be written between nurse and client to keep potassium levels low through diet adherence. Sheckel (1980) used graphs of potassium levels posted at the foot of the beds of dialysis clients as one way to reinforce diet selections. Thus, potassium levels can be one evaluative tool of effective teaching. (Table 5–8 lists foods particularly high in potassium.)

Risk for Injury Related to Subsequent Development of Hypokalemia

If the high serum levels of potassium are caused by metabolic shifts in acidosis, the potassium shifts back into the cells when the pH returns to normal, and clients may have a serum deficit. Also, if the serum potassium level increases because of cell damage, the potassium lost from injured cells results in a total body deficit. Always consider the possibility that the hyperkalemia of today could result in hypokalemia tomorrow.

TABLE 5–8. FOODS HIGH IN POTASSIUM AND CORRESPONDING SODIUM CONTENT

Potassium at Least 10 mEq or More by Serving	Sodium (mg)
Avocado, ½	5
Banana, 1 medium	1
Cantaloupe, 1 cup	19
Dates, 10	1
Figs, 5	10
Molasses, 2 tbsp	3
Orange juice, 1 cup	2
Potato, 1 baked	2
Prunes, 10 (high calories)	9
Salt substitutes (varies, but may be 30–40 mEq in a tsp)	Varies. Check label
Soybeans, ½ cup	2
Tomato juice, canned, 1 cup	486 (not good if on low-sodium diet)

The American Heart Association has patient information cards as well as pamphlets about potassium content in foods. Slawson and Slawson (1985) lists sodium and potassium content for many over-the-counter drugs, including salt substitutes. Narins et al. (1985) discuss renal retention of potassium from fruit.

Decreased Serum Potassium Levels (Hypokalemia)

Clinical Significance. Because potassium is not conserved well in the body, an inadequate intake results in a low serum level. However, as the daily need of potassium for an adult is only about 80 mEq, insufficient oral intake is usually not the cause for a low potassium unless the person is not taking anything at all by mouth. Even in fasting states, the serum potassium level may not drop immediately, because the breakdown of cells for energy causes the release of potassium.

More commonly, hypokalemia results from an excessive loss of potassium. Any loss of fluid from the gastrointestinal tract causes a loss of potassium. Almost all diuretics cause an increased excretion of potassium, except spironolactone (Aldactone), amiloride (Midamor), and triamterene (Dyrenium). Certain hormonal changes also contribute to an excessive excretion of potassium. The corticosteroids cause sodium retention and potassium excretion. Certain tumors may produce hormones that act much like the steroids and thus increase potassium excretion. (See Chapter 15 on ectopic hormone production.) Drugs that cause excessive beta-sympathetic stimulation, such as epinephrine, can cause a transient hypokalemia (Struthers et al., 1983).

An alkalotic serum pH (pH greater than 7.4) is another reason for a lowered serum potassium level. In alkalosis, hydrogen ions shift out of the cell in an attempt to lower the pH of the serum to normal. When hydrogen shifts out of the cell, more potassium shifts into the cell to replace the missing positive ions. Conversely, a low serum potassium level also contributes directly to the development of an alkalotic state because, when serum potassium levels are low, the kidneys must excrete more hydrogen ions in exchange for the reabsorption of sodium by the distal tubule. So either alkalosis may be the cause of hypokalemia, or hypokalemia may contribute to the development of metabolic alkalosis. The role of hypokalemia in the development of metabolic alkalosis is covered in Chapter 6 in the section on bicarbonate changes in acid–base balance.

▼ POSSIBLE NURSING DIAGNOSES RELATED TO HYPOKALEMIA

Altered Cardiac Output Related to Development of Arrhythmias

Hypokalemia can cause bradycardia or paroxysmal tachycardia, premature ventricular contractions (PVCs), and other arrhythmias. Therefore, potassium levels are usually not allowed to drop below 4.0 mEq for clients with cardiac problems. For clients taking digitalis, hypokalemia is quite dangerous because the toxic effects of digitalis are more likely to occur when the serum potassium level drops quickly. The typical ECG in a client with hypokalemia has prominent U waves, and the T waves are flat with eventual ST depression (Raimer, 1994).

(*continued*)

▼ POSSIBLE NURSING DIAGNOSES RELATED TO HYPOKALEMIA (*continued*)

Risk for Injury Related to Development of Muscle Weakness

Nurses need to be aware of clients who may be having extra losses of potassium so they can assess for potential hypokalemia (Toto, 1987). Although certain clinical symptoms are caused by hypokalemia, these symptoms can also be caused by other clinical abnormalities. Clients with a low serum potassium level may have anorexia, muscle weakness, a decrease in bowel sounds, and abdominal distention due to decreased peristalsis (ileus). Ileus and lethargy are key symptoms of hypokalemia in newborns. Flaccid paralysis may develop with more severe hypokalemia, as well as with hyperkalemia, because both potassium imbalances alter the resting potential of muscle cells. It is a paradox that hypokalemia can be a cause of tetany (Ault and Geiderman, 1992). Low serum potassium levels may make respiratory effort difficult.

Assisting with Potassium Replacement. Depending on the severity of the hypokalemia, potassium may be replaced in three ways: (1) intravenously, (2) by oral supplements, or (3) by diet.

Risk for Injury Related to Use of Intravenous Potassium

Most preparations of potassium chloride (KCl) for intravenous use are marketed as 2 mEq/mL. Thus, for a dose of 40 mEq, the nurse would add 20 mL to the intravenous fluid. Potassium must *always be diluted.* Potassium chloride is never given directly by intravenous push no matter how severe the deficiency. Usually no more than 40 mEq of potassium is added to 1,000 mL of intravenous fluids, although sometimes as much as 80 mEq is added to a liter. Clients should usually not be given more than 10 mEq in an hour, although some authorities say 20 mEq/hr is safe in severe deficiencies (Deglin and Vallerand, 1995). If the intravenous solution with the potassium must be slowed down because of a burning sensation, the solution must be made more dilute or a central catheter should be used. Potassium in high concentrations is irritating to the vein wall.

Any client who is receiving potassium must have adequate urinary output. In adults, "adequate" means at least 30 mL/hr. Newborns should produce 1 mL of urine per kilogram per hour. Thus a newborn who weighs 4 kg (8.8 lb) should produce about 4 mL/hr. In older children, 1–2 mL/kg per hour is a minimum output. The urinary output should always be assessed before potassium is added to an intravenous infusion. Once the intravenous infusion is begun, nurses must continue to make sure that urinary output remains adequate. Otherwise hyperkalemia can develop rapidly.

Knowledge Deficit Related to Oral Potassium Supplements

Oral preparations of potassium chloride may come marked in various strengths, such as 10% or 20% solutions, or as so many milligrams per teaspoon. On the bottle, however, the dosage in milliequivalents is also given, and this is the dosage form that should be used. One teaspoon of potassium chloride elixir is not as precise as 20 mEq. Every client should be told the dosage exactly in milliequivalents, not simply to take a certain amount by volume.

The oral preparations of potassium come in various forms of elixirs, capsules, and tablets, some that fizz when mixed with juice. Most potassium supplements also contain chloride, which may be a needed replacement in metabolic alkalosis (see Chapter 6). The most important problem with oral supplements of potassium is the gastrointestinal upsets they can cause; therefore nurses should teach clients not to take potassium supplements on an empty stomach. Liquids should be diluted. Orange juice is a good vehicle, because it has a high potassium level. Overdoses of oral potassium supplements are not common, but it is important that the urinary output always be adequate.

Potassium replacement can also be accomplished with a relatively inexpensive salt substitute that contains potassium chloride. Many salt substitutes contain more than 50 mEq of potassium per teaspoon (4 mL) (Slawson and Slawson, 1985). The client should consult the physician about the use of salt substitutes.

Knowledge Deficit Related to Dietary Sources of Potassium

The dietary intake of potassium is usually about 40–80 mEq for adults. For clients who take diuretics or who for other reasons need a higher intake of potassium, it may be wise to assess their dietary habits to see if they can gain extra potassium by dietary intake. Table 5–8 shows the amount of potassium in some common foods. By including potassium-rich foods, clients may be able to reduce or eliminate the need to take potassium supplements. However, Narins et al. (1985) observed that supplements are usually needed. The serum potassium levels for clients undergoing long-term diuretic therapy should be checked periodically to make sure dietary intake of potassium is adequate to balance an increased potassium loss. Clients changed to thiazides who have continued problems with hypokalemia may be given one of the potassium-sparing diuretics, which are more expensive (Licht et al., 1983).

▼ URINE POTASSIUM

The amount of potassium in the urine varies with the diet. It also varies with an increased amount of serum aldosterone or cortisol, which causes an increased excretion of potassium. Further, extra potassium is lost in diabetic acidosis and with thiazide diuretics, but a serum potassium is a better measurement of the need for replacement after diuresis. Renal failure causes a decreased excretion of potassium.

The primary use of a 24-hr urine potassium is to assess hormonal functioning and to determine if hypokalemia is of renal or nonrenal origin. Excretion of less than 20 mEq/day in the presence of hypokalemia is evidence that the hypokalemia is not from renal loss. (See Chapter 15 on aldosterone and cortisol levels.) Urine potassium levels are also used sometimes in research studies as one indication of the stress level of the body.

Preparation of Client and Collection of Sample

See Chapter 3 for 24-hr urine collections. No preservative is needed.

REFERENCE VALUES FOR URINE POTASSIUM
25–125 mEq/24 hr (varies with diet)

▼ SERUM AND URINE CHLORIDE

Chloride, the principal negative ion in the extracellular fluid, is important, in combination with sodium, for maintaining osmotic pressure in the serum. A loss or a gain of chloride is often due to the factors that also cause a loss or gain of sodium. Chloride is found in a variety of foods, usually in combination with sodium. A diet restricted in sodium also causes a reduction of chloride intake but not to an inadequate level. The kidneys selectively secrete chloride or bicarbonate ions, depending on the acid–base balance. In some types of renal failure, chloride excretion may be impaired. Chloride can be measured in the urine with sodium and potassium as part of a 24-hr specimen (see Chapter 3).

REFERENCE VALUES FOR SERUM CHLORIDE	
All age groups	100–108 mEq
Falls little, if at all, in pregnancy	

REFERENCE VALUES FOR URINE CHLORIDE	
Adult	110–250 mEq/24 hr
Child	15–40 mEq/24 hr
Infant	2–10 mEq/24 hr

Varies greatly with chloride intake. Chloride dipsticks estimate total sodium intake (Luft et al., 1984).

Increased Serum Chloride Level (Hyperchloremia)

Clinical Significance. *Hyperchloremia* is a term that is rarely used clinically. An increase in chlorides in the serum is not a primary focus because the increase must always be evaluated in relation to (1) an increase in sodium levels or (2) a decrease in the serum bicarbonate level.

Aldosterone, a mineral corticosteroid, causes retention of both sodium and chloride. In most cases, a proportional increase in water retention makes the electrolytes in the serum appear not to be increased. For the sodium and chloride levels to be elevated, there must be a deficit of water or a large intake of sodium chloride. Because, in these situations, the chloride level parallels the rise or fall of the sodium level, the sodium level is used to monitor fluid deficits.

In some clinical situations, the rise in chlorides may be even greater than the rise in sodium levels. In some types of renal failure, the kidneys are unable to excrete chlorides properly; this inability leads to a type of acidosis called *renal hyperchloremic acidosis*. Chlorides may also be greatly increased in the bloodstream if large amounts of normal saline solution (0.9% NaCl) are infused over several days. "Normal saline" is not really normal in relation to the sodium and chloride content of the serum, even though it is classified as an isotonic solution. Normal saline contains 154 mEq of sodium ions and 154 mEq of chloride ions per liter. This is a little higher than the serum level of 135–145 mEq for sodium ions and a great deal higher than the 100–106 mEq for serum chloride (Metheny, 1990).

Chloride levels are increased in some types of acidosis because the chloride is needed to replace the loss of another negative ion, bicarbonate, from the serum. If the metabolic acidosis is due to an increase of other negative ions, such as ketoacids, the chlorides are not increased—and may actually decrease—because of diuresis. The changes in the bicarbonate level, in the chloride level, and in the unmeasured negative ions (the anion gap) give useful information about what is causing the acidotic state. The most important thing to remember about the relation between a high serum chloride level and acidosis is that if the chlorides are higher than normal, this condition causes a drop in the serum bicarbonate level because there is room for only a set amount of negative ions. If the serum bicarbonate level drops first, chlorides may be increased to keep the correct number of negative ions in the serum. Increased chloride levels can be either a cause or a result of metabolic acidosis.

▼ POSSIBLE NURSING DIAGNOSES RELATED TO HIGH CHLORIDE LEVELS

Because changes in chloride levels always take place in combination with changes in other electrolytes, assessments depend on nurses' understanding of the reason for the increased chloride level. For example, if the chloride level is

(*continued*)

▼ POSSIBLE NURSING DIAGNOSES RELATED TO HIGH CHLORIDE LEVELS (*continued*)

related to an increased sodium level, the nursing diagnoses for sodium are to be followed. If the increased chloride level is causing, or was caused by, acidosis, the symptoms exhibited are those of acidosis. (Care of clients with metabolic acidosis is covered in the section on bicarbonate levels in Chapter 6.)

Decrease in Serum Chloride Level (Hypochloremia)

Clinical Significance. Decreases in the serum chloride level are commonly due to loss from vomiting, gastric suction, diarrhea, and the use of diuretics.

Because sodium, hydrogen, and potassium ions are usually lost with the chlorides, a chloride drain is only part of a larger problem. For example, the loss of chlorides from the serum means that more bicarbonate must be retained to replace the lack of negative ions, thus contributing to the development of metabolic alkalosis. The loss of potassium or of hydrogen ions also contributes to the development of metabolic alkalosis. Conversely, alkalotic states can cause a low chloride level. In any alkalotic state, the bicarbonate level in the serum increases, so the other principal negative ion, chloride, must decrease in the bloodstream. (By now the inverse relation between the negative ions bicarbonate and chloride should be clearly apparent.)

As explained in Chapter 6, clients with chronic lung disease often have high serum bicarbonate levels to balance an increased P_{CO_2} in the bloodstream. This chronically elevated serum bicarbonate level also causes a decreased serum chloride level. This condition would be considered a normal compensation in clients with chronic lung disease.

▼ POSSIBLE NURSING DIAGNOSES RELATED TO LOW CHLORIDE LEVELS

Altered Nutrition Related to Chloride Losses

Nurses need always to be aware of clients who may be losing abnormal amounts of chlorides, so that replacement therapy can begin before alkalotic states develop. For example, clients who are undergoing gastrointestinal suctioning are losing not only chlorides but also potassium and hydrogen ions. All three losses contribute to the development of metabolic alkalosis. Because potassium supplements contain chloride, the use of potassium chloride is one way that lost chlorides are replaced. If necessary, the physician may order normal saline solution (0.9% NaCl) to be given intravenously to replace large chloride losses. The use of oral electrolyte solutions for infants or salty broths for adults to replace sodium losses already has been mentioned. Nurses must always keep in mind that a loss of electrolytes usually involves several electrolytes and never just chlorides alone.

▼ SERUM BICARBONATE OR CARBON DIOXIDE

Serum bicarbonate levels are routinely part of both electrolytes and arterial blood gases. Note that the carbon dioxide (CO_2) combining power or total carbon dioxide is often used as an indirect measurement of serum bicarbonate. This indirect measurement is usually about 2 mmol/L or mEq/L more than the actual bicarbonate level, which makes up 95% of the total CO_2 combining power (Kaplan et al., 1995). The carbon dioxide is different from P_{CO_2}, which is a measure of blood gas. (Both are discussed in Chapter 6.) Because changes in serum bicarbonate level always signify some changes in acid–base balance, the relation between bicarbonate and carbonic acid is important. A bicarbonate-to-carbonic acid (as measured by the P_{CO_2}) ratio of 20:1 is the most important buffer in the serum. The 20:1 ratio is fundamental to understanding the clinical significance of changes in serum bicarbonate levels. The next chapter includes a summary of this ratio and a discussion of how serum bicarbonate levels decrease and increase in acid–base imbalances.

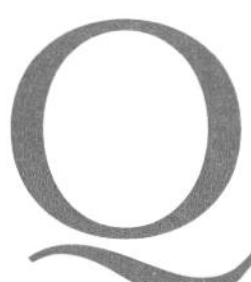

1. The home care nurse is making a visit to Mr. Brown, an elderly man who is taking digoxin and a diuretic for treatment of congestive heart failure (CHF). The nurse should be the most concerned about which of the following laboratory results? A serum level of

   a. Na^+ = 130 mmol/L **b.** K^+ = 3.0 mmol/L
   c. Cl^- = 95 mmol/L **d.** HCO^- = 29 mmol/L

2. Given the fact that 39 mg of K^+ equals 1 mEq, compute how many milligrams of K^+ are needed to give a dose of 40 mEq.

   a. 1.56 g or 1,560 mg **b.** 0.56 g or 560 mg
   c. 3.9 g or 3,900 mg **d.** 1.4 g or 1,400 mg

3. Hydrogen ions (H^+) shift into the cell when serum potassium (K^+) levels drop, because as more K^+ diffuses out of the cell

   a. The fluid balance changes unless electrolytes are shifted into the cell
   b. Another positive ion must enter the cell to keep the electrical charges neutral
   c. The acid–base balance must be maintained by decreasing serum H^+ ions
   d. There is a lack of positive ions to be excreted by the kidney

4. When the total amount of serum Na^+ and K^+ ions (cations) are compared with the total amount of serum Cl^- and HCO_3^- ions (anions), there are fewer anions. This "anion gap" is due to which of the following facts?

   a. There are always more cations (positive ions) than anions (negative ions) in the serum
   b. Some anions, such as organic acids, are not measured
   c. The electrical balance is not always neutral in acid–base imbalances
   d. The loss of electrolytes decreases the total number of anions in the serum

5. When a client has an abnormal serum sodium (Na^+) report, the most useful nursing assessment to help explore the reason for the sodium imbalance would be which of the following?

   a. Dietary intake pattern of salt and sodium-containing foods
   b. Intake and output records and daily weights
   c. Vital signs during past 24 hr
   d. Record of all medications given

6. A laboratory report of an increased serum sodium level would most likely be part of the clinical findings for a client

   a. With severe congestive heart failure who has pitting edema of the ankles
   b. Undergoing corticosteroid therapy for several months for rheumatoid arthritis
   c. Having diarrhea and unable to take fluids by mouth
   d. Receiving maintenance intravenous fluids of dextrose 5% in 0.2% sodium chloride for several days after an operation

7. A laboratory report of a slightly low serum sodium (Na^+) is *least* likely for which of the following conditions?

   a. Diet containing no more than 2.3 g (100 mEq) of sodium daily
   b. Maintenance intravenous solutions of 5% dextrose in water (D_5W) for several days
   c. Drinking large amounts of water after strenuous exercise
   d. Use of a diuretic that is an aldosterone-blocking agent

8. A characteristic assessment expected for a client with a high serum sodium (Na^+) level caused by a water deficit would include

   a. Hypertension b. Thirst
   c. Weight gain d. Subnormal temperature

9. A characteristic assessment for a client with a low serum sodium (Na^+) level caused by total body sodium depletion would be

   a. Confusion b. Hypertension
   c. Weight gain d. Flaccid paralysis

10. An increase in serum sodium (Na^+) levels is usually an indication that the client needs which of the following?

    a. Less sodium in the diet b. Less fluid intake
    c. More fluid intake d. Both sodium and water restrictions

11. Which of the following clients is the *least* likely to have an elevated serum K^+ level?

    a. Mary Burden, who is experiencing renal failure
    b. Baby Lois, who suffered extensive burns today
    c. Candy Phillips, who is in metabolic alkalosis
    d. Jack Brown, who has Addison's disease

12. A low serum potassium (K^+) is most likely to be a problem for

    a. Mr. Rhodes, who is undergoing long-term diuretic therapy with thiazides
    b. Mary Rogers, who has mild morning sickness
    c. Jackie, age 8, who is undergoing chemotherapy as part of treatment of leukemia
    d. Mrs. Cabrillo, who has a severe respiratory infection and who is not taking much fluid

13. Which of the following signs or symptoms is the most suggestive of hyperkalemia?

    a. Paralytic ileus (lack of bowel sounds)
    b. Peaked T waves on the cardiac monitor
    c. Skeletal muscle cramps
    d. Depressed T waves on the cardiac monitor

14. Mrs. Forrest, who is scheduled for a laparoscopic cholecystectomy tomorrow, has a serum K^+ of 2.3 mEq. (She has been taking thiazide diuretics.) The nurse is to monitor the potassium replacement, which Mrs. Forrest is to receive intravenously. Which of these guidelines about potassium is correct?

    a. Urine output should be at least 100 mL/hr
    b. No more than 10–20 mEq of KCl should be given in an hour
    c. No more than 10 mEq of KCl should be added to 1,000 mL of intravenous fluids
    d. KCl is given IV push only in extreme cases in which the serum K^+ is less than 2.5 mEq

15. Mrs. Forrest is going home and has been given a prescription for hydrochlorathiazide as part of the treatment of hypertension. The physician has prescribed a potassium chloride (KCl) supplement to be taken in liquid form three times a day. The nurse should instruct the client to

    a. Dilute the KCl in water, but not in juice
    b. Never take the KCl at the same time as any other medicine

c. Not take the KCl on an empty stomach
d. Keep the KCl in the refrigerator

16. Mrs. Forrest asks the nurse about foods that are high in potassium. What item does not contain at least 10 mEq of potassium?

a. Orange juice, 1 cup b. Cranberry juice, 1 cup
c. Instant coffee, 3 g d. Potato, 1 baked

17. Which one of the following clients is the *least* likely to have low serum chloride (Cl^-) levels?

a. Mr. Hagan, who has an elevated serum bicarbonate (HCO_3^-) level caused by ingestion of baking soda
b. Baby Raggio, who has had severe vomiting
c. Mrs. Rhodes, who is taking loop diuretics and a low-sodium diet
d. Mrs. Nicholls, who is experiencing renal failure

▼ REFERENCES

Ault, M.J., and Geiderman, J. (1992). Hypokalemia as a cause of tetany. *Western Journal of Medicine, 157* (1), 65–67.

Bongard, F.S., and Sue, D.Y. (1994). *Current critical care diagnosis & treatment.* Norwalk, CT: Appleton & Lange.

Cerrato, P. (1985). Hypertension: Salt isn't the only culprit. *RN, 48* (9), 74–76.

Culpepper, M., et al. (1986). Why is the serum sodium low? *Patient Care, 20* (7), 94–110.

DeCherney, A.H., and Pernoll, M.L. (1994). *Current obstetric & gynecologic diagnosis & treatment.* (8th ed.). Norwalk, CT: Appleton & Lange.

Deglin, J.H., and Vallerand, A.H. (1995). *Davis's drug guide for nurses.* (4th ed.). Philadelphia: F.A. Davis.

Don, B.R., Sebastian, A., Cheitlin, M., et al. (1990). Pseudohyperkalemia caused by fist clenching during phlebotomy. *New England Journal of Medicine, 322* (18), 1290–1291.

Goldstein, C., et al. (1983). Idiopathic syndrome of inappropriate antidiuretic hormone secretion possibly related to advanced age. *Annals of Internal Medicine, 99,* 185–188.

Hay, W.W., Groothuis, J.R., Hayward, A.R., and Levin, M.J. (1995). *Current pediatric diagnosis & treatment.* (12th ed.). Norwalk, CT: Appleton & Lange.

Kaplan, A., Jack, R., Opheim, K.E., et al. (1995). *Clinical chemistry. Interpretation and techniques.* (4th ed.). Baltimore: Williams & Wilkins.

Katzung, B. (1995). *Basic and clinical pharmacology.* (6th ed.). Norwalk, CT: Appleton & Lange.

Licht, J., et al. (1983). Diuretic regimens in essential hypertension: A comparison of hypokalemic effects, blood pressure control, and cost. *Archives of Internal Medicine, 143,* 1694–1699.

Luft, F., et al. (1984). Influence of home monitoring on compliance with a reduced sodium intake. *Archives of Internal Medicine, 144* (10), 1963–1965.

Lutomski, D.M., and Bower, R.H. (1994). The effect of thrombocytosis on serum potassium and phosphorus concentrations. *American Journal of Medical Science, 307* (4), 255–258.

McElroy, D., and Davis, G. (1986). SIADH and the acutely ill child. *MCN: American Journal of Maternal Child Nursing, 11* (3), 193–196.

Metheny, N. (1990). Why worry about IV fluids? *American Journal of Nursing, 90* (6), 50–57.

Narins, R., et al. (1985). Renal retention of potassium in fruit. *New England Journal of Medicine, 319* (9), 582–583.

Raimer, F. (1994). How to identify electrolyte imbalances on your patient's E.C.G. *Nursing 94, 24* (6), 54–58.

Ravel, R. (1995). *Clinical laboratory medicine: Clinical application of laboratory data.* (6th ed.). St. Louis: Mosby–Year Book.

Regan, W. (1981). Nursing malpractice: A giant leap in damages. *RN, 43* (12), 69.

Rinard, G. (1989). Water intoxication. *American Journal of Nursing, 89* (12), 1635–1638.

Sandifer, M. (1983). Hyponatremia due to psychotropic drugs. *Journal of Clinical Psychiatry, 44*, 301–303.

Schwartz, M. (1987). Potassium imbalances. *American Journal of Nursing, 87* (10), 1292–1299.

Sheckel, S. (1980). Contracting with patient-selecting reinforcers. *American Journal of Nursing, 80* (9), 1596–1599.

Slawson, M., and Slawson, S. (1985). Problem ingredients in OTCs. *RN, 48* (4), 53–61.

Stanley-Tilt, C. (1989). Recognizing the psychiatric water intoxicator. *American Journal of Nursing, 89* (12), 1636–1637.

Struthers, A., et al. (1983). Prior thiazide diuretic treatment increases adrenalin-induced hypokalemia. *Lancet, 1*, 1358–1360.

Toto, K. (1987). When the patient has hypokalemia. *RN, 50* (3), 38–41.

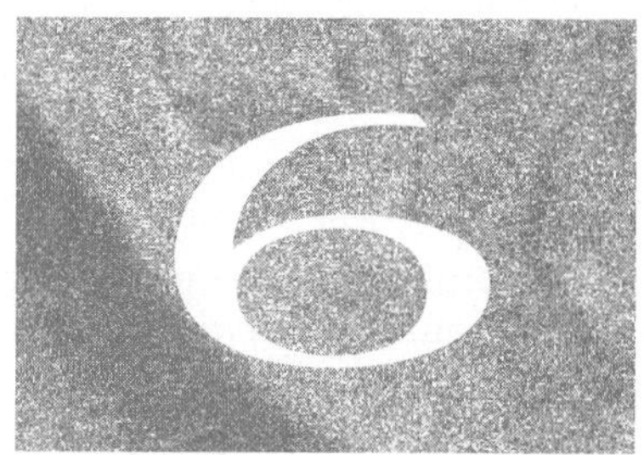

ARTERIAL BLOOD GASES

- pH of the Blood
- Partial Pressure of Carbon Dioxide
- Serum Bicarbonate and Total Carbon Dioxide Content
- Partial Pressure of Oxygen
- Oxygen Saturation
- Lactic Acid or Blood Lactate

OBJECTIVES

1. Demonstrate the four-step sequence in interpreting the meaning of arterial blood gas (ABG) reports to determine the four primary acid–base imbalances.
2. Explain how the buffering system, the lungs, and the kidneys maintain the serum bicarbonate–to–carbonic acid ratio of 20:1.
3. Describe the nurse's role when ABGs are drawn.
4. Explain how reference values for blood gases are altered in pregnancy and in the newborn period.
5. Explain the physiologic basis for the symptoms of acidosis and alkalosis, both metabolic and respiratory in origin.
6. Identify possible nursing diagnoses for clients with increased and decreased P_{CO_2} (respiratory alkalosis and acidosis).
7. Identify the possible nursing diagnoses for clients with increased or decreased serum bicarbonate levels (metabolic alkalosis and acidosis).

8. Explain how electrolytes alter and are altered by changes in the acid–base balance.
9. Explain the concept of the anion gap in relation to the various kinds of metabolic acidosis.
10. Explain why high concentrations of oxygen may be dangerous for a client with a low PO_2 and a high PCO_2.
11. Compare and contrast how PO_2 and PCO_2 levels are used by the nurse to assist with treatment of respiratory problems.
12. Describe the basic pathologic process that produces increased lactic acid in the serum.

This chapter begins with an introductory section about acid–base imbalances. Several tables help to show the fundamental differences in the four primary acid–base imbalances. After this general discussion, pH, PCO_2, and bicarbonate tests are presented because of their significance in acid–base imbalances. The last part of the chapter discusses PO_2 and oxygen saturation and measurement of lactic acid as an assessment of dangerous hypoxia at the cellular level.

Each laboratory measurement is discussed as a separate test so that the reader can better understand the clinical significance of both increases and decreases in each value. As in other chapters, possible nursing diagnoses for each change in laboratory test are discussed after the clinical significance.

PURPOSE OF BLOOD GASES

The *P* before the O_2 and CO_2 stands for the partial pressure of the gases. The respiratory gases include nitrogen, oxygen, carbon dioxide, and water vapor. Dalton's *law of partial pressure* states that the total pressure exerted by a mixture of gases is the sum of the individual partial pressure. Table 6–1 shows the percentage of gases in the blood and how this determines the partial pressure of each.

Blood gases are used to determine the respiratory status or the acid–base balance of the client. If the primary focus is to evaluate the respiratory status of the client, then the PO_2, PCO_2, and pH levels, as well as the oxygen saturation, are the most important to evaluate. If the primary focus is to evaluate a metabolic acid–base

TABLE 6–1. FOUR GASES IN ARTERIAL BLOOD AT SEA LEVEL

Gas	Percentage of Gas	Partial Pressure (mm Hg)
Nitrogen (not measured)	75.5	574
Oxygen	13.0	99—venous drops to 40 mm Hg
Carbon dioxide	5.3	40—venous rises to 46 mm Hg
Water vapor (not measured)	6.2	47
Totals	100.00	760

The total pressure exerted by a mixture of gases is the sum of the individual partial pressures. At altitudes above sea level, the partial pressures of gases are less because the total atmospheric pressure is less than 760 mm Hg.

imbalance, the Po_2 has little significance. By looking first at the pH, then the Pco_2, and then the bicarbonate level, one can figure out whether the acidosis is respiratory or metabolic in origin. In some confusing clinical situations, clients may have a combination of acid–base disorders, but this chapter focuses on the four basic types. Table 6–2 summarizes the way to interpret blood gas results to determine the primary acid–base imbalance. The last part of the chapter discusses hypoxic states that are not directly related to acid–base imbalances.

SUMMARY OF ACID–BASE BALANCE

The normal pH of arterial blood is between 7.35 and 7.45, with 7.4 taken as the average. Varying from this narrow range can be disastrous. Many chemical reactions in the body do not function normally if the pH of the blood is not in the normal range. If the pH is less than 7.35, the condition is called *acidosis*. If the pH is greater than 7.45, it is called *alkalosis*. As demonstrated in Table 6–2, if the increased or decreased pH is due to a marked change in Pco_2, the acid–base imbalance is respiratory in origin; all other acid–base imbalances are considered metabolic.

Understanding how Pco_2 and bicarbonate (HCO_3^-) function in the buffering system of the body is necessary if one is to be able to interpret the meaning of abnormal blood gas values. Buffer systems act as chemical sponges, which can give off or absorb hydrogen ions. There are minor buffers in the bloodstream, such as phosphates and proteins, but these are not measured in evaluating the acid–base balance. The main buffer system is the carbonic acid–bicarbonate buffer system. The carbonic acid level is measured indirectly with Pco_2 level and the bicarbonate level with bicarbonate level or the total carbon dioxide content. This carbonic acid–bicarbonate buffer system is often referred to as the *20:1 ratio,* which means one part of carbonic acid for each 20 parts of bicarbonate.

Note that although the carbonic acid level is not measured directly, it can be calculated because it is always 3% of the Pco_2. Hence a Pco_2 of 40 mm Hg indicates 1.2 mEq of carbonic acid in the serum, which must be balanced by 20 parts of bi-

TABLE 6–2. FOUR STEPS TO DETERMINE THE FOUR PRIMARY ACID–BASE IMBALANCES

Step 1: *Look at pH*	Is the pH > 7.45? If so, the client is alkalotic. Go to Step 2. Is the pH < 7.35? If so, the client is acidotic. Go to Step 3.
Step 2: When the pH is elevated	Is the $Pco_2 < 40$ mm Hg? If so, the alkalosis is respiratory in origin. Is the $Pco_2 > 40$ mm Hg or in the normal range? If so, the alkalosis is not respiratory in origin. Look for metabolic causes. Go to step 4.
Step 3: When the pH is decreased	Is the $Pco_2 > 40$ mm Hg? If so, the acidosis is respiratory. Is the $Pco_2 < 40$ mm Hg or normal? If so, the acidosis is metabolic in origin. Go to Step 4.
Step 4: Looking at the bicarbonate in relation to the pH	Note that in metabolic acidosis, both the pH and the bicarbonate level are decreased. In metabolic alkalosis, both the pH and the bicarbonate are elevated. (See Table 6–4 for compensation.)

Anderson (1990); Stringfield (1993); and Tasota and Wesmiller (1994) include several case studies as practice for determining acid–base imbalances by looking at laboratory reports in a systematic manner.

carbonate or 24 mEq (Table 6–3). As long as this ratio is maintained, whether it is 40:2 or 10:0.5, the pH of the blood stays in the normal range. Thus if the carbonic acid level changes, the kidneys try to compensate by changing the bicarbonate level. For example, because a P_{CO_2} of 34 mm Hg reflects a carbonic acid level of 1 mEq (34 times 3% equals 1.02), the bicarbonate level must drop to 20 mEq to keep a 20:1 ratio. If the bicarbonate level changes, the lungs change the P_{CO_2} and carbonic acid level, but this type of compensation is limited because the lungs must continue to function for oxygen exchange.

Only the lungs control the regulation of P_{CO_2}. In the bloodstream, carbon dioxide combines with water to form carbonic acid. If more P_{CO_2} is retained, this condition results in more carbonic acid and hence the person tends toward acidosis. If more carbon dioxide is expired (hyperventilation), there is less carbonic acid in the bloodstream and the person tends toward alkalosis. By this mechanism, the lungs can shift the pH of the blood in just a few minutes.

The kidneys are also instrumental in the regulation of the pH of the bloodstream. The kidneys not only constantly excrete hydrogen ions but also control the serum bicarbonate level and retain or excrete sodium, potassium, and chloride ions. For substantial corrective shifts, it may take the kidneys several days to restore the pH to normal.

If all these regulatory mechanisms—buffer systems, lungs, and kidneys—are not successful in restoring the pH, the condition progresses with varying speeds to acidosis, leading to coma and death, or alkalosis, with irritability, tetany, and sometimes death. As a general rule, acidotic states are usually more life-threatening than alkalotic states.

By looking at three laboratory tests, one can usually determine whether the acid–base imbalance is respiratory or metabolic in origin. Table 6–4 shows the laboratory findings for each of the four basic types of acid–base imbalance *before* compensation occurs and how compensation changes the laboratory tests. In the actual clinical situation, because the client may have more than one imbalance, a chart does not always pinpoint the origin of the difficulty.

TABLE 6–3. THREE LABORATORY TESTS THAT MEASURE THE BICARBONATE–CARBONIC ACID BUFFER SYSTEM

$CO_2 + H_2O$	$\rightleftarrows$	H_2CO_3	$\rightleftarrows$	H	+	HCO_3^-
↓		↓		↓		↓
Carbon dioxide measured by P_{CO_2} (40 mm Hg) Test 2		Carbonic acid not measured directly but is always 3% of P_{CO_2} or 3% × 40 mm Hg = 1.2 mEq		Concentration of hydrogen ions measured by pH (7.35–7.45) Test 1		Bicarbonate level measured by serum bicarbonate (24 mEq) Test 3
P_{CO_2} controlled by lungs				Hydrogen, bicarbonate, and other electrolytes controlled by kidneys		

Test 1: pH; Test 2: P_{CO_2}; Test 3: serum bicarbonate

A bicarbonate level of 24 mEq and P_{CO_2} of 40 mm Hg (carbonic acid of 1.2 mEq) is the desirable 20:1 ratio that maintains the pH of the serum between 7.35 and 7.45. See text on use of total CO_2 content as an indirect measurement of the bicarbonate level.

TABLE 6–4. CHANGES IN pH, P_{CO_2}, AND HCO_3^- AND THE COMPENSATORY MECHANISMS IN ACID–BASE IMBALANCES

	pH	PCO_2	HCO_3^-	Compensation
Respiratory alkalosis	↑	↓	Normal until compensation	Kidneys eventually reduce HCO_3^-. Takes few days to complete.
Metabolic alkalosis	↑	Normal unless lungs compensate	↑	Lungs try to increase PCO_2 slightly. Can do it quickly.
Respiratory acidosis	↓	↑	Normal until kidneys compensate	Kidneys eventually retain more HCO_3^-. Takes a few days to complete.
Metabolic acidosis	↓	Normal until lungs compensate	↓	Lungs usually reduce PCO_2 Can do it quickly.

See text for full explanation. Note that (1) in respiratory alkalosis and respiratory acidosis, the pH and P_{CO_2} vary inversely; (2) in metabolic alkalosis and metabolic acidosis, the pH and HCO_3^- rise or fall together; (3) the kidneys try to compensate for respiratory imbalances, but the compensation takes several days; and (4) the lungs try to compensate for metabolic imbalances, and their compensation is accomplished in a few minutes, but it is limited.

Table 6–4 makes the fundamental difference between respiratory and metabolic acid–base imbalances easy to see. If there is a marked increase or decrease in PCO_2, the acid–base imbalance is respiratory in origin. Otherwise, the imbalance is metabolic, and the change in the bicarbonate level has shifted the pH. Table 6–5 summarizes the common reasons for each type of acid–base imbalance.

TABLE 6–5. COMMON REASONS FOR ACID–BASE IMBALANCES

Primary Acid–Base Imbalance	Description of Imbalance	Common Reasons for Imbalance
Respiratory alkalosis	Decrease in PCO_2 caused by hyperventilation	Anxiety Fever, pain, hypoxia Improperly adjusted respirator
Respiratory acidosis	Increase in PCO_2 caused by hypoventilation	Chronic lung disease that causes CO_2 retention Respiratory depression from drugs or anesthesia
Metabolic alkalosis	Increase in serum bicarbonate (HCO_3^-) caused by increased intake of bicarbonate or increased loss of chlorides, hydrogen, or potassium ions	Vomiting or gastric suctioning, which causes loss of hydrogen, chloride, and potassium ions Ingestion or infusion of soda bicarbonate
Metabolic acidosis	Decrease in serum bicarbonate level caused by excess acid production, loss of bicarbonate, or increase in serum chloride levels	Excess acids such as ketone bodies in diabetic acidosis or lactic acid in cardiac arrest Loss of bicarbonate via intestines Increase in serum chloride level—renal failure

See text for explanations and Ravel (1995) for more details.

If the acidosis or alkalosis is metabolic in origin or if the respiratory problem is chronic enough for the kidneys to be involved, it is also important to look at the laboratory tests for electrolytes. (Refer to Chapter 5 to review (1) the inverse relation between chloride (Cl^-) and the bicarbonate ions, (2) the concept of anion gap, and (3) why hyperkalemia is associated with acidotic states and hypokalemia with alkalotic states. Chapter 3 describes the changes in urine pH in the different types of acidosis and alkalosis.) Table 6–6 shows the usual electrolyte abnormalities for each of the four primary types of acid–base imbalances.

ARTERIAL BLOOD GASES IN GENERAL

Preparation of Client and Collection of Sample

A physician or other clinician skilled in arterial puncture must collect the blood sample, which can be drawn from the radial, brachial, or femoral arteries. In most hospitals only physicians are allowed to perform femoral punctures, whereas nurses with special training may perform radial or brachial punctures.

Sumner (1980) gave nurses tips on how to perform arterial punctures. The site must be disinfected and allowed to dry. Clients need to be told that the puncture is momentarily painful. If they are very afraid of the procedure or if the attempt to obtain a specimen is prolonged, clients may hyperventilate because of anxiety, which can thus alter test results. If arterial blood samples are needed frequently, clients usu-

TABLE 6–6. POSSIBLE CHANGES IN ELECTROLYTES AND URINE pH FOR ACID–BASE IMBALANCES

	Sodium (Na^+)	**Potassium (K^+)**	**Chloride (Cl^-)**	**Urine pH**
Respiratory alkalosis	Usually not changed	May be low if alkalosis persists	Increased when HCO_3^- decreases for compensation	High if chronic problem
Metabolic alkalosis	Usually not changed	Low	Low	High or, paradoxically, pH may continue low
Respiratory acidosis	Usually not changed	May be a little increased	In compensation, the increase in HCO_3^- causes decrease in Cl^-	Low. Many H^+ ions excreted.
Metabolic acidosis	Total Na^+ is low if diuresis as in diabetic acidosis, serum levels may be normal in some states	May be high although cellular deficit of K^+. Serum potassium raises about 0.6 mEq/L for each 0.1 decrease in pH	May increase to replace lost HCO_3^-. If unmeasured anions are high, Cl^- may decrease or be normal	Very low pH as kidneys try to excrete H^+ ions

Note: See Chapter 5 for discussion on electrolytes and anion gap and Chapter 3 for urine pH.

ally have an arterial catheter in place. Nurses usually obtain specimens from an arterial line. In neonates, arterial sampling can be performed with an umbilical catheter.

After being collected in an airtight, heparinized syringe, the blood must be packed in ice for transport to the laboratory. The airtight container and the ice help prevent loss of gases from the sample. Special care units may have facilities for testing the sample immediately in the unit. Biswas et al. (1982) demonstrated that it is necessary to expel all air bubbles within 2 min and put the sample on ice if the test is not completed within 10 min of collection.

The amount of blood needed for ABGs depends on the technique used. Although some blood gas analyzers can test less than 0.5 mL of blood, accuracy is more assured with a minimum of 3 mL. If a prepackaged ABG kit is not available, 0.5–1.0 mL of heparin can be used to coat the inside of a glass syringe (Carroll, 1987). Preusser et al. (1989) found that a 2-mL discard of blood is needed for withdrawal of blood from a heparinized line with 1 mL of dead space. Too much heparin with a small sample causes inaccurate results.

After the sample is drawn, continuous pressure should be applied to the puncture site for at least 5 min if the radial artery is used and 10 min for the femoral. If the client has any bleeding problems, the pressure dressing should be taped on and left for several hours.

It is important to record on the laboratory slip whether the client was receiving oxygen at the time the sample was drawn, because there may be quite a difference in PO_2 if the client is undergoing oxygen therapy as opposed to breathing room air. The nurse should record how long the client has been receiving a specific amount of oxygen, such as "25 min on 2 L by nasal cannula." If the client is undergoing assisted ventilation, the settings for the respirator should be recorded in case changes have to be made later. The temperature of the client should also be noted because a fever increases metabolic rate.

If arterial blood cannot be obtained, capillary blood samples may be used. The area should be warmed for 5 min before the sample is taken. The warmed ear site is used in children and adults, whereas the warmed heel is used for infants. (See Chapter 1 for the heel stick technique.)

Other Methods of Monitoring Blood Gases and Oxygen Saturation

Transcutaneous electrodes can be used to monitor PO_2 and PCO_2 levels. Since the 1970s, these monitors have been useful for newborns because an infant's skin is thin with little subcutaneous fat as compared with an adult's (Dingle et al., 1980). The system is calibrated by a standard ABG sample each time the electrodes are moved because a change of position affects the readings. Electrodes in adults are used only to measure local skin and tissue hypoperfusion (Bongard and Sue, 1994).

A pulse oximeter measures oxygen saturation rather than the PO_2. The oximeter, which is very easy to use, is discussed in the section on oxygen saturation. A more sophisticated instrument, used with a pulmonary catheter, can give continuous oxygen saturation from mixed venous blood. These various types of readings reduce the number of ABGs needed for monitoring a client with possible hypoxia. These instruments are also useful in nursing research studies (Shively and Clark, 1986).

▼ pH OF THE BLOOD

The pH test measures the alkalinity or acidity of the blood. For chemical solutions, a pH of 7 is the neutral point; greater than 7 is alkaline and less than 7 is acid. For blood pH, the neutral point is 7.4. It is critical that blood pH remain within a narrow range because many enzymes and other physiologic processes do not function normally when the pH is altered.

REFERENCE VALUES FOR pH

Adult	7.35–7.45 (arterial) 7.30–7.41 (venous)
Newborn	7.3–7.4 (arterial)

See speciality texts for fetal blood sampling. For fetal scalp blood sampling, if the pH is above 7.25 the fetus is usually not compromised. Fetal umbilical samples are about 7.24 ± 0.07 for arterial samples and 7.32 ± 0.06 for venous samples in term nulliparous pregnancies (DeCherney and Pernoll, 1994).

Increased pH of Arterial Blood (Alkalosis)

Clinical Significance. An increased serum pH indicates that the client is in a state of alkalosis. To determine whether the alkalosis is respiratory or metabolic in origin, it is necessary to look at the P_{CO_2} and the serum bicarbonate level. If the alkalosis is respiratory in origin, the P_{CO_2} is markedly decreased. If the alkalosis is metabolic in origin, the serum bicarbonate level is markedly elevated. The common clinical situations that cause these changes and the reference values are discussed in the sections on P_{CO_2} and serum bicarbonate tests.

▼ POSSIBLE NURSING DIAGNOSES RELATED TO ALKALOTIC STATES

Risk for Injury Related to Neuromuscular Irritability and Possible Tetany

Specific nursing implications depend on whether the alkalosis is respiratory or metabolic in origin. Some general symptoms of both types of alkalosis include tingling in the extremities or nose, facial twitching, light-headedness, muscle tremors, and tetany. The neuromuscular irritability in alkalotic states occurs because calcium is less soluble in an alkaline medium. Many of the symptoms of alkalosis are those of hypocalcemia. (See Chapter 7 on hypocalcemia.) Clients must be protected from falls and assessed for convulsive movements.

Altered Breathing Pattern

In respiratory alkalosis the respiratory rate is high because hyperventilation is the cause of the alkalosis. Factors that cause hyperventilation and possible nursing interventions are discussed in the section on P_{CO_2} levels. In metabolic alkalosis, the respiratory rate is normal to slightly depressed, with slow and shallow breaths. The depressed respiration in metabolic alkalosis is an attempt by the lungs to retain more P_{CO_2} to balance the increased serum bicarbonate level. The effect on the breathing pattern is of minimal importance as discussed in the section on increased bicarbonate levels.

Decreased pH of Arterial Blood (Acidosis)

Clinical Significance. A decreased serum pH indicates that the client is in a state of acidosis. To determine whether the acidosis is respiratory or metabolic in origin, it is necessary to look at the P_{CO_2} and the serum bicarbonate level. In respiratory acidosis, the P_{CO_2} is increased; in metabolic acidosis, the serum bicarbonate level is lower than normal. Each type of acidosis is covered in the discussion about P_{CO_2} and serum bicarbonate levels. Note in Table 6–7 that newborns with low Apgar scores tend to have a proportionately low pH.

TABLE 6–7. RELATIONSHIP OF APGAR SCORES TO pH LEVEL IN NEWBORN

Sign	Score 0	Score 1	Score 2
Heart rate	Absent	Less than 100 beats/min	More than 100 beats/min
Respiratory rate	Absent	Low, irregular, hypoventilate	Good, crying lustily
Muscle tone	Flaccid	Some flexion of extremities	Active motion, well-flexed
Reflexes	No response	Cry, some motion, grimace	Vigorous cry
Color	Blue, pale	Body pink, hands and feet blue	Completely pink

APGAR SCORE	ESTIMATE OF pH
7 or greater	7.27
6 or less	7.22

Note: Apgar score is a simple and practical method to assess the overall physical status of the infant immediately after delivery. It is assessed 1 min and 5 min after birth. Although it is usually assumed that this score reflects the degree of neonatal asphyxia, DeCherney and Pernoll (1994) caution that recent studies suggest that there is poor correlation between Apgar scores and the degree of acidosis, particularly in premature infants. Asphyxia should be diagnosed only after cord blood determinations.

▼ POSSIBLE NURSING DIAGNOSES RELATED TO ACIDOTIC STATES

Risk for Injury Related to Change in Level of Consciousness

Specific nursing implications depend on whether the acidosis is respiratory or metabolic in nature. General symptoms for both types of acidosis include headaches, weakness, lethargy, and confusion. The level of consciousness is depressed as the acidotic state worsens. Unless the acidotic state is corrected, drowsiness leads from a stuporous state to coma and eventually to death.

Altered Breathing Patterns

As with alkalotic states, the respiratory patterns are opposites for the two types of acidosis. In respiratory acidosis, the respiratory rate is decreased because hypoventilation is the cause of respiratory acidosis. An ineffective breathing pattern is the focus of care. In metabolic acidosis, the respiratory rate is faster and deeper than normal (Kussmaul's respirations) because the lungs are trying to compensate for the decreased serum pH by expiring more carbon dioxide. Because the rate is a compensatory one, the breathing pattern is not a focus of care.

▼ PARTIAL PRESSURE OF CARBON DIOXIDE

The P_{CO_2} test measures the partial pressure of carbon dioxide in the arterial blood. As noted earlier, when carbon dioxide is transported in serum, much of it is combined with water to form carbonic acid ($H_2CO_3^-$), which dissociates into bicarbonate (HCO_3^-) and hydrogen (H^+) ions. The actual carbonic acid level in the serum is not measured, but it can always be determined by multiplying the P_{CO_2} by 3%. A P_{CO_2} of 40 mm Hg is 1.2 mEq of carbonic acid (40 × 3%). Because the end result is an increase in the amount of free hydrogen ions, an increase in P_{CO_2} causes blood pH to drop to less than 7.35.

REFERENCE VALUES FOR P_{CO_2}	
Adult	35–45 mm Hg (arterial) 41–51 mm Hg (venous) Values are slightly lower in women
Pregnancy	Values may be 30 mm Hg by the end of the second trimester. 30–37 mm Hg is normal for pregnancy because of hyperventilation. The kidneys compensate by excreting more bicarbonate, so the pH of about 7.4 is maintained
Altitude	At higher altitudes the atmospheric pressure is lower, so the P_{CO_2} is proportionately reduced. (See discussion of P_{O_2} values)

Increased P_{CO_2} (Hypercarbia or Hypercapnia)

Clinical Significance in Respiratory Acidosis. An increased P_{CO_2} indicates that the normal amount of carbon dioxide is not being expired. Any situation that causes hypoventilation, such as a drug overdose that results in respiratory depression, causes an elevated P_{CO_2}. Higher-than-normal P_{CO_2} levels are also present in certain chronic lung conditions in which the exchange of carbon dioxide and oxygen is impaired. Clients with chronic obstructive pulmonary disease (COPD) may have both hypoxia and hypercarbia (elevated P_{CO_2}), although the latter is not always associated with hypoxia. Some acute lung dysfunctions, such as pneumonia, may cause hypoxia but not an elevated P_{CO_2}. Hypoxia does not always lead to a retention of carbon dioxide for two basic reasons. First, carbon dioxide diffuses more readily across alveolar surfaces than does oxygen, so an impairment of respiratory function results in a decrease in P_{O_2} before the P_{CO_2} changes. Second, hypoxia is a stimulus for breathing. If the lungs can respond to the low oxygen level by increasing the respiratory rate, the carbon dioxide level may stay normal or drop below normal because of the hyperventilation.

The type of hypoventilation that causes an increased P_{CO_2} can be transitory and self-limiting, such as when the breath is held. The resultant high level of P_{CO_2} cannot be maintained because it becomes an overpowering stimulus for taking a breath—one cannot commit suicide by holding one's breath. Clients with chronic lung disease who have high carbon dioxide levels no longer use carbon dioxide as a stimulus for breathing. Instead, hypoxia becomes the primary stimulus for breathing, and the kidneys compensate for the gradual increase in P_{CO_2} by increasing the serum bicarbonate level. The normal blood pH is maintained as long as the kidneys can keep the 20:1 ratio of bicarbonate to carbonic acid. It takes the kidneys several days to compensate for increasing P_{CO_2}, so a quick increase in P_{CO_2}, or acute respiratory failure, leads to respiratory acidosis.

Clinical Significance in Metabolic Alkalosis. In metabolic alkalosis, the P_{CO_2} is usually more than 40 mm Hg because the lungs are attempting to reestablish the bicarbonate–carbonic acid ratio by increasing the carbonic acid to match the increased serum bicarbonate. This compensatory hypoventilation is not effective because the respiratory rate cannot be depressed appreciably without causing hypoxia.

▼ POSSIBLE NURSING DIAGNOSES RELATED TO HYPERCAPNIA

Altered Sensory-Perceptual Awareness Related to Change in Level of Consciousness

Nurses must always be aware of the early signs of increasing P_{CO_2} levels. The term *CO_2 narcosis,* another name for respiratory acidosis, gives a clue that carbon dioxide can be a central nervous system depressant. Early signs of in-

(*continued*)

▼ POSSIBLE NURSING DIAGNOSES RELATED TO HYPERCAPNIA (*continued*)

creased Pco_2 may be headache, dizziness, and confusion. The confusion may progress to decreasing levels of consciousness until the patient is comatose. The treatment of respiratory depression may include assisted ventilation until the underlying pathophysiologic condition can be treated. Nursing interventions are geared toward improving respiratory status. Frequent ABGs help to monitor the improvement of the client and ensure that increasing carbon dioxide levels are not occurring.

The seriousness of an elevated Pco_2 can be evaluated only in relation to the amount of compensation that has occurred. For example, clients with chronic lung disease may have a higher-than-normal Pco_2 with a higher-than-normal bicarbonate level and a resulting normal pH. Chronic hypercapnia is usually well tolerated (Ferguson and Cherniack, 1993). However, a drug that depresses the respiratory center or a respiratory infection, may throw such compensated clients into respiratory acidosis, or CO_2 narcosis.

Risk for Injury Related to Use of Oxygen and Sedatives in Clients with Chronic Obstructive Pulmonary Disease

High doses of oxygen can be lethal for clients who have a chronically high Pco_2 because hypoxia has become the respiratory stimulus for the client. The medullary center no longer responds to high levels of Pco_2, which is normally the primary stimulus for respiration, because the chronically elevated Po_2 has made the center insensitive to carbon dioxide as a stimulus for breathing. The only stimulus for breathing is hypoxia. For clients with advanced emphysema, a Po_2 of 50–60 mm Hg is "normal." The client's color may improve as the hypoxia is eliminated, but respirations become slower and slower because the client no longer has a stimulus to breathe. If these clients are not stimulated to breathe, Pco_2 rises even higher, and they may die in respiratory acidosis. Goldstein et al. (1984) found that supplemental oxygen could be given at night to clients who have *stable* but severe COPD to prevent a fall of Po_2 with sleep.

Very small doses of drugs, such as morphine or some sedatives, can depress respiration to a serious degree, because the response to hypoxia is depressed. (See the discussion of Po_2 on ways to assess and intervene for hypoxia in clients with acute or chronic respiratory problems.)

Decreased Pco_2

Clinical Significance in Respiratory Alkalosis. Just as hypoventilation leads to an increased Pco_2, hyperventilation leads to a decreased Pco_2. (The terms *hypocarbia* or *hypocapnia* are sometimes used.) Often hyperventilation is due to severe anxiety.

Hysterical or semihysterical people tend to breathe rapidly and deeply, with a lot of sighing. Physical conditions, such as fever, pain, or hypoxia, also can cause hyperventilation. No matter what the stimulus, the end result is that if enough carbon dioxide to lower the PCO_2 is expired, the client experiences respiratory alkalosis.

Some people may have a slightly low PCO_2 most of the time, but usually this form of chronic hyperventilation is not noticed until the client has an acute anxiety attack (Waites, 1978). It is unusual to see compensation for respiratory alkalosis, because severe hyperventilation typically does not last long enough for the kidneys to begin to excrete extra bicarbonate. An exception, however, is a client using a respirator: An improperly adjusted respirator can be responsible for hyperventilation that continues over a long time.

Clinical Significance in Metabolic Acidosis. A lower-than-normal PCO_2 can be a compensatory mechanism for metabolic acidosis. For example, clients in diabetic acidosis use up much of the bicarbonate buffer in their bloodstream to buffer the ketone bodies. The lungs try to restore the 20:1 ratio by reducing the PCO_2 and hence the carbonic acid part of the ratio (Kussmaul's respirations), but this compensation cannot offset the severe metabolic acidosis.

▼ POSSIBLE NURSING DIAGNOSES RELATED TO HYPOCAPNIA

Altered Comfort Related to Neuromuscular Irritability

Most of the symptoms that result from a lowered PCO_2, which can be alarming to the client and to the nurse, can be explained by the effect of an alkaline pH on serum calcium levels. Because calcium is less soluble in an alkaline medium, less ionized calcium is available when the blood pH rises above normal. Hence the client has symptoms of hypocalcemia. (See Chapter 7 for the symptoms of hypocalcemia.) There may be tingling of the fingers, twitching, muscle tremors, carpopedal spasms, and even tetany. The person may feel light-headed and dizzy. If the hyperventilation is less severe and more of a chronic problem, the person may have only symptoms such as chronic exhaustion or diffuse weakness.

Nurses in emergency departments or outpatient clinics are the ones most likely to see clients who are seeking treatment because of hyperventilation. Recognizing that the client is hyperventilating is easy, but assessing whether it is due to anxiety or to physical causes may not be so easy. Ruling out fever, pain, or hypoxia as the reason for the hyperventilation is important. (If the hyperventilation is due to an underlying metabolic acidosis, there will be no symptoms of alkalosis because the pH remains acid from the metabolic problem.)

(continued)

▼ POSSIBLE NURSING DIAGNOSES RELATED TO HYPOCAPNIA (*continued*)

Anxiety Related to Unknown Factors

If the hyperventilation is due to functional anxiety, nursing interventions can be instrumental in stopping the hyperventilation. The client needs to be reassured that slower breathing will decrease the symptoms. Breathing into a paper bag helps to increase the $P{CO_2}$ level. The nurse needs to maintain a calm, soothing environment so the client can gain control and reduce the feeling of anxiety. Hyperventilating may be a recurring problem that warrants a referral for counseling to help the client learn ways to deal with anxiety. If the anxiety level is high, the physician may order drugs to reduce the anxiety. Sometimes the client may need to be taught the proper method of diaphragmatic breathing. The long-term goal is to help the client deal with the anxiety and to see how the anxiety has caused the breathing problem.

Ineffective Breathing Pattern Related to Hypoxia and Other Causes

The nurse needs to be aware of other situations in which hyperventilating may occur. For example, a client in labor may not be performing her breathing exercises correctly and thus may experience respiratory alkalosis. Also, clients using respirators need careful monitoring to make sure that the ventilation rate is not too fast. If hyperventilation is due to a stimulus such as fever, therapeutic measures to reduce the fever eliminate the hyperventilation. The most likely cause of respiratory alkalosis, other than anxiety, is hypoxia. (See the discussion of $P{O_2}$ levels.) Paper bag rebreathing can reduce oxygen levels sufficiently to endanger hypoxic clients (Callahan, 1989).

▼ SERUM BICARBONATE AND TOTAL CARBON DIOXIDE CONTENT

Bicarbonate functions as an important buffer in the bloodstream. To keep the pH in the bloodstream between 7.35 and 7.45, the bicarbonate in it is kept at a 20:1 ratio to carbonic acid. The section on $P{CO_2}$ explained how changes in $P{CO_2}$ cause changes in bicarbonate level. Also, because bicarbonate and chloride are both negative ions in the serum, an increased retention of serum chloride means less retention of bicarbonate. Thus serum bicarbonate measurements are useful in both acid–base imbalances and electrolyte imbalances, and they are therefore a routine part of laboratory tests for either electrolytes or arterial blood gases.

Direct and Indirect Methods to Measure Bicarbonate

Several different laboratory methods measure serum bicarbonate level. Some laboratories may perform direct measurements of the bicarbonate and report it as such.

One indirect method involves measuring the total carbon dioxide content of the serum and calculating the bicarbonate level from this figure. An older method involves measuring the carbon dioxide combining power of the serum.

Nurses do not need to understand the technicalities of how these various tests are performed, but it is important to use the reference values that correspond to the exact method used by a specific laboratory. There is less standardization of bicarbonate measurement than with the other electrolytes. If a laboratory report does not have an item marked *bicarbonate,* look for *total carbon dioxide content* or *carbon dioxide capacity,* which reflects the bicarbonate component of the blood. This carbon dioxide content is different from the P_{CO_2} in a blood gas measurement.

Meaning of "Base Excess" or "Base Deficit"

Most laboratories also measure the total buffer base of the body and report this as a *base deficit* or a *base excess.* The *buffer base* refers to all the buffer ions in the serum, including not only bicarbonate but also phosphates, hemoglobin (hgb), and plasma proteins. The total buffers are usually about 50 mEq/L, but the laboratory reports only so many minus or plus milliequivalents. The normal would be a −2 mEq to a +2 mEq. More than a −2 mEq means a *base deficit,* which correlates to a decrease in bicarbonate levels. A result of more than 2 mEq signifies a *base excess,* which correlates with an increased bicarbonate level. The base excess may be a better indicator of metabolic status than the bicarbonate level (Anderson, 1990).

REFERENCE VALUES FOR BICARBONATE	
Adult	24–30 mEq/L
Pregnancy	Falls early in pregnancy by an amount consistent with the fall in P_{CO_2}. A P_{CO_2} of 34 mm Hg is balanced with a bicarbonate of about 20 mEq to keep the pH about 7.4
Newborn	20–26 mEq/L (Premature infants may have even lower reference values)
Children	Slightly lower references than those for adults
Base excess or base deficit	−2 to +2 mEq/L

Bicarbonate levels measured by carbon dioxide content.

Increased Serum Bicarbonate Level (Base Excess)

Clinical Significance in Metabolic Alkalosis. The loss of hydrogen, potassium, and chloride ions all contribute to the development of metabolic alkalosis. First, any loss of hydrogen ions causes a proportional increase in the bicarbonate side of the bicarbonate–carbonic acid buffering system. Second, as discussed in Chapter 5, when potassium is low in the serum, the kidneys are unable to excrete bicarbonate normally. Third, when chloride, a negative ion, is decreased in the bloodstream, another negative ion is needed to keep the positive and negative ions balanced in the serum. Thus the kidneys cause a retention of bicarbonate to replace the missing chloride.

The most common reason for an increase in the bicarbonate level is a loss of gastric contents. Clients who vomit or who have nasogastric suctioning without proper potassium chloride replacement (KCl) are prone to have high bicarbonate levels. Clients taking diuretics may also lose abnormal amounts of chloride and potassium and thus experience metabolic alkalosis.

An increase in the serum bicarbonate level can also occur with the ingestion of large amounts of sodium bicarbonate. As a home remedy, clients may take baking soda (soda bicarbonate), which is systemically absorbed. Commercial antacids, such as Maalox, are usually not systemically absorbed, so they do not cause alkalosis, but they may contribute to metabolic alkalosis if there is inadequate renal function. Alkalosis can also occur from overdosage with intravenous soda bicarbonate to treat acidosis. In the past, sodium bicarbonate was considered one of the primary drugs for cardiac arrest. Now the American Heart Association (1992) considers it acceptable only for types of acidosis that are bicarbonate-responsive. Bicarbonate is not recommended for most cardiac arrests, which are most likely hypoxic lactic acidosis. (See the discussion of lactic acid at the end of this chapter.)

Clinical Significance in Respiratory Acidosis. An increased serum bicarbonate level is a compensatory mechanism for the elevated P_{CO_2} of a client with chronic lung disease. The increased bicarbonate level is necessary to keep the pH of the serum normal.

▼ POSSIBLE NURSING DIAGNOSES RELATED TO ELEVATED BICARBONATE LEVELS

Risk for Injury Related to Neuromuscular Irritability

Usually clients with metabolic alkalosis do not have many symptoms directly related to the acid–base imbalance. Their respiration may be slow because their lungs are trying to compensate by conserving carbon dioxide. The change in respiratory rate is usually too slight to be clinically significant. Observable symptoms are related to the decreased solubility of calcium in an alkaline pH. As with respiratory alkalosis, clients may experience neuromuscular irritability, tingling in the fingers, twitching of the nose or lips, and even tetany or convulsions if the alkalosis is not corrected. Safety measures should be instituted.

Risk for Altered Cardiac Output Related to Arrhythmias

Because hypokalemia is associated with metabolic alkalosis, the client must be monitored for cardiac arrhythmias and will most likely need both potassium and chloride replacement (Table 6–5). Nursing implications for potassium chloride administration are covered in Chapter 5. The client may be given isotonic solutions intravenously to replenish the loss of chlorides. Fruit juices and broth may be given in less severe depletions of chloride and potassium.

Knowledge Deficit Related to Danger of Sodium Bicarbonate

If the client has a history of increased intake of soda bicarbonate, stopping the ingestion is usually enough to correct the base excess. Clients need to be taught that baking soda is not a desirable antacid because it is absorbed into the bloodstream.

Decreased Serum Bicarbonate Level (Base Deficit)

Clinical Significance in Metabolic Acidosis. Unless the client has a low P_{CO_2}, and thus a low serum bicarbonate level as compensation, a decrease in the serum bicarbonate level is an indication that the client has metabolic acidosis. The severity of the acidotic state depends on how low the blood pH has dropped. The decrease in serum bicarbonate level that occurs in metabolic acidotic states can be due to

1. Utilization of the bicarbonate to buffer acids, such as excessive lactate, ketone bodies, or other toxic metabolics, that contain hydrogen ions (the most common type of metabolic acidosis seen clinically)
2. A primary loss of bicarbonate
3. An increase in serum chloride level

Increased Production of Acids. In a normal state of health, as acids are produced or introduced into the body, they are neutralized by the bicarbonate–carbonic acid buffering system and eventually excreted by the kidneys. With a sudden increase in acids in certain pathologic states, the kidneys do not have enough time to excrete the acids or enough bicarbonate to neutralize them.

1. In diabetic acidosis, the acids produced are the ketone bodies
2. In shock, the tissue hypoxia results in an excessive buildup of lactic acid (see test for lactic acid at end of chapter)
3. In renal failure or in severe dehydration, the kidneys can no longer excrete hydrogen ions or acids such as the phosphates and sulfates
4. In cardiac arrest, there is an immediate buildup of lactic acid (as well as a high P_{CO_2}, so the client has both respiratory and metabolic acidosis)
5. Aspirin overdose floods the system with an acid. (Initially the acetylsalicylic acid [ASA] acts as a respiratory stimulant that causes respiratory alkalosis, but the end result may be acidosis)

Concept of Anion Gap. The lactates, phosphates, ketone bodies, and other acids that can cause metabolic acidosis are negative ions (anions) in the bloodstream. So an increase in these acids increases the anion gap, which is the amount of unmeasured negative ions or anions in the bloodstream (see Chapter 5). It is determined by comparing the total amount of positive ions in the serum (primarily sodium and potassium) with the total amount of negative ions in the serum (primarily chloride and bicarbonate). When the total positive and the negative ions are compared in the bloodstream, there is a gap because one type of negative ion, namely, the acids, are not measured. Usually, the unmeasured acids account for about 8–16 mEq of the total negative ions (Ravel, 1995).

In metabolic acidosis, the increase in the negative ions of ketoacids, lactate, phosphate, sulfate, or other acids makes the anion gap larger because more unmeasured negative ions are present in the bloodstream. The anion gap may be as high as 25 mEq/L in severe ketoacidosis or lactic acidosis (Kaplan et al., 1995). The anion gap is useful in differentiating this first type of metabolic acidosis from the other two types because in them there is no increase in the acids that comprise the unmeasured negative ions and therefore no increase in the anion gap.

Primary Loss of Bicarbonate. A primary loss of bicarbonate can occur with gastrointestinal losses below the pylorus because the intestinal tract and pancreatic secretions are rich in bicarbonate. (As a rule, gastrointestinal losses above the pylorus, such as vomiting or gastric suctioning, tend to cause alkalosis because of the loss of hydrogen, potassium, and chloride ions. So alkalosis is related to vomiting and acidosis to diarrhea. However, dehydration from either vomiting or diarrhea is likely to result in acidosis because of the inability of the kidney to excrete acid byproducts.) The primary loss of bicarbonate (a negative ion) leads to an increased chloride level to keep the positive and negative charges balanced in the serum. The anion gap does not increase.

Increase in the Serum Chloride Level. A primary increase in the serum chloride level means that another negative ion, bicarbonate, must be proportionally decreased. The lowering of serum bicarbonate level keeps the electrical charges of the serum electrolytes balanced, but it causes acidosis because the buffering ability of the serum is decreased.

This third type of metabolic acidosis (hyperchloremic acidosis) is a much less common clinical occurrence than the first two types. High doses of chlorides in intravenous infusions may raise the serum chloride level. Also, some types of renal failure result in an inability to excrete chloride ions properly.

▼ POSSIBLE NURSING DIAGNOSES RELATED TO LOW SERUM BICARBONATE LEVELS

Risk for Injury Related to Altered Sensory Perceptions and Level of Consciousness

It is important for nurses to recognize early symptoms of acidosis, because severe acidosis can be life-threatening. When a client has a lowered serum bicarbonate level that is causing metabolic acidosis, one of the key symptoms is hyperventilation. This deep and rapid respiration (Kussmaul's respirations) is an attempt to restore the 20:1 bicarbonate–carbonic acid ratio by decreasing the carbonic acid in the blood. (Recall that 3% of the PCO_2 is carried in the bloodstream as carbonic acid.) These fast and deep respirations may look like the client has "air hunger," but they really reflect an attempt to expire extra PCO_2. This increased respiratory rate may be one of the first clues that the pH is dropping. As the pH drops lower, the client begins to exhibit signs of confusion, lethargy, and eventually coma. (A diabetic coma is a form of severe metabolic acidosis.) Newborn infants can experience severe metabolic acidosis if they are not kept warm and given sufficient calories. Acidosis can develop immediately, such as with a cardiac arrest, or slowly, as in a client with renal failure. Some clients with diabetes who do not take their insulin may go into a coma within a day or so. A young child with diabetes may go into acidosis very quickly, whereas an adult with diabetes may not experience ketoacidosis until after several days have elapsed. The important thing is to know the type of situation that can lead to metabolic acidosis so any changes can be detected early.

The most important goal of treatment is to eliminate the cause of the acidosis. A cold-stressed newborn must be warmed and fed. A client with diabetes requires insulin so that glucose, rather than fats, can be used as the primary source of energy. Clients in shock must have increased oxygen perfusion at the cellular level to replace the anaerobic metabolism that has caused a buildup of lactic acid (see lactic acid measurement at end of this chapter).

Risk for Injury Related to Intravenous Use of Sodium Bicarbonate

Although the goal of treatment is to eliminate the cause of the acidosis, the client may need sodium bicarbonate administered intravenously to bring the serum pH back to normal immediately. Sodium bicarbonate may be given in direct intravenous push or in a continuous intravenous infusion. Other drugs should not be mixed with the bicarbonate solution because they may precipitate in an alkaline pH. For example, calcium precipitates in a strongly alkaline pH.

The respiratory rate is one objective assessment of the effectiveness of therapy. When clients with acidosis are given sodium bicarbonate, the hyperventilation decreases as the pH of the blood returns to normal. Sometimes the client may be given enough sodium bicarbonate to produce rebound metabolic alkalosis. Monitoring laboratory tests can prevent this. In an acute emergency, such as a cardiac arrest, it is essential that someone, usually the nurse, keep a detailed record of all the medications given the client.

Altered Fluid and Electrolyte Balance Related to Acidosis

Close monitoring of the intake and output for clients in acidosis is essential to prevent severe dehydration and further electrolyte imbalances. During acidotic states, more hydrogen ions go into the cells, and potassium ions are

(*continued*)

▼ POSSIBLE NURSING DIAGNOSES RELATED TO LOW SERUM BICARBONATE LEVELS (*continued*)

forced out. Hyperkalemia is associated with acidotic states. The potassium that leaves the cells is eventually excreted by the kidneys so that the aftermath of metabolic acidosis is a depletion of total body potassium. As discussed earlier in the section on anion gap, chloride levels increase in some type of acidosis. Sodium may also be depleted, particularly in diabetic acidosis in which diuresis has been a prominent feature. A nurse caring for a client who is recovering from metabolic acidosis must be aware of all the nursing implications for changes in each of these electrolytes, each of which is discussed in Chapter 5.

▼ PARTIAL PRESSURE OF OXYGEN

The Po_2 measures the amount of oxygen dissolved in the blood. The partial pressure is calculated by multiplying the amount of gas in a solution (%) by the total pressure (mm Hg, or millimeters of mercury). Hence the laboratory reports the Po_2 as "so many millimeters of mercury (mm Hg)." In a healthy young person, arterial blood may have about 13% oxygen dissolved in the plasma. At sea level, the Po_2 is 13% times 760 mm Hg or 98.8 mm Hg. As can be seen by the reference values, breathing pure oxygen, moving to a high altitude, or simply aging makes quite a difference in the partial pressure of oxygen in the bloodstream.

REFERENCE VALUES FOR Po_2

Adult	75–100 mm Hg while breathing room air. May be greater than 225 mm Hg if breathing 40% oxygen (with normal lungs)
Newborn	60–70 mm Hg are usually given as maximum reference values, or 40–60 mm Hg in some laboratories
Aged[a]	The Po_2 drops about 3–5 mm Hg for each decade after 30 years of age. After 70 years of age a Po_2 of about 85 mm Hg is the maximum reference value
Location	In high altitudes, such as Denver, where the atmospheric pressure is 670 mm Hg, the maximum reference value for a person younger than 30 years is about 87 mm Hg

[a]**The relation between age and Po_2 can be approximated by the formula**

$$Po_2 = 104 - [\text{age} \times 0.27]$$

Increased Po_2

Clinical Significance. The only clinical situation that creates a high Po_2 is the administration of high doses of oxygen. One hundred percent oxygen may increase the Po_2 to more than 500 mm Hg (Sculley, 1986). Whether high oxygen pressures in the blood can alter certain bodily conditions, such as aging, is a controversial subject that is being explored.

▼ POSSIBLE NURSING DIAGNOSES RELATED TO ELEVATED Po_2

Risk for Injury Related to Prolonged Use of High Levels of Oxygen

Retinopathy of prematurity (ROP), formerly called retrolental fibroplasia, is associated with prolonged exposure to high blood concentrations of oxygen. Oxygen alone was once thought to be the culprit for retrolental fibroplasia, but recent studies indicate that high oxygen blood levels are but one of the factors in ROP (DeCherney and Pernoll, 1994). Prolonged use of oxygen for clients of all ages can cause drying of the airways and even permanent lung damage (Nielson, 1980). In adults, oxygen toxicity in the lungs is related not to its concentration or to the Po_2 but to the partial pressure of inspired oxygen (Bongard and Sue, 1994).

The nurse should question any order for the prolonged use (>8 hr) of 100% oxygen. In severe and complicated cases of hypoxia, the client may have to receive high concentrations of oxygen for an extended period. Frequent monitoring of blood gases is necessary to evaluate whether the oxygen therapy is satisfactory and whether lower concentrations of oxygen can be used. D'Agostino (1983) noted that the general rule is to use the lowest possible amount of inspired air, that is oxygen (FIo_2), to keep the Po_2 no more than 90 mm Hg unless special circumstances, such as carbon monoxide intoxication, require higher Po_2 levels. Toxicity to oxygen rarely develops if the FIo_2 is kept less than 40%. (See the section on elevated Pco_2 for the special dangers of oxygen therapy for some clients with obstructive disease.)

Decreased Arterial Po_2

Clinical Significance. Many different conditions can cause hypoxia, which is usually defined as a Po_2 of less than 70 mm Hg in adults. With atelectasis or emphysema there may be ventilation to blood flow abnormalities so that oxygen does not reach the bloodstream. Hypoventilation, such as in a client who has taken a respiratory depressant, causes hypoxia. Anatomic defects, such as when arterial and venous blood intermix, cause hypoxia. In essence, any situation that interferes with CO_2-O_2 exchange leads to a lowered Po_2.

Because the Pco_2 may be elevated, normal, or decreased with a decreased Po_2, it is important to look at the laboratory reports for both Pco_2 and pH when evaluating the clinical significance of a low Po_2. With many types of hypoxia, the Pco_2 may remain normal because carbon dioxide can diffuse much more readily than oxygen can across alveolar surfaces. If the hypoxia state is causing marked hyperventilation, the P_{CO_2} may actually drop below normal. For example, with pneumonia, both the P_{O_2} and P_{CO_2} may be lower than normal. The infection in the lungs interferes with oxygen exchange more than with carbon dioxide exchange. The hypoxia leads to hyperventilation in an attempt to increase oxygen. The hyperventilation causes more expiration of carbon dioxide, so the P_{CO_2} becomes lower than normal (respiratory alkalosis). In respiratory depression, such as that caused by general anesthesia, lowered P_{O_2} levels cannot stimulate increased respiration, so the P_{CO_2} level rises (respiratory acidosis). In chronic lung disease, hypoxia may occur alone or with an increase in P_{CO_2} as the lung damage becomes worse. The clinical significance of hypoxia, compounded by hypercapnia (high P_{CO_2}), is quite different from that of hypoxia alone, as noted earlier.

▼ POSSIBLE NURSING DIAGNOSES RELATED TO HYPOXIA OR LOW P_{O_2} LEVELS

Altered Tissue Perfusion Related to Hypoxia

The nurse may be instrumental in preventing serious complications from hypoxia by detecting it before cyanosis occurs, which is a late symptom of hypoxia. Peripheral cyanosis that occurs in the nailbeds reflects poor peripheral perfusion, but not necessarily an extremely low P_{O_2}. Tissue hypoxia is not synonymous with arterial hypoxia. Central cyanosis is best assessed by looking at the tongue. In adults, the P_{O_2} is less than 50 mm Hg by the time central cyanosis occurs. The blue of central cyanosis denotes at least 5 g of unoxygenated hgb in the arterial blood—or more than one-third of the total hgb in the blood. The nurse needs to look for early symptoms of hypoxia, such as tachycardia and restlessness. By the time this one-third or more of the hgb is unsaturated, the client may be in distress. Lack of oxygen to the myocardium can alter cardiac output and produce arrhythmias.

Assessing for Cyanosis in Dark-Skinned Clients. Because cyanosis is difficult to assess in dark-skinned clients, nurses must become familiar with the client's precyanotic color. When cyanosis is suspected, nurses can press on the skin to produce pallor. In cyanotic tissue the color returns slowly by spreading from the periphery to the center. Also the lips and tongue become ashen gray in a black client with cyanosis (Bloch and Hunter, 1981).

Risk for Injury Related to Use of Oxygen

When oxygen is ordered for a client with hypoxia, nurses must make sure that the safety and comfort of the client are maintained. Clients and family need clear instructions about the danger of smoking. Discontinuing oxygen for just a few minutes may cause a considerable drop in the P_{O_2} of some clients, and it may take as long as 20 min to restore the previous level (Felton, 1978). Because hypoxia can contribute to the development of severe cardiac arrhythmias, 100% oxygen may be given before and after suctioning. However, rather than providing hyperoxygenation by increasing the inspired oxygen concentration, one can use a double-lumen oxygen insufflation catheter to continue the flow of oxygen during endotracheal suctioning (Dam et al., 1994). The nurse may also use the pulse oximeter, discussed later, to determine whether oxygen therapy can be interrupted for oral temperatures, feedings, or other procedures. Some clients with a chronically low Po_2 may have home oxygen, so they need instructions on the safety measures needed for long-term oxygen therapy. The most objective assessment of the need for continual oxygen therapy is the blood gas report. A client using a ventilator may have blood gases drawn frequently to assess if the ventilator is properly adjusted. (See the section on elevated Po_2 for the danger of a prolonged high Po_2.) Clients who have chronic hypoxia may often be undergoing oxygen therapy at home. The goal is usually to keep the oxygen saturation above 90% or a Pao_2 of 60 mm Hg, which is slightly higher than the standard criteria of 88 or 89% or a Pao_2 of 55 mm Hg for reimbursable oxygen therapy (Ferguson and Cherniack, 1993). Clients may need to try several methods of oxygen delivery to determine what is therapeutic and cost effective.

Impaired Gas Exchange Related to Factors Other than Simple Hypoxia

For some clients with hypoxia, oxygen may not be the primary need. For example, if the hypoxia is due to mucous plugs blocking some of the airways, coughing, deep breathing, and maybe suctioning need to be instituted. If hypoxia is due to an acute condition, such as an asthmatic attack, hydration and bronchodilation are as important as oxygenation. When a client is allowed to stay in one position, not all areas of the lungs are equally ventilated; so some unoxygenated blood goes back to the left atrium. This is called *physiologic shunting.* By changing the client's position frequently, physiologic shunting does not add to the problem of hypoxia. However, if the hypoxia is due to poor cardiac output, changing positions often may be tiring to the client and not a top priority. It is important to understand the reason for the hypoxic state so that nursing measures are geared to help the client use oxygen effectively and conserve energy so that oxygen need is not increased.

The possible nursing implications for clients with a low Po_2 and a high Pco_2 are covered in the section on Pco_2. It is essential for the nurse to understand the danger of giving high concentrations of oxygen to clients who have hypoxia coupled with a chronically increased Pco_2. Recall that a client with chronic emphysema who has an elevated Pco_2 and a "normal" Po_2 of 50–60 mm Hg is using the hypoxia as a stimulus for breathing.

(*continued*)

▼ POSSIBLE NURSING DIAGNOSES RELATED TO HYPOXIA OR LOW Po_2 LEVELS (*continued*)

Anxiety Related to Dyspnea

Some clients, such as those with lung cancer or other destructive lung diseases, may have continual problems with dyspnea because their Po_2 is chronically low and oxygen therapy is of limited use. Maxwell (1985) suggested that nurses can help these clients recognize their anxiety and how it contributes to their breathlessness. Specific items taught to help restore control and power over the shortness of breath (SOB) include controlled breathing through pursed lips, relaxation techniques, work simplification measures, and breathing techniques to use in activities of daily living. Research is continuing on factors that promote functional performance in clients with COPD (Leidy, 1995).

▼ OXYGEN SATURATION

Because the Po_2 measures the amount of dissolved oxygen in the blood, not the amount of oxygen carried by the hgb, one must determine the oxygen saturation of the blood to evaluate its total carrying capacity. If hgb is carrying the normal amount of oxygen, the oxygen saturation is close to 100%. The oxygen saturation of the hgb is affected by the partial pressure of oxygen, by the temperature, by the pH, and by the chemical and physical structure of the hgb itself. Unless there is substantial change in the last three factors, the oxy–hgb dissociation curve can be used to compute the oxygen-carrying capacity of the blood.

REFERENCE VALUES FOR OXYGEN SATURATION

96–100% (arterial sample)
Comparison with Po_2 values (normal pH and temperature):
- 98% = Po_2 of 100 mm Hg
- 95% = Po_2 of 80 mm Hg
- 89% = Po_2 of 60 mm Hg
- 84% = Po_2 of 50 mm Hg
- 35% = Po_2 of 20 mm Hg

Venous blood has about 70–75% oxygen saturation.

Decrease in the Oxygen Saturation

Clinical Significance. Shunting of blood from the venous to the arterial system causes decreased oxygen saturation. The oxygen saturation is also low with carbon monoxide poisoning because carbon monoxide combines with hgb more than 200 times faster than oxygen does. The additional information from the oxygen saturation test is usually part of the assessment of a client who is having cardiac catheterization studies (see Chapter 26). The oxygen saturation is a measurement of the reserve of oxygen in the hgb that can be used to replenish the oxygen dissolved in the plasma (i.e., the Po_2 measured as the blood gas). As noted in the reference values, decreases in oxygen saturation correlate with a decrease in Po_2 although not in a linear manner. Clients with oxygen saturation less than 90% have an increased mortality, so studies are underway to determine which clients are likely to benefit most from pulse oximetry monitoring (POM). For example, severe decreases in saturation are unlikely when clients have normal chest radiographs (Bowton, et al., 1994).

Use of Pulse Oximeter to Monitor Oxygen Saturation

Although blood gases, with oxygen saturation as one component, are the most accurate way to assess for hypoxemia, the pulse oximeter, less costly and more convenient, has become an important tool for nurses to use in many clinical settings. Using a pulse oximeter has been called taking the "fifth vital sign."

Pulse oximeters are noninvasive devices that monitor the oxygen saturation of arterial blood by measuring the amount of light absorbed by hgb in red blood cells. A light-emitting sensor sends beams of light through the tissue, and a light-detecting sensor records the amount of light absorbed by the oxygenated hgb. (The pulse oximeter is called a *pulse* oximeter because it senses arterial blood by pulsation.) A computer converts the absorption rate to a percentage of oxygen saturation, which is displayed on a digital readout along with the pulse rate. Recent advances include built-in indicators of arterial flow that display the strength of the blood flow and a pulse bar that indicates the relative strength of the pulse (Ehrhardt and Daleiden, 1994). Most pulse oximeters store information that can be printed as hard copy.

Capnographs. The end tidal (expired) levels of carbon dioxide can be measured with a carbon dioxide sensor called a *capnograph*. Some pulse oximeters are combined with this feature. A digital display of the oxygen saturation of arterial blood (Sao_2), carbon dioxide level, pulse, and respiratory rates are provided on a bedside monitor.

Preparation of Patient. The pulse oximeter probes must be placed on a site with good circulation. Fingers, earlobes, toes, and the bridge of the nose are all possible sites. Some probes are disposable and must be taped in place. Nondisposable probes use clips. Before attaching the probe to a client, test the functioning of the machine by attaching the probe to a healthy person. If possible, let the client hear the alarm so he or she will be prepared for the sound. Reassure him or her about what steps might be taken if oxygen saturation is too low. Also let the client know that if the probe becomes dislodged, the alarm will go off.

Technical difficulties with the equipment and inadequate blood flow to the extremity can cause false alarms. Changes in hgb levels, the presence of contrast medium (see Chapter 21), and the presence of bright lights may also produce inaccurate readings (Ehrhardt and Graham, 1990).

If a capnograph is an addition to the pulse oximeter, special airway adapters are used to measure end tidal CO_2.

REFERENCE VALUES OF PULSE OXIMETER

Specific orders should be written concerning the lower reference value for the alarm. For example, a saturation of 92% may be desirable for one client, whereas a saturation of 89% is considered permissible for another client. A number lower than the preset range would alert the nurse to assess for the reason for hypoxia and begin appropriate interventions as discussed in the section on low Po_2. A saturation of 100% may indicate more than adequate oxygen therapy because the machine can only register to 100%.

▼ LACTIC ACID OR BLOOD LACTATE

Lactic acid is produced by anaerobic glycolysis and is a normal byproduct of strenuous exercise. Dangerous levels of lactic acid can develop from pathologic conditions that cause prolonged hypoxia. Liver disease can also cause a buildup. (Lactic acidosis is the first type of metabolic acidosis discussed in the section on decreased serum bicarbonate levels.) Lactic acidosis can develop in a short time and almost immediately with a cardiac arrest. Lactic acidosis can also coexist with other types of acidosis such as those brought on by diabetes, dehydration, or renal failure. Lactic acidosis is a probability in any stuporous or comatose client who has a large anion gap (Kaplan et al., 1995) (see Chapter 5 on the anion gap). Lactic acidosis can be idiopathic in a seriously ill client and can be fatal within a short time. Treatment involves taking measures to eliminate cellular hypoxia. A prospective study of the clinical course of lactic acidosis in adults noted most of the causes, such as sepsis, were refractory to care. Most clients had more than one organ failure. Only 17% survived and were discharged from the hospital (Stacpoole et al., 1994).

Gross hemolysis depresses results. Falsely low values occur with high lactic dehydrogenase (LDH) levels. Elevations of lactate may occur with exercise, epinephrine, alcohol, glucose, and sodium bicarbonate infusions.

Preparation of Client and Collection of Sample

Venous or arterial blood is collected in either a gray-topped or green-topped container, depending on the laboratory method. Arterial blood may be more reliable (Ravel, 1995). Note on the laboratory slip whether the blood is arterial or venous, because values differ. The specimen should be packed in ice and analyzed within 15–30 min after collection.

REFERENCE VALUES FOR LACTIC ACID

Venous	1.5–2.2 mEq/L	(0.5–19.8 mg/dL)
Arterial	0.6–1.8 mEq/L	(5.4–16.2 mg/dL)

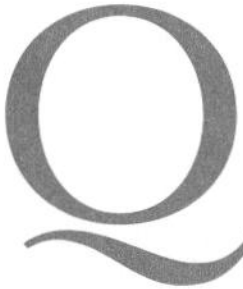

1. In a client with no previous metabolic acid–base imbalances, hyperventilation results in which of the following?

   a. ↓ P_{CO_2} and ↓ pH of serum b. ↓ P_{CO_2} and ↑ pH of serum
   c. ↑ P_{CO_2} and ↑ pH of serum d. ↑ P_{CO_2} and ↓ pH of serum

2. In a client with chronic lung disease, the kidneys can compensate for an elevated P_{CO_2} by which of the following?

   a. Retaining additional HCO_3^- (bicarb)
   b. Excreting more Na^+ and K^+ ions
   c. Excreting carbonic acid
   d. Retaining H^+ ions to balance the P_{CO_2}

3. When a client has blood drawn from the radial artery for arterial blood gases (ABGs), the nurse should

   a. Pack the blood sample in ice for transport to the laboratory
   b. Keep pressure on the puncture site for at least 1 min
   c. Transfer the blood sample to a heparinized test tube
   d. Draw a second sample in 10 min

4. Mrs. Candy is admitted in a diabetic coma. The nursing student reports to the RN that on admission, Mrs. Candy's respirations are rapid (30 per minute) and seem very deep. The RN should do which of the following?

   a. Recheck the respirations because it is unusual to have such a high rate with a coma
   b. Check for signs of infection because this is probably causing the increased rate
   c. Notify the physician that the client is having dyspnea
   d. Ask the students about their understanding of acid–base balance

5. Which of the following assessments by the nurse supports the possibility that a client is going into metabolic acidosis?

   a. Twitching b. Irritability
   c. Slow, shallow breaths d. Difficulty being aroused

6. Michael, a 7-lb newborn, has an Apgar score of 7 (the normal is 10). He lost points for heart rate, respiratory rate, and color. The meperidine (Demerol) given to his mother before delivery has resulted in the newborn having a slight

   a. Metabolic alkalosis (bicarbonate excess)
   b. Respiratory alkalosis (low P_{CO_2})

c. Metabolic acidosis (bicarbonate deficit)
d. Respiratory acidosis (high PCO_2)

7. In a normal pregnancy, blood gases are which of the following?

   a. The same as in the nonpregnant state
   b. A lower PCO_2 and a lower HCO_3^-
   c. A higher PCO_2 and a higher HCO_3^-
   d. A lower PCO_2 and a higher HCO_3^-

8. High concentrations of oxygen may be dangerous for a client with a chronically elevated PCO_2 because the client

   a. May experience respiratory distress because of oxygen toxicity
   b. No longer has hypoxia as a stimulus for breathing
   c. Depends on the PCO_2 as a stimulus for breathing
   d. Has a high PCO_2, not a low PO_2

9. Respiratory alkalosis (low PCO_2) could result from which one of the following situations?

   a. Hypoxia b. Hypokalemia c. Infection d. Narcotic overdose

10. Which *one* of the following clients should be observed for possible signs of tetany if the calcium levels are borderline normal?

    a. Mr. Vick, who had a cardiac arrest yesterday
    b. Ms. Rona, who tends to hyperventilate when she is anxious
    c. Mrs. Degas, who was hypotensive after her delivery today
    d. Baby Fong, who is in respiratory distress

11. Deborah, age 18, is in the emergency department. She says she is having an "anxiety" attack. She complains of feeling light-headed and "shaky" all over. Which action by the nurse would be most appropriate in this situation?

    a. Have Deborah practice taking rapid, deep breaths
    b. Provide a pamphlet on anxiety attacks
    c. Help Deborah identify what has made her so anxious now
    d. Ask Deborah to breathe into a paper bag

12. Which type of loss from the gastrointestinal tract contributes to the development of metabolic alkalosis (high serum bicarbonate)?

    a. Draining fistula from pancreatic cyst b. Gastric suctioning
    c. Diarrhea d. Ileostomy drainage

13. Which one of the following conditions causes a decrease in serum bicarbonate HCO_3^- level?

a. Prolonged increase in PCO_2
b. Increased serum chloride level
c. Markedly increased serum sodium level
d. Increased serum potassium level

14. Jimmy, age 6, has lost an abnormal amount of chlorides because of vomiting. The loss of chlorides contributes to which of the following?

a. Respiratory alkalosis (low PCO_2)
b. Respiratory acidosis (high PCO_2)
c. Metabolic alkalosis (base excess)
d. Metabolic acidosis (base deficit)

15. Betty Parker was admitted to the hospital with severe vomiting of pregnancy. She has been unable to retain any meals or liquids. Her dehydrated and near-starvation state may lead to which of the following?

a. Metabolic acidosis (base deficit)
b. Metabolic alkalosis (base excess)
c. Respiratory acidosis (high PCO_2)
d. Respiratory alkalosis (low PCO_2)

16. Rhonda, a 6-lb 2-oz (2.7 kg) newborn, had a normal Apgar score. A half-hour after birth, her rectal temperature is 96.8°F (36.3°C). She must burn extra calories because she is cold-stressed. Unless she is warmed and fed, she is likely to experience which of the following?

a. Metabolic acidosis (base deficit)
b. Respiratory acidosis (high PCO_2)
c. Metabolic alkalosis (base excess)
d. Respiratory alkalosis (low PCO_2)

17. The anion gap is increased (i.e., the unmeasured negative ions are increased) in which one of these types of acidosis?

a. Primary loss of serum bicarbonate
b. Increase of lactic acid
c. Increase of chlorides
d. Increase of CO_2

18. Mrs. Landino has been receiving sodium bicarbonate intravenously for metabolic acidosis. The nursing assessment that indicates the sodium bicarbonate has restored the blood pH to normal is which of the following?

a. Blood pressure is in normal range
b. Urine output has increased
c. Irritability and muscle spasms decreased
d. Respirations have returned to normal

19. Blood gases drawn on a client reveal a normal PO_2, a slightly low PCO_2, and a slightly high pH. Which of the following clients would most likely have these blood gas results?

a. Mr. Emory, who has chronic emphysema
b. Bobby Black, who is in diabetic acidosis

c. Mrs. Calhoun, who is recovering from anesthesia and has received a considerable amount of muscle relaxants

d. Mrs. Delgado, who has been using breathing exercises during her labor contractions

20. Mr. Cope has been admitted with a diagnosis of respiratory acidosis caused by a chronic lung condition. In his laboratory data, which of the following would be indicative of his acid–base difficulty? (Assume some compensation has occurred.)

a. High blood pH, low P_{CO_2}, high HCO_3^-
b. Low blood pH, high P_{CO_2}, high HCO_3^-
c. High blood pH, low P_{CO_2}, low HCO_3^-
d. Low blood pH, high P_{CO_2}, low HCO_3^-

21. Bill Phillips is using a respirator because of a drug overdose. Which of the following sets of blood gases would be an indication that the respirator needs to be set at a lower rate?

a. P_{CO_2} 60 mm Hg; P_{O_2} 100 mm Hg, pH 7.32; HCO_3^- 28 mEq
b. P_{CO_2} 40 mm Hg; P_{O_2} 80 mm Hg, pH 7.42; HCO_3^- 25 mEq
c. P_{CO_2} 30 mm Hg; P_{O_2} 98 mm Hg, pH 7.56; HCO_3^- 26 mEq
d. P_{CO_2} 45 mm Hg; P_{O_2} 110 mm Hg, pH 7.42; HCO_3^- 29 mEq

▼ REFERENCES

American Heart Association. Emergency Cardiac Care Committee and Subcommittees. (1992). Guidelines for cardiopulmonary resuscitation and emergency cardiac care. *JAMA, 268* (16), 2172–2183.

Anderson, S. (1990). ABGs: Six easy steps to interpreting blood gases. *American Journal of Nursing, 90* (8), 42–45.

Biswas, C., et al. (1982). Blood gas analysis: Effect of air bubbles in syringe and delay in estimation. *British Medical Journal, 284,* 923–927.

Bloch, B., and Hunter, M. (1981). Teaching physiological assessment of black persons. *Nurse Educator, 6,* 24–27.

Bongard, F.S., and Sue, D.Y. (1994). *Current critical care: Diagnosis & treatment.* Norwalk CT: Appleton & Lange.

Bowton, D.L., Scuderi, P.E., and Haponik, E.F. (1994). The incidence and effect on outcome of hypoxemia in hospitalized medical patients. *American Journal of Medicine, 97,* 38–46.

Callahan, M. (1989). Hypoxic hazards of traditional paper bag rebreathing in hyperventilating patients. *Annals of Emergency Medicine, 18* (6), 1989.

Carroll, P. (1987). More arterial blood sampling tricks. *RN, 50* (3), 37.

D'Agostino, J. (1983). Set your mind at ease on oxygen toxicity. *Nursing 83, 13* (7), 55–56.

Dam, V., Wild, M.C., and Baun, M.M. (1994). Effect of oxygen insufflation during endotracheal suctioning on arterial pressure and oxygenation in coronary artery bypass graft patients. *American Journal of Critical Care, 3* (3), 191–197.

DeCherney, A.H., and Pernoll, M.L. (1994). *Current obstetric & gynecologic diagnosis and treatment.* (8th ed.). Norwalk, CT: Appleton & Lange.

Dingle, R., et al. (1980). Continuous transcutaneous O_2 monitoring in the neonate. *American Journal of Nursing, 80* (5), 890–893.

Ehrhardt, B.S., and Daleiden, J. (1994). Pulse oximeters. *Nursing 94, 24* (8), 32 v–32 x.

Ehrhardt, B.S., and Graham, M. (1990). Pulse oximetry: An easy way to check oxygen saturation. *Nursing 90, 20* (3), 50–54.

Felton, C. (1978). Hypoxemia and oral temperatures. *American Journal of Nursing, 78* (1), 56–57.

Ferguson, G.T., and Cherniack, R.M. (1993). Management of chronic obstructive pulmonary disease. *New England Journal of Medicine, 328* (14), 1017–1022.

Goldstein, R., et al. (1984). Effect of supplemental nocturnal oxygen on gas exchange in patients with severe obstructive lung disease. *New England Journal of Medicine, 310* (7), 425–429.

Kaplan, A., Jack, R., Opheim, K.E., et al. (1995). *Clinical chemistry interpretation and techniques.* (4th ed.). Baltimore: Williams & Wilkins.

Leidy, K.L. (1995). Functional performance in people with chronic obstructive pulmonary disease. *Image, 27* (1), 23–24.

Maxwell, M. (1985). Dyspnea in advanced cancer. *American Journal of Nursing, 85* (6), 673–677.

Nielson, L. (1980). Pulmonary oxygen toxicity and other hazards of oxygen therapy. *American Journal of Nursing, 80* (12), 2213–2215.

Preusser, B. (1989). Quantifying the minimum discard sample required for accurate arterial blood gases. *Nursing Research, 38* (5) 276–279.

Ravel, R. (1995). *Clinical laboratory medicine: Clinical application of laboratory data.* (6th ed.). St. Louis: Mosby–Year Book.

Sculley, R. (1986). Normal reference values. *New England Journal of Medicine, 314* (1), 41.

Shively, M., and Clark, A. (1986). Continuous monitoring of mixed venous oxygen saturation: An instrument for research. *Nursing Research, 35* (1), 56–58.

Stacpoole, P.W., Wright, E.C., Baumgartner, T.G., et al. (1994). Natural history and course of acquired lactic acidosis in adults. *American Journal of Medicine, 97,* 47–54.

Stringfield, Y. N. (1993). Back to basics: Acidosis, alkalosis, and ABGs. *American Journal of Nursing, 93* (11), 43–44.

Sumner, S. (1980). Refining your technique for drawing arterial blood gases. *Nursing 80, 10* (4), 65–69.

Tasota, F.J., and Wesmiller, S. W. (1994). Assessing ABGs: Maintaining the delicate balance. *Nursing 94, 24* (5), 34–44.

Waites, T. (1978). Hyperventilation: Chronic and acute. *Archives of Internal Medicine, 138* (11), 1700–1701.

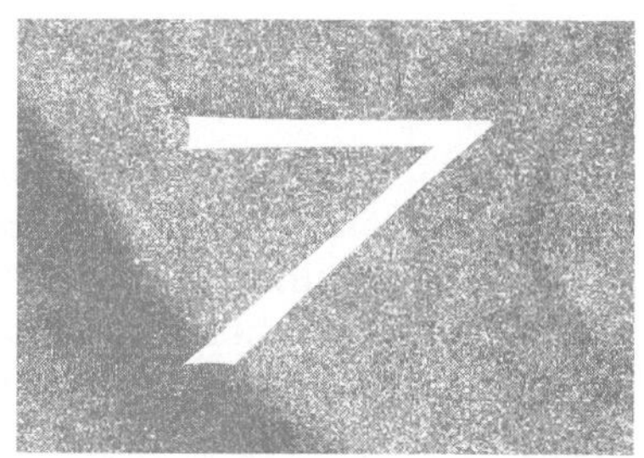

THREE LESS COMMONLY MEASURED ELECTROLYTES

- Serum Calcium
- Urinary Calcium
- Serum Phosphorus or Phosphates
- Urinary Phosphorus or Urine Phosphates
- Serum Magnesium

OBJECTIVES

1. Explain the relation between parathyroid hormone (parathormone) and serum and urine levels of calcium and phosphorus.
2. Identify nursing assessments useful in detecting hypercalcemia or hypocalcemia.
3. Plan appropriate nursing interventions to decrease the harmful effects of hypercalcemia.
4. Analyze clinical situations to determine which clients are likely to have changes in serum phosphorus or calcium levels.
5. Identify potential nursing diagnoses for clients with calcium and phosphorus imbalances.
6. Prepare teaching plans for clients who must decrease or increase calcium and phosphorus intake.
7. Identify nursing assessments useful in detecting serum magnesium excess and deficiency.
8. Identify potential nursing diagnoses for clients with magnesium excess or deficiency.

This chapter covers three electrolytes or minerals that appear in small amounts in the serum: calcium, phosphorus, and magnesium.

Both calcium and phosphorus serum levels are controlled by parathyroid hormone (parathormone or PTH). The end results of an increased secretion of PTH are an increased serum calcium and a decreased serum phosphorus level. Although the serum calcium level often varies inversely with the phosphorus level caused by this hormonal control, both calcium and phosphorus may be increased or decreased together in other clinical situations. Calcium and phosphorus are discussed in separate sections, but the reader needs to be aware that both tests are useful in assessing an imbalance of either electrolyte. In addition, urinary tests for both may give additional information about their overall metabolism. Methods of testing for calcium and phosphorus in the urine are discussed after each section on the electrolytes.

Magnesium is less well understood than the other two electrolytes. It is known that a marked increase in serum magnesium has been shown to decrease the release of PTH and that aldosterone causes a decrease of serum magnesium as it does of potassium. The section on magnesium discusses the interrelationship of magnesium and calcium and potassium in deficiency states.

Unlike the more commonly measured electrolytes discussed in Chapter 5 (Na^+, K^+, Cl^-, HCO_3^-), the three electrolytes in this chapter are not always measured in milliequivalents (see Chapter 5 for a definition of milliequivalent). Because a particular laboratory may use either *milligram* or *milliequivalent,* reference values using both systems are presented. In addition, some laboratories may use the SI units discussed in Chapter 1. For Na, K, Cl, and HCO_3^-, the SI and the milliequivalent figures are the same. But with Ca, P, and Mg, the SI figures are different from the milliequivalent. (See Appendix A and the inside cover for the SI equivalents.)

▼ SERUM CALCIUM

Calcium (Ca^{2+}), a positively charged ion, circulates in the bloodstream both in the free or ionized state and bound to plasma proteins. Some authorities strongly recommend measurement of the ionized calcium rather than the total, but this is a more difficult and time-consuming procedure (Kaplan et al., 1995). The bound calcium, carried chiefly by albumin, is about half of the total calcium in the bloodstream. Because most laboratories measure the total calcium level, not just the ionized calcium, a change in serum albumin level means a change in the total serum reference values. A decrease of 1 g of albumin means that the serum total calcium level is about 0.8 mg less. Because the free, or ionized, calcium affects neuromuscular function, a low calcium level caused by a low albumin level does not cause symptoms of hypocalcemia. Factors that cause decreased serum albumin levels are discussed in Chapter 10.

The amount of calcium in the serum is quite small compared with that present in the teeth and bones. The bones contain a tremendous reservoir of calcium that can be used if needed to keep the serum calcium level normal. Two hormones control serum calcium levels. Calcitonin, a hormone secreted by the thyroid gland, protects against a calcium excess in the serum. PTH, secreted by the parathyroid gland, keeps a sufficient level of calcium in the bloodstream; an increase in PTH not only increases the serum calcium level but also decreases phosphorus levels. Thus, for many types of serum calcium imbalance, it is important to evaluate the serum phosphorus level, too. The relation between phosphorus and calcium is discussed in detail in the section on serum phosphorus levels.

Calcium is obtained in several food sources, of which milk products are the best: 1 cup (240 mL) of milk, for example, contains 236 mg of calcium. Other sources that contain a fairly large amount of calcium include vegetables such as turnip greens, collard greens, white beans, and lentils (Table 7–1). Intestinal cells need vitamin D, a unique vitamin made entirely in the body from cholesterol and a photochemical reaction, to absorb calcium. Thus sunlight and a diet adequate in fat are important to ensure proper levels of vitamin D. Protein is also required for the proper utilization of calcium. Chronic nutritional deficiencies of calcium, vitamin D, and protein eventually result in lowered serum calcium levels. Yet, because of the vast reservoir of calcium in the bones, dietary deficiencies do not immediately cause lowered serum calcium levels.

Infants require 360–540 mg of calcium, depending on age. Children and adults require about 800 mg of calcium. Adolescents, as well as pregnant and lactating women, have the greatest requirement for calcium, which is about 1,200 mg (Kaplan et al., 1995). Calcium supplementation to a total intake of about 1,500 mg a day has been shown to inhibit age-related bone loss in postmenopausal women (Holm and Walker, 1990). In 1984 only one calcium supplement was on the market. After the National Institutes of Health (NIH) issued a report about osteoporosis and calcium, the market was flooded with products boasting their calcium content.

TABLE 7–1. EXAMPLES OF FOODS HIGH IN CALCIUM OR PHOSPHORUS

Food in 100-g Portions	Calcium (mg)	Phosphorus (mg)
Swiss cheese	925	563
Cheddar cheese	750	478
Brick cheese	730	455
American cheese	697	771
Turnip greens	246	58
Almonds	234	504
Collard greens	203	63
Beans, white	144	425
Milk (100 g = scant 1/2 cup [120 mL])	118	93
Frankfurter	32	603
Bologna	32	581
Peanuts	69	401
Whole wheat flour	41	372
Liver	8	352

Modified from Linkswiler and Zemel (1979), with permission.

Excess calcium is excreted in the urine. The measurement of urinary calcium is covered after the discussion on serum calcium levels.

REFERENCE VALUES FOR SERUM CALCIUM (TOTAL)	
Adult	Calcium levels tend to be slightly higher in men 8.5–10.5 mg/dL, or 4.3–5.3 mEq/L[a,b]
Pregnancy	Falls gradually to a level at term about 10% below non-pregnant level. Consistent with the fall in albumin
Newborn	7.4–14 mg/dL or 3.7–7 mEq
Children	Slightly higher in children—may be up to 12 mg

[a]Some laboratories measure the ionized calcium, which is usually 3.5–5.2 mg/dL.
[b]Each 1-g drop in serum albumin decreases the total calcium by 0.8 mg, and each 0.1-drop in pH below 7.4 decreases the total calcium by 0.01 mg (Calloway, 1987).

Preparation of Client and Collection of Sample

One milliliter of serum is needed. Some laboratories require a fasting state, although water is allowed. Remember that if the serum albumin level drops 1 g, the total serum calcium level drops 0.8 mg, even though the ionized calcium remains the same. Always interpret calcium levels in relation to serum albumin levels.

Increased Serum Calcium Level (Hypercalcemia)

Clinical Significance. As with many other tests, dehydration gives a falsely high reading of serum calcium level. An increased level of PTH causes a persistently elevated serum calcium level. Because adenomas of the parathyroid gland can cause the gland to produce additional amounts of PTH, the physician may order several other tests, including an assay of PTH levels to rule out the possibility that a parathyroid tumor is responsible for hypercalcemia. Often the client may have no symptoms even though the laboratory report shows a higher-than-normal serum calcium level. In borderline cases, the test may be repeated several times during a period of weeks or months, in addition to other diagnostic studies, such as the PTH assay (discussed in Chapter 15). If the high serum calcium level is due to parathyroid dysfunction, the client may need surgical intervention to remove part of the parathyroid gland.

There are several other common reasons for the serum calcium level being higher than normal (Table 7–2). The most common is the release of calcium in metastatic bone disease as bone is destroyed. Also, some of the hormonal changes in malignant states may contribute to raising the serum calcium level. Some tumors produce PTH-like substances. (See Chapter 15 for a discussion on ectopic hormone production.) Long-term immobilization may result in increased serum calcium levels because the lack of normal bone stress causes the release of calcium from bone.

TABLE 7–2. COMMON CAUSES OF HYPERCALCEMIA AND HYPOCALCEMIA

- **HYPERCALCEMIA** (serum Ca^{2+} levels > 10.5 mg/dL or see values for specific laboratory)
  - False-rise caused by dehydration
  - Hyperparathyroidism (serum P level decreased)
  - Malignant tumors
  - Immobilization
  - Thiazide diuretics
  - Vitamin D intoxication (serum P level increased)
- **HYPOCALCEMIA** (serum Ca^{2+} levels < 8.5 mg/dL or see values for specific laboratory) Infants have lower values to 8 or 7.5 mg/dL
  - False-decrease caused by low albumin levels
  - Hypoparathyroidism (serum P level increased)
  - Early neonatal hypocalcemia
  - Chronic renal disease (serum P level increased)
  - Pancreatitis
  - Massive blood transfusions
  - Severe malnutrition (serum P level decreased)
  - Symptoms of hypocalcemia when client is alkalotic although total serum calcium is normal (see text)

Serum phosphorus levels help with interpretation of serum Ca level.

Thiazide diuretics are another reason for hypercalcemia. Excessive milk intake (at least 3 quarts [2.8L] of milk a day) is a less frequent cause of hypercalcemia. Vitamin D intoxication can also result in hypercalcemia. Hypercalcemia and elevated serum vitamin D levels may persist for months after use of the vitamin D supplements is discontinued (Butler et al., 1985).

▼ POSSIBLE NURSING DIAGNOSES RELATED TO HYPERCALCEMIA

Altered Fluid Requirements Related to Risk for Injury from Formation of Renal Stones

An increased serum calcium level almost always means increased calcium excretion by the kidneys. Thus, insofar as a high concentration of calcium in the urine may lead to the formation of renal stones (*calculi*), it is very important that a client with hypercalcemia stay well-hydrated. Some authorities suggest that the urine volume needs to be greater than 2,500 mL in 24 hr. Health teaching for the client at home should include information on how to make sure the urine is never concentrated; the client must be aware of the importance of drinking fluids at bedtime and also during the night. A home care nurse can help make out a schedule for the client or for a member of the family to follow.

Calcium is more likely to precipitate in an alkaline urine. Yet, because the urine pH is normally acid (~6), precipitation may not be a threat unless a uri-

(*continued*)

▼ POSSIBLE NURSING DIAGNOSES RELATED TO HYPERCALCEMIA (*continued*)

nary tract infection develops, which may make the urine alkaline. Measures, such as the intake of cranberry juice, to change an alkaline urine to acid are discussed in Chapter 3.

For emergency treatment of hypercalcemia, forced diuresis with intravenous normal saline solution is usually used because calcium excretion improves when sodium supplementation is provided. The standard saline solution infusion rate is 200–300 mL/hr (Boyer, 1993). The nurse must monitor daily weights and intake and output records to avoid overload. Furosemide (Lasix) may be given. Thiazide diuretics are never used with hypercalcemia because they exacerbate the condition.

Risk for Injury Related to Slowing of Reflexes

The client with an increased serum calcium level may demonstrate some slowing of reflexes. Because increased serum calcium levels decrease the permeability of nerve cell membranes to sodium, the depolarization process is affected, and the nerve fibers have a decreased excitability. This condition may result in some lethargy or a general sluggish feeling. Other possible problems are anorexia and constipation. Confusion may develop and lead to a comatose state. Mahon (1987) found that changes in mental status were the most evident clue of hypercalcemia. For example, clients could not recall their phone numbers.

Risk for Altered Cardiac Output

An elevated serum calcium level also tends to slow the heart, and arrhythmias may develop. If the client is taking digoxin, a high serum calcium level may be particularly dangerous because it potentiates the effect of the digoxin.

Risk for Injury and Impaired Mobility Related to Development of Pathologic Fractures

If the hypercalcemia is a result of loss of calcium from the bones, the client becomes very susceptible to fractures. These types of fractures are referred to as *pathologic fractures* because the bone is made fragile by a pathologic process. Clients who are prone to pathologic fractures must be handled very gently. The nurse must be alert to any vague symptoms of bone pain. Sometimes just turning in bed can cause a fracture. If the client can walk, weight bearing can help minimize loss of calcium from the weight-bearing bones. A walker or other supportive device is essential for safety. Walking helps maintain skeletal integrity (Krall and Dawson-Hughes, 1994).

Knowledge Deficit Related to Drug Therapy for Hypercalcemia

Several drugs may be used to reduce high serum calcium levels after rehydration with saline solution and diuresis with furosemide (Katzung, 1995). With all these drugs the client must remain well-hydrated at all times, including during the night.

1. Calcitonin (Calcimar) is a synthetic preparation of the hormone produced by the thyroid gland. Clients with Paget's disease may take calcitonin injections daily over a long period of time. Often the nurse must teach the client how to perform the injections at home. Allergic reactions can occur.
2. Gallium nitrate (Ganite) is given intravenously for 5 days. Nephrotoxicity may occur so assess for renal function (Chapter 4).
3. Plicamycin, an antineoplastic drug, is also sometimes used to reduce high serum calcium levels in clients with malignant neoplasms. A single dose may reduce elevated serum calcium levels for several days. However, thrombocytopenia, along with many toxic side effects, may result from the use of this drug.
4. Glucocorticosteroids, such as prednisone and some others, reduce serum calcium levels, but they may take a week to 10 days to do so. The nurse and the client must be aware of the potential side effects from the use of corticosteroids. (See Chapter 15 on hormones.)
5. Etidronate (Didronel) and other biphosphonates (given orally or intravenously) may not produce immediate improvement in the serum calcium level but improvement may continue for months after use of the drug is stopped (Walpert, 1990).

Altered Nutrition Related to Possible Dietary Restrictions

Depending on the underlying pathophysiologic condition, the dietary restriction of foods high in calcium may be used to control hypercalcemia. The concept that a higher dietary calcium intake increases the risk for kidney stones has been questioned because a high intake of calcium may reduce urinary excretion of oxalate. A prospective study of a large group of men with no history of kidney stones showed a high dietary calcium intake decreased the risk for kidney stones (Curhan et al., 1993). Because hypercalcemia may be due to complex pathologic processes, the value of diet restriction must be evaluated in relation to the particular medical problem that exists. For hypercalcemia related to malignant conditions, it is usually *not* necessary to avoid foods high in calcium (Coward, 1985). Table 7–1 gives examples of foods high in calcium.

Decreased Serum Calcium Level (Hypocalcemia)

Clinical Significance. Because much of serum calcium is bound to albumin, it is important to make sure that the lowered serum calcium level is not due to a lowered serum albumin level.

Just as *hyper*parathyroidism causes *hyper*calcemia, *hypo*parathyroidism causes *hypo*calcemia, because PTH controls serum calcium levels. Hypoparathyroidism, or a lack of PTH, can be due to accidental damage to the parathyroid glands during operations on the thyroid. The hypocalcemia may be more severe from surgical removal of the parathyroid glands than from the other causes of hypoparathyroidism.

Early neonatal hypocalcemia is a clinical condition experienced by some infants in the first 24–48 hr of life. Neonatal hypocalcemia may occur either early, in the first 2 days of life, or later, in the first week or two. Early onset is associated with prematurity, sepsis, respiratory distress, and maternal diabetes. Late-onset hypocalcemia has been linked to a high intake of phosphates in feedings (Hay et al., 1995).

Hypocalcemia is also commonly seen in clients with renal failure when elimination of acid phosphates is impaired. The increase in phosphates in the serum causes a decreased calcium level because of the inverse relation between these two levels. (See the beginning of the chapter for an explanation of this interrelation caused by PTH control.) Also in chronic renal disease, because the kidney is unable to finish the process of making vitamin D chemically active, calcium absorption is impaired. The tubules of the kidney are responsible for the final active form of vitamin D, which functions as calcitrol, a hormone necessary for calcium absorption. Vitamin D is the only vitamin known to be converted to a hormonal form. Children who have chronic renal disease may have rickets because of the lowered serum calcium level.

Serum calcium level also can be lowered because calcium is being deposited in tissues. In pancreatitis, the fatty acids that are released can bind up calcium. The pancreas may actually become calcified in areas of necrotic tissue. In massive blood transfusions, the serum calcium level may drop because the calcium ions in the blood are bound by the citrate the blood bank uses as an anticoagulant. The liver removes the citrate from the circulation, but it may not be able to do so fast enough when a large amount of blood is infused.

Severe malnutrition may eventually lead to hypocalcemia, but, because of the vast reserves of calcium in the bones, a calcium-deficient diet does not immediately cause a drop in serum calcium levels. Hence a pregnant or lactating woman who does not consume enough calcium continues to have a normal serum calcium level as she loses calcium from the teeth and bones. Children and elderly people who have calcium-deficient diets usually retain normal serum calcium levels, too. But rickets develops in the child, and osteomalacia, or a softening of the bones develops in the older person. Osteoporosis, a health problem for many postmenopausal women, may be related to a lack of calcium intake that existed for many years.

Severe malnutrition that includes a lack of vitamin D and protein eventually causes a lowered serum calcium level when calcium cannot be released from the bones or teeth.

The nurse should bear in mind the effect of pH on calcium solubility. In alkalotic states, even though the total serum calcium does not change, the amount of ionized calcium is less because calcium is less soluble in an alkaline medium. A decrease in the ionized portion of serum calcium causes symptoms of hypocalcemia even though the laboratory test looks normal. (Recall that the serum calcium level measures both bound calcium and ionized calcium.)

When a client is in an acidotic state, the total serum calcium level may be low, but the client has few symptoms as long as he or she is in the acidotic state because more calcium is in the ionized state. When the pH returns to normal, there is less ionized calcium and the symptoms of hypocalcemia become apparent. Thus acidotic states may mask true hypocalcemia.

▼ POSSIBLE NURSING DIAGNOSES RELATED TO HYPOCALCEMIA

Risk for Injury Related to the Development of Tetany

The symptoms of hypocalcemia vary depending on how low the serum calcium level drops and on how abruptly it drops. Hypocalcemia causes muscle twitching and cramps, which may lead to generalized muscle spasms called *tetany*. These cramps in the muscles are due to the neuromuscular irritability from the lack of calcium ions. In a client with a low serum calcium level, a tapping of the jaw causes a facial spasm (Chvostek's sign). Some clients, particularly women, may exhibit this sign even though the calcium level is normal. Another assessment of low serum calcium levels is to look for carpopedal spasms (spasms in the hands and feet). Spasms may be elicited when the arm becomes a little ischemic. For example, when the nurse takes the blood pressure, the client's hand may twitch when the cuff is left inflated for a couple of minutes (Trousseau's sign). Subtle signs of neuromuscular irritability caused by hypocalcemia, such as a twitching of the nose, may be overlooked unless the nurse is aware that any neuromuscular irritability should be watched for in a client who may experience hypocalcemia. In the newborn the symptoms may include twitching or convulsions. The symptoms of hypocalcemia often coincide with hypoglycemia in the newborn. (See Chapter 8 for a discussion on hypoglycemia in the newborn.)

Because clients with the potential for hypocalcemia may have a convulsive state, the nurse must be prepared for such a possibility. Calcium gluconate for intravenous administration should be on an emergency cart. After operations on the thyroid or parathyroid gland, an ampule of calcium gluconate is usually kept at the bedside. Clients at risk for hypocalcemia usually have their serum calcium levels measured daily. Untreated hypocalcemia can lead to laryngeal spasms and death.

Special Emphasis for Symptoms of Hypocalcemia in Alkalosis. If a client is having symptoms of tetany because less calcium is in an ionized state, the client is not given calcium as treatment. In alkalosis, the symptoms arise from a lack of ionized calcium, not from a *true lack* of calcium. When the pH returns to normal, the calcium is once again ionized in the correct amount for neuromuscular

(*continued*)

▼ POSSIBLE NURSING DIAGNOSES RELATED TO HYPOCALCEMIA (*continued*)

functioning. (The possible nursing implications for the client in alkalosis are covered in Chapter 6.)

Risk for Injury Related to Replacement of Calcium

The treatment of hypocalcemia depends on the underlying cause. For prevention of tetany and convulsions, the serum calcium level must be raised quickly to normal. If the signs of tetany are severe, the physician orders calcium to be given intravenously. Several different salts of calcium are available, but usually calcium gluconate is given for fast replacement. For tetany, 10 mL of 10% calcium gluconate is given intravenously over 15–30 min (Lockhart, 1988) or longer than 5 min (Walpert, 1990). The medication may give the client a feeling of warmth because of the vasodilation that occurs along with a drop in the blood pressure or arrhythmias for which the client must be monitored.

In less acute situations—when the client is having few symptoms—an ampule of calcium gluconate may be added to a bottle of intravenous fluid. Because calcium precipitates in an alkaline medium, calcium salts can never be added to intravenous fluids with an alkaline pH. Most dextrose and saline solutions are acid in pH, but this point must be carefully checked because an intravenous infusion may also contain sodium bicarbonate.

Because calcium has a profound effect on the heart, some physicians may choose to have the client use a cardiac monitor the entire time calcium is being replaced. This precaution is most likely if the client is also taking digoxin, because calcium increases the possibility of digitalis toxicity.

Knowledge Deficit Related to Use of Oral Calcium Supplements

For mild hypocalcemia, and in chronic states, the client may be given various oral preparations of calcium salts. Newborns may be given oral supplements, once feedings are tolerated. The nurse needs to find out whether the particular preparation being used should be taken while the stomach is empty. With some preparations, alkaline foods and milk tend to decrease the absorption of calcium. The calcium of other preparations may have a bitter taste or cause gastrointestinal irritation, so it is better tolerated with food. Some preparations may be constipating. Clients taking calcium supplements should not take tetracyclines at the same time because calcium interferes with the absorption of this type of antibiotic. Metabolites of vitamin D, such as calciferol or calcitrol, are used to increase serum calcium levels. The use of vitamin D supplements requires careful monitoring of serum calcium levels because vitamin D has a cumulative effect. An inexpensive source of calcium carbonate is some antacid tablets, so clients should discuss with their physician the best type of calcium replacement for them.

Altered Nutrition Related to Calcium Requirement

Calcium requirements are best met by having adequate calcium in the diet. So the nurse must assess the dietary habits of individual clients to determine whether their calcium intake is adequate. If the client does not like milk or cheese (which, as dairy products, are among the best sources for calcium), powdered milk can be added to many dishes without changing their taste. A tablespoon of powdered milk contains nearly 50 mg of calcium (Table 7–1). Foods high in oxalates and phosphates, such as spinach, rhubarb, and asparagus, tend to decrease calcium absorption. Also, a lack of protein decreases calcium utilization, but a diet with excess protein wastes calcium. Elderly clients may have a decrease in gastric hydrochloric acid, which decreases calcium absorption. A form of oral glutamic acid hydrochloride (Acidulin) may be used to improve calcium absorption (Cerato, 1985).

Knowledge Deficit Related to Phosphate Binders

Another way to help raise the serum calcium level is to reduce the amount of phosphate intake. (The relationship of high phosphorus levels to low serum calcium levels is discussed next in the section on phosphorus.) Oral antacids that contain magnesium or aluminum (Aludrox) are sometimes ordered with meals to help bind phosphates so that more calcium can be absorbed. If the low serum calcium level related to a high serum phosphorus level is due to renal failure, medications containing aluminum, not magnesium hydroxide, are prescribed to lower the serum phosphorus level because magnesium is not excreted well in renal dysfunction.

▼ URINARY CALCIUM

Preparation of Client and Collection of Sample

All urine for 24 hr is collected in a special bottle that contains 10 mL of hydrochloric acid (HCl). The hydrochloric acid is to keep the pH of the urine low (pH 2–3) because calcium tends to precipitate in an alkaline medium. The client consumes the usual diet. Any increased intake of protein by the client should be noted because more calcium is excreted on a high-protein diet. (See Chapter 3 for general instructions about 24-hr urine collections.)

REFERENCE VALUES FOR URINARY CALCIUM	
Adult	50–300 mg/dL, depending on dietary intake
Children	Range is about 5 mg/kg of body weight if on normal dietary intake of calcium

Clinical Significance. Normally up to 99% of the calcium filtered by kidneys is reabsorbed. An increased urinary calcium level is almost always due to an elevated serum calcium level. The amount of calcium being excreted in the urine may differ for various types of hypercalcemia, so the 24-hr urine collection may give extra diagnostic clues. For example, a highly elevated urine calcium does not usually accompany primary hyperparathyroidism because the increased amount of PTH promotes additional reabsorption of calcium. In other types of hypercalcemia, such as with malignant tumors, the urine calcium level may be as high as 800 or 900 mg in 24 hr. In conditions in which there is a low serum calcium level, such as in primary hypoparathyroidism, the urinary excretion of calcium is very low.

▼ SERUM PHOSPHORUS OR PHOSPHATES

Laboratories may report phosphorus levels as phosphorus (P) or phosphate (PO_4) levels, as phosphorus is one component of phosphate. Whereas potassium is the main intracellular *cation,* phosphorus is the main intracellular *anion.* So phosphorus is in bone tissue and skeletal muscle, and phosphates regulate many enzymatic actions critical for energy transformations. Because phosphorus has a close relation to calcium, the phosphorus level is usually more useful as a diagnostic tool when evaluated in relation to the serum calcium level.

The phosphate electrolyte is the only electrolyte that is markedly different in values for children and adults. (The bicarbonate ion discussed in Chapter 5 does have slight variations with age.) The marked increase in phosphate ions in young children is partially explained by the increased amount of growth hormone present until puberty.

The recommended dietary allowances for phosphorus, except in infancy and lactation, is a one-to-one ratio to calcium. Thus an adult requires about 800 mg of phosphorus a day. In infants and lactating women, the need for calcium exceeds the need for phosphorus. In most United States diets, however, the intake of phosphorus is probably twice that of calcium: The average calcium intake may be about 700 mg, whereas the average phosphorus intake is about 1,500 mg. This higher phosphorus intake occurs for two reasons. First, phosphorus is abundant not only in dairy products but also in many natural foods. Second, many food additives contain substantial amounts of phosphates. Linkswiler and Zemel (1979), in a detailed discussion of the additional source of phosphorus from food processing, concluded that there are no data to suggest harm from the extra phosphates in the diet. Processed meat, cheese, and soft drinks are three sources that are quite high in phosphates. Table 7–1 lists other foods that are high in calcium or phosphates.

Like calcium, phosphorus is controlled by PTH. Increases in the level of PTH cause a decrease in the serum level of phosphorus and an increased secretion of phosphorus by the kidney.

Additional phosphates are excreted by the kidney. Some phosphate is also excreted in the feces. Drugs, such as aluminum hydroxide, can increase fecal excretion of phosphates.

Preparation of Client and Collection of Sample

One milliliter of serum is needed. Some laboratories require the fasting state, although water is allowed. Because increased carbohydrate metabolism lowers serum phosphorus levels, the client should not have intravenous solutions of glucose running before the test. If an intravenous infusion of glucose is being administered, record it on the laboratory slip. The serum needs to be sent to the laboratory as soon as possible because the laboratory must quickly separate the serum from the cells.

REFERENCE VALUES FOR SERUM PHOSPHORUS

Adult	3.0–4.5 mg/dL or 1.8–2.6 mEq/L
Pregnancy	Slightly lower in pregnancy
Newborn	5.7–9.5 mg/dL. May be higher in premature infants and for a few days after birth
Children	4–6 mg. Levels decline with maturity
Aged	May be slightly lower in the aged

Increased Phosphate Level (Hyperphosphatemia)

Clinical Significance. The clinical significance of an elevated phosphorus level is always evaluated in relation to the serum calcium levels to get a clear idea of what may be a very complicated pathologic process (Table 7–3):

1. When the phosphorus level is elevated and the serum calcium level is low, hypoparathyroidism may be the reason. The lack of PTH decreases the renal excretion of phosphates.
2. In some types of renal dysfunction, the kidneys cannot excrete phosphate ions. A high phosphate level in the serum then depresses the serum calcium level through several hormonal actions.

TABLE 7–3. COMMON REASONS FOR CHANGES IN SERUM PHOSPHATE LEVELS

- **HYPERPHOSPHATEMIA** (serum phosphorus > 4.5 mg/dL in adult)
  - Hypoparathyroidism (serum Ca^{2+} decreased)
  - Renal failure (serum Ca^{2+} decreased)
  - Increased growth hormone
  - Vitamin D intoxication (serum Ca^{2+} increased)
- **HYPOPHOSPHATEMIA** (serum phosphorus < 3 mg/dL in adult)
  - Hyperparathyroidism (serum Ca^{2+} increased)
  - Diuresis
  - Malabsorption; or malnutrition (serum Ca^{2+} decreased)
  - Increased glucose metabolism—carbohydrate loading
  - Antacid abuse

Serum calcium (Ca^{2+}) helps in interpretation.

3. Diseases of childhood may sometimes involve an increase in the production of growth hormone and an increase in the serum phosphates. In such a case, the serum calcium level is not elevated.
4. If the phosphates in the serum are elevated because of vitamin D intoxication or the excessive intake of milk, the serum calcium level also is most likely elevated.
5. In certain malignant conditions, the serum phosphate level may either remain normal or be somewhat elevated when serum calcium is elevated.

▼ POSSIBLE NURSING DIAGNOSES RELATED TO ELEVATED PHOSPHATE LEVELS

Altered Nutrition Related to Calcium and Phosphorus Requirements

If the underlying problem is due to hypoparathyroidism, replacement with calcium and vitamin D corrects the problem. If the phosphorus and calcium levels are both elevated, clients may be instructed to moderately reduce calcium and phosphorus in their diet by limiting dairy products (see the discussion of hypercalcemia diets). If the serum phosphorus level is increased and the serum calcium is normal or decreased, the restriction of dairy products must be countered by calcium supplements. It is difficult to reduce the serum phosphorus level with diet alone because phosphorus is abundant in many more foods than is calcium. Some medications also may contain large amounts of phosphates. For example, sodium phosphate enemas are contraindicated if hyperphosphatemia is possible (Biberstein and Parker, 1985).

Knowledge Deficit Related to Use of Phosphate Binders

If the phosphorus level is high and the calcium level is low, as often happens in renal failure, the client needs information about the medication used to reduce the phosphate level. Aluminum hydroxide gels (Alu-Caps or Aludrox), given by mouth, unite with the phosphates present in food to form insoluble aluminum phosphate. These insoluble phosphate compounds are then excreted in the feces. Constipation may become a problem. Magnesium hydroxide also binds phosphates, but the additional magnesium intake is contraindicated in renal failure. Aluminum hydroxide is continued even after dialysis is started because dialysis cannot efficiently reduce serum phosphate levels.

Decreased Serum Phosphorus Level (Hypophosphatemia)

Clinical Significance. Moderate hypophosphatemia can result from a variety of conditions (Table 7–3):

1. Hyperparathyroidism results in a high serum calcium level and a low phosphorus level.
2. Diuretics may cause a low phosphorus level.
3. Phosphates can be lost in large amounts in some types of renal diseases, although phosphate retention is more common.
4. Drugs that bind phosphate, such as aluminum or magnesium gels, can cause phosphate deficiency. However, diets are usually high in phosphates, so this pharmacologic binding of antacids is usually not a concern.
5. Malabsorption syndromes may eventually lead to low serum phosphorus levels.

Other clinical conditions in which serum phosphorus concentrations may decrease are alcoholic withdrawal, diabetes mellitus, the recovery diuretic phase after severe burns, hyperalimentation therapy, and nutritional recovery syndrome. Baker (1985) noted that hypophosphatemia is the most frequent and dangerous electrolyte disorder that occurs with hyperalimentation. The most striking examples of rapid drops in serum phosphorus levels occur with the treatment of ketoacidosis and the refeeding syndrome (Bongard and Sue, 1994). It is known that when glucose metabolism is increased (carbohydrate loading), the phosphorus ions become tied up. A decrease in serum magnesium ions or a shift in potassium ions tends to produce hypophosphatemia (Knochel, 1985).

▼ POSSIBLE NURSING DIAGNOSES RELATED TO LOW PHOSPHORUS LEVELS

Risk for Injury Related to Neuromuscular Deficits

It is hypothesized that lowered serum phosphorus levels produce central nervous system symptoms such as irritability and confusion. Hence nurses must be aware that clients with any altered electrolyte may not be able to function normally; safety precautions become important. Plasma phosphate levels can plunge rapidly when a malnourished client resumes a normal diet (Cummings et al., 1987).

Risk for Injury Related to Replacement Therapies

Therapy for low serum phosphate levels may include administration of phosphate salts in oral or intravenous form. Because clients likely to experience low phosphorus levels may also experience low potassium and low magnesium levels, the nurse must be familiar with all the replacements being used. Potassium phosphate should be given at no more than 10 mEq/hr (Baker, 1985). The greatest hazard of giving large amounts of phosphates is that hypocalcemia may result.

(*continued*)

▼ POSSIBLE NURSING DIAGNOSES RELATED TO LOW PHOSPHORUS LEVELS (*continued*)

Altered Nutrition

If the client can tolerate oral feedings, milk is a good source of phosphorus. Long-term health teaching about phosphorus intake usually is not necessary because in a conventional diet phosphates are abundant. The concern for a client who has a low serum phosphorus level is to correct the often complex metabolic problem that has caused the deficiency in the serum.

▼ URINARY PHOSPHORUS OR URINE PHOSPHATES

Preparation of Client and Collection of Sample

All urine is collected over a 24-hr period. There is no need for a preservative in the bottle, and the urine does not have to be iced. (Note that for urine calcium, a preservative is needed. When both calcium and potassium are to be collected, the preservative does not interfere with the test for phosphorus.)

REFERENCE VALUES FOR URINARY PHOSPHORUS	
All groups	0.4–1.3 g in 24 hr. Varies with intake. Average is 1 g in 24 hr

Clinical Significance. Urinary phosphorus levels usually reflect the amount of both organic and inorganic phosphates in the diet. Because PTH decreases renal reabsorption of phosphorus, hyperparathyroidism causes an increased urinary phosphorus level 70–75% of the time (Ravel, 1995). In renal failure, the excretion of phosphates may be impaired so that the urinary phosphorus level is decreased. However, testing the urine in renal failure usually does not provide additional clinical information. The urinary phosphorus test is most often used when there is a complex metabolic problem, such as an endocrine disturbance or malnutrition problems, and when a very complete investigation of all electrolyte disturbances must be performed to monitor the progress of the client.

▼ SERUM MAGNESIUM

Primarily an intracellular ion, magnesium (Mg^{2+}) appears in the bloodstream only in very small amounts. The bulk of magnesium is combined with calcium and phosphorus in the bones. Magnesium is essential for neuromuscular function and for activation of some enzymes. Changes in serum magnesium levels affect other serum ions, too, such as potassium, calcium, and phosphorus. Thus magnesium deficiency is not usually seen alone. Evidently the body can store magnesium, because deficiencies usually develop in chronic conditions and not in acute conditions.

Because magnesium is present in a variety of foods, a conventional diet supplies the recommended daily allowances. Approximately 6 mg/kg a day of magnesium is required for a normal magnesium balance (Bongard and Sue, 1994).

Magnesium is excreted primarily by the kidney. The hormone aldosterone causes an increased excretion of magnesium as it does of potassium. Compared with the facts known about potassium, much is still to be learned about how magnesium functions in the body. (See Chapter 5 for a detailed discussion of the effect of aldosterone on potassium levels.) Magnesium is given not only for replacement but also as therapy for preeclampsia, preterm labor, and an expanding array of medical conditions, including ischemic heart disease and arrhythmias (McLean, 1994). Unlike potassium, magnesium supplements are not likely to cause a dangerous clinical state unless the client has impaired renal function (Owens, 1993).

Preparation of Client and Collection of Sample

The client does not have to be fasting. One milliliter of serum is needed. Calcium gluconate may interfere with some test methods. Hemolysis of the specimen must be avoided because magnesium is primarily an intracellular ion. Lowered albumin levels cause lower magnesium levels.

REFERENCE VALUES FOR SERUM MAGNESIUM

Adult	1.5–2.0 mEq/L or 1.4–1.9 mg/dL
Pregnancy	Gradual fall of about 10–20%
Children	1.54–1.86 mEq/L
Aged	No reported difference

Some laboratories use 1.2 or 1.3 mg/dL as the lower level. Values are highly method-specific.

Increased Serum Magnesium Level (Hypermagnesemia)

Clinical Significance. Renal failure is the most common reason for magnesium excess, because the kidneys are unable to excrete magnesium normally. If renal output is not adequate, an increased magnesium level may result from the administration of medications containing magnesium, such as milk of magnesia (Table 7–4). Also, severe cases of hypermagnesemia have been reported because of incorrect use of magnesium replacements. One such case led to respiratory failure (Hoffman et al., 1989).

TABLE 7–4 COMMON REASONS FOR CHANGES IN SERUM MAGNESIUM LEVEL

- **HYPERMAGNESEMIA** (serum Mg^{2+} level > 2 mEq/L)
  Renal failure
  Intravenous administration of $MgSO_4$ for toxemia
- **HYPOMAGNESEMIA** (serum Mg^{2+} < 1.5 mEq/L)
  Chronic malnutrition (e.g., alcoholism)
  Diarrhea or draining gastrointestinal fistulas
  Diuretics
  Diabetes
  Hypercalcemia or other complex metabolic disorders

Obstetric clients may receive magnesium parenterally as treatments of the hypertensive disorders of pregnancy and for premature labor (DeCherney and Pernoll, 1994). Therapeutic levels may need to be as much as 4 times the usual reference values, but this is almost never in a toxic range (Weaver, 1987). However, nursing assessments are important.

▼ POSSIBLE NURSING DIAGNOSES RELATED TO ELEVATED MAGNESIUM LEVELS

Risk for Injury Related to Altered Neuromuscular Functioning

Higher-than-normal levels of serum magnesium produce sedation, depression of the neuromuscular system, and reduction in blood pressure. If a mother was given $MgSO_4$, the newborn may have lethargy and respiratory depression. Whether the excess magnesium is due to renal failure or intravenous therapy for toxemia, an excess of magnesium can lead from muscle weakness to muscle paralysis, so that deep tendon reflexes are weak or absent. In severe hypermagnesemia (>10 mEq/L), paralysis of voluntary muscles produces flaccid quadriplegia and respiratory failure. Severe hypotension occurs. The electrocardiogram shows prolonged PR and QT intervals (Raimer, 1994). Thus nursing assessments for a client who is at risk for serum magnesium excess should include (1) frequent blood pressure and pulse monitoring, (2) assessment of level of consciousness, (3) presence of normal reflexes such as knee jerk, and (4) careful intake and output records.

In addition to muscle weakness, the client may be confused and thus less aware of the surrounding environment. The nurse must take whatever measures are necessary to protect the client from injury. If the magnesium excess is causing acute problems, the physician may order calcium gluconate or calcium chloride to be given intravenously because calcium is the antidote for magnesium excess.

Knowledge Deficit Related to Hidden Sources of Magnesium

Clients with chronic renal failure should not be given any medications that contain magnesium. The nurse needs to provide client teaching because several over-the-counter drugs contain magnesium. For example, antacids used should be those that contain aluminum hydroxide gels, not magnesium hydroxide. A popular cathartic, epsom salts, is a compound of magnesium sulfate. Many other laxatives contain magnesium, and those pose a special threat to elderly people with decreased renal function. The dietary restriction of magnesium intake is not a focus for teaching because most foods contain only a trace of this mineral.

Decreased Serum Magnesium Level (Hypomagnesemia)

Clinical Significance. A decrease in serum magnesium is usually due to a chronic problem involving a low intake of dietary magnesium over a period of time (Table 7–4). For example, people who use alcohol as the primary source of calories may become deficient in magnesium. Deficiencies may also result from impaired absorption, such as that associated with a draining intestinal fistula or with heavy use of diuretics. Other drugs, such as the aminoglycosides, cyclosporine, and cisplatin, may also cause hypomagnesemia. Chernow et al. (1989) found hypomagnesemia to be common in postoperative clients in a surgical intensive care unit. Cohen and Kitzes (1983) noted that a normal serum magnesium level does not rule out the possibility that a digitalis-toxic arrhythmia is being caused by a magnesium deficiency. One study revealed that clients taking digitalis were twice as likely to have a deficit of magnesium as a deficit of potassium (Whang et al., 1985). Clients with low magnesium levels may also have unexplained hypocalcemia and hypokalemia, which causes complex electrolyte imbalances (McLean, 1994).

▼ POSSIBLE NURSING DIAGNOSES RELATED TO HYPOMAGNESEMIA

Altered Nutrition: Less than Body Requirements

An assessment for magnesium deficiency is appropriate for clients who have to be fed by artificial means or who are chronically malnourished. A normal serum value does not contraindicate supplementation (Owens, 1993). Nurses should be aware of the need for replacement therapy of magnesium for any client who has poor nutrition over an extended period of time. Also the combination of diuretics and digioxin can lead to digioxin toxicity if the magnesium level is low in the cells.

(continued)

▼ POSSIBLE NURSING DIAGNOSES RELATED TO HYPOMAGNESEMIA (*continued*)

Altered Comfort Related to Neuromuscular Irritability

Early symptoms of a lack of magnesium are related to neuromuscular irritability: The client may have tremors, muscle cramps, and insomnia. The nurse should assess for any involuntary movements or twitching by the client. (See the section on hypocalcemia on how to check for a positive Chvostek's sign and a positive Trousseau's sign.) The client may eventually show symptoms that look very similar to the tetany of hypocalcemia. Often the client may have several deficiencies so the clinical signs and symptoms are not so simple. Laboratory tests have to be performed to identify exactly which electrolyte imbalances coexist. A low calcium or a low potassium that is unresponsive to treatment may be due to a coexisting low magnesium, so interventions may focus on replacements of multiple electrolytes.

Risk for Injury Related to Magnesium Replacements

Magnesium deficits are corrected by the use of magnesium sulfate. One gram of $MgSO_4$ is equal to 8.12 mEq, or 4.06 mmol. Usually 8–24 mEq may be given daily in divided doses. The dosage for children is calculated on the basis of weight. If magnesium is being given intravenously, the nurse must assess carefully for the signs and symptoms of magnesium excess discussed in the section on hypermagnesemia. The intravenous infusion should be stopped if there is a sharp decrease in blood pressure, extreme sedation, or weak reflexes. The importance of assessing for the patellar reflex (knee jerk) has been discussed. Intramuscular injections may be painful, so they must be made deeply in the gluteal muscle (Calloway, 1987; Owens, 1993). Oral replacements may cause diarrhea.

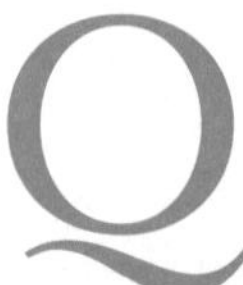

1. A home care nurse is visiting Mrs. Johnson, an elderly woman who lives alone and who does her own cooking. She considers milk to be "for babies." If she does not wish to drink milk or use it in cooking, which alternative foods would offer the highest calcium intake?

   a. Fresh greens, beans, whole wheat products

   b. Rice, liver, and chicken

c. Apples, oranges, and other citrus fruits
d. Potatoes, shellfish, and cornmeal

2. A nursing diagnosis of "risk for injury related to hypercalcemia" would be most likely for

   a. Jack Jones, who is beginning dialysis because of chronic renal failure
   b. Baby Terry, whose mother has diabetes
   c. Helen Simpson, who has metastatic breast cancer
   d. Dawn Penrod, who experiences respiratory alkalosis from hyperventilating

3. A nurse is caring for a client who is receiving normal saline solution intravenously followed by furosemide (Lasix) as treatment of hypercalcemia. As a next step the nurse may need to monitor which of the following drugs to further lower the hypercalcemia?

   a. Aluminum hydroxide b. Thiazide diuretic
   c. Magnesium sulfate d. Plicamycin

4. Which nursing action is the most important to prevent complications for clients with a high serum calcium level?

   a. Keeping the pH of the urine alkaline
   b. Checking for signs of tetany
   c. Making sure the client is well-hydrated
   d. Checking for tachycardia

5. A lactating mother who drinks only one or two glasses of milk a day will most likely continue to have a normal serum calcium level for which of the following reasons?

   a. Two glasses of milk supply the minimum calcium requirements for lactation
   b. Calcium is also available in most meat products and leafy green vegetables
   c. Lactation causes a decrease in parathyroid hormone
   d. Calcium is being drawn from the reservoir in the bones and teeth

6. Which of the following is a characteristic symptom of a low serum calcium level?

   a. Flank pain b. Carpopedal spasms
   c. Bradycardia d. Constipation

7. Which of the following clients has little possibility of experiencing symptoms of hypocalcemia?

   a. Baby Lynn, a premature infant born this morning
   b. Mrs. Thomas, who had a subtotal thyroidectomy today
   c. Mrs. Rhoades, who has metastatic cancer of the liver
   d. Jack Benson, who has acute pancreatitis

8. Which of these clients is the most likely to have decreased serum calcium and serum phosphorus levels?

a. Mr. Lamb, who takes a lot of antacids and milk

b. Mr. Babiloni, who is in renal failure

c. Jane, age 15 months, who eats a low-fat diet and who is never taken outdoors

d. Mrs. Candy, who is in a diabetic coma and who is being treated with glucose and insulin

9. Mr. Jacobs is undergoing therapy to reduce his serum phosphorus level. Which of the following foods is not high in phosphorus content and would thus be allowed on his diet?

a. Processed luncheon meat **b.** Skim milk

c. Soft drinks **d.** Apples

10. In a client with chronic renal failure, aluminum hydroxide may be useful in lowering serum phosphorus levels because the drug

a. Causes precipitation of insoluble phosphates in the intestine

b. Increases secretion of phosphorus in the urine

c. Counteracts the effect of parathyroid hormone

d. Balances the pH of the serum

11. Which of the following clients is the least likely to have a magnesium deficiency?

a. Sally, age 5, who has had vomiting and diarrhea for 24 hr

b. Mrs. Leandro, who is undergoing hyperalimentation therapy

c. Mr. White, who has a long history of alcohol abuse

d. Mrs. Warzenkiak, who has a chronic problem with a draining gastrointestinal fistula

12. Mr. Olino is an elderly man who has had poor nutritional habits over an extended period of time. The home care nurse suspects that magnesium deficiency may be one of his problems. Which of the following symptoms would be least indicative of a low serum magnesium?

a. Leg and foot cramps **b.** Tremors

c. Irritability **d.** Unusual amount of sleeping

13. Mrs. Long is receiving magnesium sulfate ($MgSO_4$) intravenously as treatment for preeclampsia. Which of the following nursing assessments is an indication that Mrs. Long may be experiencing a serum magnesium excess?

a. Rise in pulse and blood pressure

b. Exaggerated patellar reflex (knee jerk)

c. Sedation

d. Seizure activity

14. An antidote for high serum magnesium levels is the administration of which of the following?

    a. Potassium chloride **b.** Calcium gluconate
    c. Aluminum hydroxide **d.** Calcitonin

▼ REFERENCES

Baker, W. (1985). Hypophosphatemia. *American Journal of Nursing, 85* (9), 999–1003.

Biberstein, M., and Parker, B. (1985). Enema-induced hyperphosphatemia. *American Journal of Medicine, 79,* 645.

Bongard, F.S., and Sue, D.Y. (1994). *Current critical care diagnosis and treatment.* Norwalk, CT: Appleton & Lange.

Boyer, C.L. (1993). Three cancer complications that can't wait. *Nursing 93,23* (10), 34–41.

Butler, R., et al. (1985). Calcinosis of joints and periarticular tissues associated with vitamin D intoxication. *Annals of Rheumatic Disease, 44* (7), 494–498.

Calloway, C. (1987). When the problem involves magnesium, calcium, or phosphate. *RN, 50* (5), 30–36.

Cerrato, P. (1985). Hidden malnutrition in geriatric patients. *RN, 48* (7), 60–62.

Chernow, B., et al. (1989). Hypomagnesemia in patients in post-operative intensive care. *Chest,* 95 (2), 391–397.

Cohen, L., and Kitzes, R. (1983). Magnesium sulfate and digitalis: toxic arrhythmias. *JAMA, 249* (20), 2808–2810.

Coward, D. (1985). Knowledge of hypercalcemia in patients at risk to develop cancer-induced hypercalcemia. *National Symposium of Nursing Research Abstracts.* San Francisco: Stanford University Hospital.

Cummings, A., et al. (1987). Refeeding hypophosphatemia in anorexia nervosa and alcoholism. *British Medical Journal, 295,* 490.

Curhan, G. C., Willett, W.C., Rimm, E.B., et al. (1993). A prospective study of dietary calcium and other nutrients and the risk of symptomatic kidney stones. *New England Journal of Medicine, 328* (12), 833–838.

DeCherney, A.H., and Pernoll, M.L. (1994). *Current obstetric & gynecologic diagnosis & treatment* (8th ed.). Norwalk, CT: Appleton & Lange.

Hay, W.W., Groothuis, J.R., Hayward, A.R., and Levin, M.J. (1995). *Current pediatric diagnosis & treatment* (12th ed.). Norwalk, CT: Appleton & Lange.

Hoffman, R., et al. (1989). An "amp" by any other name: The hazards of intravenous magnesium dosing (Letter to the editor). *JAMA, 261,* 557.

Holm, K., and Walker, J. (1990). Osteoporosis: Treatment and prevention update. *Geriatric Nursing, 11* (3), 140–142.

Kaplan, A., Jack, R., Opheim, K.E., et al. (1995). *Clinical chemistry interpretation and techniques* (4th ed.). Baltimore: Williams & Wilkins.

Katzung, B. (1995). Basic and clinical pharmacology (6th ed.). Norwalk, CT: Appleton & Lange.

Knochel, J. (1985). The clinical status of hypophosphatemia: An update. *New England Journal of Medicine, 313* (7), 447–449.

Krall, E.A., and Dawson-Hughes, B. (1994). Walking is related to bone density and rates of bone loss. *American Journal of Medicine, 96* (1), 20–26.

Linkswiler, H., and Zemel, M. (1979). Calcium to phosphorus ratios. *Contemporary Nutrition, 4,* 1–2.

Lockhart, J. (1988). Action stat: Tetany. *Nursing 88, 18* (8), 33.

McLean, R.M. (1994). Magnesium and its therapeutic uses: A review. *American Journal of Medicine, 96* (1), 63–76.

Mahon, S. (1987). For the research record: Symptoms as clues to calcium levels. *American Journal of Nursing, 87* (3), 354–356.

Owens, M.W. (1993). Keeping an eye on magnesium. *American Journal of Nursing, 93* (2), 66–67.

Raimer, F. (1994). How to identify electrolyte imbalances on your patient's E.C.G. *Nursing 94, 24* (6), 54–58.

Ravel, R. (1995). *Clinical laboratory medicine: Clinical application of laboratory data* (6th ed.). St. Louis: Mosby–Year Book.

Walpert, N. (1990). Calcium metabolism disorders. *Nursing 90, 20* (7), 60–64.

Weaver, K. (1987). Magnesium and its role in vascular reactivity and coagulation. *Contemporary Nutrition, 12* (3), 1–2.

Whang, R., et al. (1985). Frequency of hypomagnesemia in hospitalized patients receiving digitalis. *Archives of Internal Medicine, 145* (5), 655.

TESTS TO MEASURE THE METABOLISM OF GLUCOSE AND OTHER SUGARS

- Fasting Blood Sugar
- Postprandial Blood Sugar, or 2-hr p.c. Blood Sugar
- Blood Glucose Finger Sticks
- Glucose Tolerance Test
- Glycohemoglobin and Hemoglobin A_{1c}
- Serum Acetone or Ketones
- Islet Cell Autoantibodies
- Sugars Other than Glucose in Urine
- Lactose Tolerance Test
- Serum Test for Galactosemia

OBJECTIVES

1. Describe the hormonal control of serum glucose levels.
2. Compare the client preparation, usefulness, and limitations of the various tests of glucose to detect diabetes.
3. Contrast the expected laboratory findings and related assessments in HHNK and ketoacidosis.
4. Identify appropriate nursing diagnoses for clients with hyperglycemia of varying severity.
5. Compare and contrast the assessment of hypoglycemia in adults, children, newborns, and the elderly.
6. Determine the priority nursing and medical interventions for various types of hypoglycemia, including reactive hypoglycemia.

7. Identify nursing assessments that would indicate the possibility of a rebound effect from insulin (Somogyi effect).
8. Develop a teaching plan to inform clients about glucose tests performed at home.
9. Analyze the similarities and differences in galactose and lactose intolerances, along with the laboratory tests used to identify each abnormality.

FBS, FPG, PPFG, RBS, GTT, and S and A's—these abbreviations should all be familiar to the nurse because they represent common measurements of the glucose in the blood and urine. Clinicians may use several of these tests both to diagnose and to evaluate therapy for diabetes mellitus, as well as for other conditions involving an elevated blood sugar level (hyperglycemia) or a low blood sugar level (hypoglycemia).

Normally, all complex carbohydrates, including sugars and starches, are eventually broken down to glucose. In some metabolic abnormalities, sugars such as lactose and galactose are present in the serum and urine. The tests that may be performed to detect these abnormal sugars are described in the last part of this chapter.

SUMMARY OF GLUCOSE METABOLISM

Although most glucose comes from the dietary intake of carbohydrates, the liver can convert fats and protein into glucose when not enough glucose is available for the cells. The liver also stores extra glucose in the form of glycogen. With an excess of glucose intake, the glucose that is not stored as glycogen is converted into adipose (fat) tissue. Several hormones influence serum glucose levels:

1. *Insulin,* secreted by the β cells of the pancreas, is essential for the transport of glucose (and potassium) into the cells. A lack of insulin causes an increase in blood glucose level and a potassium imbalance because glucose and potassium cannot get into the cells.
2. *Glucagon,* secreted by the α cells of the pancreas, elevates blood glucose levels by promoting the conversion of glycogen to glucose. The role of glycogen in the treatment of hypoglycemia is explained in the section on hypoglycemia.
3. Other hormones that cause an elevation of blood glucose levels are the *corticosteroids, epinephrine,* and *growth hormone.* The hyperglycemic effects of these hormones are discussed under the section on the clinical significance of hyperglycemia.
4. In pregnancy, *human placental lactogen* (HPL) promotes increased blood glucose levels. Other hormones in pregnancy, *progesterone, estrogens,* and *prolactin,* are insulin antagonists.

Table 8–1 summarizes the effect of hormones on glucose metabolism.

For most people, the renal threshold for glucose is about 160–190 mg/dL (i.e., glucose is not spilled into the urine until the blood glucose level is greater than

TABLE 8–1. EFFECTS OF HORMONES ON SERUM GLUCOSE LEVELS

Promote Hyperglycemia	Promote Hypoglycemia
Growth hormone	Insulin
Glucocorticoids	
Epinephrine and norephinephrine	
Glucagon	
Human placental lactogen (HPL)	
Estrogen	
Progesterone	
Thyroxin	

See Chapter 15 for detailed discussion of the tests for hormones.

160–190 mg/dL). For some people, however, the renal threshold may be higher or lower. For example, in elderly people with a high renal threshold, glucose may not be excreted by the kidney even though the blood glucose is elevated above normal limits. Urine sugar levels need to be compared with blood glucose levels to determine the specific renal threshold for an individual.

In clinical practice the more general term *blood sugar* is often used interchangeably with the more precise term *plasma glucose.* Whole blood glucose is about 10–15% lower than plasma values because the red blood cells (RBCs) are not as rich in glucose as is the plasma. Plasma glucose levels are measured in the laboratory, and whole blood samples are used for finger sticks. Laboratories used to use both chemical and enzymatic methods to determine glucose levels so this made an even greater difference in reported values. Now all laboratories use enzyme methods, so nonenzymatic methods, such as the Nelson–Somogyi or the Folin-Wu are only of historical interest (Kaplan, et al., 1995).

▼ FASTING BLOOD SUGAR

A fasting plasma glucose (FPG) greater than 140 mg/dL on two occasions probably indicates diabetes. Borderline results may be followed by a carbohydrate loading test for a definitive diagnosis of diabetes. Although the FPG has the best screening properties, the glycohemoglobin test (discussed later) has shown promise as a screening tool. The choice of a particular method may depend on cost, convenience, and availability (Hanson et al., 1993).

Preparation of Client and Collection of Sample

For a fasting blood sugar (FBS) or FPG test, the client may not eat for at least 4-hr before the test, but water intake may continue. If the client has an intravenous infusion that contains dextrose, the test is not valid. If the client has diabetes and is being treated with insulin, both food and insulin are withheld until the specimen is drawn.

The blood is collected in a tube with an EDTA-fluoride mixture as a glycolytic inhibitor. (Gray-topped vacuum tube is usually used, but check with the laboratory for the specific method.)

REFERENCE VALUES (SERUM VALUES, NOT WHOLE BLOOD VALUES) FOR FPG

Adult	70–110 mg/dL
Newborn	Less than 40 mg may be hypoglycemia (Beckmann, 1990)
Pregnancy	Slightly lower values than in nonpregnant state
Aged	Reference values may be slightly higher with aged, particularly with glucose tests other than FPG. The FPG increases only 1–2 mg per decade.

▼ POSTPRANDIAL BLOOD SUGAR OR 2-HR P.C. GLUCOSE

Purpose of Test and Preparation of Client

Postprandial, or *post cibum* (p.c.), means after a meal. Sometimes the client is given a meal consisting of a standard amount of carbohydrate, or the laboratory draws the blood after a conventional meal. The purpose of the postprandial test is to see how the body responds to the ingestion of carbohydrates in a meal.

The timing of the blood specimen drawing must be accurate. All the factors that affect the glucose tolerance test results may also affect the postprandial blood sugar (PPBS) levels.

REFERENCE VALUES FOR PPBS

Normal is less than 120 mg/dL. A value greater than 120 but less than 200 mg/dL may necessitate further study. Levels greater than 200 mg/dL are considered indicative of diabetes. Because the 2-hr value rises about 5 mg/dL for each decade of life, a person 60 years of age has a 2-hr PPBS about 15 mg higher than a person 30 years of age.

▼ BLOOD GLUCOSE FINGER STICKS

In the past, most clients with diabetes were monitored by self-testing of urine and occasional blood glucose levels obtained by means of venipuncture by health professionals. (See Chapter 3 on urine tests for glucose.) A "revolution" occurred when self-monitoring of blood glucose became possible with reagent strips and monitors.

Frequent monitoring by finger sticks is needed to maintain tight control of blood glucose levels. The Diabetes Control and Complications Trial Research Group (1993) found that intensive therapy does delay the onset and slow the progression of diabetic retinopathy, nephropathy, and neuropathy in clients with insulin-dependent diabetes mellitus (IDDM). Although self-monitoring of blood glucose levels is much more desirable than urine glucose testing, which Miller (1986) called meaningless, Carr (1990) noted that some clients may have difficulty with finger sticks because of a lack of manual dexterity, the status of the peripheral circulation, or diminished memory or coping ability. Thus, nurses need to evaluate if urine testing may be a better option for the *few* clients who cannot perform satisfactory return demonstrations of self-monitoring of blood glucose. Also note that testing of urine for ketones continues to be important in ketoacidosis, as discussed later in this chapter.

Preparation of Client and Collection of Sample

A drop of capillary blood is obtained by means of a finger stick, an earlobe stick, or in the case of an infant, a heel stick. The extremity should be warm to encourage vasodilation. (See Chapter 1 on the procedure for heel and finger sticks.) For routine monitoring at home, clients may use soap and water rather than alcohol to clean the site. Several different companies make test strips, so it is crucial to follow the manufacturer's recommendations for a certain product. General guidelines are as follows:

1. Cover the entire reagent pad with a drop of blood. Newer monitors require less blood. Don't let the finger touch the pad, because oils from the finger may affect the results.
2. If using a strip alone, begin timing when the blood touches the pad. Check to see if the blood should be wiped off. Some strips do not require blotting.
3. Compare the strip with the color chart on the bottle in which the strip arrived. Each color chart is batch-specific. Most strips have a range from 20 to 40 mg to 800 mg or more. The color pads are in 20–40-mg increments. If the sample is between two colors, estimate the result.
4. If using a meter, calibrate the machine to each new batch of strips as instructed by the manufacturer. Test the meter once a week by using a control solution.
5. Use the meter, immediately before or after a plasma glucose measurement is performed by the laboratory. A meter value should register within 15% of the lab result (Bogosian, 1994).
6. Regular insulin may be given to cover the glucose. Guidelines for coverage may be 180 mg/dL, no insulin; 240 mg/dL, 2–6 units; 400 mg/dL, 5–16 units; 800 mg/dL, 13–26 units. Also clients can learn to fine-tune their own insulin dosages.

The American Diabetes Association (1995) listed 20 different meters, six types of reagent strips, and many brands of equipment for self-sticks. For the visually impaired, there are meters that speak (Herget and Williams, 1989). Glucose meters with built-in timers and digital readouts can be used with memory chips that record each determination so that when they are connected to a microcomputer, a data base is available for decision making. Although glucose photometers or reflectance meters were originally designed for use with capillary blood samples, venous or arterial blood samples may also be used. Research by nurses (Pressly et al., 1990) suggested that obtaining a specimen from a preexisting arterial line rather than using a finger stick is just as accurate and may be preferable for both the nurse and the client in an acute care setting.

Although meters do make blood glucose monitoring easier, clients with diabetes should be confident in just reading the strips. For example, some diabetes camps may encourage the children not to always use a meter so they can "travel light" on a backpacking trip or do a quick check in a variety of other settings in which carrying a monitor may be cumbersome. Newer monitors are very small so portability is less of an issue. Nurses need to assess if clients are using both the visual strips and the monitors correctly.

The Joint Commission on Accreditation of Health Care Organizations (JCAHCO) requires each nurse who uses a meter to demonstrate competency once a month, so it is important that nurses have a voice in selecting the monitors for a particular setting (Juchniewicz, 1993). On the horizon are noninvasive blood glucose monitors that detect glucose with a laser, so finger sticks will not be needed (Kestel, 1994).

▼ GLUCOSE TOLERANCE TEST

Purpose of Test

The oral glucose tolerance test (GTT) used to be considered the best way to diagnose diabetes mellitus. Yet because so many factors can render the test invalid, the current trend is to rely more on FBS levels and PPBS, unless the purpose is to assess for transitional gestational glucose intolerance. Bed rest, infections, and trauma—as well as drugs such as diuretics, birth control pills, or cortisone—all cause an abnormal GTT. Even stress can alter the results. In fact, most clinicians consider a GTT useless when a client is in the hospital because the client is always under some type of stress that makes the test results questionable.

Another objection to the GTT is that normally no one ever sits down and eats pure glucose. Hence the response to the oral glucose load may not reflect a normal response.

Preparation of Client and Collection of Sample

The client must eat a conventional diet for several days before the GTT is performed. The test is usually scheduled for early morning after the client has been fasting all night. Water may be consumed.

At the start of the test, blood is drawn for a FPG, and urine is obtained for testing for glycosuria. The client is then given 75 or 100 g of glucose dissolved in water. The glucose drink may be flavored with lemon juice to make it more palatable. To assess for gestational diabetes, 50 g of glucose is given at 24 and 48 weeks gestation. If the 1-hr glucose is greater than 140 mg, a 3-hr test is completed after an overnight fast (Weiss, 1988; Jackson and Bash, 1994).

Blood samples of glucose are collected at 1-, 2-, and 3-hr intervals. (Some laboratories may collect in half-hour intervals, and others may continue the test for up to 5 hr.) Urine samples may or may not be collected. Although the client may not eat anything during the test, he or she should continue to drink plenty of water so that all the urine samples can be obtained.

The results of all the samples are plotted on a graph to see how long it takes the blood sugar to return to normal. People with diabetes may either take longer to return to baseline readings or never return to fasting levels. Blood sugar in clients with reactive hypoglycemia may drop to subnormal levels in response to the glucose load. The meaning of the curve must be carefully interpreted by the physician. The sample reference values that follow are based on information from several sources, and they show some of the differences that may be expected in GTT results.

REFERENCE VALUES FOR GTT

	Range of Values Before Age 55	Average After Age 75	Pregnancy (upper limits)
FBS	80–110 mg/dL	110 mg	105 mg
Blood sugar in 1 hr	120–160 mg/dL	200 mg	190 mg
Blood sugar in 2 hr	80–110 mg/dL	150 mg	165 mg
Blood sugar in 3 hr	80–110 mg/dL	140 mg	145 mg

See Ravel (1995) for more details.

▼ GLYCOHEMOGLOBIN AND HEMOGLOBIN A_{1c}

With prolonged hyperglycemia, the hemoglobin (hgb) in RBCs remains saturated with glucose as glycohemoglobin (GHB) for the life of the RBC, about 120 days. However, the GHB level is not a simple average of the blood glucose level for 4 months, because RBCs are continually being replaced. The blood glucose levels for the last month count the most, about one-half the total amount (Goldstein, et al., 1994). Hence the test is a weighted average of the glucose level over the last few months.

Beyond 6 months of age, at least 90% of hgb is hgb A. The glycolated part of hgb is designated A_1, or as three subunits—A_{1a}, A_{1b}, and A_{1c}. Hgb A_{1c} is the most abundant of the three and some laboratories report only the finding for A_{1c}. However, other laboratories measure all hgb A_1 as GHB. It is important to know which components are being measured because GHB A_1 is always 2–4% higher than A_{1c}.

The GHB, first introduced in the 1980s, has become part of the standard follow-up care of all people with diabetes. Minimum testing is twice a year, but for clients taking insulin or who have poor control, four times a year is recommended (Ryan, 1994). The GHB is also being investigated as a screening test for diabetes (Hanson et al., 1993).

Preparation of Client and Collection of Sample

Usual diet and medications are taken, including insulin or oral hypoglycemic agents. (People with diabetes may believe they must fast as they do for other routine tests for blood glucose levels.) A 5-ml specimen of venous blood is collected in a lavender-topped (EDTA) tube, put on ice, and sent promptly to the laboratory.

REFERENCE VALUES FOR hgb A_{1C} AND GHB

Hemoglobin A_{1c} (only measures one component of hgb A: A_{1c})

2.2–4.8%	Nondiabetic adult
1.8–4.0%	Nondiabetic child
2.5–5.9%	Good diabetic control
6.0–8.0%	Fair diabetic control
>8.0%	Poor diabetic control

Glycosylated Hemoglobin (measures three components of hgb A: A_{1a}, A_{1b}, A_{1c})

7.5% or less	Good diabetic control
7.6%–8.9%	Fair diabetic control
9.0% or more	Poor diabetic control

Pregnancy results in a lower "normal" range. A variety of methods are used to measure glycated hemoglobins, so values may vary. Also, various factors may affect results, including interference by hemoglobin F with the automated electrophoretic method (Cox et al., 1993).

▼ POSSIBLE NURSING DIAGNOSES RELATED TO ELEVATED GHB

Impaired Home Maintenance Management

An elevated GHB may help motivate clients to reconsider the way they are managing diabetic control. Clients may take more interest and responsibility for their management of diabetes when they see their present regimen is resulting in poor control. Newman et al. (1990) used the GHB to assess if clients were using self-monitoring of glucose to achieve better glucose levels. A high GHB is definitely a risk for diabetic complications, so helping clients understand and use the results of the test is crucial (Ryan, 1994).

Elevated Blood Glucose Level (Hyperglycemia)

Clinical Significance. The most common reason for a persistently elevated blood glucose is diabetes mellitus, in which the relative lack of physiologically active insulin results in an increased blood glucose level and can lead to acidosis and a comatose state.

1. In mild diabetic acidosis, the blood glucose level is usually about 300–450 mg/dL.
2. In moderate diabetic acidosis, the blood glucose is about 450–600 mg/dL.
3. In severe diabetic coma, the blood glucose is usually greater than 600 mg/dL.

Hyperglycemia from other causes may not be as pronounced as the hyperglycemia in diabetic acidosis. In addition, the test for plasma acetone (discussed in the next section) is positive in diabetic acidosis and not in other types of hyperglycemia. Clients with IDDM, or Type I diabetes, are at much greater risk for diabetic ketoacidosis than are clients with non-IDDM or Type II diabetes.

In clinical conditions in which certain hormones are elevated, hyperglycemia may be present.

1. The *glucocorticoids,* for example, tend to raise blood glucose levels because of the breaking down of protein to form new glucose (neoglucogenesis). Clients with Cushing's syndrome or clients taking high doses of cortisone may have higher-than-normal blood glucose levels.
2. Because *epinephrine* increases serum glucose levels, any stress such as shock, burns, or trauma may produce an elevated blood glucose level.
3. *Growth hormone,* secreted by the pituitary gland, produces an elevated blood glucose level by making the cells more resistant to insulin. Tumors or other factors may cause abnormal functioning of the pituitary gland (see Chapter 15).
4. During pregnancy, several hormones tend to cause some hyperglycemia. The placenta secretes HPL, or *human chorionic somatomammotropin,* which tends to raise the blood glucose level. In addition, the increased levels of *estrogen* and *progesterone* may cause some hyperglycemia.

Hormonal changes in pregnancy may make some women less sensitive to the effects of insulin. See the section on the GTT. Transient gestational carbohydrate intolerance (GCI), previously known as gestational diabetes, develops during the second half of the pregnancy and resolves after delivery. However, it may be a precursor to later development of IDDM (Doshier, 1995).

▼ POSSIBLE NURSING DIAGNOSES RELATED TO HYPERGLYCEMIA

Anxiety Related to Potential Diagnosis of Diabetes

Clients with newly elevated blood glucose levels may be very anxious while further testing is being completed. The possibility of diabetes may be particularly frightening if a client knows someone who has numerous complications of the disease. Assessments may indicate the need for health teaching while the client is undergoing an evaluation for diabetes.

1. Excess glucose in the blood can be deposited in the lenses of the eyes, causing blurred vision. It may be several weeks before the sugar deposits are cleared from the lenses. Thus eye examinations for fitting glasses should not be performed until the hyperglycemia is controlled.
2. Talking about a specific diabetic diet during testing would be premature. But if the client is overweight, diet counseling may be appropriate if aimed at motivating the client to shed extra pounds.
3. The importance of exercise in helping the body use glucose can be discussed.
4. Because an elevated blood sugar level makes the client more susceptible to infections, good hygiene becomes very important.

Risk for Fluid Volume Deficits and Electrolyte Imbalances

Two of the most important nursing implications for clients with elevated blood sugar levels are (1) to keep them from becoming dehydrated and (2) to assess for electrolyte imbalances. Glucose in high concentrations in the bloodstream functions as an osmotic diuretic because it makes the plasma hypertonic (Table 8–2). Extra water is pulled into the vascular system from the interstitial spaces and even from the cells if the hyperglycemia is severe and long-lasting. As excess glucose is excreted by the kidneys, so are enormous

TABLE 8–2. EFFECT OF ELEVATED GLUCOSE ON SERUM OSMOLALITY

For an estimate of serum osmolality, the formula is

2(Na + K) + BUN/2.8 + blood glucose/18 = estimate of serum osmolality

Use of formula with normal lab values

2(135 + 4.5) + 15/2.8 + 120/18

279 + 5.36 + 6.67 = 291

Change of values with HHNK

2(146 + 5.0) + 28/2.8 + 300/18

302 + 10 + 16.67 = 329

Note: Reference values for serum osmolality are 282–295 mOsm/kg H_2O, and the values for a calculated one should be within ± 9 or 10 mOsm. See Chapter 4 for a discussion of the precise measurement of serum osmolality. Sometimes K is not used in the formula.

amounts of water. Thus the key symptoms of hyperglycemia are thirst (polydipsia) and increased urination (polyuria).

As long as the client can drink large amounts of water, dehydration may not occur, but the continued diuresis causes a loss of potassium and sodium. The loss of these electrolytes leads to some of the specific problems discussed in Chapter 5.

If the hyperglycemia is due to a lack of insulin, the other two cardinal signs of diabetes, polyphagia and weight loss, eventually occur, because the cells are literally starving for glucose.

When dehydration becomes pronounced, the client has characteristic signs and symptoms, such as the loss of skin turgor, flushed warm skin, and soft eyeballs. The soft eyeballs are due to lack of fluid in the interstitial tissue of the eyeball.

Interventions for Hyperosmolar Hyperglycemic Nonketotic Coma. The progression of the foregoing symptoms is called *hyperosmolar hyperglycemic nonketotic coma* (HHNK). A hyperglycemic coma can occur as a result not only of diabetes but also of any pathologic condition that entails a persistently high blood sugar that causes severe dehydration and electrolyte imbalance. The coma is called *nonketotic* because ketones are not part of the pathologic problem; the serum ketones (see the test for plasma acetone) do not increase. Therapy is geared to reducing the blood sugar level by replacing fluids and perhaps by giving some insulin to help the body use the excess sugar. Because thromboembolic episodes can occur, caused by the increased viscosity of the blood, nurses should institute measures to decrease the chance of venous thrombi. HHNK can be a complication of hyperalimentation therapy if glucose levels are not closely monitored. (See Chapter 3 on urine sugar levels in hyperalimentation therapy.)

Interventions for Diabetic Coma Related to Ketoacidosis. In diabetes, the three levels of glucose intolerance are hyperglycemia, ketosis, and ketoacidosis. Diabetic coma is caused by severe dehydration and by the acidosis resulting from the buildup of ketone bodies. When glucose is not available for the cells because of the lack of insulin, fats and sometimes protein are converted to glucose and used as the source of energy. The incomplete oxidation of fats and proteins leads to the buildup of ketones in the bloodstream (ketosis). Eventually the ketones, which are acid, exhaust the buffering capacity of the blood, and ketoacidosis occurs. The serum bicarbonate level is decreased. Ketoacidosis, as one type of metabolic acidosis, is discussed in Chapter 6 in the section on decreased serum bicarbonate levels. (Note also that the P_{CO_2} level decreases in an attempt to compensate for an overwhelming acidotic state.) Table 8–3 provides a summary of some of the symptoms of hyperglycemia and of hypoglycemia. Table 8–4 shows the laboratory reports used for diabetic ketoacidosis.

(*continued*)

▼ POSSIBLE NURSING DIAGNOSES RELATED TO HYPERGLYCEMIA (*continued*)

Nursing interventions for ketoacidosis include the careful regulation of intravenous fluid and electrolyte replacements, as for HHNK. Electrolytes must be carefully monitored during the acute stages of diabetic coma. Isotonic saline solution (0.9% NaCl) is usually administered, at a rapid rate, as the first infusion. When the blood glucose falls to 250 or 300 mg/dL, the physician may change the intravenous fluid orders to include dextrose 5% so hypoglycemia will not occur later (McCarthy, 1985; Reising, 1995a). Potassium levels are high in the serum because insulin is needed for optimal transportation of potassium into the cells. Potassium also leaves the cell as more hydrogen ions go into it. (See Chapter 5 on the effect of acidosis on the potassium level.) When the acidosis is corrected, hypokalemia may occur if adequate replacement is not given, and hyponatremia may result from the loss of sodium by diuresis. Because dehydration may cause a pseudo-elevation of serum sodium levels, osmolality tests of serum and urine (Chapter 4) are useful to assess the magnitude of the dehydration.

TABLE 8–3. OUTSTANDING SIGNS AND SYMPTOMS OF HYPERGLYCEMIA AND HYPOGLYCEMIA

■ **HYPERGLYCEMIA** (most of the symptoms are due to dehydration, occurs gradually)

- Frequent urination (positive for sugar)
- Thirst, dry mouth, and poor skin turgor
- Soft eyeballs
- Nausea, vomiting, abdominal pain
- Weakness, confusion, blurred vision
- Severe dehydration and electrolyte imbalance
- Possible coma
- Urine positive for ketones[a]
- Kussmaul's respirations[a]
- Acetone breath[a]
- See Table 8–4 for laboratory tests in diabetic ketoacidosis

■ **HYPOGLYCEMIA** (many of the symptoms are due to release of epinephrine, also due to lack of sugar for central nervous system, happens quickly)

- Diaphoresis (see exceptions for newborns and elderly)
- Tachycardia, anxiety
- Weakness, hunger
- Irritability, confusion, behavioral changes
- Tremors or convulsions
- Coma
- Urine negative for sugar
- Low blood sugar

[a]Present only if ketosis and ketoacidosis develop and not present in HHNK.

TABLE 8–4. LABORATORY TESTS USED IN DIABETIC KETOACIDOSIS

	Ketoacidosis		
	"Mild"	"Moderate"	"Severe"
Serum glucose	300–450 mg/dL	450–600 mg/dL	600 mg/dL +
Plasma ketones	4+ in undiluted sample	4+ in 1:1 diluted sample	4+ in 1:2 diluted sample
Serum bicarbonate (see Chapter 6)	More than 15 mEq/L	10–15 mEq/L	Less than 10 mEq/L
pH (see Chapter 6)	More than 7.3	7.2–7.3	Less than 7.2
BUN (see Chapter 4)	Less than 25 mg/dL	25–40 mg/dL	40–100 mg/dL
Urine glucose (see Chapter 3)	2%	2%	2%
Urine acetone (see Chapter 3)	Small	Moderate	Large

See Chapter 4 on osmolality.

Administering Insulin. Regular insulin is the only type of insulin used in treating elevated serum glucose levels that may fluctuate every few hours. It is also used to control glucose blood levels during labor and delivery or during surgical procedures, when the unusual stress causes unpredictable levels of hyperglycemia. The intermediate insulins (NPH and Lente) or longer-acting insulins (Ultralente) are begun when the severe hyperglycemia in ketoacidosis has been corrected and the client is in a more stabilized condition. The nurse must carefully monitor blood sugar levels because additional units of regular insulin are usually ordered on the sliding scale format, as noted in the earlier section on blood glucose reagent strips.

Knowledge Deficit Related to Management of a Chronic Disease

Education for clients who have just received a diagnosis of diabetes is critical. Many health care settings have registered nurses who are certified diabetes educators. However, all nurses in contact with a client with newly diagnosed diabetes can be instrumental in helping the client become proficient in monitoring glucose levels and, if required, insulin injections. Because the dietary regimen is so important, the nurse can reinforce and expand on the information given by the dietician. Some clients may be unaware that "sugar-free" foods may have sweeteners such as sorbitol that have as many calories as sucrose or table sugar (Crapo and Powers, 1990). Education also needs to focus on possible ways to prevent long-term complications. A six-step program of CHANGE is recommended (Colwell and Jewler, 1990) to lower the risk for vascular disease:

- Cholesterol and lipid control (see Chapter 9)
- Hypertension control
- Appropriate weight management

(*continued*)

▼ POSSIBLE NURSING DIAGNOSES RELATED TO HYPERGLYCEMIA (*continued*)

- No smoking
- Glycemic control
- Exercise

The Diabetes Control and Complications Trial Research Group (1993) performed the first important study to demonstrate that intensive therapy effectively delays the onset and slows the progression of three severe complications—diabetic retinopathy, nephropathy, and neuropathy in clients with IDDM.

Clients with Type I (insulin-dependent) diabetes have an increased frequency of thyroid disease. (See Chapter 15 on thyroid tests.) The American Diabetes Association has excellent resources, including several monthly publications, for both the general public and professionals who want to be as up-to-date as possible about management of diabetes and related problems. Call 1-800-232-3472 for more information on the latest standards of care for diabetes.

▼ SERUM ACETONE OR KETONES

When glucose is not available to the cells and the body mobilizes fat and protein as sources of energy, ketone bodies (acetoacetic acid, acetone, and β-hydroxybutyric acid) are the byproducts. The acidity of these ketone bodies causes the ketoacidosis that results from uncontrolled diabetes mellitus or starvation.

When ketoacidosis is suspected, the laboratory can quickly test a blood sample to determine the relative amount of ketones in the blood. Some laboratories may test acetoacetic acid and acetone rather than just ketones. The report for ketone bodies should be *negative*. Various laboratories use slightly different techniques to estimate the presence of ketone bodies, and consequently they report serum ketone or acetone levels in different ways.

Preparation of Client and Collection of Sample

The laboratory usually needs about 2 mL of blood to complete any form of these tests, and there is no special preparation of the client. The tablets used for urine testing of ketones can also be used to test ketones in serum or blood. For serum testing, the color of the tablet is evaluated 2 min after a drop of serum is placed on it. If whole blood is put on the tablet, the clot is removed after 10 min, and the tablet is compared with the chart. Except when laboratory facilities are not readily available, such as during a home visit or in a camp, it is better to let the laboratory measure serum acetone under controlled conditions in which serum can be separated from whole blood and properly diluted.

REFERENCE VALUES FOR SERUM KETONES	
Acetoacetate plus acetone levels	0.3–2.0 mg/dL
Serum ketone levels:	
Undiluted sample	4+ is considered mild ketoacidosis
1:1 diluted sample	4+ is considered moderate ketoacidosis
1:2 diluted sample	4+ is considered severe ketoacidosis

Some laboratories may simply report abnormal results as small, moderate, or large amounts of ketones.

Positive Test for Ketones in Serum and Urine

Clinical Significance. The presence of large amounts of ketones in the serum is diagnostic of ketoacidosis. More often, the presence of ketones is assessed by frequent urine testing because ketones are excreted by the kidney. Urine ketone levels are very important in helping the person with diabetes manage minor illnesses at home (Mackowiak and McCarthy, 1989). (The specific procedure for testing urine for ketones is described in Chapter 3.) As ketones enter the bloodstream, the excess is excreted by the kidneys so that the urine test is positive *before* the buildup in the serum is excessive. However, in severe ketoacidosis, the dehydrated state may cause oliguria, so obtaining urine for testing is difficult. Also, when the acidosis is coming under control with therapy, the serum level is more reflective of the current status of the client because the serum levels begin to drop while the urine level remains high. The serum acetone level is thus the more useful as an immediate indicator of the amount of ketones in the bloodstream. When clients have a continuing positive serum acetone level, the nurse may note a fruity odor to their breath similar to the odor of nail polish remover. The odor is due to the excretion of acetone by the lungs.

Low Blood Glucose Level (Hypoglycemia)

Clinical Significance of Hypoglycemia in a Diabetic Client. Hypoglycemia in a diabetic client is caused by (1) too much insulin or, less frequently, by too high a dose of oral hypoglycemic agents; (2) too little food; or (3) increased exercise without additional food intake. Less insulin is needed for the utilization of glucose when the body's activity is increased by work or exercise. In stressful events, such as infection or trauma, more insulin is needed to control hyperglycemia. Hence, if bouts of hyperglycemia and hypoglycemia are to be prevented, a client with well-controlled diabetes must have a balance among diet, medication, and exercise, plus a lack of stress.

In pregnant women, hypoglycemia is most likely to occur at two times during the pregnancy. During the first 3 months, because the growing fetus requires additional glucose, the mother may experience some periods of low blood sugar. During labor, the extra exertion may make the woman prone to hypoglycemia. There is wide variation in the change of insulin requirements in pregnant women with Type I diabetes (Steel et al., 1994).

Hypoglycemia is always a potential problem in infants whose mothers have diabetes. During uterine life, the infant's pancreas secretes large amounts of insulin because of the high blood glucose levels in the mother. Glucose crosses the placental barrier, but insulin does not. After birth, the infant's pancreas may continue to secrete large amounts of insulin even though the blood glucose levels are much less than in utero. Usually glucose levels drop the most an hour or two after birth, reach a plateau in 2–4 hr, and then gradually increase. Infants who are premature or who have a low birth weight are also prone to hypoglycemia caused by a lack of glycogen reserves in the immature liver. Beckmann (1990) found that postterm infants were not at high risk for hypoglycemia even though the blood glucose level did drop in the first 4 hr of life.

Clinical Significance of Hypoglycemia in Nondiabetic Clients. Hypoglycemia in nondiabetic clients is not well understood. Two main groups of hypoglycemia are classified as *fasting* and *postprandial*. Fasting hypoglycemia is likely to suggest serious organic disease. In a few clients a low blood sugar level can be traced to a tumor of the pancreas, to a lack of cortisone (Addison's disease), to extensive liver disease, or to pituitary hypofunction (see Chapter 15 on growth hormone). Alcohol-induced fasting hypoglycemia can cause death if not identified and corrected.

Most cases of hypoglycemia, however, are termed *functional* because their exact cause cannot be attributed to organic abnormality. Sometimes this type of hypoglycemia is termed *reactive* because the hypoglycemia attack may follow a meal high in carbohydrates, particularly one with a large amount of sugar. Sometimes this functional hypoglycemia may be related to anxiety and stress. The diagnosis of "reactive hypoglycemia" usually refers to a blood glucose level of 50 mg/dL or less, which occurs 2–5 hr after ingestion of food (Palardy et al., 1989).

▼ POSSIBLE NURSING DIAGNOSES RELATED TO HYPOGLYCEMIA

Risk for Injury Related to Lack of Glucose for Normal Cellular Function

For clients who are likely to experience hypoglycemia because of too much insulin, the key nursing implication is to assess for early symptoms of hypoglycemia so that treatment is given quickly. Hypoglycemia occurs rapidly and can lead to coma if it is not treated. (In contrast, the coma of hyperglycemia usually takes much longer to develop as the person becomes progressively more dehydrated and as the ketones build in the bloodstream.)

One of the most outstanding symptoms of hypoglycemia in many adults and children is diaphoresis (excessive sweating). Because infants do not perspire, however, this clinical sign is not useful in the newborn nursery. The diaphoresis, along with tachycardia, dizziness, and tremors, is the result of an increased surge of epinephrine to raise the blood sugar level. Clients taking β-blockers do not exhibit tachycardia.

If the brain is deprived of glucose for more than a few minutes, the client begins to experience irritability, confusion, and behavioral outbursts. These behavioral changes may resemble an intoxicated state. The onset of hypoglycemia in the elderly may not show the signs and symptoms of increased epinephrine usually seen in the young. As a result, the episodes of confusion or other cerebral dysfunctions may be wrongly attributed to cerebral arteriosclerosis.

Interventions to Raise the Blood Sugar Level. Clients may be given 4 ounces (120 mL) of orange juice (10 g simple carbohydrate) or other sugar-containing beverage or candy to treat mild hypoglycemia. At home, 2 ounces of cake-decorating gel supplies the 10 g of simple sugar. Cake gel may be less tempting than candy to keep as a reserve (Lumley, 1988). Basic safety requires that a fast-acting sugar must always be readily available when clients are taking insulin. For example, counselors and nurses in diabetes camps are instructed to *always* carry sugar cubes or gel in their pockets because the additional exercise encouraged by an outdoor setting often causes hypoglycemia. Glucose can be given intravenously. In settings where the client is unable to swallow and intravenous access is not possible, glucagon, discussed next, can be used. Honey or cake-decorating gel can be put under the tongue if the client cannot swallow. After the initial sugar to treat the acute hypoglycemia, food with protein and complex carbohydrates should be given if the next meal is more than 30 minutes away (Reising, 1995b).

Assessing and Treating Hypoglycemia in the Newborn. In newborn infants, the symptoms of hypoglycemia are tremors, listlessness, apnea, cyanosis, a shrill cry, changes in muscular tone, and an unstable temperature. When an infant has hypoglycemia, the resultant release of glucagon stimulates the secretion of calcitonin from the thyroid, which may cause a rapid decrease in serum calcium, which causes tetany. (See Chapter 7 for a discussion of hypocalcemia.) Usually the newborn of a mother with diabetes is fed early with 10–20% glucose by a bottle, by gavage, or by intravenous infusion if necessary. Blood glucose levels are frequently measured (see the procedure for reagant strips discussed earlier in this chapter). Any infant prone to hypoglycemia is usually kept in a special care nursery for close observation.

Assessing for Hypoglycemia When Clinical Symptoms Are Not Obvious. Clients who have experienced hypoglycemia are usually aware of the beginning of symptoms and take some orange juice or candy to offset the reaction. For some people the early symptoms of hypoglycemia may not be obvious, or the hypoglycemia may occur during sleep. For example, with the intermediate-acting insulins (NPH and lente), the peak action is 8–12 hr after administration and the duration is about 24 hr. Headache and weakness may be the only symptoms.

(*continued*)

▼ POSSIBLE NURSING DIAGNOSES RELATED TO HYPOGLYCEMIA (*continued*)

Knowledge Deficit Related to Use of Glucagon as Treatment of Hypoglycemia

Some physicians may order the hormone glucagon as treatment of an insulin reaction when it is not feasible to give intravenous glucose immediately. The hormone, available in 1-mg ampules, is injected the same way as insulin, and it should be effective in raising the blood sugar in 5–15 min (Katzung, 1995). Glucagon, secreted by the α cells of the pancreas, stimulates the formation of glucose from glycogen stores. So it is not effective for a client who is malnourished and who thus has little stored glycogen. A member of the family needs to be instructed on how to give glucagon when the client has an insulin reaction that does not respond to oral sugar. If glucagon is used, the client needs a feeding of combined simple and complex carbohydrates to replenish the glucose.

Altered Nutrition Related to Changes in Activity

The nurse and the diabetic client receiving insulin need to be aware that unusual exercise increases the chance of hypoglycemia. Because active muscular exercise increases the utilization of carbohydrates, the client requires more food intake or less insulin. When a person is in the hospital, the stress of the hospitalization and the lack of normal muscular activity both contribute to increasing the blood sugar level. When the person is discharged, the stress is less and normal muscular activities are resumed. So the insulin requirement may be decreased. Sometimes in pediatric units, children are taken to a park or playground a few times before they are discharged from the hospital so that the insulin maintenance dose matches the food intake and exercise level of the child. This may be very helpful in preventing hypoglycemic attacks after the child is at home.

Knowledge Deficit Related to Insulin Rebound

The Somogyi effect, named after the man who first described the phenomenon, is the occurrence of insulin rebound. After a period of hypoglycemia, several hormones (epinephrine and the glucocorticosteroids) are released to raise serum glucose levels. So repeated episodes of slight hypoglycemia may have theend result of making the client hyperglycemic, which may partially explain why some clients who take insulin have fluctuations of blood sugar levels that are not directly related to food intake. On the basis of this theory, a plan for reducing the insulin dose may bring about a more stable blood sugar level because there is no longer the rebound effect from the periods of slight hypoglycemia.

Unrecognized hypoglycemia most often occurs at night, so the early morning glucose may be higher than normal. However, the *dawn phenomenon,* a term coined in 1984, may also cause a rise in early morning glucose (Lodewick, 1993). The dawn phenomenon refers to the surge of growth hormone that may cause blood glucose to rise. To determine if the client needs more or less insulin, 3 AM glucose tests are performed for a week. If these nighttime results are elevated, more insulin is needed at bedtime. If the 3 AM results are low, less insulin at bedtime prevents insulin rebound.

Altered Nutrition Related to Functional Hypoglycemia

In contrast to a client who has hypoglycemia caused by an insulin reaction, a client with functional hypoglycemia does not have symptoms that progress to a coma. The light-headedness, sweating, and palpitations may be relieved by the intake of a carbohydrate. For the long-term management of hypoglycemic attacks, the client is usually advised not to eat concentrated sugars at all because they may cause a surge of insulin in the bloodstream. The diet usually is a high-protein, low-carbohydrate diet with frequent feedings. For example, the client should eat cottage cheese and maybe some fruit for a mid-morning snack rather than pastry or a doughnut and coffee. Stimulants such as caffeine should be avoided because the caffeine may cause a sudden rise in blood sugar that stimulates insulin production.

Anxiety Related to Functional Hypoglycemia

The relation of diet, stress, and anxiety to functional hypoglycemia still is not well understood. The nurse needs to evaluate the potential stress in the environment because this may be a contributing factor for the development of hypoglycemic symptoms. Emphasis is placed not on the symptoms but on eradicating the stimulus for the symptoms—be it food indiscretions, anxiety, or an undetected organic abnormality. Measuring blood glucose during a hypoglycemic attack at home may be helpful in documenting the physiologic nature of the symptoms and differentiating them from anxiety symptoms.

▼ ISLET CELL AUTOANTIBODIES

Type I diabetes, which usually develops before the age of 30 years, involves a destruction of the islet cells in the pancreas. Close relatives of people with diabetes can be screened with a blood test for islet cell autoantibodies (ICA) to see if they are at risk for diabetes. The Diabetes Prevention Trial for Type I (DPT-1), started in early 1994, is a 5-year national, multicenter clinical trial being sponsored by the National Institutes of Health (NIH). Volunteers who are ICA-positive and meet the criteria for the study are enrolled into one of two different forms of insulin therapy (Ryan, 1994). Although Type I prevention strategies are experimental, clients at risk can undergo an ICA screening and talk to their physicians about the current status of the research to prevent Type I diabetes. Information and a blood screening kit can be obtained by calling the DPT-1 at 1-800-425-8361.

▼ SUGARS OTHER THAN GLUCOSE IN URINE

As discussed in Chapter 3, using the copper-reduction technique (Clinitest), rather than the enzyme method, is important if the presence of sugars other than glucose is to be assessed. Lactose, fructose, and galactose can be detected only with the reduction method. In newborns, metabolic abnormalities caused by genetic defects can cause various sugars to be present in the urine. The excretion of abnormal sugars begins after the baby begins a milk diet. Thus testing for abnormal sugars must not be performed when the baby is still taking just glucose and water. Most of the sugars, such as lactose (discussed next), are fairly benign. The most important other sugar to detect in the urine is galactose, because its presence is a potentially dangerous condition.

▼ LACTOSE TOLERANCE TEST

Lactase, an enzyme found only in the small intestine, is important for digestion of lactose, a sugar found in milk. Because of genetic and other factors, some people, particularly black and Asian people, may have a deficiency of lactase (Savaiano and Kotz, 1988).

A lack of this enzyme leads to an intolerance for milk because the lactose in the milk cannot be converted to a simple sugar. (One glass (8 oz or 240 mL) of milk contains 12 g of lactose). The stools are sour and have a low pH, rather than an alkaline pH, because of the presence of undigested milk. The test for lactose tolerance is to give a measured amount of lactose and then test the blood *glucose* level at various intervals. An increase of less than 20 mg of glucose, associated with gastrointestinal symptoms (bloating or diarrhea) is strongly suggestive of lactase deficiency. Most of the hydrogen from the undigested lactose is passed as flatus, but some is absorbed into the bloodstream and expelled. A breath sample can be analyzed for hydrogen. The treatment is to remove all sources of dietary lactose until the client is symptom-free and then gradually increase lactase until a tolerance level is identified (Englert and Guillory, 1986). Several different commercial lactase formulations are available for replacement of the endogenous lactase. Ramierez et al. (1994) found that lactase preparations differ in ability to improve both breath hydrogen excretion and symptoms. Clients need to investigate what is most effective for them.

▼ SERUM TEST FOR GALACTOSEMIA

Galactosemia is an inherited disorder in which galactose cannot be converted to glucose because of a lack of the enzyme galactose-1-phosphate-uridyl transferase or two other enzymes (Ravel, 1995). The galactose is wasted in the urine. Once galactose has been detected in the urine, the test for these enzymes verifies that there is a genetic defect in metabolizing galactose. To prevent mental retardation and other complications, a diet containing no milk products should be instituted within the newborn period. If milk is not eliminated from the diet, cataracts may appear within 1 month and any neurologic defects may be permanent.

All parents, especially those who deliver the baby at home, need to be aware of the importance of early detection of the presence of any sugar in the urine or any intolerance to milk. Galactosemia is one of the tests sometimes mandated by law for newborns. (See Chapter 18 on genetic screening tests.) Vomiting, liver enlargement, and jaundice are often the earliest signs of the disease. Galactosemia should be considered in any infant with jaundice because of the benefits of early dietary restriction of galactose. The RBC levels of galactose or its metabolites may be used as a monitor to gauge adherence to the diet.

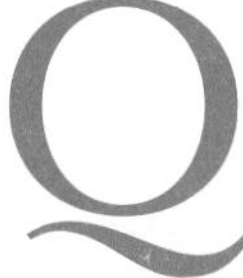

1. Blood glucose levels are the least affected by

   a. Growth hormone b. Cortisone
   c. Testosterone d. Epinephrine

2. In comparing the tests for fasting blood sugar (FBS), postprandial blood sugar (PPBS), and glycohemoglobin (GHB), which statement is the most accurate?

   a. The client must not take anything by mouth before all three tests are performed
   b. An abnormality of any two of the tests indicates diabetes mellitus
   c. GHB gives the most accurate assessment of carbohydrate metabolism
   d. The exact timing of drawing of the specimen is most critical for PPBS

3. A nurse working in an ambulatory center should be familiar with the oral glucose tolerance test to assess transient glucose intolerance if the clients are

   a. Newborns b. Pregnant women
   c. Women approaching menopause d. Elderly men and women

4. Which of the following statements is correct about glucose tests in the elderly client (older than 65 years)?

   a. The curve for a glucose tolerance test for the elderly should return to baseline as soon as the curve for a person younger than 50 years
   b. The renal threshold for glucose is usually decreased in the elderly
   c. The postprandial glucose level in the elderly tends to be higher than postprandial glucose levels for young adults
   d. Normal values for fasting glucose tests tend to border on hypoglycemia in the elderly

5. The plasma acetone level is

a. Increased in both diabetic coma and hyperosmolar hyperglycemic nonketotic coma (HHNK)
b. Decreased in both diabetic coma and HHNK
c. Unchanged in either diabetic coma or HHNK
d. Increased in diabetic coma and not changed in HHNK

6. Mrs. Forini is a diabetic client in labor. She is on sliding-scale insulin coverage for blood glucose greater than 240 mg/dL. Which type of insulin is usually used to control hyperglycemia in acute situations such as labor and delivery?

a. Regular insulin **b.** Lente insulin
c. NPH insulin **d.** Semi-Lente insulin

7. Jack Vinson has just received the diagnosis of IDDM. He asks the nurse what he should do if his blood sugar is always 240 mg/dL before breakfast. The nurse tells him he can find out more information by

a. Testing his blood sugar at 3 AM to see if it is high or low
b. Restricting fluids because he may be overhydrated
c. Verifying the reading by performing a urine test for glucose
d. Keeping a record of his daily caloric intake

8. The risk for injury related to hyperglycemia is the most likely for

a. Baby Tell, born 4 hr ago to a mother with diabetes who is using sliding-scale coverage
b. Ms. Fannin, who is in her first trimester of pregnancy and has insulin-dependent diabetes (Lente 20 units)
c. Mr. Lord, whose diabetes has been controlled on NPH 40 units, but who now is undergoing bed rest because of an infected toe
d. Mr. Sloan, with a possible diagnosis of functional hypoglycemia, who has just eaten two candy bars to "tide him over" until mealtime

9. A characteristic symptom of hypoglycemia in *both* the adult and newborn is which of the following?

a. Diaphoresis **b.** Tremors
c. Shrill cry **d.** Bradycardia

10. The night nurse discovers Mr. Riley, a client with newly diagnosed diabetes, wandering about in his room. He says he has a headache. He appears flushed and warm. The nurse knows that Mr. Riley had 55 units of Lente insulin in the morning and 10 units of regular insulin at bedtime to cover a blood glucose of 240 mg/dL. Which action would be the most appropriate for the nurse to perform first?

a. Get Mr. Riley back to bed and check to see if he has an order for pain relief for the headache

b. Call the intern to check Mr. Riley for possible diabetic acidosis
c. Obtain a finger stick for a blood glucose and then give Mr. Riley a glass of orange juice if his blood sugar is low
d. Assess vital signs, particularly temperature and blood pressure, and wait to see if the client is becoming diaphoretic

11. Glucagon, a hormone from the α cells of the pancreas, is sometimes used to do which of the following?

a. Treat mild cases of diabetes
b. Counteract the effect of epinephrine
c. Help promote conversion of glycogen to glucose
d. Reduce the blood sugar level in newborns

12. A client who has functional or reactive hypoglycemia needs to be taught to avoid a diet that includes

a. Concentrated sugar **b.** High protein
c. Low fats **d.** Frequent small feedings

13. Sarah, age 8, and her parents are in a class for families who have a child with diabetes. Which of the following points should be emphasized to the parents?

a. Recent research has confirmed that tight glucose control lessens the onset and severity of diabetic retinopathy, nephropathy, and neuropathy.
b. Regular exercise is important, but extra insulin must be given
c. Urine ketone testing should be performed if the blood glucose level is greater than 400 mg/dL
d. The glycohemoglobin (GHB) is used to assess for glucose control over the past week

14. Which of the following conclusions is *incorrect* in comparing galactose and lactose intolerances and the tests completed for each?

a. Both galactose and lactose can be detected in the urine with Clinitest tablets
b. Galactose intolerance is a more serious defect than lactose intolerance
c. A nonmilk diet in the infant eliminates the symptoms of both lactose intolerance and galactose intolerance
d. The blood glucose level is abnormally elevated in both conditions

▼ REFERENCES

American Diabetes Association. (1995). Buyer's guide update. *Diabetes Forecast, 48* (1), 66–69.

Beckmann, C. (1990). Postterm pregnancy: Effects on temperature and glucose regulation. *Nursing Research, 39* (1), 21–24.

Bogosian, J. (1994). Meter mysteries solved! *Diabetes Forecast, 47* (10), 26–28.

Carr, P. (1990). Home blood glucose monitoring: It's not for everyone. *Nursing 90, 20* (10), 50.

Colwell, J., and Jewler, D. (1990). Lowering the risk. *Diabetes Forecast, 43* (2), 57–62.

Cox, T., Hess, P.P., Thompson, G.D., et al. (1993). Interference with glycated hemoglobin F may be greater than is generally assumed. *American Journal of Clinical Pathology, 99,* 137–141.

Crapo, P., and Powers, M. (1990). Alias sugar. *Diabetes Forecast, 43* (3), 59–63.

Diabetes Control and Complications Trial Research Group. (1993). The effect of intensive treatment of diabetes on the development and progression of long-term complications in insulin-dependent diabetes mellitus. *New England Journal of Medicine, 329* (14), 977–986.

Doshier, S. (1995). What happens to the offspring of diabetic pregnancies? *MCN: American Journal of Maternal Child Nursing, 20* (1), 25–28.

Englert, D., and Guillory, J. (1986). For want of lactase. *American Journal of Nursing, 86* (8), 902–906.

Goldstein, D., Rife, D., Derrick, K., et al. (1994). The test with a memory. *Diabetes Forecast, 47* (5), 23–25.

Herget, M., and Williams, A. (1989). New aids for low-vision diabetics. *American Journal of Nursing, 89* (10), 1319–1322.

Hanson, R. L., Nelson, R.G., McCance, D.R., et al. (1993). Comparison of screening tests for non-insulin dependent diabetes mellitus. *Archives of Internal Medicine, 153,* 2133–2140.

Jackson, P., and Bash, D.M. (1994). Management of the uncomplicated pregnant diabetic client in the ambulatory setting. *Nurse Practitioner, 19* (12), 64–73.

Juchniewicz, J. (1993). Selecting a QA glucose meter. *American Journal of Nursing, 93* (4), 81–82.

Kaplan, A., Jack, R., Opheim, K.E., et al. (1995). *Clinical chemistry interpretation and techniques.* (4th ed.). Baltimore: Williams & Wilkins.

Katzung, B. (1995). *Basic and clinical pharmacology.* (6th ed.). Norwalk, CT: Appleton & Lange.

Kestel, F. (1994). Blood glucose meters. *Nursing 94, 24* (8), 32P–32R.

Lodewick, P.A. (1993). Is it brittle diabetes or the Somogyi effect? *Diabetes Forecast, 46* (1), 34–36.

Lumley, W. (1988). Controlling hypoglycemia and hyperglycemia. *Nursing 88, 18* (10), 34–41.

Mackowiak, L. and McCarthy, R. (1989). Managing diabetes on "sick days." *American Journal of Nursing, 89* (7), 950–951.

McCarthy, J. (1985). The continuum of diabetic coma. *American Journal of Nursing, 85* (8), 878–882.

Miller, V. (1986). Diabetes: Let's stop testing urine. *American Journal of Nursing, 86* (1), 54.

Newman, W., et al. (1990). Impact of glucose self monitoring on glycohemoglobin values in a veteran population. *Archives of Internal Medicine, 150,* 107–110.

Palardy, S., Havrankora, J., Leogo, R., et al. (1989). Blood glucose measurements during symptomatic episodes in patients with suspected postprandial hypoglycemia. *New England Journal of Medicine, 321* (21), 1421–1425.

Pressly, K., et al. (1990). Use of arterial blood for glucose measurement by reflectance. *Nursing Research, 39* (6), 371–373.

Ramierez, E.C., Lee, K., and Graham, D.Y. (1994). All lactase preparations are not the same: Results of a prospective, randomized, placebo-controlled trial. *American Journal of Gastroenterology, 89* (4), 566–570.

Ravel, R. (1995). *Clinical laboratory medicine: Clinical application of laboratory data* (6th ed.). St. Louis: Mosby–Year Book.

Reising, D.L. (1995a). Acute hyperglycemia: Putting the lid on the crisis. *Nursing 95, 25* (2), 33–40.

Reising, D.L. (1995b). Acute hypoglycemia: Keeping the bottom from falling out. *Nursing 95, 25* (2), 41–48.

Ryan, C. (1994). Magnificent seven. *Diabetes Forecast, 47* (1), 37–39.

Savaiano, D., and Kotz, C. (1988). Recent advances in the management of lactose intolerance. *Contemporary Nutrition, 13* (9), 1–4.

Steel, J.M., Johnstone, F.D., Hume, R., et al. (1994). Insulin requirements during pregnancy in women with Type I diabetes. *Obstetrics and Gynecology, 83* (2), 253–258.

Weiss, B. (1988). Guidelines for using five new prenatal tests. *Postgraduate Medicine, 83* (7), 63–64.

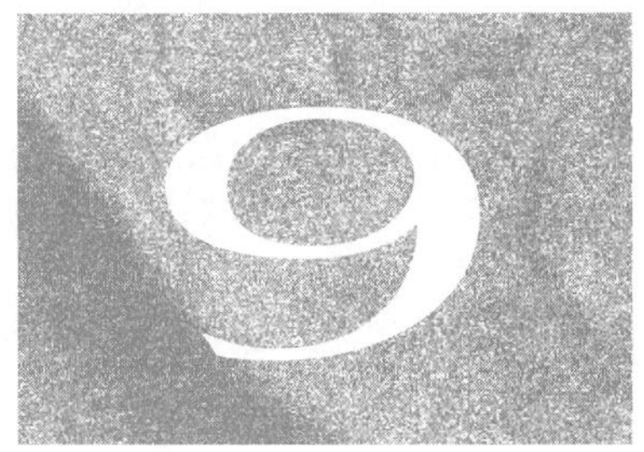

TESTS TO MEASURE LIPID METABOLISM

- ► Serum Cholesterol
- ► Serum Triglycerides
- ► Lipoprotein Electrophoresis and Lipid Profiles
- ► High-density Lipoprotein Cholesterol
- ► Low-density Lipoprotein Cholesterol

OBJECTIVES

1. Define hyperlipidemia and discuss factors that seem to contribute to its development.
2. Describe the client preparation necessary for tests of serum cholesterol and serum triglyceride levels.
3. Discuss the controversial aspects of the relation of serum cholesterol and serum triglyceride levels to the development of cardiovascular disease.
4. Plan a diet low in cholesterol and saturated fats.
5. Identify nursing diagnoses that may be useful for clients with elevated serum cholesterol levels.
6. Identify assessments that might indicate a lack of essential fatty acids in the diet.
7. Give examples of how serum triglyceride levels are used as an evaluation tool.
8. Describe how the research findings on high-density lipoprotein (HDL) and low-density lipoprotein (LDL) cholesterol have been applied to clinical situations.

Hyperlipidemia is a broad term that means high plasma concentrations of cholesterol, triglycerides, or the complex lipoproteins. Lipoproteins transport triglycerides and cholesterol in the plasma. Other lipids found in the serum include the phospholipids, such as lecithin and sphingomyelin. Lecithin and sphingomyelin comprise the basis of the L/S ratio, a test performed on amniotic fluid to evaluate the maturity of the fetus (see Chapter 28).

Serum cholesterol levels and, less frequently, triglyceride levels are measured to evaluate risk for the development of atherosclerosis. According to current knowledge, the serum cholesterol level and the HDL cholesterol are the screening tests for hyperlipidemia.

In addition to the use of these two tests to evaluate hyperlipidemia, lipoprotein electrophoresis may be carried out to evaluate rarer types of lipid abnormalities. Lipoproteins are complex protein molecules that contain several protein and lipid components. Lipoprotein molecules can be separated into four different bands on a strip of paper by using an electric current to cause migration of the molecules.

▼ SERUM CHOLESTEROL

Cholesterol, a natural constituent of the serum, is essential for the production of bile salts, for the manufacture of many of the steroid hormones, and for the composition of cell membranes. Cholesterol is manufactured from saturated fats in the diet. The liver esterifies cholesterol by combining it with a fatty acid. Most of the cholesterol is present in the bloodstream in the esterified form. Cholesterol levels seem to differ greatly depending on variables such as age, diet, geographic location, and genetic influences. Values in the United States used to be considered normal up to about 335 mg, depending on age. Many authorities questioned whether these "normal" values of cholesterol were ideal for optimal health (Kannel, 1976). And a statement by the National Institutes of Health (NIH) Consensus Development Panel (1985) noted moderate-to-high risk for cardiovascular disease when cholesterol levels are greater than 200 mg/dL.

A report written by an expert panel on the detection, evaluation, and treatment of high blood cholesterol in adults (National Cholesterol Education Program Expert Panel, 1988) spurred many organizations to focus on educating the public about the health risk of high cholesterol levels. Nurses have been involved in an extensive program to educate other nurses about the care and treatment of hypercholesteremia (LaRosa and Somelofski, 1990). The average for serum cholesterol levels has lowered in the last few years, but many people in the United States still have levels greater than 200 mg/dL. The National Cholesterol Education Program Expert Panel (1993) recommended (1) emphasizing weight loss and exercise, as well as dietary changes, for the primary prevention of high blood cholesterol, (2) delaying drug therapy for young adult men and premenopausal women who have no other risk factor except a LDL cholesterol in the range of 160–220 mg/dL, and (3) measuring HDL cholesterol, along with total cholesterol, for regular check-ups.

Two approaches have been recommended to deal with the problem of high cholesterol in the United States public. One approach is to identify people at high risk (case-finding approach) so they can receive treatment. Almost all authorities agree that high cholesterol should be treated first with diet and only with drugs if intensive dietary management is not successful. A second approach, the recommendation that *all* people older than 20 years follow a diet low in cholesterol and saturated fats is a public health or population-strategy approach. Continuing debate occurs on the most prudent approach to the "cholesterol problem" and the role of a prudent diet (Mauer, 1987; McNamara, 1987; Hassel, 1990; Durrington, 1994; Reece, 1995). Roberts (1993) noted that even cardiologists are not always enthusiastic about primary prevention programs to lower cholesterol levels.

Preparation of Client and Collection of Sample

The client should consume conventional foods with no dieting for several days. Fasting is not needed unless the cholesterol is part of a lipid profile (e.g., triglycerides, HDL cholesterol, and LDL cholesterol, which are discussed later). Because cholesterol can fluctuate considerably from day to day, at least two samples should be drawn if the first level is 200 mg/dL or greater. If the second level is within 30 mg of the first level, the average of the two can be used. If the first two samples vary more than 30 mg, a third sample is needed, and the average of the three is used to guide the treatment plan. The two or three samples should be drawn within a period of 1–8 weeks. Because some studies have suggested that volume responses to posture can affect cholesterol, the client should be sitting for at least 5 min before the blood is drawn. The venous blood test usually requires 0.5 mL in a tube with no anticoagulant. If plasma is collected (EDTA tube), the blood must clot for 30 min before the test can be performed. Finger sticks can be used for initial screening when an automated analyzer is used. Some drugs, such as vitamin E, phenytoin, or steroids, may cause false elevations, whereas other drugs, such as some antibiotics, may cause falsely low readings.

Home Testing for Serum Cholesterol

In 1993, a blood cholesterol test became available for home use by consumers. The test, available without a prescription, requires one drop of blood to be placed on a test strip within a cassette. Results take 10–15 minutes. Package labeling for the test includes detailed instructions for proper use, a discussion of the test's limitations, and a toll free number (1-800-927-7776) for additional information from Chemtrak, 929 East Arques Avenue, Sunnyvale, CA 94086.

REFERENCE VALUES FOR SERUM CHOLESTEROL

Adults, 20 years and older	
Desirable	<200 mg/dL
Borderline high	200–239 mg/dL

High	≥240 mg/dL
Pregnancy	Increases should return to baseline in about 1 month
Children	<170 mg/dL
Aged	Levels >200 mg/dL may not be a concern

Increased Serum Cholesterol Level

Clinical Significance. For most clients, the reason for a high cholesterol level is not known. Much research is being conducted to determine to what extent genetic, dietary, or other environmental factors contribute to high cholesterol levels. Three recognized genetic disorders lead to hyperlipidemia: (1) familial hypercholesterolemia, (2) familial combined hyperlipidemia, and (3) familial hypertriglyceridemia. Although these three disorders affect 0.5–1% of the population and are the most common genetic diseases, they do not cause most of the high cholesterol levels seen in adults.

In some clinical situations, the cause of the increased serum cholesterol level can be identified. For example, liver disease with biliary obstruction, hypothyroidism, and pancreatic dysfunction all cause increased cholesterol levels. Some drugs, such as corticosteroids, may cause an increased cholesterol level, but the clinical significance of this increase is not known. Although cholesterol levels are normally high in pregnancy, they rise even higher in preeclampsia. The cholesterol level also may increase in nephrotic syndromes.

Recommendations for Follow-up on Total Cholesterol and HDL

The National Cholesterol Education Expert Panel (1993) advised that all clients older than 20 years undergo a serum cholesterol test and a HDL cholesterol. If the results are in the desirable range, the client should undergo another test in 5 years. The public health approach, discussed earlier, mandates that even these clients be given general dietary and risk reduction education. As noted earlier, emphasis on physical activity and any needed weight loss is as important as dietary instruction. Clients with borderline high cholesterol who do not have any evidence of coronary heart disease (CHD) or two other of the risk factors in Table 9–1 should be given the

TABLE 9–1. RISK FACTORS FOR CORONARY HEART DISEASE (CHD)

Male sex[a]
Family history (CHD before 55 yr of age in parent or sibling)
Smoking (more than 10 cigarettes per day)
Hypertension
Low HDL (<35 mg/dL at repeated measurements)
Diabetes mellitus
History of cerebrovascular or occlusive peripheral vascular disease

Information from the *National Cholesterol Education Program Expert Panel* (1993).
[a]Women have an increased risk after menopause (Matthews et al., 1989).

TABLE 9–2. COMPONENTS OF STEP I DIET FOR TREATMENT OF HIGH BLOOD CHOLESTEROL

Nutrient	**Percentage of Total Calories**
Total fat	<30
Saturated fatty acids	<10
Polyunsaturated fatty acids	≤10
Monosaturated fatty acids	10–15
Carbohydrates	50–60
Protein	10–20
Cholesterol	<300 mg/day
Total calories	To achieve and maintain desirable weight

Figures are from National Cholesterol Education Program Expert Panel (1988 and 1993).
Note that a Step II diet has the added limitations of up to 7% saturated fatty acids and only 200 mg of cholesterol per day. Step II is added if Step I does not achieve a desirable cholesterol level in 3–6 months.

dietary information in Table 9–2 and reevaluated in 1 year. Clients with borderline high cholesterol levels who already have evidence of CHD or two or more of the risk factors in Table 9–1 should undergo a thorough medical evaluation. The discussion of LDL cholesterol describes the importance of decreasing this component of the total cholesterol. If an intensive dietary plan, including Step II as noted in Table 9–2, does not bring the levels of cholesterol down to more acceptable limits in 6 months, drug therapy may be started.

▼ POSSIBLE NURSING DIAGNOSES RELATED TO HYPERLIPIDEMIA

Knowledge Deficit Related to Alterations in Diet

Once a client has been definitely identified as having elevated cholesterol, the first recommendation is to decrease the amount of fat in the diet and to replace saturated fats with polyunsaturated fats. Vegetable oils tend to be high in polyunsaturated fats, whereas animal fats are high in saturated fats and cholesterol. Meat, egg yolks, and dairy products are the main sources of cholesterol in the United States diet (Table 9–3). A fat-controlled diet may have other health benefits. The National Research Council's study on diet, nutrition, and cancer supports a total fat intake not more than 30% of the total calories because of the association between high-fat diets and some types of cancer (O'Connor, 1985).

As noted in Table 9–2, the difference between Step I and II diets is that there is 100 mg less of cholesterol and 3% less saturated fatty acids. Even while consuming a Step I diet, many clients can reduce both the total cholesterol and the LDL cholesterol by 10–15% (Stoy, 1989a). Earlier studies (Rifkind and Segal, 1983) involving 12 lipid research clinics reported reductions of serum

(*continued*)

TABLE 9–3. SOURCES OF CHOLESTEROL AND SATURATED FATS IN DIET

	Approximate Amount of Cholesterol (mg)	Approximate Amount of Saturated Fat (g)
Liver	370	2.5
Egg, one	275	1.7
Veal	86	4.0
Pork	80	3.2
Hot dog	75	9.9
Lean beef	73	3.7
Chicken: Light meat	72	1.7
Dark meat	82	2.7
Ice cream, 1 cup	59	8.9
Fish	59	0.3
Lobster	46	0.07
Whole milk, one glass	33	5.1
Cheese, 1 ounce	30	6.0
Butter, 1 tablespoon	31	7.1
Coconut oil	0	11.8
Palm oil	0	6.7
Olive oil	0	1.8
Corn oil	0	1.7
Safflower oil	0	1.2

Note: All meat is 3-ounce servings. Oils is 1 tbsp.
Values collected from several sources published by American Heart Association and others.

▼ POSSIBLE NURSING DIAGNOSES RELATED TO HYPERLIPIDEMIA (*continued*)

cholesterol by at least 7% with diet. The use of soluble fiber, such as oat bran, may be used to implement but not replace the overall dietary plan. Studies continue to see if certain foods, such as boiled but not filtered coffee, increase cholesterol (Bak and Grobbee, 1989). Commercial interpretation of the effects of food on cholesterol level may be confusing to both the client and the nurse. Registered dieticians are an excellent resource for evaluating the scientific foundation of many of the claims made about the effects of various foods on serum cholesterol levels. However, much research is still far from conclusive (Hassel, 1990; Durrington, 1994).

Risk for Noncompliance Related to Need for Long-term Changes in Dietary Patterns

When a client has a high serum cholesterol level, the nurse's role in diet teaching may be crucial. Rather than emphasizing a diet based on restrictions (no eggs, no steak, no ice cream, no butter), it may be better to take a positive approach and emphasize the foods to choose. Thus the client can be encouraged to choose fish, chicken, and lean beef, polyunsaturated margarine rather than butter, and fresh fruit. Clients should also be aware of the food served in "fast food" places, which specialize in selling food that contains high amounts of fats and calories. However, in the past few years several fast food chains have decreased the calorie, fat, and sodium content of their food (Roberts, 1992).

Phillipson et al. (1985) reported that some fatty acids in fish oil may actually protect against cardiovascular disease. The client must read current findings on diet changes because research continues on the role of dietary fatty acids in lowering plasma lipid levels (Grundy, 1989). The American Heart Association has excellent material for teaching clients about low-fat diets. Many authorities have suggested that as early as the second year of life, American children should eat the modified low-fat diet described for adults (Glueck, 1986; Reese, 1995).

Knowledge Deficit Related to Drug Therapy

If dietary changes are not sufficient to lower cholesterol levels after 6 months, the physician may order medications such as those listed in Table 9–4. Cholestyramine (Questran) is also used to lower an elevated direct bilirubin because it binds bile salts. (See Chapter 11 on direct bilirubin.) Some of the most popular drugs for treating hyperlipedemia are hydroxymethylglutaryl–coenzyme A (HMG-CoA) reductase inhibitors, which block an enzyme needed for cholesterol production. The HMG-CoA inhibitors, such as lovastatin and

(*continued*)

TABLE 9–4. DRUGS USED TO TREAT HYPERLIPIDEMIA

Drug	Decreases in LDL Cholesterol (%)	Comments
Cholestyramine (Questran)	15–30	Can increase triglyceride levels. Alters absorption of other drugs and can cause gastrointestinal (GI) symptoms
Colestipol (Colestid)	15–30	Rash, GI symptoms
Nicotinic acid	15–30	Need to test for hyperuricemia (Chapter 4), hyperglycemia (Chapter 8), and liver enzymes (Chapter 12)
Lovastatin (Mevacor)	25–40	Check liver enzymes and for skeletal myopathy
Gemfibrozil (Lopid)	5–15	Not used with gallbladder disease
Probucol (Lorelco)	10–15	Lowers HDL but clinical significance not known Prolongs Q-T interval (Chapter 24)

Percentages based on National Cholesterol Education Program Expert Panel (1988). See also Stoy (1989b); Katzung (1995); and Wilson (1994) for more details on other assessments needed.
Note that after 65 years of age, diet may be the therapeutic approach rather than drugs (Wagner, 1989) because of unwanted effects of drugs in the elderly.

▼ POSSIBLE NURSING DIAGNOSES RELATED TO HYPERLIPIDEMIA (*continued*)

several newer drugs, are effective, but some clinicians believe they should be reserved for clients at high risk whose condition cannot be managed with other drugs (Wilson, 1994).

Nurses must be aware of the information about the specific drug chosen for the client. With most of the drugs, the serum level of cholesterol may not drop for 1–2 months. The client needs encouragement to continue whatever diet has been prescribed and to report any side effects of the drug. Gradually increasing the dosage has been found to decrease side effects (Stoy, 1989b).

Altered Nutrition: Less than Body Requirements

Any plan for diet restriction must be evaluated in relation to the total nutritional needs of the client. A client following a diet very restricted in saturated fats faces the possibility of vitamin E deficiency. If a client does not like skim milk, a calcium deficiency can occur (see Chapter 7). Iron deficiency also may occur with low cholesterol diets, and may be of concern for premenopausal women (Worthington-Roberts, 1987).

Ineffective Individual Coping Related to the Need to Adopt Healthier Lifestyle

The nursing implications for a client with a high serum cholesterol level are broader than simply teaching about diet and drug therapies because cholesterol seems to be only one of the risk factors for cardiovascular disease. Thus, it is important to identify the other risk factors that may be present, such as lack of exercise, obesity, hypertension, stressful environments, and cigarette smoking (NIH Consensus Development Panel, 1985). All these risk factors seem to be interrelated, along with other factors such as glucose levels. For example, hypertension may be a critical factor in the development of atherosclerosis because atheromatous plaques do not develop in low-pressure areas of the circulation, although bathed in the same lipid-laden blood, as they do in arteries that have the highest pressures (Kannel, 1976). Obesity and stress both contribute to the development of hypertension. For each 5 lb (2.25 kg) of extra weight, the diastolic pressure rises about 1 mm Hg. It is not enough to tackle just one of the risk factors, because all are part of a still *poorly understood* pathophysiologic condition.

Hence a nurse skilled in health teaching and counseling can help clients with a high serum cholesterol level to find ways to achieve a healthier lifestyle. A cardiovascular nurse interventionist is an emerging new role (Engler and Engler, 1994). It is essential that clients know both what is known and what is still not known about the role of serum cholesterol and other risk factors in the development of vascular disease. Clients can then make choices about what can be changed in their style of living to reduce some of or all the risk factors.

Altered Health Maintenance Related to Need for Family Follow-up Care

Although the influence of genetics cannot be controlled by the person, it is important to consider genetic implications in counseling a client with an elevated serum cholesterol level. Because severe hyperlipidemia may sometimes be partly genetically based, the family members of clients with diagnosed hyperlipidemia need to be screened for the same condition. It is usually considered advisable to screen close relatives when a parent or sibling has a coronary event before the age of 55 years. Children whose parents are known to have a blood cholesterol of 240 mg/dL or higher should also be screened (Reece, 1995). If familial hyperlipidemia is suspected and a child's lipid levels are normal, rescreening every 3–5 years is recommended. Most authorities believe the prevention of hyperlipidemia, particularly in young people, begins with basic changes in health practices for the entire family. Williams et al. (1986) offered evidence that men with familial hypercholesterolemia can avoid early coronary death by controlling the known risk factors.

Decreased Serum Cholesterol Level

Clinical Significance. Common conditions that cause low serum cholesterol levels include (1) *hyperthyroidism,* in which the increased metabolism accounts for an increased utilization of fat; (2) *severe liver damage,* after which the liver can no longer manufacture cholesterol; and (3) *malnutrition,* which eventually leads to a deficiency of cholesterol caused by the lack of fats in the diet. Chronic anemia, cortisone therapy, and acquired immunodeficiency syndrome (AIDS) also cause lowered cholesterol levels. If the low serum cholesterol level is the result of a disease process, treatment is geared toward the particular pathophysiologic condition. The low serum cholesterol level, by itself, is not of specific concern.

If the client is following a diet or taking drugs to reduce cholesterol levels, a gradual lowering of the serum cholesterol levels is an indication of the effectiveness of therapy.

▼ SERUM TRIGLYCERIDES

Triglycerides, like cholesterol and the phospholipids, are lipids that are normally present in the serum. The more precise chemical term for this group of lipids is *tri-*

acylglycerols, but the laboratory test is called *triglycerides*. The triglycerides, the most abundant group of lipids, are neutral fat and oils that come from both animal fat and vegetable oils. A heavy meal or alcohol causes a transient increase in serum triglyceride level. Excess triglycerides, which are useful for energy, are stored in the body as adipose tissue. The triglyceride test is useful in identifying some types of hyperlipidemia and is used as one factor in determining the LDL cholesterol.

Preparation of Client and Collection of Sample

The test should be performed in the fasting state, but the client should consume a conventional diet before the fasting begins. The laboratory needs 2 mL of serum. Because there is much variation in what is considered normal, the client should undergo the test two or three times in a 1- to 8-week period as discussed for serum cholesterol. Certain drugs such as thiazide diuretics, β-adrenergic blockers, estrogen, and corticosteroids may increase the levels of triglycerides.

REFERENCE VALUES FOR TRIGLYCERIDES

Adult	40–150 mg/dL. Age- and diet-related. Women slightly lower[a]
Pregnancy	Level rises progressively during pregnancy Note that oral contraceptives also cause an increase
Newborn	Less than 40 mg at birth but rises to 55–60 mg/dL
Children (aged 10–14)	Boy, 65 mg/dL; girl, 75 mg/dL
(aged 15–19)	Man, 80 mg/dL; woman, 75 mg/dL
Aged (older than 65)	130–135 mg/dL

[a]See Rifkind and Segal (1983) for specific breakdown for all age groups. Note that triglyceride levels as great as 250 mg/dL may be considered normal if the serum cholesterol level is normal. Definite hypertrigliceridemia is defined as greater than 500 mg/dL (National Cholesterol Education Program Expert Panel, 1988; 1993).

Increased Serum Triglyceride Levels

Clinical Significance. Many of the clinical conditions that cause an increase in serum cholesterol levels also cause increases in triglyceride levels. Thus clients with nephrotic syndrome, pancreatic dysfunction, diabetes, toxemia of pregnancy, and hypothyroidism have elevated triglyceride levels. Pancreatitis may cause a very high elevation of triglycerides. Fatty meals and alcohol always raise the triglyceride level for a while. The serum triglyceride level peaks about 5 hr after a fatty meal. An increase of serum triglycerides is sometimes associated with certain abnormal patterns of lipid metabolism that are probably genetic in origin.

▼ POSSIBLE NURSING DIAGNOSES RELATED TO ELEVATED TRIGLYCERIDE LEVELS

Knowledge Deficit Related to Diet and Possible Drug Therapy

Clients need the same instructions on diet discussed in the section on cholesterol levels. Often weight reduction and a low-fat diet can lower the serum triglyceride level. Some of the drugs used to lower cholesterol may affect triglyceride levels, as noted in Table 9–4.

Risk for Ineffective Coping Related to Unhealthy Lifestyle

The reduction of hyperlipidemia needs to be done in conjunction with other measures to improve the total health of the person. Authorities consider cigarette smoking, hypertension, and cholesterol the three main risk factors for cardiovascular disease. The elevated serum triglyceride level is not as firmly established as cholesterol as a risk factor. Because alcohol causes secondary hyperlipidemia, the possibility of alcohol abuse should be investigated when there are unexplained high levels of triglycerides. Alcohol should be avoided. Fish oils may help lower triglyceride levels (Phillipson et al., 1985).

Risk for Injury Related to Use of Fat Emulsions

Clients who are deficient in fatty acids can be given fat emulsions intravenously. Because the usual hyperalimentation fluids contain only glucose and amino acids, the fat is given as a separate solution. The fat used for intravenous replacement is composed of soybean oil emulsions and purified egg phosphatides in glycerol and water. This lipid emulsion (Intralipid, Liposyn) can be given via a peripheral vein. Maintaining the stability of the emulsion before and during infusion, as well as watching for untoward reactions, is the responsibility of the nurse. Specific instructions about how to administer the emulsion are included with the bottle of solution. The client's ability to use lipid emulsions is evaluated by testing the serum triglyceride levels. Within 18 hr after the lipid infusion, the serum triglyceride levels should return to baseline. If the serum triglyceride level remains elevated longer than 18 hr, the client should not be given more fat emulsions.

Decreased Serum Triglyceride Levels

Clinical Significance. A decreased triglyceride level is rarely seen as a clinical problem. Some rare genetic defects may cause low serum triglycerides, and severe malnutrition may lead to low levels. Although hypothyroidism may cause an abnormally high triglyceride level, hyperthyroidism does not contribute to a low level. If the low serum triglyceride level is due to an exhaustion of the body's store of essential fatty acids, the client may have sparse hair growth, scaly and dry skin, poor wound healing, and a decrease in blood platelets, which may lead to some bleeding. The nurse should look for these signs when clients are not getting enough fat in their diet.

▼ LIPOPROTEIN ELECTROPHORESIS AND LIPID PROFILES

Lipoproteins are complex molecules that contain lipids, such as cholesterol and triglycerides, in combination with various proteins. Researchers have been able to make some broad classifications of these lipoproteins based on the varying density of their molecules: HDL, which weigh the most, LDL, and very low-density lipoproteins (VLDL). Electrophoresis can separate these types with an electric current to cause migration of the molecules. The direction of the different protein molecules is based on size and electrical charge. After the lipoproteins have separated into distinct layers, the layers make a distinct pattern that shows the relative distribution of four bands of lipoproteins: (1) chylomicrons (particles representing dietary fat in transport), (2) pre-β lipoproteins (VLDL), (3) β lipoproteins (LDL), and (4) α lipoproteins (HDL).

A classification system developed by Fredrickson et al. (1967) used lipoprotein electrophoresis to classify hyperlipidemia into six types (Types I through V, Type II having an a and b part). For many years, diet and drug therapy was based on this classification system. Some research projects may still use information based on these broad lipoprotein patterns. However, the lipid profile, which includes serum cholesterol, triglycerides, and the HDL and LDL cholesterols, has replaced the older lipoprotein electrophoresis as the clinical assessment of risk for coronary disease.

▼ HIGH-DENSITY LIPOPROTEIN CHOLESTEROL

The cholesterol component of HDL (α lipoproteins) is measured as part of a lipid profile. Normally about 20% of cholesterol is HDL cholesterol. Data from the Framingham study, a longitudinal study of the cardiovascular risk for a population in Massachusetts, have supported the theory that low levels of HDL are associated with an increased incidence of CHD. In 1993, the National Cholesterol Education Program Expert Panel recommended that HDL cholesterol be measured when total cholesterol is screened.

Lafferty and Fiske (1994) reported that the mean serum LDL cholesterol was 21% lower and the HDL cholesterol 37% higher in women receiving estrogen replacement than in women who served as controls.

Preparation of Client and Collection of Sample

The client should fast overnight. Water is allowed. The client should not have had weight changes in the past few weeks. Because many drugs may affect the pattern, drugs should be withheld for 24–48 hr, if possible. Radiologic contrast agents interfere with the test. See notes on total cholesterol for timing of repeat samples.

REFERENCE VALUES FOR HDL CHOLESTEROL
Levels below 35 mg/dL are considered a positive risk factor for CHD
Levels above 60 mg/dL are considered a negative risk factor for CHD

Rifkind and Segal (1983) reported percentile reference values for various age groups. The average for men was 44–45 mg/dL and for women was 55 mg/dL.

▼ LOW-DENSITY LIPOPROTEIN CHOLESTEROL

LDLs carry cholesterol in the plasma. Because this type of LDL cholesterol has been associated with coronary arterial atherosclerosis, it is called "bad" cholesterol. HDL cholesterol is the "good" cholesterol. The laboratory can determine the amount of LDL by use of the following formula:

$$\text{LDL cholesterol} = \text{total cholesterol} - [\text{HDL cholesterol} + (\text{triglycerides}/5)]$$

For example:

$$\text{LDL cholesterol} = 200 - \left(55 + \frac{100}{5}\right)$$

$$200 - 75 = 125$$

The formula is not valid for specimens with chylomicrons present or if triglyceride levels are greater than 400 mg/dL (Kaplan et al., 1995).

Preparation of Client and Collection of Sample

The client should consume a stable diet for at least 2 weeks before lipid profiles are performed. Fasting is required 12 hr before the test. (See notes on total cholesterol levels, since LDL can be calculated from other blood work. Some laboratories may do a direct test of LDL so check for amount of blood needed for the single test.)

REFERENCE VALUES FOR LDL CHOLESTEROL	
Desirable range for adults[a]	<130 mg/dL
Borderline	130–159 mg/dL
High risk	>160 mg/dL

[a]Until menopause, women have considerably lower ranges than men. Rifkind and Segal (1983) gave percentiles for all age groups.

▼ POSSIBLE NURSING DIAGNOSES RELATED TO HDL AND LDL CHOLESTEROL LEVELS

Altered Health Maintenance Related to Low Levels of HDL Cholesterol or High Levels of LDL Cholesterol

Clients with high LDL cholesterol or low HDL cholesterol may want to know what else besides diet and drugs may help them decrease the risk of cardiovascular disease. Several studies have suggested that alcohol may increase the amounts of HDL cholesterol, but the National Cholesterol Education Program does not recommend alcohol because of the other health hazards that can occur from overuse. Genetics cannot be changed, but other factors that are related to less of the good HDL cholesterol and more of the bad LDL cholesterol are obesity and lack of exercise. These factors and smoking are under the control of the person, although making changes does often require professional support. However, being at risk for coronary artery disease can be a strong motivation for clients to evaluate the effect of their total lifestyle on their health. Computer programs are available to help with the assessment of risk factors. Pilon and Renfroe (1990) evaluated one such computerized health assessment program managed by occupational health nurses. Their findings suggested that nursing interventions of focused, written feedback about risk factors as well as counseling and classes in risk reduction helped a large number of hospital employees reduce diastolic blood pressure, smoking, and serum cholesterol levels.

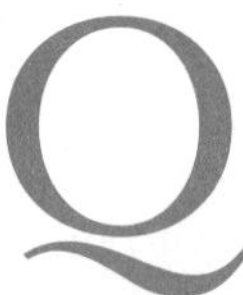

1. In women, serum cholesterol levels tend to remain at relatively low levels

   a. During the menstrual cycle **b.** During pregnancy
   c. After menopause **d.** With hypothyroidism

2. Which one of the following meals contains the least amount of cholesterol?

   a. Steak, baked potato with sour cream, roll and butter, tossed salad with French dressing, and coffee
   b. Lobster, rice, salad with Thousand Island dressing, milk, and apple pie with cheese slice

c. Chicken, mashed potatoes, green beans, salad with blue cheese dressing, wine, and strawberries with powdered sugar
d. Liver, rice, peas, cole slaw, tea, and ice cream

3. For clients with hyperlipidemia, the nurse needs to help assess whether the lifestyle contains other high risk factors for the development of coronary heart disease (CHD). Which one of the following has the least impact on development of CHD?

a. Alcoholic beverages b. Cigarette smoking
c. Hypertension d. Obesity

4. Mr. Riley, 44 years of age, has started drug therapy for a high serum cholesterol level that did not respond to diet and weight control. Which of the following information about hyperlipidemia and drug therapy is appropriate to use to teach Mr. Riley about his disease and drug therapy?

a. Serum cholesterol levels should drop in a week or two after drugs are begun
b. Drug therapy eliminates the need for dietary restrictions
c. Drug therapy always reduces both cholesterol and triglyceride levels
d. Family members of Mr. Riley should undergo screening for abnormal lipid levels because they may need treatment

5. Which one of the following lipid-lowering drugs is also used to treat jaundice?

a. Niacin or nicotinic acid b. Cholestyramine (Questran)
c. Lovastatin (Mevacor) d. Gemfibrozil (Lopid)

6. Serum triglyceride levels would be the least useful for

a. Evaluating the effect of intravenous fat emulsions
b. Assessing the presence of hyperthyroidism
c. Evaluating the effectiveness of some drugs used to control hyperlipidemia
d. Assessing the type of hyperlipidemia that may be present

7. According to data from the Framingham study, the type of lipoproteins that may offer some protection against the development of cardiovascular disease is which of the following?

a. Chylomicrons
b. Pre-β (very low-density) lipoproteins (VLDL)
c. β (low-density) lipoproteins (LDL)
d. α (high-density) lipoproteins (HDL)

8. A factor that tends to increase the level of HDL cholesterol is which of the following?

a. Losing weight if obese b. Eating meat
c. Eliminating alcohol from the diet d. Lack of exercise

▼ REFERENCES

Bak, A., and Grobbee, D. (1989). The effect on serum cholesterol levels of coffee brewed by filtering or boiling. *New England Journal of Medicine, 321* (21), 1432–1437.

Durrington, P.N. (1994). Can any agreement be reached on cholesterol lowering? *British Heart Journal, 71,* 125–128.

Engler, M.B., and Engler, M.E. (1994). Cardiovascular nurse interventionist: An emerging new role. *Nursing & Health Care, 15* (4), 198–202.

Fredrickson, D.S., et al. (1967). Fat transport in lipoproteins: An integrated approach to mechanisms and disorders. *New England Journal of Medicine, 276* (4), 215–224.

Glueck, C. (1986). Pediatric primary prevention of atherosclerosis. *New England Journal of Medicine, 314* (3), 175–176.

Grundy, S. (1989). Recent research on dietary fatty acids: Implications for future dietary recommendations. *Food and Nutrition News, 61* (5), 29–31.

Hassel, C. (1990). An examination of diet, blood cholesterol and coronary heart disease. *Food and Nutrition News, 62* (2), 12–14.

Kannel, W. (1976). Some lessons in cardiovascular epidemiology from Framingham. *American Journal of Cardiology, 37* (2), 269–282.

Kaplan, A., Jack, R., Opheim, K.E., et al. (1995). *Clinical chemistry interpretation and techniques* (4th ed.). Baltimore: Williams & Wilkins.

Katzung, B. (1995). *Basic and clinical pharmacology* (6th ed.). Norwalk: Appleton & Lange.

Lafferty, F.W., and Fiske, M.E. (1994). Postmenopausal estrogen replacement: A long-term cohort study. *American Journal of Medicine, 97,* 66–77.

LaRosa, J., and Somelofski, C. (1990). Cholesterol education program for nurses. *Transitions: Council on Medical-Surgical Nursing Practice, 8* (1), 3.

Matthews, K., et al. (1989). Menopause and risk factors for coronary heart disease. *New England Journal of Medicine, 321* (10), 99–103.

Mauer, A. (1987). Dietary cholesterol recommendations for children. *Contemporary Nutrition, 12* (5), 1–2.

McNamara, D. (1987). The diet-heart question: How good is the evidence? *Contemporary Nutrition, 12* (4), 1–2.

National Cholesterol Education Program Expert Panel (1988). Report of the national cholesterol education program expert panel on detection, evaluation, and treatment of high blood cholesterol in adults. *Archives Internal Medicine, 148* (1), 36–69.

National Cholesterol Education Program Expert Panel. (1993). Second report of the expert panel on detection, evaluation, and treatment of high blood cholesterol in adults. Executive Summary. U.S. Department of Health and Human Services. NIH Publication No. 93–3096.

National Institutes of Health Consensus Development Panel (1985). Lowering blood cholesterol to prevent heart disease. *Consensus Development Conference Statement 5* (7). Bethesda: U.S. Department of Health and Human Services.

O'Connor, T. (1985). Dietary fat, calories and cancer. *Contemporary Nutrition, 10* (7), 1–2.

Phillipson, B., et al. (1985). Reduction of plasma lipids, lipoproteins, and apoproteins by dietary fish oils in patients with hypertriglyceridemia. *New England Journal of Medicine, 312,* 1210–1216.

Pilon, B., and Renfroe, D. (1990). Evaluation of an employee health risk appraisal program. *AAOHN Journal, 38* (5), 230–235.

Reece, S. M. (1995). Toward the prevention of coronary heart disease: Screening of children and adolescents for high blood cholesterol. *Nurse Practitioner, 20* (2), 22–35.

Rifkind, B., and Segal, P. (1983). Lipid research clinics program reference values for hyperlipidemia and hypolipidemia. *JAMA, 250* (14), 1869–1872.

Roberts, W.C. (1992). More on fast foods and quick plaques. *American Journal of Cardiology, 70,* 268–270.

Roberts, W.C. (1993). Getting cardiologists interested in lipids. *American Journal of Cardiology, 72,* 744–745.

Stoy, D. (1989a). Controlling cholesterol with diet. *American Journal of Nursing, 89* (12), 1625–1627.

Stoy, D. (1989b). Controlling cholesterol with drugs. *American Journal of Nursing, 89* (12), 1628–1633.

Wagner, J. (1989). Cholesterol screening in the elderly. *JAMA, 262* (4), 454.

Williams, R., et al. (1986). Evidence that men with familial hypercholesterolemia can avoid early coronary death. *JAMA, 255* (2), 219–224.

Wilson, B.A. (1994). Understanding management of hyperlipidemia. *MEDSURG Nursing, 3* (4), 319–321.

Worthington-Roberts, B. (1987). Dietary guidelines and lipid profiles of young women. *Food and Nutrition News, 59* (5), 75–78.

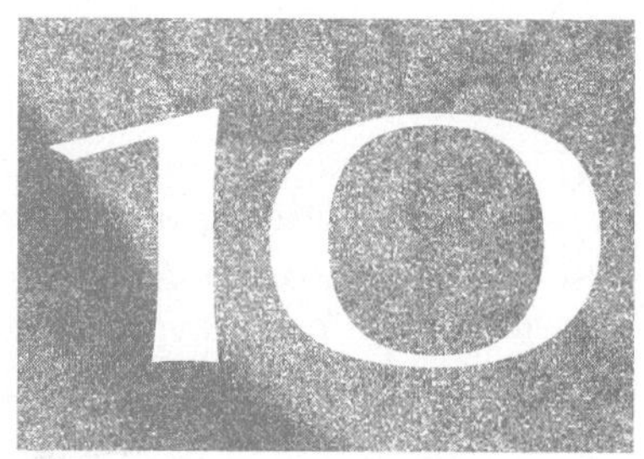

TESTS RELATED TO SERUM PROTEIN LEVELS

- Serum Protein Electrophoresis
- Serum Albumin
- Pre-albumin
- Alpha-1-antitrypsin or Alpha-1-proteinase Inhibitor
- Gamma Globulins
- Immunoelectrophoresis and Quantification of Serum Proteins: IgG, IgA, IgM, IgD, and IgE
- Urine Protein Electrophoresis and Immunoelectrophoresis
- Serum Ammonia
- Alpha-fetoprotein
- Tumor Markers
- Carcinoembryonic Antigen
- CA 125 Antigen
- CA 50
- Prostate-specific Antigen

OBJECTIVES

1. Identify the serum proteins measured by electrophoresis and immunoelectrophoresis.
2. Illustrate how cellular and humoral immunity are assessed by specific laboratory tests.
3. Identify nursing diagnoses for clients with low serum albumin levels (hypoalbuminemia).

4. Explain the general clinical significance of various aclonal, monoclonal, and polyclonal patterns of immunoglobulins in serum and urine.
5. Identify basic nursing interventions for clients who have an abnormal pattern or deficiency of γ-globulins.
6. Describe how the radioallergosorbent (RAST) test is used in the assessment of allergies.
7. Identify the types of medications and food that must be withheld when a client has an elevated serum ammonia level.
8. Describe the clinical usefulness of AFP, CEA, CA 125, CA 50, and PSA as tumor markers.

This chapter focuses on the most common tests used to measure proteins in the serum, including some tumor markers. The difference between serum and plasma proteins is that plasma proteins include those involved in the clotting of the plasma. (The plasma proteins, fibrinogen and prothrombin, are discussed in Chapter 13.)

The two serum proteins measured in the test for total proteins are albumin and globulin. Albumin is a singular type of protein that is either in the serum in sufficient amounts or is not. The tests for globulins are more complex because there are five types of globulins (α-1 and -2, β-1 and -2, and γ-globulins). In addition, there are many singular types of proteins in each of these main classes.

The exact amounts of albumin and of the five main globulin types are determined with a procedure called *electrophoresis*. If certain of the γ-globulins are shown to be abnormal, a further test, *immunoelectrophoresis,* is performed to separate the five main types of γ-globulins. Electrophoresis uses an electrical current to separate the six protein fractions, whereas *immunoelectrophoresis,* involves, as an added step, the use of antiserum to cause precipitation of the five γ-globulins. Immunofixation uses a similar technique. The proteins identified by these tests are shown in Table 10–1. These tests can be performed not only on serum but also on urine and spinal fluid.

FUNCTIONS OF ALBUMIN IN THE SERUM

Albumin, produced only by the liver, is essential in maintaining the oncotic pressure in the vascular system. A lack of albumin in the serum allows fluid to leak out into the interstitial spaces and into the peritoneal cavity. Albumin is also very important in the transportation of many substances in the bloodstream. For example, when the serum albumin level is less than normal, the total serum calcium level is depressed. (See Chapter 7 on how albumin affects the interpretation of serum calcium levels.) Many drugs, lipids, hormones, and toxins are bound to albumin while they are circulating in the bloodstream. Once the drug or other substance reaches the liver, it is detached from the albumin and converted to a water-soluble form that can be excreted. (See Chapter 11 for further discussion about the role of albumin in the conjugation process of bilirubin.) Albumin is also one of the buffers that function to maintain acid–base balance in the bloodstream, as discussed in Chapter 6.

TABLE 10–1. TESTS OF SERUM PROTEINS

Measured as Total Proteins (TP)	Measured with Protein Electrophoresis (PEP)	Measured with Immunoelectrophoresis (IEP) or Quantitative Analysis	
Serum proteins 6.0–8.0			
Albumin (3.1–4.3 g/dL) 52–68%			
Globulins[a] 2.6–4.1 g/dL	α-1 globulins (4.2–7.2%)		
	α-2 globulins (6.8–12%)		
	β-1 globulins (3–10%)		
	β-2 globulins (1–9%)	IgG	75%
	γ-globulins (13–23%)	IgA	10–15%
		IgM	7–10%
		IgD	<1%
		IgE	<1%

Values are approximate values for adults. See text for variations across life span.
[a]Note that many of the α- and β-globulins can be measured by individual tests for α-1-antitrypsin, α-fetoprotein, and so on.

FUNCTIONS OF GLOBULINS IN THE SERUM

As can be seen in Table 10–1, the globulins are a very complex and diversified group of serum proteins, for which both the α and the β types are synthesized in the liver:

1. α-*1 globulins* contain various lipoproteins, glycoproteins, antitrypsin, and other proteins such as thyroxine-binding globulin.
2. α-*2 globulins* contain macroglobulins, haptoglobulin, ceruloplasmin, and hormones such as erythropoietin.
3. β-*1 globulins* contain hormones, fat-soluble vitamins, transferrin, and plasminogen, in addition to other lipoproteins.
4. β-*2 globulins* contain most of the various components of the complement system and other proteins.

Nurses need not necessarily remember which specific proteins belong with which type of α- or β-globulin. The point is that the globulins are composed of many types of proteins. Liver dysfunction is a common reason for overall changes in α- and β-globulins. Diseases that change an individual α- or β-globulin, such as the lack of erythropoietin in renal disease, do not cause a substantial change in the broad grouping of serum globulins. (Some of the individual tests for the various components of the complement system, as well as other serologic tests involving protein reactions, are described in Chapter 14.) Lipoprotein electrophoresis, which measures specific α- and β-globulins involved in fat (lipid) transport, is used to detect some types of hyperlipidemia. (Lipoprotein electrophoresis is discussed in Chapter 9.)

Unlike the α- and β-globulins, γ-globulins, now called *immunoglobulins,* are not synthesized by the liver. They are made by B lymphocytes in response to a stimulus from an antigen. Classified as five main types that are designated by the letters IgG, IgA, IgM, IgD, and IgE, these five immunoglobulins are changed considerably in different types of immunologic responses. To understand the clinical significance of testing for immunoglobulins, one must recall some facts about the concepts of cellular and humoral immunity.

Immune System

Optimal immunologic defense depends on interactions between cellular and humoral immunity, but much is still to be learned about the interaction between these two systems.

Cellular Immunity

Cellular immunity and delayed hypersensitivity are functions of the T lymphocytes controlled by the thymus. The presence of adequate cellular immunity can be demonstrated by a positive response to various skin tests. Clients with negative tests for all the antigens on a skin test panel have anergy, the inability to mount an immune response. Anergy panel testing has become much more common with the growing threat of tuberculosis and the continuing threat of human immunodeficiency virus (HIV) infection (Calianno and Pino, 1995). Blood lymphocyte phenotyping (Chapter 2) helps assess the adequacy of T lymphocytes for cell-mediated immunity and for assisting with humoral immunity.

Humoral Immunity

Because the immunoglobulins secreted by the B lymphocytes are found in the bloodstream and in other secretions, such as saliva, tears, and colostrum, this type of immunity is called *humoral.* Humoral immunity is the type directly measured by assessment of the circulating antibodies in serum and in other body fluids. The *B* stands not for blood but for bursa, because earlier research discovered this type of lymphocyte in the bursae of chickens. In humans, the B lymphocytes are thought to be matured in the lymphoid tissue at various locations. The B lymphocytes produce the IgM class of antibodies as a first response to a potential infection. As the response proceeds, the B lymphocytes can be switched to produce other isotypes such as IgG, IgA, or IgE (see the section on immunoglobulins). Isotype switching requires collaboration between the B lymphocytes and the helper CD4+ T lymphocytes. Knowledge of both congenital and acquired immune deficiencies is increasing as researchers explore the genetic basis of immunoglobulin class switching (Geha and Rosen, 1994).

The complement system contains several proteins that are classified by the letter C and a number (e.g., C2, C4). The complement system enhances the antibody–antigen reaction of the humoral system. The tests involving the complement system are discussed in Chapter 14.

▼ SERUM PROTEIN ELECTROPHORESIS

In serum protein electrophoresis, the laboratory uses an electrical current to separate normal human serum into six distinct protein fractions, through a migration of protein molecules. Various protein molecules, after separating out in a gel mixture or on a coated film, are fixed on a sheet of paper. Albumin, the largest component, has the greatest mobility, so it moves the farthest away from the point of the electrical current. The α-globulins line up next, then the β-globulins. Because the γ-globulins migrate the least from the electrical point, this group makes the last large, distinct band on the paper. Once the six protein fractions have been separated on the strip of paper, the sheet is stained to identify the pattern.

This pictorial representation of the amounts of each protein type is useful as a screening device because changes in the patterns can be seen and further testing carried out if deemed necessary by the clinician. For example, protein electrophoresis is a screening test for multiple myeloma. The pathologist is usually the one to compare the pattern with known abnormal patterns seen in various disease states. The strip of paper, or electrophorectogram, can be put into a machine that quantifies the six serum protein fractions and reports the amount in percentages. This report in percentages can be read by the nurse, who can compare the numbers with reference values for each type of protein fraction.

Preparation of Client and Collection of Sample

The client should be fasting but can have water. One milliliter of whole blood is ample for total protein (TP) and serum protein electrophoresis (SPEP). Fresh samples are ideal, but older samples can be used.

REFERENCE VALUES FOR SPEP

Essentially the same for all people. Variations noted for electrophoresis results are as follows:

Total serum protein	6.0–8.0 g/dL	
Serum albumin	3.1–4.3 g/dL	
Serum globulins	2.6–4.1 g/dL	

Electrophoresis (reported as a percentage of total protein):

Adult	Albumin	52–68%
	Globulins	
	α-1	4.2–7.2%
	α-2	6.8–12%

	β-1	3–10%	(some laboratories report β together as 9.3–15%)
	β-2	1–9%	
	γ	13–23%	
Newborn	See details about γ-globulins in text.		
Pregnancy	Albumin falls quickly the first few months and then more slowly during rest of pregnancy. Overall decrease is about 1 g/dL with a return to normal within 8 weeks postpartum.		
Children	Tend to have slightly lower amounts of albumin until 4 years of age or later. Types and amounts of γ-globulins depend on age. See text.		
Aged	The γ-globulins, or at least the immunologic response, decreases with age. Albumin levels gradually decrease.		

See Hay et al. (1995) for details on newborn and pediatric values.

▼ SERUM ALBUMIN

Elevated Serum Albumin Level

Clinical Significance. No pathologic conditions cause the liver to produce extra amounts of albumin. So an increased value of albumin on a laboratory report is a reflection of dehydration. (Recall that many tests can be falsely elevated by dehydration.) The inclusion of excess amounts of protein in the diet does not raise the serum albumin level, because protein is first broken down into amino acids and then used for various purposes, including storage as adipose (fat) tissue.

Decreased Serum Albumin Level

Clinical Significance. Because albumin is totally synthesized by the liver, liver dysfunction is a common reason for a decreased serum albumin level (hypoalbuminemia). Reduced albumin levels are not seen in acute liver failure because it takes several weeks of lack of production before the albumin level drops. The most common reason for a lowered level is chronic liver dysfunction caused by cirrhosis. Clients with acquired immunodeficiency syndrome (AIDS) have hypoalbuminemia (Kotler, 1990). A loss of albumin in the urine caused by renal dysfunction (nephrotic syndrome) can also cause a decrease of albumin in the serum. Clients with low albumin levels undergoing dialysis have higher death rates (Owen, et al., 1993). Although a drop of about 1 g/100 mL is normal in pregnancy, there is even more of a drop with preeclampsia. (Albuminuria, or albumin in the urine, is a sign of both renal disease and eclampsia. See Chapter 3.) Severe burns, with related damage to capillaries and blood vessels, result in a large loss of serum proteins, including albumin. The increased capillary permeability caused by the burn damage may cause a continual leak of serum proteins out of the vascular system. Also, the long-term depression of protein synthesis after a burn may last for a couple of months.

If there is inadequate intake of protein, the body begins to break down muscles (catabolism) to obtain enough amino acids for the continuing synthesis of serum albumin. Thus albumin levels do not drop in fasting states or in malnutrition until the condition is severe. Protein requirements may be greatly increased during stress, infection, or injury. The client is in a negative nitrogen balance when the catabolic process is greater than the anabolic process. (See Chapter 4 on the test for urinary urea nitrogen as a test for negative nitrogen balance.) Although albumin normally has a long half life, the serum albumin may fall within 3–5 days in a critically ill client. The degree of decrease reflects the severity of the illness (Marik, 1993).

▼ PRE-ALBUMIN

Pre-albumin, also known as thyroxin-binding pre-albumin, has a half life of only 2 days. Because of its short half life, pre-albumin is a sensitive indicator of recent changes in catabolism (Kaplan, et al., 1995). This test is used for nutritional assessment. Other test results that indicate malnutrition are a low transferrin level and a low lymphocyte count (see Chapter 2).

REFERENCE VALUE FOR PRE-ALBUMIN
10–40 mg/dL

▼ POSSIBLE NURSING DIAGNOSES RELATED TO HYPOALBUMINEMIA

Impaired Skin Integrity Related to Development of Edema

Because albumin is responsible for the oncotic pressure in the vascular system, a reduction in serum albumin causes edema. Edema occurs when the albumin level falls to 2.0–2.5 g/dL. Without adequate albumin in the bloodstream, fluid leaks out into the interstitial spaces and into the peritoneal cavity. Unlike the edema caused by too much volume in the vascular space, this type of edema is not found primarily in dependent areas. For example, clients with an increased volume caused by congestive heart failure have edema in the feet if they are sitting up or in the sacral area if in bed. In contrast, clients with edema caused by a lack of albumin may also have puffy eyelids or hands and a swollen abdomen caused by leakage of fluid into the peritoneal cavity. (A client with cirrhosis who has hypoalbuminemia is also likely to have portal hypertension that intensifies the collection of fluid in the peritoneal cavity.) In addition to weighing these clients and checking their ankles and sacral area for edema, the

(*continued*)

▼ POSSIBLE NURSING DIAGNOSES RELATED TO HYPOALBUMINEMIA (*continued*)

nurse should also measure the abdominal girth to check the progression of edema. Besides causing edema, the lack of protein also escalates the risk of decubitis ulcers because cellular nutrition is inadequate (Cerrato, 1986). Skin breakdown is always a potential problem. These clients need superb skin care. Serum albumin levels may be used to predict risk for pressure sores in the elderly (Norvell et al., 1988).

Assisting with Interventions to Decrease Edema. A collection of fluid in the peritoneal cavity may make it impossible for the client to breathe comfortably in a reclining position. Sometimes a paracentesis must be performed to take the pressure off the diaphragm. (See Chapter 25 for a description of paracentesis.) The disadvantage of a paracentesis is that proteins are lost in the peritoneal fluid. Diuretics, along with some restrictions of fluids and sodium, may be ordered because an increased amount of aldosterone may also be contributing to the formation of edema. (See Chapter 5 for a discussion of hypernatremia.)

Altered Nutrition Related to Protein Requirement

The primary treatment of edema caused by a lack of serum albumin is to increase the albumin level. If the liver can still synthesize albumin, a diet with adequate protein is appropriate for long-term therapy. The recommended daily allowance for protein for various ages is shown in Table 10–2.

Often the clients who need the protein the most can tolerate it the least because their livers are unable to handle the ammonia that results from protein breakdown. (See the test for serum ammonia at the end of this chapter.) If protein is well-tolerated, however, eggs, cheese, fish, and meat are excellent sources, along with a correct mixture of nuts, grains, and vegetables. If protein must be increased in the diet, one egg or 1 ounce (28 g) of cheese supplies

TABLE 10–2. REQUIREMENTS OF PROTEIN ACROSS LIFE SPAN

Age	Protein (g/kg)
0–6 months	2.2
6–12 months	2.0
1–3 years	1.8
4–6 years	1.5
7–10 years	1.2
11–14 years	1.0
15–18 years	0.84 girls 0.85 boys
19 and older	0.8[a]

[a]A 70-kg man would need (70 × 0.8) 56 g of protein each day and a 50-kg woman (50 × 0.8) only 40 g.

about 7 g of protein. One 8-ounce (240 mL) glass of milk made from dried milk powder supplies 8 g of protein without increasing the cholesterol intake (see Chapter 9). Dried milk is economical and can be added to many foods and beverages. Commercially made protein supplements can be used. If the client is also deficient in minerals and vitamins, these liquid diets may ensure a higher level of many necessary nutrients. The client must have plenty of calories from carbohydrates, so that protein is not used as an energy source. See Table 10–3 for a comparison of the protein content in various foods.

Risk of Injury Related to Intravenous Albumin Replacement

For a client who needs albumin replacement immediately, albumin can be given intravenously. Albumin is also used as a plasma expander. Some albumin, which is collected from human donors, is obtained from placental blood, which is important because the infusion of some albumins causes a rise in alkaline phosphatase level. (See Chapter 12 for this enzyme test.) Albumin does not need to be refrigerated as does whole blood. It does not have any preservatives added, so it must be used soon after it is opened.

Albumin comes in a 5% and a 25% concentration. The 25% solution is usually given at a rate no faster than 1 mL/min. The 5% solution can be given at a rate of about 2–4 mL/min. The intravenous infusion must be given slowly because of the danger of circulatory overload. Vital signs must be monitored.

As the oncotic pressure returns to normal, edematous fluid is pulled back into the vascular system. The mobilization of edema from the tissues causes increased urine output. The albumin remains in the bloodstream for several

(*continued*)

TABLE 10–3. FOODS HIGH IN PROTEIN

Food Item	Protein (g)
■ **COMPLETE PROTEINS**	
1 egg	7.0
1 oz (28g) meat or fish	7.0–8.0
1 oz (28g) cheese	6.0–7.0
8 oz (240 mL) milk	8.5
1 tbsp dried milk	1.6
■ **INCOMPLETE PROTEINS**[a]	
1 tbsp peanut butter	4.0
2 slices wheat bread	4.0
1 cup nuts	7.0–8.0
3 oz lentils	7.0
1/4 cup garbanzo beans	10.0

Estimates are from various food labels and nutritional pamphlets.

[a]Consult a nutrition text on how incomplete vegetable proteins can be balanced to supply all needed amino acids.

▼ POSSIBLE NURSING DIAGNOSES RELATED TO HYPOALBUMINEMIA (*continued*)

days, but with a severe albumin deficiency, the client may need repeated infusions over time. Marik (1993) noted that not all clients with hypoalbuminemia benefit from albumin replacements, so sometimes this expensive and limited supply is misused.

Risk for Infection Related to Associated Lymphopenia

Protein malnutrition in the hospitalized elderly may greatly increase the risk for infection (Lipschitz, 1990). Severe protein malnutrition inhibits lymphocyte and antibody synthesis. Thus a client who has a decreased serum albumin level may have a low lymphocyte count. In fact, lowered albumin levels and a lowered lymphocyte level ($<1{,}500\ mm^3$) are two markers of malnutrition that are used in research on nutrition. Poor nutrition may also lead to impaired neutrophil functioning (Cerrato, 1990). Nursing interventions should be geared to protect the client from infection, as discussed in Chapter 2 (lymphocytes and neutrophils) and Chapter 16 (culture and sensitivity tests) and to promote a healthful diet.

▼ ALPHA-1-ANTITRYPSIN OR ALPHA-1-PROTEINASE INHIBITOR

α-1-Antitrypsin (AAT) is an example of a special α-globulin that can be measured. A decrease or near-absence of AAT can be a factor in chronic obstructive pulmonary disease (COPD). The role of antitrypsin is to inhibit the damaging effects of proteolytic enzymes released by bacteria and phagocytes in the lung. The relation of antitrypsin to the liver is not well understood, but a lack of this protein is found in young children with liver disease. Clients with lung or liver dysfunctions undergo screening for a lack of this α-protein, which occurs in several genetic variants. The most useful screening test is SPEP (discussed earlier) because the α-1-globulin peak is absent or nearly absent in homozygotes. In heterozygous clients the α-1-globulin peak may look normal. Immunoassay is used to confirm an electrophoretic finding (Ravel, 1995). Specific phenotyping can be performed. Because ATT deficiency is an inherited disease, relatives of the client should undergo testing for the gene and be offered genetic counseling. The deficiency is found primarily in Europeans and those of European ancestry. AAT deficiency can also be assessed by amniocentesis (Chapter 28).

Preparation of Client and Collection of Sample

No special preparation of the client is necessary. The laboratory needs 10 mL of blood.

REFERENCE VALUE FOR AAT

85–213 mg/100 mL

▼ POSSIBLE NURSING DIAGNOSIS RELATED TO DECREASED ALPHA-1-ANTITRYPSIN

Risk for Impaired Health Maintenance Related to Development of Chronic Lung Disease

People with a moderate deficiency of AAT whose environment is healthful may live a normal life span, but those who smoke or live in a polluted environment may develop lung disease and die at an early age. Lung transplantation is an option for some clients. Hence, clients need information on how to protect themselves from air pollutants and need referrals to stop-smoking programs if needed.

In the late 1980s, human alpha$_1$ protinease inhibitor (Prolastin) became available as replacement therapy for clients with severe AAT deficiencies. At present, the replacement is given intravenously every few weeks. Studies are ongoing about the long-term effects of replacement therapy. The National Association for AAT, in Minneapolis, has current information on treatment options and information on local chapters and support groups. A phone number, sponsored by the Florida chapter, is 1-(800)-4-ALPHA-1.

Risk for Impaired Health Management Related to Liver Dysfunction

Some clients with AAT deficiency may develop cirrhosis. Treatment is supportive, as discussed in the section on low albumin levels. The American Liver Foundation has information on this condition. The phone number is 1-(800)-223-0179. Liver transplantation has been successful for children who have AAT deficiency (Hay et al., 1995).

▼ GAMMA GLOBULINS

Clinical Significance. There may be an increase either of various types (polyclonal) or of only one type (monoclonal), or there may be an absence (aclonal) of γ-globulins. The use of the term *clonal* refers to the origin of the globulins from a particular *clone* of plasma cells.

Polyclonal Patterns. This pattern is a reflection of an overproduction of almost all the immunoglobulins in response to antigens. Several different clones of plasma cells produce increased amounts of various immunoglobulins. The result is general hypergammaglobulinemia, a characteristic response to infections (the inflammatory response). Autoimmune diseases and some liver diseases also cause a generalized increase.

Monoclonal Patterns. In this pattern, only one type of γ-globulin is increased. Patterns of this sort may be diagnostic because they involve a spike of a single globulin, which can be closely examined by means of immunoassay to detect paraproteins or abnormal variants of an immunoglobulin. Monoclonal patterns are found in a number of situations:

1. Most clients with multiple myeloma have a peak of a paraprotein or abnormal globulin. (The discussion on immunoelectrophoresis explores paraproteins.)
2. Sometimes the elderly have a monoclonal pattern that appears to be more the result of the aging process than of a specific disease, but some clients who show a monoclonal pattern may eventually have multiple myeloma.
3. Macroglobulinemia, an increase in IgM, is characterized by an increase in only one type of immunoglobulin.
4. Malignant lymphomas and other tumors may cause an increase in only one type of immunoglobulin.

Aclonal Patterns. In aclonal patterns, or hypogammopathies, some of the γ-globulins are absent or markedly decreased.

1. The lack of γ-globulins may be congenital. Infants with an aclonal pattern may appear to have a normal pattern at birth because of the presence of immunoglobulins from the mother. But then frequent and severe infections begin to occur when the passive immunity from the mother no longer exists.
2. Acquired hypogammaglobulinemia is most often seen with chronic lymphocytic leukemia, malignant lymphomas, or other diseases that affect the bone marrow.
3. Drugs, such as corticosteroids and cytotoxic drugs used for treatment of malignant tumors, may reduce γ-globulin levels or at least make the γ-globulins ineffective.
4. Radiation therapy and toxins in the environment can produce an acquired lack of γ-globulins.

▼ POSSIBLE NURSING DIAGNOSES RELATED TO ABNORMAL GAMMA GLOBULINS

High Risk for Infection Related to Ineffective Immune Response

A person with either fewer γ-globulins or abnormal γ-globulins is susceptible to diseases caused by opportunistic pathogens. Bacterial pneumonia is often the cause of death. The client must be protected from others who have upper respiratory infections. Sometimes it may be necessary to initiate reverse isolation to protect the client, particularly infants who have a severe immunodeficiency disorder. With older clients, meticulous handwashing is most important, because reverse isolation, with its extra cost, still does not protect people from the bacteria on their own skin or from the bacteria in food. An effort should be made to keep the environment relatively free of pathogens. Because the main defense against invading organisms is intact skin and mucous membranes, the nurse must promote good skin care. Proper nutrition with adequate protein is important for the production of immunoglobulins and lymphocytes. (See the discussion on albumin for ways to ensure adequate protein intake.)

Risk for Injury Related to Injections of Gamma Globulins

γ-Globulin may be administered to increase immunoglobulin levels temporarily. Immune serum globulin may prevent serious infection if circulatory levels of IgG (discussed next) are kept at about 200 mg/dL. However, immune globulin may not prevent chronic infections of the secretory tissues, such as those of the respiratory tract. The γ-globulin, may be needed every 3–4 weeks. Because serum globulin injections can cause anaphylaxis, the client should be observed for 20–30 min after the injection. Intravenous therapy may also be used if larger doses of passive immunity are needed; repeated injections are painful and time-consuming (Katzung, 1995).

Knowledge Deficit Related to Technical Aspects of Therapy

In addition to the replacement of normal γ-globulins, there may also be an attempt to remove abnormal proteins from the bloodstream by pheresis. *Pheresis* is the process by which a specific plasma constituent is separated from other blood constituents and removed from the client's plasma. If the client has an excessive amount of abnormal IgM (see the discussion on macroglobulinemia), this protein can be filtered out of the blood by the pheresis machine. Another therapeutic alternative is bone marrow transplantation, but there may not be a histocompatible donor. Identification of specific markers, such as those for x-linked hyper-IgM immunodeficiency, can be used for prenatal diagnosis and may lead to new types of therapeutic interventions (DiSanto, et al., 1994).

▼ IMMUNOELECTROPHORESIS AND QUANTIFICATION OF SERUM PROTEINS: IgG, IgA, IgM, IgD, AND IgE

Immunoglobulins are defined as proteins of animal origin that are endowed with known antibody activity. Although there are only five main groups of immunoglobulins (IgG, IgA, IgM, IgD, and IgE), 40 or more fractions can be differentiated by researchers. This discussion is limited to general knowledge about the five main types of immunoglobulins.

The laboratory uses antiserum preparations to cause a precipitation of each of the five main types of immunoglobulins. For electrophoresis the precipitations may be carried out in a gel or on a glass slide and then transferred to a sheet of paper. The final result is a pattern of bands that have a certain curvature, position, and intensity of color. Abnormalities in any of the immunoglobulins cause the band for that precipitation to be displaced, bowed, lighter in color, thicker than normal, or absent. The laboratory can also quantify each type of immunoglobulin.

Preparation of Client and Collection of Sample

A fresh sample is the sample of choice, but aged serum or plasma can be used. Depending on the technique, only 1 mL of blood may be needed. Any blood transfusions or blood component therapy within the past 6 weeks, as well as any immunizations or vaccines within the past 6 months, should be recorded on the laboratory requisition.

REFERENCE VALUES FOR IMMUNOGLOBULINS

Adult	IgG	639–1,349 mg/dL (usually about 75% of total)
	IgA	70–312 mg/dL (10–15%)
	IgM	56–352 mg/dL (7–10%)
	IgD	0.5–3 mg/dL (<1%)
	IgE	0.01–0.04 mg/dL (<1%)
Newborn	IgG	640–1,250 mg/dL
	IgA	0–11 mg/dL
	IgM	5–30 mg/dL
	IgD	—
	IgE	—
Children	Depends on age. By 6 months to 1 year of age, levels begin gradual increase. Adult values may be reached by late teens.	
Pregnancy	Evidently IgE falls somewhat during pregnancy, but the others show no significant change.	
Aged	Even healthy older people may show abnormal patterns with increase of paraproteins (Lipschitz, 1990). In response to a challenge, such as an infection, immunoglobulin production is likely to be reduced or a less vigorous response.	

Changes in Immunoglobulins

Clinical Significance. The exact significance of changes in immunoglobulins may be determined only in conjunction with other tests such as urine immunoelectrophoresis and perhaps bone marrow studies. Following is a brief summary of the general characteristics of changes in each component of the immunoglobulins. One way to remember which one is the most abundant and which is the least is to think of *GAMDE,* because G is the most abundant and E the least abundant in the adult.

IgG. This immunoglobulin, which makes up about three-fourths of the total immunoglobulins, is the only one that crosses the placenta. Hence infants have a high level, which shows a decrease until about 6 months to 1 year, when the infant begins production of IgG.

IgG protects against viruses, bacteria, and toxins. It is more for a secondary response. Thus specific IgG antibodies against infections such as hepatitis or rubella indicate past exposure and probable immunity (see Chapter 14). In the newborn, IgG levels indicate passive immunity. A lack of IgG causes severe immunodeficiency. Injections of immune serum globulin contain primarily IgG.

IgA. The second most common immunoglobulin in the bloodstream, IgA is also present in other fluids and in surface secretions, such as saliva, tears, and colostrum. These immunoglobulins are thought to be the first line of defense against organisms invading the respiratory, gastrointestinal, or urinary tracts. The infant begins producing IgA after a few months. Deficiencies of IgA may be combined with other deficiencies or occur alone.

IgM. In the bloodstream in slightly lower levels than IgA, IgM does not cross the placenta, but the infant begins synthesizing IgM sooner than IgA. IgM is the most important component in a primary immune response. IgM antibodies are indicators of an active infection. IgM activates the complement system, its level remaining high as long as the antigen is present. The antibodies to blood group antigens are in the group of IgM immunoglobulins. (See Chapter 14 for discussion of IgM antibodies for hepatitis and rubella.)

Because IgM has a high molecular weight, abnormal increases are called *macroglobulinemia*. These immunoglobulins tend to make the blood highly viscous. Normal viscosity of blood is 1.4–1.8 compared with the viscosity of water. The increase of macroglobulins also makes the client very sensitive to cold. As discussed earlier, pheresis therapy may be used to remove abnormal immunoglobulins.

IgD. This immunoglobulin is in the bloodstream in very small amounts. The exact functions of IgD are unclear at present.

IgE and the RAST. IgE, which is in the bloodstream in very small amounts, increases in allergic states and in the event of parasitic infestation. Evidently IgE is responsible for severe hypersensitivity reactions. A measurement of specific IgE antibodies in the serum helps establish the diagnosis of allergic disease by identifying which allergens are causing clinical symptoms such as hay fever, asthma, or skin rashes.

A RAST measures the quantity of antigen-specific IgE in the serum. Antibodies to a variety of pollens, such as animal dander or food, can be quantified. For example, the RAST may be used to test for latex allergy, but the test is less sensitive and more expensive than skin pricks or interdermal testing (Gold, 1994). An advantage of the RAST is no risk of triggering anaphylaxis.

IgE antibodies are used in a rapid, easy-to-use dipstick that has 10 allergens common to an area. This allergy screen has the advantage of being performed quickly without the trained technician and instrumentation needed for the RAST (Nalebuff and Prasad, 1990).

▼ URINE PROTEIN ELECTROPHORESIS AND IMMUNOELECTROPHORESIS

The techniques of electrophoresis and immunoelectrophoresis (IEP) of urine are similar to those of serum testing. If an abnormal amount of protein is detected in the urine, these tests can identify exactly which kinds of proteins are being excreted. (See Chapter 3 for the screening technique for proteinuria.) Normally, a 24-hr urine has a protein content of about 40–150 mg, with no more than 10 mg in a random specimen. The dipstick used for screening registers 1+ when there are about 30 mg in the specimen; less than 30 mg causes a trace showing.

The dipstick method of screening for proteinuria tests for albumin, so a dipstick for protein is not reliable as a screening test for proteins other than albumin. The laboratory uses other methods to screen for abnormal proteins, such as Bence Jones protein, which may occur with multiple myeloma. Bence Jones protein in the urine is now called light-chain disease. Light chains are the polypeptide chains that compose immunoglobulins. Immunoelectrophoresis and immunofixation are being used with increasing frequency to identify light chains in the urine (Kaplan et al., 1995).

REFERENCE VALUES FOR URINE PROTEIN ELECTROPHORESIS

Three main types of pathologic pattern may be identified by separating the protein fractions in urine.

1. There may be a marked increase in the albumin fraction and some increase in α- and β-globulins. This signifies increased glomerular permeability such as that seen in some renal diseases and in eclampsia.
2. There may be a marked elevation in α- and β-globulins with a decrease in albumin. This most likely signifies tubular damage.
3. There may be various abnormal proteins or paraproteins, such as those found in multiple myeloma or in other disorders of the γ-globulins. This is considered a prerenal pattern. Just as in the serum, quantitative assay and, if needed, IEP can be used to identify exactly which globulins are present.

▼ SERUM AMMONIA

The liver normally converts ammonia (NH_3), a byproduct of protein metabolism, into urea, which is excreted by the kidneys. When the liver is unable to convert ammonia to urea, toxic levels of ammonia accumulate in the bloodstream. In severe liver failure, the blood urea nitrogen (BUN) drops as the ammonia level rises. (See Chapter 4 on the use of the BUN as a test for renal function.)

Preparation of Client and Collection of Sample

Some laboratories may require a fasting state; water is allowed. One milliliter of either venous or arterial blood can be used. The blood is put into a heparinized tube (green-topped vacuum tube) and packed in ice for transport to the laboratory. The specimen is stable for about 20 min. If the client is on antibiotics (such as neomycin) for treatment of hepatic coma, record this fact on the laboratory slip.

REFERENCE VALUES FOR SERUM AMMONIA

Adult	35–65 μg/dL
Newborn	90–150 μg/dL
Children	45–80 μg/dL

Values may vary considerably from laboratory to laboratory.

Increased Ammonia Level

Clinical Significance. Increased ammonia levels, which occur in liver dysfunction, may be due either to blood not circulating through the liver well or to actual hepatic failure. Clients with cirrhosis who have portacaval shunts performed to relieve portal hypertension may have increased ammonia levels after the operation because blood is shunted away from the liver. Reye's syndrome, which sometimes occurs with viral infections, leads to elevated ammonia levels. The prognosis is related to the depth of the coma and the peak of the serum ammonia levels. The number of reported cases of Reye's syndrome has decreased in the past few years, perhaps because salicylates are no longer given to young children who have viral infections (Hay et al., 1995).

▼ POSSIBLE NURSING DIAGNOSES RELATED TO INCREASED AMMONIA LEVELS

Risk for Injury Related to Sensory-Perceptual Alterations

Although high levels of ammonia occur in hepatic coma (hepatic encephalopathy), the ammonia may not be the only factor that causes the neurologic symptoms. Most likely, many toxins in hepatic failure cause the symptoms of disorientation and tremors seen in hepatic encephalopathy. Increased intracranial pressure may accompany severe liver failure, and a bioartificial liver may help bring down serum ammonia levels and other toxins until a transplant is possible (LePage, et al., 1994). The client should be checked for a certain kind of tremor of the hand called *liver flap* or *asterixis* (which can also be caused by

(*continued*)

▼ POSSIBLE NURSING DIAGNOSES RELATED TO INCREASED AMMONIA LEVELS (*continued*)

high levels of uremia or other central nervous system toxins). Ask the client to extend his or her arms out in front of the body, spread the fingers, and hold the hands in a dorsiflexed position. Clients who have a high level of ammonia in their blood and in whom hepatic encephalopathy is developing cannot hold their palms up in a steady manner. The hands flap. Asking the client to write his or her name or to draw a star are other ways to assess the neurologic dysfunction. The nurse may often be the first one to notice subtle changes in the client's ability to perform simple tasks that require coordination and mental alertness. The lack of mental alertness and coordination may progress to a coma unless treatment is begun. Renal failure (see Chapter 4) is often associated with liver failure, but the reasons are unclear. The development of hepatorenal syndrome carries an extremely poor prognosis (Young, 1993).

Altered Nutrition Related to Need to Reduce All Sources of Ammonia from Protein Breakdown

Because a rising serum ammonia level indicates an inability of the liver to handle the breakdown of protein, the client should have limited protein intake until the ammonia level returns to normal. An enteral amino acid formula may be used to prevent muscle breakdown. If the patient in hepatic failure has gastrointestinal bleeding, the progression to hepatic coma accelerates because ammonia is produced when the blood proteins in the intestine are digested. Enemas and gastric lavage may be needed to get as much of the blood out of the gastrointestinal tract as possible. Because intestinal bacteria produce ammonia by breaking down protein, the amount of bacteria may be reduced with administration of neomycin, a nonsystemic antibiotic, which may be given orally or by means of enemas.

Resuming Protein Intake. When the ammonia level returns to normal, protein is cautiously put back into the diet in increasing amounts. The diet may be limited to only 20 g of protein per day for awhile. (See Table 10–3 for a list of the protein content of foods.) As the protein level in the diet is increased, the nurse must watch carefully for any signs of hepatic encephalopathy. Serum ammonia levels are useful in evaluating the ability of the liver to handle protein once again. Lactulose, an ammonia detoxicant, may be given orally or rectally to help reduce ammonia levels. Oral lactulose may be continued as long-term treatment.

Risk for Injury Related to Use of Sedatives and Diuretics

In addition to the amount of protein in the diet, other factors that contribute to the development of hepatic coma include hypokalemia and the use of sedatives and narcotics. The body is less able to handle ammonia when the potassium level is low or when alkalosis is present. Thus diuretic therapy (which often causes potassium loss) may be contraindicated when the client has an increased ammonia level. In addition, the failing liver is unable to detoxify many drugs, including sedatives and narcotics. When a client has a rising ammonia level, all previous drug orders need to be reevaluated to see if they are still appropriate in respect to the change in the client's condition.

▼ TUMOR MARKERS

Tumor markers are substances associated with malignant growths. An example already discussed was the paraprotein found in the serum or urine of clients with multiple myeloma. Hormones, such as human chorionic gonadotropin (HCG) (Chapter 15), are sometimes tumor markers. The appearance of fetal proteins such as carcinoembryonic antigen (CEA) or α-fetoprotein (AFP) in some types of malignant tumors in adults gives support to the theory that cancer somehow arises from very primitive cells. The oncofetal antigens discussed later in this chapter have been used to assess some tumors. Other tumor antigens or antibodies are designated simply by numbers such as CA 125 or CA 50. A more tissue specific antigen, such as prostate specific antigen (PSA), is also a tumor marker. Researchers are continuing to refine the specificity and sensitivity of these tests so they can be even more useful as screening tests and for evaluating treatment outcomes.

▼ ALPHA-FETOPROTEIN

Normally this globulin, formed only in the yolk sac and liver of the fetus, disappears from the bloodstream after birth, except for trace amounts. The test for AFP is performed on amniotic fluid to detect specific congenital defects (see Chapter 28) and on the serum of pregnant women and other adults to detect pathologic conditions.

The serum AFP, recommended since 1985, has the distinction of being the first maternal serum test to screen for a genetic defect in the fetus. In the fetus, if the neural tube fails to close properly, enormous amounts of fetal protein leak into the amniotic fluid throughout the pregnancy. In the pregnant woman, levels greater than the usual reference values for a particular gestational age may indicate a neural tube defect in the fetus. The AFP is also used with two other tests, estriol and HCG, to assess for Down syndrome. See Chapter 18 for the discussion of these three tests.

In a nonpregnant adult, a markedly increased AFP level is associated with primary carcinoma (hepatoma) of the liver and some types of testicular cancer (Ostchega and Culnane, 1985). Metastatic cancer to the liver does not cause such a rise. Very small amounts of AFP are present in some nonmalignant liver diseases in children and adults.

Preparation of Client and Collection of Sample

There is no special preparation of the client for a serum sample. The laboratory needs 1 mL of clotted blood.

REFERENCE VALUES FOR AFP	
Men and nonpregnant women	<20 ng/mL or <10 IU/mL
Pregnancy	Serum levels increase during pregnancy (see Chapter 18)

▼ CARCINOEMBRYONIC ANTIGEN

CEA, a glycoprotein that circulates at a high level during fetal life, is detectable in only tiny amounts in the blood of healthy adults. CEA is elevated in malignant tumors, such as colonic cancer and metastatic breast disease, and thus is useful as a tumor marker. Most clients with colonic cancer have elevated CEA levels. Although CEA may be used as part of a diagnostic evaluation for cancer of the colon, the CEA is most useful as a marker to determine the effectiveness of treatment. For example, CEA levels usually return to normal about 6 weeks after a malignant tumor of the colon is surgically removed (Ostchega and Culnane, 1985). A CEA that begins to rise after treatment is an indication of a return of the tumor. CEA is helpful but not conclusive and is thus of little value in a diagnostic evaluation for cancer of the colon because (1) not all people with cancer of the colon show elevated CEA levels and (2) several conditions other than colonic cancer may cause elevated CEA levels. Other conditions that cause elevated CEA levels are heavy cigarette smoking, cirrhosis, ulcerative colitis, diverticulitis, rectal polyps, peptic ulcer disease, pancreatitis, and many malignant tumors (Fletcher, 1986; Ravel, 1995).

Preparation of Client and Collection of Sample

Venous blood is collected in a lavender-topped tube. The specimen must be sent on ice.

REFERENCE VALUE FOR CEA
0–2.5 ng/mL

Smokers may have values as high as 5.0 ng/mL or even higher (Kaplan et al., 1995).

▼ CA 125 ANTIGEN

Like other tests discussed in this section, CA 125 is a tumor marker. This test uses an antibody against an antigen tissue culture of cells of an ovarian carcinoma. CA 125 antigen is not specific enough to be used to screen all clients for ovarian cancer, because other cancers and nonmalignant conditions such as cirrhosis, peritonitis, and endometriosis may also cause an increase. Women at high risk for this disease because of a history of ovarian cancer in the family may undergo the test and intra-abdominal or transvaginal ultrasonography on a routine basis. The CA 125 test is positive in about 80% of women with epithelial ovarian cancer (Dillon, 1994). The test is used to follow clients once they have been diagnosed as having ovarian cancer. As many as 90% of clients with persistent CA 125 elevations after surgical intervention do have residual tumor. Unfortunately 50–61% of clients who have undergone treatment of ovarian cancer and have a normal level of CA 125 may also have recurrent or persistent tumor (Ravel, 1995). Thus the test is usually most predictive if there is a change from normal to abnormal or if there is a rising titer.

Preparation of Client and Collection of Sample

One milliliter of serum is needed in a serum separator tube (SST).

REFERENCE VALUE FOR CA 125
<35 U/mL

▼ CA 50

CA 50 is a tumor marker used in the evaluation and follow-up assessment of some cancers of the digestive tract. It frequently produces false-positive results if the client has any pancreatic or hepatobiliary disease. Several cutoff levels for normal are based on the diagnosis and the level of bilirubin (Collazos et al., 1993).

▼ PROSTATE-SPECIFIC ANTIGEN

Unlike the other tumor markers, PSA is relatively specific for both benign and malignant prostate epithelium. For men with symptoms, the PSA and the digital rectal examination are commonly used for diagnostic purposes and as follow-up assessment after therapy. The question remains if the PSA should be used as a screening tool for men without symptoms (Walsh, 1993). Controversy exists over whether early diagnosis is useful because early treatment may have no added benefit for some very slow-growing tumors. Another concern is the rate of false-positive results that lead to unnecessary follow-up tests with the associated anxiety and cost. Because the net benefit of widespread screening is unclear, a randomized, prospective study of the effect of screening on prostate cancer mortality was initiated by the National Cancer Institute (Kramer et al., 1993). For this study, men are screened once a year for 4 years, which is similar to the screening intervals that showed a benefit for mammography for breast cancer. Some medical centers now offer all men older than 50 years the option of PSA screening, and this measure is supported by the American Cancer Society.

Preparation of Client and Collection of Sample

Several commercial kits are available (Ravel, 1995), so check with the laboratory for specific instructions on collecting serum.

REFERENCE VALUE FOR PSA
0–4 ng/mL

Reference varies with type of testing.

▼ POSSIBLE NURSING DIAGNOSES RELATED TO ELEVATION OF TUMOR MARKERS

Risk for Ineffective Coping Related to Severity of Malignant Condition and Possible Need for More Treatment

AFP, CEA, CA 125, CA 50, and PSA are tumor markers, so persistent or rising levels indicate that the tumor is still active and prognosis is thus less favorable than if the levels remain normal. Additional treatments may be needed, and the client and family may need help in coping with the less than favorable news from the physician. Fletcher (1986) noted the importance of whether information about a bad prognosis is humanely used. Nurses often help clients deal with unpleasant news and can be very effective in helping clients use their coping skills.

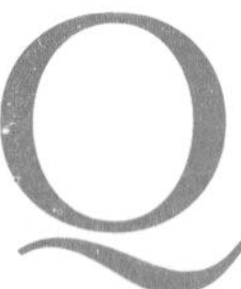

1. Sarah Nicholson is caring for her sister who has advanced ovarian cancer. She asks the home care nurse the name of the test being used to monitor her sister's response to treatment. The nurse explains that the test is

   a. CA 50 **b.** PSA
   c. CEA **d.** CA 125

2. The only clinical condition that creates an elevated serum albumin level is which of the following?

   a. Early liver dysfunction **b.** Increased protein intake over a long period
   c. Dehydration **d.** Kwashiorkor

3. A nursing diagnosis of altered nutrition related to hypoalbuminemia would be most likely for

   a. Mrs. Lehman, who is in her last trimester of pregnancy and is expecting twins.
   b. Tommy, aged 6, who has severe asthma.
   c. Mr. Buber, who has advanced cirrhosis
   d. Shirley, aged 17, who has been on a very restricted diet (only juices) for the past 8 days

4. The most important clinical manifestation of a lowered serum albumin level is which of the following?

   a. Decreased susceptibility to infection
   b. Edema
   c. Loss of weight
   d. Tendency to bleed

5. Mr. Buber is receiving a 25% solution of albumin intravenously because his serum albumin level was 2 g/100 mL. Which of the following nursing actions is appropriate?

   a. Run the solution no faster than 10 mL/min
   b. Observe the client frequently for possible circulatory overload
   c. Tell Mr. Buber he will probably have decreased urination over the next several hours
   d. Keep the albumin refrigerated until 30 min before it is hung

6. For a client who can tolerate oral feedings, the most efficient and economical way to increase protein intake is to do which of the following?

   a. Use commercially prepared protein mixtures or powders
   b. Add extra tablespoons of powdered milk to foods and beverages
   c. Increase meat consumption
   d. Reduce carbohydrate intake so the person can eat more protein

7. The principal nursing diagnosis for a client who is deficient in α-1-antitrypsin is which of the following?

   a. Risk for injury related to smoking
   b. Knowledge deficit related to dietary changes
   c. Altered cardiac output related to fluid volume excess
   d. Impaired skin integrity related to edema

8. Which of these clients is the *least* likely to have low levels of immunoglobulins?

   a. Baby Federini, a premature infant born yesterday
   b. Mrs. Patch, who is a month pregnant and diabetic

c. Mr. Regoni, who is undergoing corticosteroid therapy and is malnourished
d. Mrs. Adams, who is 85 years of age and has been admitted because of a malignant tumor

9. The single most important nursing diagnosis in caring for any client with an abnormal γ-globulin pattern is which of the following?

a. Fluid volume deficit **b.** Fluid volume excess
c. High risk for infection **d.** Impaired skin integrity

10. Which immunoglobulin crosses the placenta and provides immunity for the newborn for several months?

a. IgG **b.** IgA **c.** IgM **d.** IgD

11. The radioallergosorbent test (RAST) is useful for which of the following?

a. To measure all types of immunoglobulins in the serum
b. To differentiate between cellular and humoral immunity
c. To measure the quantity of antigen-specific IgE antibodies in the serum that increase in immediate allergic reactions
d. To discriminate the globulins of high molecular weight (macroglobulin) from other globulins

12. Mr. Buber is a client with cirrhosis who has an ammonia level greater than 100 μg/100 mL. He states he wants "something to eat." Which diet would be appropriate for Mr. Buber this morning?

a. Eggs, toast, jelly, and coffee
b. Grapefruit juice, cereal, and a glass of milk
c. Orange juice and sliced banana
d. Pancakes, syrup, butter, and coffee

13. In a nonpregnant state, what might the continuing presence of large amounts of α-fetoprotein in the serum indicate?

a. Infertility **b.** Lack of adult proteins
c. Congenital enzymatic defect **d.** Active malignant tumor

▼ REFERENCES

Calianno, C., and Pino, T. (1995). Getting a reaction to anergy panel testing. *Nursing 95, 25* (1), 58–61.
Cerrato, P. (1986). How diet helps the skin fight against pressure sores. *RN, 49* (1), 67–68.
Cerrato, P. (1990). Does diet effect the immune system? *RN, 53* (6), 67–70.

Collazos, J., Genolla, J., and Ruibal, A. (1993). Serum levels of CA 50 in nonmalignant liver diseases: A clinical and biochemical study. *American Journal of Gastroenterology, 88* (3), 409–412.

Dillon, P. (1994). Ovarian cancer: Confronting the silent killer. *Nursing 94, 24* (5), 66–69.

DiSanto, J.P., Markiewicz, S., Gauchat, J.F., et al. (1994). Brief report: Prenatal diagnosis of X-linked hyper-IgM syndrome. *New England Journal of Medicine, 330* (14), 969–973.

Fletcher, R. (1986). Diagnostic decision: Carcinoembryonic antigen. *Annals of Internal Medicine, 104* (1), 66–73.

Geha, R.S., and Rosen, F.S. (1994). The genetic basis of immunoglobulin-class switching. *New England Journal of Medicine, 330* (14), 1008–1009.

Gold, J. (1994). Ask about latex. *RN, 57* (6), 32–34.

Hay, W.W., Groothuis, J.R., Hayward, A.R., and Levin, M.J. (1995). *Current pediatric diagnosis & treatment* (12th ed.). Norwalk, CT: Appleton & Lange.

Kaplan, A., Jack, R., Opheim, K.E., et al. (1995). *Clinical chemistry interpretation and techniques* (4th ed.). Baltimore: Williams & Wilkins.

Katzung, B. (1995). *Basic and clinical pharmacology* (6th ed.). Norwalk, CT: Appleton & Lange.

Kotler, D. (1990). Nutritional considerations in AIDS. *Contemporary Nutrition, 15* (4), 1–2.

Kramer, B.S., Brown, M.L., Prorok, P.C., et al. (1993). Prostate cancer screening: What we know and what we need to know. *Annals of Internal Medicine, 119* (9), 914–923.

LePage, E.B., Rozga, J., and Rosenthal, P., et al. (1994). An artificial liver used as a bridge to liver transplantation. *American Journal of Critical Care, 3* (3), 224–227.

Lipschitz, D. (1990). Impact of nutrition on the age-related decline in immune and hematologic function. *Contemporary Nutrition, 15* (2), 1–2.

Marik, P.E. (1993). The treatment of hypoalbuminemia in the critically ill patient. *Heart & Lung, 22* (2), 166–170.

Nalebuff, D., and Prasad, K. (1990). Comparison of Quidel allergy screen with modified RAST. *Immunology and Allergy Practice, 12* (1), 17–20.

Norvell, K., et al. (1988). Instant nutritional assessment as an indicator of pressure sore risk in institutionalized elderly. *Transitions, 5* (2), 1,4.

Ostchega, Y., and Culnane, M. (1985). Tumor markers. *Nursing 85, 15* (9), 49–51.

Owen, W.F., Lew, N.L., Liu, Y., et al. (1993). The urea reduction ratio and serum albumin concentration as predictors of mortality in patients undergoing hemodialysis. *New England Journal of Medicine, 329,* (14), 1001–1006.

Ravel, R. (1995). *Clinical laboratory medicine: Clinical application of laboratory data* (6th ed.). St. Louis: Mosby–Year Book.

Walsh, P.C. (1993). Using prostate-specific antigen to diagnose prostate cancer: Sailing in uncharted water. *Annals of Internal Medicine, 119* (9), 948–949.

Young, L.M. (1993). Managing the patient with liver failure. *MEDSURG Nursing, 2* (4), 275–281.

TESTS TO MEASURE THE METABOLISM OF BILIRUBIN

- Total Bilirubin
- Unconjugated (Indirect) Bilirubin
- Conjugated (Direct) Bilirubin
- Urine Bilirubin
- Urine Urobilinogen
- Fecal Urobilinogen
- Bilirubin in Amniotic Fluid
- Transcutaneous Bilirubinometer

OBJECTIVES

1. Diagram the normal pathway for bilirubin excretion and explain the five laboratory tests used as assessment tools.
2. Distinguish between prehepatic, intraheptic, and posthepatic jaundice in regard to causation, symptoms, and changes in laboratory values.
3. Compare and contrast the nursing diagnoses appropriate for elevated unconjugated and conjugated serum bilirubin levels in infants and adults.
4. Describe the role of the nurse in assisting with medical interventions for newborns with markedly elevated serum unconjugated bilirubins (BU).
5. Describe the nurse's role in assisting with medical interventions for clients with elevated serum conjugated bilirubin (BC).
6. Discuss the psychological impact of jaundice on the client and on significant others.

7. Explain the clinical significance of measuring the bilirubin content in amniotic fluid.
8. Describe the usefulness of the transcutaneous bilirubinometer in the care of the newborn.

This chapter begins with a discussion about the normal pathway of bilirubin excretion and differences between the two types of bilirubin, conjugated and unconjugated. The clinical symptom of any elevated bilirubin is jaundice, but the nursing implications are somewhat different depending on whether the jaundice is prehepatic, posthepatic, or hepatic in origin. The chapter ends with a discussion about general nursing diagnoses for any client with an elevated bilirubin (jaundice), along with more specific implications that depend on the origin of the jaundice.

PATHWAY OF NORMAL BILIRUBIN EXCRETION

When the reticuloendothelial system breaks down old or nonuseful red blood cells (RBCs), bilirubin is one of the waste products. This "free" bilirubin, which is not water-soluble, is a lipid-soluble waste product that needs to be made water-soluble to be excreted. So it is carried by albumin to the liver, where it is conjugated by the liver and made water-soluble. Only water-soluble BC can be excreted in the urine.

The liver handles bilirubin in a similar way to other poorly water-soluble compounds, such as steroids, drugs, and toxins. In general, such substances are carried by the plasma proteins (see Chapter 10) to the liver, where they are detached from the protein and made less toxic by conversion to a form that can be excreted.

An enzyme, glucuronyl transferase, is necessary for the transformation, or conjugation, of bilirubin. Either a lack of glucuronyl transferase or the presence of drugs that interfere with this enzyme renders the liver unable to conjugate bilirubin.

Urine, however, is not the most important pathway of excretion for BC, almost all of which is excreted as one of the components of bile salts. In fact, bilirubin, a vivid pigment, gives bile the characteristic bright greenish-yellow color. When the bile salts reach the intestine via the common bile duct, the bilirubin is acted on by bacteria to form chemical compounds called *urobilinogens*. Technically, the breakdown of BC in the intestine produces several other compounds, but the end product that is measured in both urine and feces is labeled *urobilinogen*. These breakdown products give feces their dark color; hence an absence of bilirubin in the intestine causes clay-colored stools. Most of the urobilinogen is excreted in the feces, but some is reabsorbed and goes through the liver again, and still another small amount is excreted in the urine. Thus tests for fecal and urine urobilinogens can detect abnormalities in bilirubin excretion.

Because the bilirubin is chemically different after it goes through the conjugation process in the liver, laboratory tests of the serum can differentiate between the bilirubin that is free (prehepatic) and the bilirubin that is conjugated (posthepatic). If the laboratory reports the test results as "direct" or "indirect" bilirubin, these older terms refer to the way the two types react to certain dyes (sometimes referred to as the Van den Bergh reaction):

1. The conjugated water-soluble (posthepatic) bilirubin reacts *directly* when dyes are added to the blood specimen.
2. The non-water-soluble, free (prehepatic) bilirubin does not react to the reagents used for the test until alcohol is added to the solution; hence their measurement is *indirect.*

A newer method of bilirubin measurement can also measure fractions of the serum bilirubin, and the results are listed as *BU* for unconjugated bilirubin and *BC* for conjugated bilirubin. Although most references use the term *conjugated,* Kaplan et al. (1995) prefer the term *esterified.* Another less common term is *delta bilirubin,* which refers to a fraction of conjugated bilirubin associated with cholestasis. Table 11–1 can be used as a quick summary of how each of the bilirubin tests is related to the normal pathway of bilirubin excretion. Table 11–2 summarizes how each of the five tests of bilirubin is changed in the three types of jaundice (prehepatic, hepatic, and posthepatic).

TABLE 11–1. RELATION OF NORMAL BILIRUBIN EXCRETION TO THE FIVE TESTS USED TO MEASURE BILIRUBIN METABOLISM

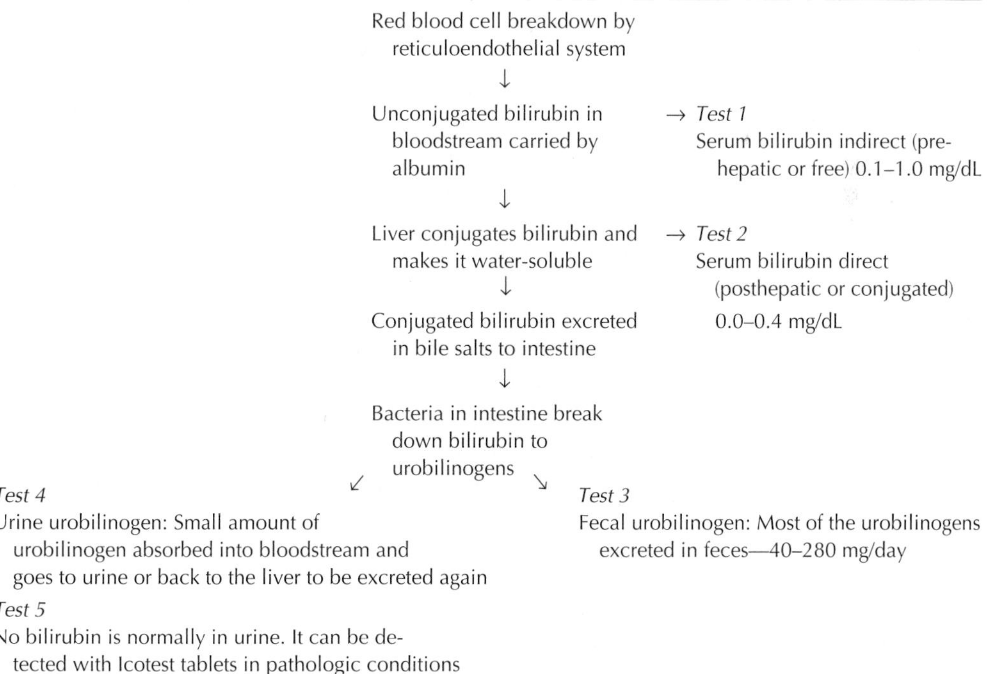
Red blood cell breakdown by reticuloendothelial system
↓
Unconjugated bilirubin in bloodstream carried by albumin → *Test 1* Serum bilirubin indirect (prehepatic or free) 0.1–1.0 mg/dL
↓
Liver conjugates bilirubin and makes it water-soluble → *Test 2* Serum bilirubin direct (posthepatic or conjugated) 0.0–0.4 mg/dL
↓
Conjugated bilirubin excreted in bile salts to intestine
↓
Bacteria in intestine break down bilirubin to urobilinogens ↙ ↘

Test 4
Urine urobilinogen: Small amount of urobilinogen absorbed into bloodstream and goes to urine or back to the liver to be excreted again

Test 3
Fecal urobilinogen: Most of the urobilinogens excreted in feces—40–280 mg/day

Test 5
No bilirubin is normally in urine. It can be detected with Icotest tablets in pathologic conditions

Note: Total bilirubin measures both unconjugated (BU) and conjugated (BC) bilirubin. See Ravel (1995) for a discussion on some of the problems with including delta bilirubin and some unconjugated bilirubin as direct bilirubin.

TABLE 11–2. CHANGES IN SERUM, URINE, AND FECES IN THREE TYPES OF JAUNDICE

	Unconjugated Serum Bilirubin	Conjugated Serum Bilirubin	Urine Bilirubin	Urine Urobilinogen	Fecal Urobilinogen
Reference values	Average 0.5 mg/dL	Average 0.1 mg/dL	None	0.4–1 mg/day	40–280 mg/day
Prehepatic jaundice (hemolytic)	Elevated usually not more than 5 mg in adults. May be >20 mg in newborns	Normal	None	Up to 10 mg	Up to 1,400 mg
Hepatic jaundice	Elevated—may be 15–20 mg in severe liver failure	Elevations depend on amount of stasis of bile	Elevated if obstruction present	Normal or increased (see text)	Normal or little decrease (see text)
Posthepatic jaundice (obstruction)	Normal in beginning	Elevated—may be 30–40 mg if obstruction complete	Elevated—urine dark and foamy	Slight decrease or normal	Absent—clay-colored stools

Ravel (1995) cautioned that the degree of bilirubinemia is not a completely reliable diagnostic criterion in differentiating types of jaundice.

▼ TOTAL BILIRUBIN

Preparation of Client and Collection of Sample

Most laboratories require the client to fast for 8 hr before the test because a large intake of fat interferes with the chemical testing. The test requires 1 mL of serum. The specimen should be protected from bright light because bilirubin is broken down by exposure to sunlight or to high-intensity artificial light. The test should not be performed for 24 hr after a dye has been used for radiographic studies. For neonatal use, blood is drawn from a heel stick by means of a capillary pipette (see Chapter 1). This "micro" bilirubin only measures totals and is appropriate for the first 10 days of life.

REFERENCE VALUES FOR SERUM BILIRUBIN

Most laboratories report only the figures for the total and the direct. The indirect is calculated by subtracting the direct from the total. Lum (1988) noted that a direct bilirubin should be done only if the total is greater than 1.0 mg/dL.

Adult and children past newborn stage

BU or indirect bilirubin	0.1–1.0 mg/dL Mean 0.5 mg	This is the prehepatic, free, or unconjugated bilirubin
BC or direct bilirubin	0.0–0.4 mg/dL Mean 0.1 mg	Posthepatic, conjugated or esterified bilirubin (water-soluble)
Total bilirubin	0.1–1.0 mg/dL	Includes both types of bilirubin

Newborn	See text for explanation of physiologic jaundice in newborns. Examples used here reflect *total* bilirubins. Check with individual laboratory for newer methods that use a layered technology for neonatal bilirubin	
Term infant	First 24 hr	<6 mg
	Up to 48 hr	<8 mg
	2–5 days	<12 mg
Premature infant	First 24 hr	<8 mg
	Up to 48 hr	<12 mg
	2–5 days	<16 mg
Pregnancy	Bilirubin levels usually remain in normal ranges, but some normal pregnancies may have increased bilirubins	

▼ UNCONJUGATED (INDIRECT) BILIRUBIN

Increased Level of BU

Clinical Significance. An increase in the BU can be caused in two different ways. First, the breakdown of RBCs can increase, causing an excess of free bilirubin in the bloodstream. Many conditions cause an increased destruction (hemolysis) of RBCs:

1. Sickle cell disease
2. Autoimmune diseases
3. Hemorrhage into a body cavity when the RBCs are broken down
4. Drug toxicity
5. Any physical or physiologic stress (a slight increase)
6. A transfusion reaction caused by incompatible blood (See Chapter 14 on transfusion reactions)
7. Rh or ABO incompatibility in an infant

The BU of a newborn with Rh incompatibility (erythroblastosis fetalis) is often greater than 20 mg. Usually the BU in an adult does not rise much above 5 mg because of hemolysis. The BU is about 6 mg with sickle cell disease.

Second, the BU can be elevated when the ability of the liver to conjugate the free bilirubin that circulates in the bloodstream is decreased. Liver dysfunction causes high elevations of BU in both adult and newborns. In severe liver disease, the BU may be greater than 20 mg. Although the most common reason for severe liver dysfunction in adults is cirrhosis, hepatitis may also make the liver less capable of conjugating bilirubin. Some infants are born with a deficiency in the enzyme glucuronyl transferase (Crigler-Najjar syndrome), which is necessary for the conjugation of bilirubin in the liver. This syndrome is rare but may be very severe. On the other hand, a relatively common, benign type of familial hyperbilirubinemia (Gilbert's syndrome) is associated with a mild decrease in enzymatic activity. Bilirubin levels increase with fasting or illness, but no treatment is needed for the fluctuating bilirubin levels. Drugs, viral diseases, and other toxins may injure the liver or interfere with enzymatic actions, so that the liver cannot conjugate bilirubin efficiently.

Jaundice in the Newborn. An increase in the total bilirubin is a physiologic occurrence in the newborn that is due both to increased hemolysis and to slower conjugation by the liver. The infant is born with a large number of fetal RBCs that have a short life span. So the hemolysis that occurs after birth is a normal adaptation to the new environment. Yet, because the newborn's liver has inadequate glucuronyl transferase, the liver takes longer to conjugate and to remove bilirubin from the bloodstream. The synthesis of the enzyme occurs a few days after birth in a full-term infant and a little longer after birth in a premature infant. Because of these events, about 50% of newborns have some physiologic jaundice that disappears in a few days.

Differentiating physiologic jaundice from any other kind is important. If the BU is markedly elevated the first day, or if it does not begin to drop after 3–5 days, the jaundice may be pathologic rather than physiologic. For example, an infant with Rh incompatibility has a high BU immediately after birth. (See Chapter 14 for other tests for Rh babies.) Lowered serum albumin levels, hypoxia, cold, stress, drugs, and other metabolic factors may also cause abnormal increases in BU by interfering with the transportation or conjugation of bilirubin (Thaler, 1977; DeCherney and Pernoll, 1994).

In a few instances, breast feeding may intensify physiologic jaundice because an enzyme present in some women's milk inhibits the action of glucuronyl transferase. Brown, et al. (1993) documented the incidence and pattern of jaundice for 155 healthy, breast-fed infants during the first month of life and noted that there is no standard of medical management for breast-feeding jaundice. Breast feeding may or may not be stopped. One of the difficulties in managing early neonatal jaundice in breast-fed infants is trying to determine if the jaundice is related to reduced milk intake. These nurse researchers emphasize the importance of helping the mother learn to be successful with breast feeding.

A newborn is particularly susceptible to environmental contaminants because the epidermis is thin and percutaneous absorption is great. Infants' fast respiratory rate also increases the intake of any environmental contaminant. For example, two epidemics of neonatal hyperbilirubinemia were linked to the use of a phenol disinfectant detergent (Wysowski et al., 1978). Several infants had very high BUs after a new detergent was used to clean bassinets.

▼ CONJUGATED (DIRECT) BILIRUBIN

Increased Level of BC

Clinical Significance. Normally the amount of BC circulating in the bloodstream is very small because the larger portion of this type of bilirubin is excreted in the bile salts into the intestine. Thus a marked increase in this type of bilirubin is a sign of obstruction in the normal flow of bile. Jaundice caused by an elevation in BC or direct bilirubin is called *obstructive jaundice*. The obstruction may be in the collecting channels in the liver, in the hepatic ducts, or in the common bile duct. For example, a gallstone lodged in the common bile duct prevents the normal excretion of bile salts (which contain the BC) into the intestine. The BC is absorbed into the bloodstream in much larger amounts than normal. In complete biliary obstruction, the BC may be as high as 30–40 mg. Another example of an obstruction is cancer of the head of the pancreas, of which jaundice is often the first symptom. Newborns with a congenital malformation in the biliary tree (biliary atresia) also have high BCs.

Sometimes the BC may be elevated even though biliary obstruction is not apparent. Some drugs, notably contraceptive steroids and some of the phenothiazines such as chlorpromazine (Thorazine), may cause stasis of bile in the liver (intrahepatic cholestasis). The bile tends to be viscous, and the small bile ducts in the liver become dilated. The BC is elevated because of this partial obstruction to the normal outflow of bile. A similar condition of stasis occurs in what is called the *benign jaundice* of pregnancy. The rise in bilirubin is an occasional occurrence in pregnancy, and the bilirubin returns to normal after delivery. Inflammation of the liver, as in hepatitis, or scarring, as in cirrhosis, may also cause partial obstruction to the flow of bile out of the liver and thereby cause an elevation of the BC.

Combination of Conjugated and Unconjugated Elevations

Although the previous discussion attempts to clarify the distinction between elevations of BC and of BU, clinical situations often entail elevations of both. Any clinical condition, any drug, or any toxic condition that causes obstruction to the flow of bile may eventually cause an increase in BU as well, because stasis of bile in the collecting ducts eventually impairs normal functioning of the liver. Intrahepatic disease, such as cirrhosis or hepatitis, and drug toxicity may cause elevations in both BC and BU. Urine bilirubin, urine urobilinogen, and less frequently, fecal urobilinogen, tests may give additional information about the nature of the jaundice. Table 11–2 summarizes the usual findings in jaundice that is prehepatic (hemolytic), intrahepatic (liver dysfunction), or posthepatic (obstruction).

For clinical jaundice, tests other than those for bilirubin and urobilinogen may be needed. For example, alkaline phosphatase and γ-glutamyl transferase (GGT) are enzymes normally excreted in the bile and are elevated in biliary obstruction. The transaminases are also elevated in most types of liver disease. (See Chapter 12 on using these enzymes in detecting liver and biliary disease.) For cholestatic jaundice ultrasonography (Chapter 23), or oral cholecystography (Chapter 20) may help detect gallstones. Transhepatic cholangiography (Chapter 20) and endoscopic cholangiography (Chapter 27) are two other diagnostic approaches to obstructive jaundice.

▼ URINE BILIRUBIN

Because only the water-soluble conjugated (direct) bilirubin can cross the glomerular filter, it is the only type of bilirubin ever found in the urine. Normally even this type of bilirubin is not in the urine in detectable amounts because it has been converted to urobilinogen in the intestine. Bilirubin becomes apparent in the urine when there is an obstruction to the normal pathway of BC. This test is therefore used to detect obstructive jaundice, and it is sometimes said incorrectly to be a test for "bile" in the urine. Because the test is likely to be positive for bilirubin before the client has signs of clinical hepatitis, it may be a screening procedure performed on populations that were known to be exposed to hepatitis. It may also be useful to screen blood donors, food handlers, and other possible carriers of the disease when controlling the spread of subclinical cases of hepatitis is imperative.

Preparation of Client and Collection of Sample

A few milliliters of freshly voided urine are needed. The urine must be fresh because oxidation affects the results, and exposure to strong lights also changes the chemical composition of the bilirubin.

Sometimes the nurse or client may test urine for bilirubin by using either a tablet or a dipstick. For the Icotest (Ames Products), 5 drops of urine are placed on a special test mat. A tablet is then placed on the mat and 2 drops of water are added. If the mat turns blue or purple within 30 sec, the test is positive for bilirubin. With the dipstick method, the positive reaction is a tan-to-purple color. The dipstick method is 2–4 times less sensitive than the tablet method. Drugs that change the color of the urine may mask the color change on the tablet or strip of paper. (See Chapter 3 for a list of drugs that cause color changes in urine, as well as for a dipstick method to check for ascorbic acid, because this may interfere with the bilirubin tests.)

REFERENCE VALUES FOR URINE BILIRUBIN	
All groups	Normally bilirubin is present in such small quantities in the urine that it is not detected with routine screening procedures

▼ POSSIBLE NURSING IMPLICATION RELATED TO BILIRUBIN IN THE URINE (BILIRUBINURIA)

Large amounts of bilirubin make urine a dark-orange color, and they also make urine foam when it is shaken (shake test). Urine does not foam or become dark if it contains only urobilinogen. Because the nurse or client may be the first to notice that the urine color is abnormal, the color of urine and stools should always be a priority assessment when an obstruction of the common bile duct is suspected. (The stools become clay-colored when complete obstruction occurs.)

▼ URINE UROBILINOGEN

Urobilinogen is formed in the intestine from the BC normally present in bile salts. Most of the urobilinogen is excreted in the feces, but a small amount that finds its way into the bloodstream either goes through the liver again or is excreted in the urine. This test may be used to detect hemolytic jaundice or early liver dysfunction.

An increase in urine urobilinogen follows hemolysis, with the increase in fecal urobilinogen even more pronounced than that in urinary urobilinogen. Because some of the urobilinogen in the feces is picked up by the portal circulation and carried to the liver again and because urinary urobilinogen excretion is increased when the liver cannot excrete the recycled urobilinogen, urinary urobilinogen can also be used to detect early liver dysfunction. The inability of the liver to handle urobilinogen occurs before bilirubin excretion is affected (Lewis, 1985).

In obstructive jaundice, the lack of bilirubin excreted into the intestine causes a decrease in the amount of urobilinogen in the urine, which is not important to measure because it is very small even in normal health. The amount of urinary urobilinogen also decreases when there is a lack of intestinal flora to convert bilirubin to urobilinogen; this effect, however, is more of academic interest than of clinical usefulness.

Preparation of Client and Collection of Sample

If a 24-hr specimen is needed, a preservative must be used. (See Chapter 3 for tips on 24-hr urine collection.) The more common procedure is to collect a 2-hr urine sample in the afternoon, because the excretion of urobilinogen is at a maximum from mid-afternoon to evening when food is being digested. The urine should be taken to the laboratory immediately after collection. Strongly acid urine may make the results inaccurate; so if a client is taking drugs, such as high doses of salicylates, record this fact on the laboratory slip. Drugs that color the urine interfere with the test. Laboratories may report in milligrams or in units.

The nurse can also check for urobilinogen by using a dipstick, which shows 0.1–1 Ehrlich units as normal. For amounts from 2 to more than 12 Ehrlich units, the color goes from dark yellow to orange when read after 45 sec.

REFERENCE VALUES FOR URINE UROBILINOGEN

All groups	0.3–1.0 Ehrlich units in a 2-hr sample (1–3 PM)
	0.5–4.0 Ehrlich units in a 24-hr sample (ask laboratory about preservative)
	0.4–1 mg/day. Use specific color chart if dipstick method is used.

▼ FECAL UROBILINOGEN

The amount of urobilinogen in the feces depends on the amount of BC excreted in the bile salts into the intestine and the presence of bacteria in the intestine. A lack of bacteria to break down the bilirubin may reduce the urobilinogen in the intestine, and thus the feces become lighter in color. For example, this may occur with antibiotic use (Lewis, 1985). The test for fecal urobilinogen is not often performed because urine and serum tests may give enough information about the cause of the impaired bilirubin excretion.

The fecal urobilinogen is increased when there is an increased breakdown of RBCs (hemolytic jaundice) because much more bilirubin is conjugated by the liver and excreted into the intestine. A lack of fecal urobilinogen occurs in obstructive jaundice because the BC cannot be excreted into the intestine. A lack of BC in the intestine is apparent to the eye because the feces are clay-colored. In infants, this condition may not be apparent because the stools are normally light-colored.

▼ POSSIBLE NURSING DIAGNOSES RELATED TO HYPERBILIRUBINEMIA

Knowledge Deficit Related to Clinical Signs of Jaundice

Although serum tests are used to monitor the exact level of the bilirubin from day to day, the nurse or client should also record color changes on a daily basis. Because clients may be the best judges of day-to-day changes in their own skin color, this source of data should never be overlooked, and clients should be instructed on changes that are important to note. An excess of serum bilirubin, either the BU or BC, gives a yellowish coloration to the sclera of the eyes, skin, and mucous membranes. The symptoms of jaundice begin to appear when the total bilirubin is about 2–4 mg in adults, or older children. In infants, jaundice may not be apparent until the total bilirubin is about 5–7 mg. Often the yellow is noted first in the sclera of fair-skinned clients. In dark-skinned clients, the inner canthus of the eye may show more change. In dark-skinned or Asian clients, the yellowish tinge also becomes apparent in the mucous membranes of the hard palate (Roach, 1977). Blanching the skin of newborns by pressing on the sternum makes the jaundice of the skin more apparent. With proper lighting, one can see jaundice on the abdomen nearly as easily as in the sclera. Observations for jaundice should be carried out in natural daylight, if possible.

In a community health setting or clinic, the nurse may be the first to notice the beginning of jaundice. In high-risk populations composed of abusers of alcohol or other drugs, inspections of the eyes and skin are especially important to detect liver damage.

Differences in BU and BC. Nurses must also know whether the BU or BC is elevated, because the nursing implications vary for each type of elevation. Some of the implications, such as changes in body image or ways to assess for jaundice, are the same for both types. However, the danger to the central nervous system (CNS), itching, discomfort, and bleeding are problems associated more with one type than the other.

Anxiety of Parents Related to Risk for Central Nervous System Damage in the Newborn

In older children and adults, an increase in BU is not in itself dangerous or uncomfortable for the client. After infancy, the blood-brain barrier prevents the BU from affecting the CNS. A high BU in newborns, however, is of grave concern. In infants, BU does leak through the vascular walls and can damage the CNS. *Kernicterus* (*kern* = kernel, *icterus* = yellow) is the term used to describe the CNS damage that results from a high BU (usually > 20 mg) in newborns.

No one figure, such as "over 20," defines the upper limits of BU that necessitate intervention in a newborn. The clinician must consider the clinical course and birthweight. Infants who weigh less than 2.5 kg may need phototherapy at low levels, whereas infants who weigh more than 2.5 kg may not need intervention until the BU is 16–20 mg/dL (DeCherney and Pernoll, 1994).

Parents are often concerned about the appearance of jaundice. A nurse may be able to alleviate some anxiety with a brief explanation of a specific protocol for newborn jaundice and the importance of frequent laboratory testing. Parents may prefer not to see the heel sticks performed to obtain blood. Anxiety may also be lessened by helping the mother be successful with breast feeding, because an adequate milk supply may be useful in reducing the level of breast-feeding jaundice.

Risk for Injury Related to Treatments to Decrease Indirect Bilirubin in Newborns

Researchers are exploring the use of protoporphrins to decrease bilirubin production (Hay et al., 1995), but the two standard treatments to decrease the indirect bilirubin in newborns are exchange transfusions and phototherapy.

Exchange Transfusions. These are used primarily for severe cases of blood-type incompatibility. (See Chapter 14 for safety needs with transfusions.)

Phototherapy. High-intensity light is used to help break down the BU to a nontoxic substance. Phototherapy converts bilirubin to derivatives that apparently can be excreted in the bile and urine without being conjugated by the liver. It is important that the baby's eyes be protected under the lights. It is also crucial to monitor the temperature to prevent hypo- or hyperthermia. Extra fluids should be given to prevent dehydration. The skin becomes lighter in the areas under the light. Evidently, turning the baby so that no areas are shaded is not important because the rapidity of the bilirubin level drop is due to the

(*continued*)

▼ POSSIBLE NURSING DIAGNOSES RELATED TO HYPERBILIRUBINEMIA (*continued*)

dose of light, not to the amount of skin illuminated (Tan, 1975), but most current protocols require turning after each feeding. Registered nurses skilled in newborn care, including heel-stick blood collection, have managed home care phototherapy for several years (Shibley, 1988).

Because the BU itself is not a danger to older children or adults, little effort is made to decrease the level itself. Theoretically, sitting in the sun would be beneficial to a child who has a high BU, but it is more important to correct the pathophysiologic process causing the elevation.

Altered Comfort Related to Pruritus

It is presumed that the severe itching (pruritus) that often accompanies an elevated BC is due to something toxic in the "bile salts" deposited in the skin. Keeping the environment cool is useful because perspiration may accentuate the pruritus. Soothing baths and lotions may give some relief. Aveeno, a colloidal oatmeal bath for irritated skin, contains no soaps or synthetics that can harm the skin. The bath soothes and cleanses naturally because of its unique adsorption action. Oatmeal baths can be used for infants as well as adults who have pruritus. Children may need to be restrained from scratching. Excess bilirubin levels may also irritate connective tissue in the sclera. Clients may have photophobia and thus a need to avoid bright lights.

Although there is no direct evidence that the pruritus is directly attributed to bile salts, the use of medications that bind bile salts may relieve the itching. Cholestyramine (Questran) is a resin that is taken orally to bind bile salts in the intestine and prevent their reabsorption (Katzung, 1995). This treatment may be helpful when the obstruction is not complete. To prevent constipation, a person taking cholestyramine needs a large intake of fluids and a diet high in fiber. Because the drug may bind other drugs, it should be given at least 1 hr before or 4 hr after other drugs. Supplements of fat-soluble vitamins may be needed if the client is undergoing long-term therapy with the drug. (Cholestyramine is also used as a drug to lower cholesterol levels [see Chapter 9].)

Risk for Injury Related to Bleeding Caused by Hypoprothrombinemia

For fats and fat-soluble vitamins to be emulsified and absorbed from the intestine, there must be adequate bile salts. For this reason, a client with an elevated BC may have a tendency to bleed. Without bile salts, fat-soluble vitamins, including vitamin K, are not absorbed from the small intestine. If vitamin K is not absorbed into the bloodstream, the liver cannot make enough prothrombin and other factors needed for normal blood clotting. Clients with obstructive jaundice thus often have increased prothrombin times. Clients with elevated prothrombin times caused by obstructive jaundice are given parenteral injections of vitamin K. Parenteral vitamin K can reach the liver because the bile salts are not needed to get the vitamin from the intestine into the bloodstream. Specific methods to prevent bleeding when the client has an increased prothrombin time are discussed in Chapter 13 on clotting tests.

Risk for Pain Related to Obstructive Jaundice

Although jaundice caused by an elevation of BU is painless, pain, other than that associated with pruritus, may or may not be associated with jaundice caused by an elevation of the BC. Because obstruction of the biliary tree by a pancreatic tumor may be painless for quite awhile, the first indications of biliary obstruction could be jaundice and a tendency to bleed. However, jaundice caused by a gallstone in the common bile duct tends to cause severe abdominal pain in the right upper quadrant. In such a case, the client may need narcotics to relieve the pain. Characteristically, the pain tends to radiate to the right shoulder, and it may be intensified by an attempt to eat fatty foods.

Altered Nutrition Related to Inability to Tolerate Fats and Other Nutrients

Clients with an elevated BC usually have marked intolerance to fatty foods. Their nutritional status must be carefully assessed so that their caloric needs are met. If indicated, an operation is performed to relieve the obstruction. Before the operation, the client may need intravenous feedings to maintain hydration and caloric intake. Fat-soluble vitamins can be added to intravenous fluids. Even with only a partial or clearing obstruction, the client may have little appetite for food, so the nurse must plan meals carefully. (As a rule, an increase in the BU does not seriously interfere with appetite unless the liver is involved, and then anorexia can be profound.)

Hepatitis, which causes cholestasis and elevations of both BU and BC, is accompanied by anorexia. Even if foods are not desired, the client should be encouraged to drink fruit juices. These provide some calories and help flush the water-soluble BC into the urine. As the client's appetite returns, food is needed to supply adequate calories and protein for liver regeneration. Protein in the diet is encouraged only if serum ammonia levels are normal (see Chapter 10). Otherwise, hepatic coma can result from too much protein. Fats can be allowed as tolerated.

Altered Self-concept Related to Changes in Body Image

A concentration on the physical aspects of care for clients with an elevated bilirubin must not overshadow their psychological needs. Nurses need to be

(*continued*)

▼ POSSIBLE NURSING DIAGNOSES RELATED TO HYPERBILIRUBINEMIA (*continued*)

aware that jaundice is a definite change in the body image of the person. Jaundice may be very upsetting not only to clients but also to their families. Some clients are afraid to look in a mirror, and others may prefer not to have any visitors. If these clients must come to a clinic, they may not want others to stare at them. (In addition, other clients may be afraid that the jaundice is contagious.) Soft, subdued lights make the jaundice less apparent while treatments are begun to reduce the bilirubin level.

Clients' reactions, of course, can also be unexpected. A young man was once admitted to the hospital with severe jaundice caused by cirrhosis. Blue dye for a lymphogram (Chapter 20) turned the man's sclera and skin from yellow to green. One might jump to the conclusion that the client would not want anyone to see him and that he would be upset by the parade of nursing students, residents, and interns who came to examine the "green man." On the contrary, the client enjoyed all the extra attention from being unique and seemed a little disappointed when his color began to return to normal. So, as with all generalizations about nursing implications, nurses must choose which ones are applicable for a certain client in a certain setting. Nurses should also recognize that a change in body image caused by a specific *external* source (such as the dye) may be quite a different experience from the change due to a longer-term and less specific *internal source* such as jaundice caused by an inoperable tumor.

▼ BILIRUBIN IN AMNIOTIC FLUID

It is not known for sure how bilirubin reaches the amniotic fluid; some of it may diffuse across the skin. The bilirubin in the amniotic fluid is the unconjugated, nonwater-soluble type and cannot be excreted in the urine of the fetus. The bilirubin content of amniotic fluid is often high during early pregnancy, but it should fall progressively after midpregnancy. (See Chapter 28 for a discussion on the procedure for amniocentesis.) The importance of measuring the bilirubin content of amniotic fluid is to determine whether the normal downward progression of bilirubin concentration in the last half of pregnancy is continuing. If the bilirubin content is not dropping or if it begins to rise for the fetus of an Rh-negative mother, medical interventions may be necessary to save the fetus. Laboratories may use either light or chemical methods to determine the amount of bilirubin in the amniotic fluid. (See Chapter 14 for Rh antibody titers and the Coombs' test, which are used to determine the need for amniocentesis.)

▼ TRANSCUTANEOUS BILIRUBINOMETER

A transcutaneous bilirubinometer is a handheld device that contains a fiber-optic probe to measure the color intensity of the skin. The probe is placed on the neonate's forehead, and a button is pressed to activate the meter. An audible click and a flash of light are emitted. Measurements of how the light travels through and reflects off the skin are converted to a digital display. The digital readings correlate with total serum bilirubin levels. Each institution must establish its own criteria for correlating the readings with approximate serum bilirubin levels and for determining a protocol for when follow-up serum bilirubin levels are indicated. For example, if the digital reading is less than a certain number, the infant may be spared the discomfort of having blood drawn. Work by Brown et al. (1990) contains a review of the literature on the reliability and validity of these meters, their care and maintenance, and their usefulness for nursing research and clinical practice.

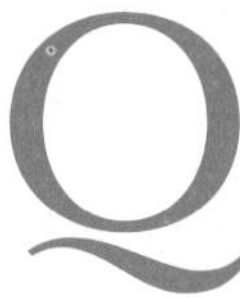

1. When the body is using the normal pathway of bilirubin excretion, which laboratory test is negative?

   a. Serum bilirubin level (indirect portion)
   b. Fecal urobilinogen
   c. Urine urobilinogen
   d. Urine bilirubin

2. Which of the following terms is a synonym for indirect bilirubin?

   a. Conjugated bilirubin b. Water-soluble bilirubin
   c. Posthepatic bilirubin d. Free bilirubin

3. The laboratory slip on Mrs. Fong's chart shows a total bilirubin of 3.0 mg and a direct bilirubin of 0.3 mg. Her indirect bilirubin is which of the following?

   a. Unknown at the present time b. 3.3 mg/dL
   c. 2.7 mg/dL d. 3.9 mg/dL

4. Mr. Sarconi has been admitted with a diagnosis of complete obstructive jaundice related to a gallstone in the common bile duct. The nurse would expect to observe for

   a. Dark stools and dark orange urine with a high specific gravity
   b. Clay-colored stools and pale yellow urine with a low specific gravity

c. Clay-colored stools and dark orange urine that foams when shaken
d. Dark stools and pale yellow urine that foams when shaken

5. In an infant, clinical jaundice becomes apparent when the total bilirubin level is about which of the following levels?

a. 3–4 mg/dL b. 5–7 mg/dL c. 7–9 mg/dL d. More than 9 mg/dL

6. In an adult, clinical jaundice becomes apparent when the serum bilirubin (total) is about which of the following levels?

a. 3–4 mg/dL b. 5–7 mg/dL c. 7–9 mg/dL d. More than 9 mg/dL

7. An elevation of the direct or conjugated bilirubin would be an expected finding for

a. Mrs. Rhoades, aged 31, who has anemia caused by a lack of iron in her diet
b. Baby Holmes, 2 days old, breast feeding and slightly jaundiced
c. Shirley, aged 7, who has been admitted to the pediatric unit in a sickle-cell crisis
d. Mr. Smith, aged 42, who has cholestatic jaundice related to drug therapy

8. An elevation of the indirect or unconjugated bilirubin would be an expected finding for

a. Mrs. Fonolini, who has gallstones in the common bile duct
b. Mr. Petersen, who is undergoing an operation (Whipple procedure) for cancer of the head of the pancreas
c. Baby Jones, who has a malformation in the biliary tree (biliary atresia)
d. Reggie, aged 7, who had a transfusion reaction caused by incompatible blood

9. Baby Jennifer has been diagnosed with breast-feeding jaundice. Which of the following points is appropriate to include in a teaching plan for the parents of this baby?

a. Breast feeding should not be continued
b. Phototherapy is usually begun if bilirubin levels are greater than 12 mg/dL
c. Inadequate milk intake may intensify the jaundice
d. Phototherapy requires the baby to stay in the hospital

10. A possible nursing diagnosis for an adult client with an elevated indirect or unconjugated bilirubin is

a. Alteration in self-concept related to changes in body image
b. Risk for bleeding related to hypoprothrombinemia
c. Altered nutrition related to intolerance for fats
d. Risk for injury related to central nervous system damage

11. The most common method used to treat high levels of bilirubin in the newborn is

a. Complete elimination of breast milk to reduce the factors that interfere with glucuronyl transferase in the liver
b. Exchange transfusions to remove toxic products from the bloodstream
c. Phototherapy with high-intensity lights to help break down the bilirubin
d. Drug therapy with phenobarbital to promote the hepatic clearance of bilirubin

12. A home care nurse is visiting Mary Brown, who is recovering from hepatitis. The nurse knows that the drug cholestyramine (Questran) is being effective if Ms. Brown states that

a. Constipation is no longer a problem
b. Itching is less
c. Appetite is better
d. Bright lights no longer hurt her eyes

▼ REFERENCES

Brown, L., Arnold L., Allison, D., et al. (1993). Incidence and pattern of jaundice in healthy breast-fed infants during the first month of life. *Nursing Research, 42* (2), 106–109.

Brown, L., Arnold, L., Chavsha, D., et al. (1990). Transcutaneous bilirubinometer: An instrument for clinical research. *Nursing Research, 39* (4), 241–243.

DeCherney, A.H., and Pernoll, M.L. (1994). *Current obstetric and gynecologic diagnosis & treatment.* (8th ed.). Norwalk, CT: Appleton & Lange.

Hay, W.W., Groothuis, J.R., Hayward, A.R., and Levin, M.J. (1995). *Current pediatric diagnosis and treatment.* (12th ed.). Norwalk, CT: Appleton & Lange.

Kaplan, A., Jack, R., Opheim, K.E., et al. (1995). *Clinical chemistry interpretation and techniques* (4th ed.). Baltimore: Williams & Wilkins.

Katzung, B. (1995). *Basic and clinical pharmacology.* (6th ed.). Norwalk, CT: Appleton & Lange.

Lewis, S. (1985). What bilirubin tests can tell you. *RN, 48* (3), 85–86.

Lum, G. (1988). Efficacy of using total bilirubin values as a guide for screening direct bilirubin requests. *American Journal of Clinical Pathology, 89* (2), 242–246.

Ravel, R. (1995). *Clinical laboratory medicine: Clinical application of laboratory data* (6th ed.). St. Louis: Mosby–Year Book.

Roach, L. (1977). Color changes in dark skin. *Nursing 77, 7* (1), 48–51.

Shibley, B. (1988). Now newborns can stay home for phototherapy. *RN 51,* (2), 69–71.

Tan, K.L. (1975). Comparison of the effectiveness of single direction and double direction phototherapy for neo-natal jaundice. *Pediatrics, 56* (4), 550–553.

Thaler, M. (1977). Jaundice in the newborn: Algorithmic diagnosis of conjugated and unconjugated hyperbilirubinemia. *JAMA, 237,* 58–62.

Wysowski, D., et al. (1978). Epidemic neo-natal hyperbilirubinemia and use of a phenolic disinfectant detergent. *Pediatrics, 61* (2), 165–170.

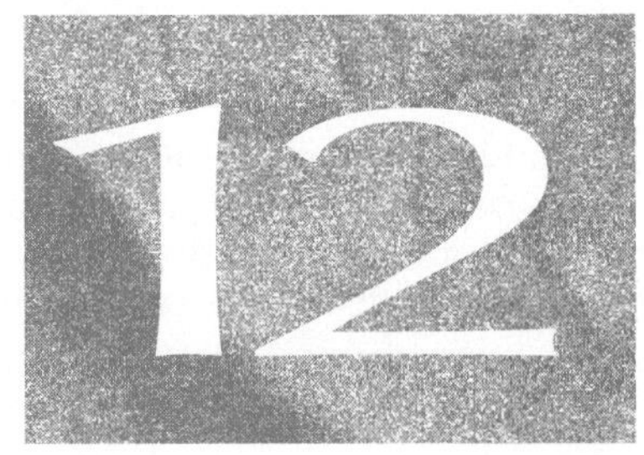

TESTS TO MEASURE ENZYME AND ISOENZYME LEVELS

- Alkaline Phosphatase
- γ-Glutamyl Transferase or γ-Glutamyl Transpeptidase
- 5′Nucleotidase
- Acid Phosphatase or Prostatic Acid Phosphatase
- Alanine Aminotransferase (Serum Glutamic-Pyruvic Transaminase)
- Aspartate Aminotransferase (Serum Glutamic-Oxaloacetic Transaminase)
- Creatine Kinase or Creatine Phosphokinase
- Lactic Dehydrogenase
- Serum Aldolase
- Serum Amylase
- Urinary Amylase
- Serum Lipase

OBJECTIVES

1. Identify factors, other than pathologic processes, that tend to cause elevations in most of the serum enzyme tests.
2. Explain the usual clinical significance of an elevated serum alkaline phosphatase (ALP) level and compare with the γ-glutamyl transferase (GGT) level.
3. Compare and contrast the use of the serum acid phosphatase level with use of the prostate-specific antigen (PSA) test.

4. Describe possible nursing diagnoses when a client has marked elevations of the transaminases, alanine aminotransferase (ALT) (formerly serum glutamic-pyruvic transaminase [SGPT]), and aspartate aminotransferase (AST) (formerly serum glutamic-oxaloacetic transaminase [SGOT]).
5. Discriminate between the cardiac enzymes—creatine kinase (CK) and lactic dehydrogenase (LDH or LD)—in relation to the onset, peak, and duration of elevation after a myocardial infarction.
6. Explain why measurements of isoenzymes of CK and LDH are more valuable than measurement of the total amounts of the enzymes.
7. Identify the most important nursing diagnosis for a client with cardiac disease who has unexpected normal levels of cardiac enzymes.
8. Plan an appropriate activity schedule for a client who has an elevated CK level or serum aldolase level caused by a muscular disorder.
9. Explain how serum amylase and lipase and urinary amylase are used as assessment tools for pancreatitis.
10. Identify the nursing diagnoses for clients who have marked elevations of serum amylase and lipase levels.

This chapter covers the most common enzymes measured in the serum. As an additional assessment, only one of the enzymes, amylase, is measured in the urine. Almost all cells contain the principal enzymes, although some types of tissue contain larger concentrations of particular enzymes. So when tissue cells are damaged, the enzymes leak into the serum.

Although the enzymes are not tissue-specific, various types of tissue have isoenzymes with different chemical and physical properties. Isoenzymes of a particular enzyme all control the same specific metabolic function even though their molecular forms vary slightly from one to another. The enzyme LDH, for example, which is abundant in most tissues, can be separated into five distinct types of isoenzymes. LDH_1 is abundant in heart tissue, whereas LDH_5 is abundant in liver tissue. Each of the five LDH isoenzymes is still not organ-specific, however, because the heart or liver may have more than one type of isoenzyme and isoenzymes may come from several different tissues. Nonetheless, the use of isoenzymes narrows the possibilities of the origin of the elevated enzyme in the serum. (The various isoenzymes are separated with electrophoresis, explained in Chapter 10 for protein electrophoresis.)

Enzymes are often named for the reaction that they catalyze. For example, lipase is an enzyme used for the reaction of a lipid or fat, and transaminases transfer amino groups in energy production. Enzymes are easy to recognize because their names almost always end in *-ase*. However, because many of the serum enzyme tests are known by initials rather than by names, there is no way to know that CPK is an enzyme test unless one sees it written out as *creatine phosphokinase,* and more recently *CPK* has become just *CK* for *creatine kinase.*

To make matters more confusing, the transaminases, which until recently were called SGPT and SGOT, are now called ALT and AST, because the new names are more correct in a chemical sense.

Enzyme levels used to be reported in Bodansky units, Somogyi units, or other units, which usually bore the name of the originator of the method. Now almost all laboratories report results as international units per liter (IU/L). Variation in techniques still produce differences in normal reference values for many of the enzymes.

Table 12–1 summarizes the most important enzyme elevations for several common pathologic conditions. With a quick glance at the table, the reader sees that none of the enzyme tests is totally specific and that many are changed by several pathologic conditions. Also, various nonpathologic factors, such as vigorous exercise, cause elevated serum enzymes. Apple and McGue (1983) found marked increases in the CK, LDH, and ALT levels of men training for marathons. Treatments such as intramuscular injections and the administration of opiates cause serum elevations of some enzymes. Improper handling of the specimens also brings about elevations caused by hemolysis.

In this chapter, each of the factors that affects a particular enzyme is discussed with the specific test. The enzymes are usually not affected by food. The exact timing of each specimen must be documented because several of these enzymes peak quickly and are of short duration, whereas others do not show up in the bloodstream until a couple of days after tissue injury. For most of the enzyme tests, only elevations of the enzymes or isoenzymes are clinically significant. However, decreased ALP levels and, very rarely, decreased transaminase levels may be clinically significant.

▼ ALKALINE PHOSPHATASE

Two types of phosphatases are measured in the bloodstream: alkaline and acid. These two types of phosphatases are so termed because their activity is best measured in a pH of about either 10 (alkaline) or 5 (acid).

The ALP is a more common clinical test because the enzyme is abundant in several organs. ALP is found in the tissues of the liver, bone, intestine, kidney, and placenta. Its three isoenzymes can be identified by electrophoresis:

1. Band I: Liver, vascular endothelium, and lung
2. Band II: Bone, kidney, and placenta
3. Band III: Intestinal mucosa

However, unlike the other isoenzymes, the isoenzymes of ALP are not commonly used in clinical evaluations of pathologic conditions.

Except in pregnancy, most of the serum ALP is made up of liver and bone isoenzymes. Because ALP is increased with new bone formation (osteoblastic activity), children have higher levels than adults, and because the placenta is a rich source of ALP, a high level of this enzyme is also normal in pregnancy. The ALP from liver tissue is normally excreted into the bile, so biliary obstruction causes an increase of ALP. The ingestion of a fatty meal also causes a temporary increase of serum ALP.

TABLE 12–1. ENZYME ELEVATIONS IN COMMON PATHOLOGIC CONDITIONS

Serum Enzymes	Eclampsia	Cancer of Prostate	Biliary Obstruction	Bone Metastasis	Malignant Tumor of Liver	Hepatitis	Cirrhosis	Myocardial Infarction	Infectious Mononucleosis	Hemolytic Disease	Pulmonary Infarction	Muscular Necrosis or Inflammation	Pancreatitis	Brain Tissue Injury
1. Alkaline phosphatase	↑	↑	(↑)	(↑)	(↑)	↑	↑		↑				↑	
2. Acid phosphatase	↑	(↑)			↑					(↑)				
3. GGT			(↑)		(↑)	↑	↑							
4. 5′Nucleotidase			(↑)		(↑)		↑							
5. ALT (SGPT)	↑		↑	↑	↑	(↑)	↑		(↑)		↑	↑	↑	
6. AST (SGOT)	↑	↑	↑	↑	↑	(↑)	↑	(↑)	(↑)	↑	↑	↑	↑	
7. CK (total)								(↑)			↑	(↑)		↑
CK-I (BB)														↑
CK-II (MB)								(↑)						
CK-III (MM)												(↑)		
8. LDH Total	↑	↑	↑	↑	↑			↑	↑	(↑)		↑	↑	↑
LDH_1								(↑)		↑				
LDH_2								(↑)		↑	↑		↑	
LDH_3									↑	↑	(↑)		↑	
LDH_4					↑	↑			↑				↑	
LDH_5			↑		↑	↑	↑		↑			↑	↑	
9. Aldolase		↑			↑	↑		↑			↑	(↑)		
10. Amylase			↑										(↑)	
11. Lipase			↑										(↑)	

↑ Clinically significant elevation. Note that any tissue injury causes *slight* increase in many of these enzymes.

(↑) Used as principal diagnostic tool. See text for elaborations.

Preparation of Client and Collection of Sample

The client should be fasting, because a fatty meal may cause an elevation. If the client is taking oral contraceptives, phenothiazines, morphine, or phenytoin, record use of the drug on the laboratory slip, because elevations in the enzyme level may be related to the drug. The laboratory needs 1 mL of serum. Some methods require immediate refrigeration of the sample.

REFERENCE VALUES FOR ALP

Adult	Men 45–115 U/L Women 30–100 U/L
Pregnancy	Levels increase because of production by placenta. Levels return to normal about 3 weeks after delivery.
Infant and Children	1.6 to 2.6 times adult levels[a]
Puberty	6 to 7 times adult levels
Aged	Values tend to increase after the age of 50 years

[a]See Hay et al. (1995) for more details.

Increased ALP Level

Clinical Significance. A markedly increased ALP level in a nonpregnant adult is a general warning of a bone or liver abnormality. If there is question whether bone or liver is the origin, other enzyme tests more specific for hepatobiliary disease may be done (see discussion on GGT, and 5′ nucleotidase [5′N]).

In Paget's disease, in which there is considerable bone destruction and bone rebuilding, the ALP level is higher than normal. Cancer metastatic to the bone also often causes an elevated ALP if the body attempts to continue to form new bone. If bone is only being broken down (osteolytic process), ALP is not elevated. However, most types of osteolytic processes are accompanied by some osteoblastic activity. A healing fracture causes a modest rise in the ALP level. Conditions such as hyperparathyroidism and vitamin D or calcium deficiencies cause an increased amount of ALP, even though bone growth may be abnormal.

Liver dysfunction is the other main reason for increased ALP levels. The elevation may be due either to actual liver tissue damage or, because ALP is excreted in the bile, to an obstruction of bile flow. Morphine sulfate and other opioids may cause some spasm of the sphincter of Oddi and thus elevate the ALP level. Conditions that cause obstructive jaundice, such as a stone in the common bile duct or cancer of the head of the pancreas, cause a markedly elevated ALP.

Certain drugs, such as the estrogens and phenothiazines, may cause a stasis of bile (cholestatic effect), thus elevating the ALP in the serum. Anticonvulsants and other drugs may induce a synthesis of increased amounts of ALP and other liver enzymes. The elevation of the ALP may be the first indication of an adverse reaction to a drug and indicates that the drug should be stopped.

In eclampsia, the ALP levels are increased above the normally high levels of pregnancy, probably because of a liver dysfunction.

Often patients with liver problems, such as cirrhosis, receive albumin intravenously. (See Chapter 10 for a discussion on albumin deficiency.) In such cases, the fact that the placenta is normally a rich source of ALP is important to remember. Administration of albumin derived from placentas causes an elevation of the serum ALP level.

Benign transient hyperphosphatasemia occurs mainly in young children but has also been observed in a few adults who have no bone or liver disease or drug toxicity. The ALP usually returns to normal within 4–8 weeks. If the ALP stays elevated, a family study is indicated to determine whether familial hyperphosphatasemia exists (Garty and Nitzan, 1994).

▼ POSSIBLE NURSING DIAGNOSES RELATED TO INCREASED ALP LEVEL

Risk of Injury Related to Pathologic Fractures

One of the most common uses of the ALP test is to screen for the possibility of bone metastasis in clients with malignant tumors. The possibility of bone metastasis is an indication that the client may be prone to pathologic fractures and thus should be handled very carefully and protected from injury. Remember that the metastatic destruction of bone causes an increase of ALP only if osteoblastic activity is occurring along with bone destruction. So not all bone metastases cause elevated ALP levels. In metastatic disease, any elevated ALP is usually followed with a bone scan (see Chapter 22) to determine the exact points of bone destruction.

Altered Comfort Related to Development of Obstructive Jaundice

If the elevated ALP is due to any type of obstruction in the common bile duct, specific nursing implications are related to the presence of obstructive jaundice. (The problems associated with obstructive jaundice are discussed in Chapter 11 in the section on conjugated bilirubin levels.)

Knowledge Deficit Related to Need to Change Therapeutic Regime

If the client is taking drugs that can cause cholestasis, such as estrogens or phenothiazines, even a small increase in the ALP level may be an indication that the client should not continue taking the drug. A client who is taking oral contraceptives that contain estrogen needs information about other forms of birth control. The physician must be consulted about any needed changes in medication regimens such as a change in tranquilizers.

Decreased ALP Level

Clinical Significance. In a child who has not yet reached puberty, a decrease in ALP indicates a lack of normal bone formation. This condition may be caused by pathologic conditions, such as hypothyroidism, celiac disease, cystic fibrosis, or chronic nephritis. A decreased ALP may also be caused by a genetic defect. Dentists may observe that these children have premature bone loss. Very low levels of ALP are seen in scurvy. Adults with a lack of bone formation caused by malnutrition or excessive vitamin D intake may have lowered ALP levels.

▼ POSSIBLE NURSING DIAGNOSIS RELATED TO DECREASED ALP LEVEL

Altered Nutrition: Less than Body Requirements
The exact nursing implications depend on the reason for a lack of normal bone formation. Usually a dietary plan is needed to ensure an adequate intake of protein, vitamins, and minerals for optimal bone growth.

▼ γ-GLUTAMYL TRANSFERASE OR γ-GLUTAMYL TRANSPEPTIDASE

Gamma-glutamyl transferase (GGT), an enzyme that is useful in amino acid transport, is found chiefly in the liver, kidney, prostate, and spleen. When ALP is elevated, the GGT may be used to assess whether the increase is due to liver and biliary involvement, because the GGT is more specific for the hepatobiliary system, whereas the ALP can be elevated in bone or liver disease. The GGT is also raised by alcohol and hepatotoxic drugs and thus is useful to monitor drug toxicity and alcohol abuse.

Preparation of Client and Collection of Sample

Some laboratories may require fasting for 8 hr, with water allowed. Serum is collected in a red-topped tube.

REFERENCE VALUES FOR GGT

Adult:	
Men	5–38 U/L
Women	5–29 U/L
Children	3–30 U/L
Newborn	Levels five times childhood values (premature infants have 10 times childhood values)

Clinical Significance. Elevated GGT levels are found in liver disease, including liver metastasis, and in biliary obstruction. Because liver damage from alcohol causes immediate increases in the GGT, this test is considered the enzyme test of choice in investigating alcohol abuse (Kaplan, et al., 1995). The GGT may also be used to monitor the course of hepatitis; a return to normal shows an excellent prognosis.

▼ 5′NUCLEOTIDASE

5′N, an enzyme used in controlling nucleic acid production, is found in high concentrations in the plasma membranes of liver cells and biliary canaliculi. Clinically significant elevations are associated with hepatobiliary disease. When the ALP is elevated (see discussion of ALP), the 5′N helps determine if the ALP elevation is due to cholestasis. Thus the 5′N is very similar in use to the tests for GGT.

Preparation of Client and Collection of Sample

Fasting is not required. Serum is collected in a red-topped tube.

REFERENCE VALUES FOR 5′N	
Adult	1–11 U/L
Pregnancy	Increased in third trimester

Increased 5′N Level

Clinical Significance. The 5′N is elevated in liver diseases but not in bone diseases. It may be useful as a follow-up test for an elevated ALP, especially in children who have high ALP levels. This test may also help confirm the diagnosis of hepatic metastases and assess the prognosis of infectious hepatitis.

▼ POSSIBLE NURSING DIAGNOSES FOR ELEVATED GGT AND 5′N

Both these enzymes are related to liver damage or biliary stasis. For diagnoses related to liver damage, see the discussion on ALT (SGPT) in this chapter. For diagnoses related to biliary stasis, see the discussion on obstructive jaundice in Chapter 11.

▼ ACID PHOSPHATASE OR PROSTATIC ACID PHOSPHATASE

Acid phosphatase is found in high concentrations in the prostate gland, erythrocytes, and platelets. Because this enzyme is excreted in the seminal fluid, a test for acid phosphatase is sometimes performed on vaginal secretions as supportive evidence for alleged rape. Because the prostatic portion of the enzyme occurs in such small amounts in the serum, the laboratory may measure the prostatic isoenzyme. The test has been a tumor marker for prostatic cancer (Ostcheya and Culnane, 1985). A newer marker for prostatic cancer is PSA, which is discussed in Chapter 10.

Preparation of Client and Collection of Sample

There is no special preparation of the client. It is important, however, that the specimen not be hemolyzed because the erythrocytes are rich in acid phosphatase. The specimen should be examined within 1 hr or stored as frozen serum. The laboratory needs 1 mL of serum. The enzyme is subject to circadian rhythm, so it should be drawn at the same time each day. Repeated measures may fluctuate from 25 to 50% (Ravel, 1995).

REFERENCE VALUES FOR ACID PHOSPHATASE

Adult	
Men	Total: 2.2–10.5 IU/L
	Prostatic isoenzyme: 0.8 U/L

Increased Serum Acid Phosphatase Level

Clinical Significance. Operative trauma or instrumentation of the prostate gland, such as cystoscopy, can cause a transient increase in the acid phosphatase level. However, the most important reason for a marked elevation in the prostatic portion of this enzyme is cancer of the prostate that has invaded the capsule surrounding the gland. Conditions that cause an increased destruction of red blood cells (RBCs), such as the various hemolytic anemias, also cause an increase of the nonprostatic portion of acid phosphatase. Acute renal impairment, liver dysfunction, and some diseases of the bone may also cause an increase in the total acid phosphatase level, but this test is not used to evaluate these conditions.

▼ POSSIBLE NURSING DIAGNOSIS RELATED TO INCREASED SERUM ACID PHOSPHATASE LEVEL

Anxiety Related to Coping with a Life-threatening Illness

The most important use of the serum acid phosphatase level is to evaluate treatment of carcinoma of the prostate gland. If the tumor is successfully

(continued)

▼ POSSIBLE NURSING DIAGNOSIS RELATED TO INCREASED SERUM ACID PHOSPHATASE LEVEL (*continued*)

treated with surgical excision, the acid phosphatase levels decrease in a few days. If estrogen therapy is used as treatment of the prostatic cancer, the levels of acid phosphatase may not return to normal for several weeks. (See Chapter 15 for nursing diagnoses related to hormone therapy.) An increasing acid phosphatase level may signal a much worse prognosis for the client. Also see PSA in Chapter 10.

▼ ALANINE AMINOTRANSFERASE (SERUM GLUTAMIC-PYRUVIC TRANSAMINASE)

Formerly known as SGPT, this transaminase is found in the largest concentration in liver tissue, but it is also present in kidney, heart, and skeletal muscle tissue. Like the other transaminase (AST or SGOT), ALT is increased in various types of tissue damage, and so it is not very specific. ALT may be used if there is a specific need to evaluate the possibility of liver tissue necrosis or liver damage from drugs. ALT has been useful in screening blood donors to reduce the incidence of non-A non-B hepatitis (now known as hepatitis C) (Apple and McGue, 1983), and its use has reduced the incidence of transfusion-borne hepatitis (Ravel, 1995). See Chapter 14 for more specific tests for hepatitis C.

Preparation of Client and Collection of Specimen

The client does not need to fast. The specimen can be refrigerated after it is clotted, but it is important that the blood not be hemolyzed. The exact time that the specimen was drawn should be recorded because serial measurements give useful information about the progression or lessening of liver damage. The laboratory needs 1 mL of blood. Various antibiotics, narcotics, and salicylates may cause false elevations of liver enzymes.

REFERENCE VALUES FOR ALT OR SGPT	
Adult	Men 10–55 U/L
	Women 7–30 U/L
Aged	Very slight increase
Newborns have higher levels.	

Elevated ALT or SGPT

Clinical Significance. In severe hepatitis, the ALT is often greater than 1,000 IU and may rise to 4,000 IU. In chronic hepatitis and cirrhosis, the levels are not so markedly elevated. Infectious mononucleosis, which often involves the liver, causes a substantial rise in ALT. (See Chapter 14 for tests for infectious mononucleosis.) Shock, Reye's syndrome, congestive heart failure, and eclampsia all cause an increased ALT because of some liver tissue damage. Hydatidiform moles also cause elevations of the ALT. (Chapter 15 discusses the diagnosis of hydatidiform moles by hormone assay.) A comparison of the ratio of AST to ALT can help to evaluate liver disease. AST levels are greater than ALT in cirrhosis and metastatic carcinoma of the liver. In acute hepatitis and nonmalignant hepatic obstruction, the AST is usually less than the ALT, but Ravel (1995) cautioned that the use of ratios may not always be helpful for individual clients.

▼ POSSIBLE NURSING DIAGNOSES RELATED TO INCREASED ALT LEVELS

Risk for Injury Related to Hepatic Failure

Because a markedly elevated ALT may be indicative of severe liver tissue damage, nurses must carefully assess for any signs of liver insufficiency, which could progress to a hepatic coma. (See Chapter 10 for the test of ammonia levels as a sign of liver dysfunction and for details of the symptoms that may be present. Chapter 11 discusses the special needs of the jaundiced patient.)

Altered Nutrition; Less than Body Requirements

The basic ingredients for the encouragement of liver tissue regeneration are the promotion of rest, the avoidance of drugs toxic to the liver, and the provision of a nutritious diet. Liver disease often causes anorexia, so meeting nutritional needs is challenging.

Activity Intolerance Related to Fatigue

Nurses may have to teach clients how to conserve energy. For clients at home, someone should be available to see that they do indeed rest. Rest is not a luxury here; it is often *the* basic therapy. Enzyme levels, tested over a period of weeks, may be used to gauge the amount of activity allowed. Boredom and depression can occur because of a long convalescent period with prolonged restrictions on usual activities.

▼ ASPARTATE AMINOTRANSFERASE (SERUM GLUTAMIC-OXALOACETIC TRANSAMINASE)

Formerly called SGOT, AST is found predominantly in heart, liver, and muscle tissue, although all tissues contain some of the enzyme. Because the transaminases are very important to energy transformation, the highest amounts of them are found in high-energy cells such as the heart, liver, and skeletal muscle. As discussed in the previous section, the highest concentration of ALT or SGPT is in the liver, and it is used primarily to detect liver necrosis. AST can also be used to detect liver necrosis, because both transaminases rise before there are any signs of jaundice. Neither the ALT nor AST is used to evaluate skeletal muscle necrosis because two other enzymes (CK and aldolase) are more specific for muscle tissue necrosis.

Preparation of Client and Collection of Sample

The client is prepared and the specimen collected in the same way and under the same conditions as for the other transaminase, ALT. Various drugs may interfere with the test.

REFERENCE VALUES FOR AST OR SGOT

Adult	Men 10–40 U/L Women 9–25 U/L
Newborn	Values are 2–3 times higher
Aged	Slight increase

Increased AST or SGOT Level

Clinical Significance. The discovery, in 1954, that SGOT increases soon after a myocardial infarction greatly accelerated research on enzymes as specific markers of injured tissue (Kaplan et al., 1995). SGOT, now called AST, was used for many years as one of the "cardiac enzymes" until the isoenzymes of LDH and CK became available. Lavie and Gersh (1990) noted that other enzymes, namely, CK isoenzymes and LDH, have replaced AST as the preferred laboratory tests.

In hepatitis, the AST may reach levels greater than 500 U/L, and it is elevated in the bloodstream even before jaundice appears. The return to normal may take weeks to months after hepatitis. Other types of liver involvement, such as that with shock, trauma, or cirrhosis, may cause lesser elevations of the AST. Reye's syndrome and pulmonary infarction are other causes of an elevated AST. The ratio of AST to ALT is useful in differentiating various types of liver disease as discussed in the section on ALT. GGT also helps identify liver involvement.

▼ POSSIBLE NURSING DIAGNOSES RELATED TO ELEVATED AST OR SGOT

Because the AST can be elevated from many different causes, nursing care must be based on the underlying pathophysiologic condition. If the AST level is due to hepatic damage, the nursing diagnoses for ALT elevations would be useful as general guidelines.

Decrease in Transaminases ALT and AST

Clinical Significance. Because the levels of transaminases are normally very low, a decrease is unlikely. In *rare* instances, both transaminases are decreased or nonexistent because the liver can no longer make the enzymes. Uremia sometimes causes a pseudodecrease, as can chronic dialysis and ketoacidosis.

▼ CREATINE KINASE OR CREATINE PHOSPHOKINASE

Creatine phosphokinase, or CK as it is now called, is very important in energy utilization and is involved in the reaction that changes creatine to creatinine. Because almost all circulating CK comes normally from muscular tissue, muscular activity and intramuscular injections are two common ways that CK values are elevated. CK can be measured as one total enzyme in the serum, or it can be separated into three different isoenzymes. The three types of CK isoenzymes are

1. CK-I (BB): Produced primarily by brain tissue and smooth muscle
2. CK-II (MB): Produced primarily by heart tissue
3. CK-III (MM): Produced primarily by muscle tissue

The isoenzymes of CK are particularly useful in detecting myocardial infarction and progressive muscular diseases that cause muscle necrosis.

Preparation of Client and Collection of Sample

The timing of the drawing for the CK is crucial because the enzyme may disappear from the bloodstream in less than 24 hr after a myocardial infarction. The laboratory needs 1 mL of serum or blood, which should be refrigerated if it cannot be sent to the laboratory immediately. If possible, intramuscular injections should be delayed until the sample is drawn.

REFERENCE VALUES FOR CK

Adult			
Women	Total: 40–150[a] U/L		
Men	Total: 60–400 U/L		
Isoenzymes	CK-I	(BB)	Brain 0–1%
	CK-II	(MB)	Heart <3% or 0–7.5 ng/mL
	CK-III	(MM)	Muscle 95–100%
Pregnancy	Levels are reduced in first half of pregnancy but rise in second half of pregnancy. Slight increase during labor and delivery. Surgical procedures, such as an episiotomy, cause more increase.		
Newborns	Higher values, which may be very high because of birth trauma		

[a]Intramuscular injections and exercise may elevate the total CK.

Increased Serum CK

Clinical Significance of Elevation of CK-II. CK, the first enzyme to be elevated after a myocardial infarction, begins to rise in 3–6 hr and may peak in the first 24 hr (Table 12–2). In some clients the CK returns to normal within 16 hr after the chest pain.

If the CK total is above normal, measurement of CK-II or CK-MB is needed. (Laboratories may only perform a CK-MB if the total CK is above normal.) When the CK-MB is reported in U/L, the laboratory may note the following:

- If less than 10 U/L, a myocardial infarction is improbable
- If 10–12 U/L, the finding is inconclusive
- If greater than 12 U/L, a myocardial infarction is probable

Other laboratories report isoenzymes in percentages. More than 3 or 4% is considered evidence of a myocardial infarction. As with all laboratory tests, the reader must use the interpretive ranges specified by the laboratory performing the test. One test of CK on admission and another within 12 hr are usually enough to diagnose or rule out a very recent infarction. Some physicians may order a third CK in 24 hr. Repeated determinations are indicated if the client has recurrence of chest pain, congestive heart failure, hypotension, or acute dysrhythmias (Lavie and Gersh, 1990). CK-II (MB) is very useful in the initial detection of an infarction, but it is not useful if the client has had chest pain for a day or two before seeking medical help. For some clients, the duration of CK may continue for about 3 days, but the peak is missed; in such cases, LDH isoenzymes are more helpful (Reis et al., 1988).

Clinical Significance of Elevation of CK-III. CPK-III (MM) elevations are never diagnostic of a specific muscular disease, but high levels are an indication for further specific testing of muscular function. In the early stages of muscular dystrophy, CK is as high as 3,000 IU/L. As the disease progresses, the CK levels drop, and by the time the client is bedridden, they may be normal. Healthy female carriers of X-linked Duchenne muscular dystrophy have raised levels of CK. Once these women are pregnant, however, the lowering of the CK in the first half of pregnancy may mask the elevation. CK-II is also used as a screening test for malignant hyperthermia (Ravel, 1995).

TABLE 12–2. TIME FRAME FOR CHANGES IN SERUM ENZYME LEVELS AFTER AN ACUTE MYOCARDIAL INFARCTION

	Appears in Serum (hr)	**Peaks (hr)**	**Duration (days)**
CK (isoenzyme II-B)	3–6	18–24	~3
LDH (isoenzyme LDH_1 and LDH_2 as a "flipped" LDH)	12–24	48–72	6–12

Note: These time frames are general approximations based on several references. Not all clients fall exactly into these patterns. See Lavie and Gersh (1990); Ravel (1995).

Elevation of CK-I. The third type of isoenzyme, CK-I (BB), may be elevated in the case of extreme shock, brain tumors, or severe cerebral accidents.

▼ POSSIBLE NURSING DIAGNOSES RELATED TO CHANGED LEVELS OF CK

Risk for Injury Related to Delayed Treatment

Nurses must be alert to have a CK performed as part of a rapid baseline assessment of a client who presents with chest pain or other symptoms of an acute myocardial infarction. The National Heart Attack Alert Program Coordinating Committee (1993) noted that emergency department nurses should have standing orders to initiate the following diagnostic interventions for clients with suspected myocardial ischemia or acute myocardial infarction: an electrocardiograph (ECG), a cardiac monitor, and laboratory tests to include CK and CK-MB, hematocrit (hct), and hemoglobin (hgb). There also should be protocols for oxygen therapy, intravenous access, and administration of aspirin and nitrates. None of these tests or procedures should delay a decision about thrombolytic therapy, which if deemed needed by the physician, should begin within 1 hour of onset of symptoms.

Altered Cardiac Output Related to Extension of Myocardial Infarction

Because this CK is the first cardiac enzyme to be increased and has a short duration in the serum, it should not be elevated after the first few days of an infarction. A sudden increase in the CK after a day or 2 should be reported to the physician immediately and the client assessed for the possibility of an extension of the infarction. If the client undergoes thrombolytic therapy, a high peak of CK followed by a dramatic drop is indicative of reperfusion (Olbrych, 1993).

Knowledge Deficit Related to Diagnostic Procedures for Muscle Necrosis

If the elevated CK is related to muscle necrosis, the client may need to undergo a battery of tests to identify the exact problem. Women who are found to be carriers of the sex-linked gene for muscular dystrophy may need to be referred for genetic counseling if they want to bear children (see Chapter 18). The enzyme aldolase is another test for muscular inflammatory diseases. Some general nursing implications for patients with myositis are covered in the section on aldolase later in this chapter.

▼ LACTIC DEHYDROGENASE

LDH is an enzyme that helps remove a water molecule from lactic acid. LDH is found in large amounts in the heart, liver, muscles, and erythrocytes. It is also present in other organs such as the kidney, pancreas, spleen, brain, and lungs. Like the enzyme CK, LDH can be separated into various isoenzymes:

1. LDH_1 is primarily from the heart and erythrocytes
2. LDH_2 comes mostly from the reticuloendothelial system
3. LDH_3 is from the lungs and other tissue
4. LDH_4 comes from the placenta, kidney, and pancreas
5. LDH_5 is largely from the liver and striated muscle

Total LDH and LDH_1 and LDH_2 are most often used in detecting a myocardial infarction. LDH is not typically used to assess liver function or muscle function, because other enzymes are more specific. (See Table 12–1 for elevations of LDH isoenzymes in various pathologic states.)

Preparation of Client and Collection of Sample

The sample must be handled carefully because any hemolysis of the RBCs falsely elevates the results. Even if the hemolysis is not enough to turn the serum pink, there is still an increased LDH. The client does not need to be fasting. The laboratory needs 1 mL of serum.

Increased Serum LDH

Clinical Significance. In myocardial infarction, the LDH begins to rise about 12–24 hr after the cardiac damage. The peak, usually about 300–800 U/L is in 2–6 days, and the enzyme remains in the bloodstream for up to 2 weeks. (See Table 12–2 for a comparison of this time frame with the other cardiac enzymes.) The measurement of isoenzymes 1 and 2 gives an even more specific indication that damaged cardiac tissue is causing the elevation. As shown in the reference values, LDH_2 is usually higher in concentration than LDH_1. In a myocardial infarction the greatest rise is in the LDH_1 isoenzyme, and thus it becomes higher than LDH_2. This change in the percentage ratio between LDH_1 and LDH_2, called a *flipped LDH,* is considered to be highly suggestive of a myocardial infarction. A flipped LDH, or the reversal of the ratio of LDH_1 to LDH_2, is apparent sooner than the rise in the total LDH. It also remains evident for 3–4 days after the total LDH returns to normal after a myocardial infarction. Immunoassay methods are also available for measurement of LDH_1 alone and may be used rather than the ratio (Ravel, 1995).

REFERENCE VALUES FOR LDH

Adult	45–90 U/L (Reference ranges highly method-dependent)
Pregnancy	Normal in pregnancy but increases slightly during labor and delivery, as with other vigorous exercise

Newborn	First week of life: 160–450 U/L	
Children	60–170 U/L (Decreases with age)	
Aged	55–102 U/L	
Isoenzymes	LDH_1 (erythrocytes, heart tissue)	17–27%
	LDH_2 (reticuloendothelial tissue, kidney)	23–28%
	LDH_3 (lungs, lymph nodes, spleen, and various other tissues)	18–28%
	LDH_4 (kidney, placenta, liver tissue)	5–15%
	LDH_5 (liver tissue, skeletal tissue, kidney)	5–15%

See Hay et al. (1995) for more age-related values.

Other possible causes of LDH elevations are as follows:

1. Hemolytic and macrocytic anemias tend to cause elevations in LDH_1 and LDH_2.
2. In pulmonary infarction LDH_3 is elevated.
3. Leukemia and malignant tumors in general cause large increases in LDH_3.
4. Liver damage increases the last two isoenzymes, LDH_4 and LDH_5. Because the last two isoenzymes make up only a small portion (10%) of the total LDH, such an increase may not change the total drastically.
5. Shock and trauma may cause an elevation of all the isoenzymes, as does cardiac operations. If a heart–lung machine is used, the LDH is 4–6 times the normal reference values.
6. In pregnancy, placental disturbances such as abruptio placentae affect an elevation in the isoenzymes.
7. Hepatitis causes a more modest increase in the total than that accompanying myocardial infarction.
8. An LDH of 2,000 IU or more is almost always due to either megaloblastic anemia or cancer. LDH is a tumor marker for non-Hodgkin's lymphoma (Ostcheya and Culnane, 1985).
9. More than 90% of clients with *Pneumocystis carinii* pneumonia (PCP) have elevations of LDH greater than 450 IU (Zaman and White, 1988).

▼ POSSIBLE NURSING DIAGNOSIS RELATED TO INCREASED CARDIAC ENZYMES

Altered Cardiac Output Related to Extension of Infarction or Other Complications

When the presence of an infarction is open to question, it is prudent to continue to treat the client as having a possible myocardial infarction until

(*continued*)

▼ POSSIBLE NURSING DIAGNOSIS RELATED TO INCREASED CARDIAC ENZYMES (*continued*)

the condition is definitely ruled out. The key nursing actions are to promote physical and mental relaxation and to watch the vital signs carefully. Ideally, such clients should be in a coronary care unit so that they can be monitored very closely. The use of a cardiac monitor does not take the place of the nurse. The nurse must be able to recognize that the client is having a potentially dangerous arrhythmia so that early treatment can be initiated. The nurse can also detect distended neck veins, crackles, or slight dyspnea as signals of fluid overload. Even a slight change in vital signs may indicate impending cardiogenic shock. This very careful watching of the client is essential any time there is a question of myocardial infarction. (See Chapter 24 for more information on monitoring.)

Understanding the Limitations of Enzymes as Assessment Tools. The real client in the clinical area is never quite as predictable as the one indicated by the textbook tables. So although the diagnostic interpretation of cardiac enzymes is the responsibility of the attending physician, a nurse caring for clients with cardiac disease needs general knowledge about standard practices when enzyme levels are puzzling. Usually, in a client with a myocardial infarction, the changes in the cardiac enzymes roughly follow the time frames given in Table 12–2. If all the enzymes, including the isoenzymes, are normal for 2 days, the client most likely has not had a myocardial infarction.

Recognizing Clinical Situations That Cause False Elevations of Myocardial Enzymes. When isoenzymes are not available, the enzyme tests may be even more likely to give a pseudomyocardial infarction pattern. For example, if the client has any disease of the biliary tract, the use of opiates, such as morphine or codeine, can cause a spasm of the sphincter of Oddi. This temporary narrowing or obstruction of the common bile duct can cause an increase in LDH. Nurses must also remember that intramuscular injections increase the total CK level.

Strenuous exercise can elevate CK and LDH. Evidently the amount of increase of these enzymes is related directly to the vigor of the exercise and inversely to the level of training before the exercise (Statland, 1979). A man in poor physical condition from a lack of training may have chest pain after a vigorous run or a handball game, and the cardiac enzymes may be elevated even though he has not had an infarction. Even men in good shape may have an elevation of LDH and CK when training for a marathon (Apple and McGue, 1983). Again the point is that the enzymes may not always be diagnostic when used alone.

Recognizing the Importance of Timing of Enzyme Determinations. Just as an elevation of serum enzymes is not always proof positive of an infarction, a lack of enzyme elevations does not always mean that an infarction can be ruled out. Table 12–2, in showing the importance of timing in relation to the serum levels of the enzymes, also demonstrates that missing the peak of the enzyme in the serum is possible. It takes at least 1 g of necrotic myocardial tissue to release enough enzymes to cause elevated serum levels. Fatal arrhythmias can result from a very small infarction or from ischemic heart tissue. Thus normal cardiac enzymes must not give nurses a false sense of security.

▼ SERUM ALDOLASE

Like most of the other enzymes in this chapter, aldolase is present in all cells. Its highest concentrations are found in skeletal muscles, heart, and liver tissue. Because damage to muscular tissue causes marked elevations of aldolase, it is a diagnostic test for some types of muscle damage. (CK, discussed earlier, is a more common test for muscular damage.)

Preparation of Client and Collection of Sample

Fasting is not necessary. Aldolase is in erythrocytes, so the specimen must not be hemolyzed. The laboratory needs 2 mL of fresh serum.

REFERENCE VALUES FOR ALDOLASE	
Adult	0–7 U/L
Children	Two times adult level
Newborn	Up to 4 times adult level

Increased Serum Aldolase Level

Clinical Significance. Muscular disorders that cause inflammation of the muscles (myositis) cause an elevation of aldolase. In the event of muscular wasting caused by a muscular disease of the central nervous system, such as myasthenia gravis or multiple sclerosis, the aldolase level is not elevated. In progressive muscular dystrophy, the level may be 10–15 times normal in the early stages of the disease, but the level subsides as muscle wasting continues. In some types of acute myositis the levels of aldolase return to normal when corticosteroid treatment is effective. Aldolase testing may be used in conjunction with more specific diagnostic measures to identify the exact reason for muscle necrosis.

▼ POSSIBLE NURSING DIAGNOSES RELATED TO INCREASED ALDOLASE SERUM LEVEL (OR CK-MM)

Self-care Deficit Related to Muscle Fatigue

The key nursing implication for a client with a skeletal muscular problem is to help the client be as independent as possible while conserving muscle strength. If the muscular disorder is due to an acute condition, the client is comforted to know that the lack of muscle strength is temporary. Return of muscle strength occurs after the enzymes return to normal. Nursing care during the acute phase may center on preventing any complications from disuse of muscles. (The other enzymes that become elevated in acute muscular myositis are the transaminases and CK.)

Risk for Ineffective Coping Related to Problems of Chronic Muscular Disease

If the muscular disorder is a chronic problem, such as muscular dystrophy, the client is faced with learning how to cope with a progressively debilitating disease. Because each case of muscle disease differs from all others, the nursing care plan must be individualized to the severity of the disease and to its effects on the client. The home care nurse may be very involved in helping clients adapt to a crippling disease by suggesting ways to be independent in doing personal care and housekeeping while using limited energy wisely. The nurse needs to emphasize to clients that a schedule that allows frequent and short rest periods is much better than one with a long rest period. Clients may be able to do much more if they are not hurrying to accomplish several activities in a limited time. In addition to emphasizing a planned exercise and rest schedule, the nurse may also need to teach about the expected effects of the prescribed medications and the necessity for follow-up diagnostic tests.

▼ SERUM AMYLASE

Amylase, an enzyme that helps with the digestion of starch, is found in high concentrations in the salivary glands and in the pancreas, each of which contains a different isoenzyme. These two isoenzymes can be separated to rule out nonpancreatic sources.

Amylase may be measured in both serum and urine. The serum amylase may be done as a stat procedure in clients with acute abdominal pain to differentiate pancreatitis from other acute abdominal problems that necessitate surgical intervention. Serum amylase is not always a good screening test for pancreatitis because it lacks specificity. Simon et al (1994), who researched the use of serum amylase tests in children noted that isoenzymes are more specific but have disadvantages as screening tests because of cost and lack of rapid results. Combining the amylase with the lipase has also been tried, but even together the tests remain imperfect

(Orebaugh, 1994). Therefore imaging the pancreas with computed tomography (CT) (Chapter 21) or ultrasonography (Chapter 22) may replace serum amylase levels in the diagnosis of acute pancreatitis (Bongard and Sue, 1994).

Preparation of Client and Collection of Sample

About 60% of the total amylase is from the salivary gland. If health workers talk over an uncovered urine or blood sample, this can falsely elevate total amylase levels. Drugs that cause spasm of the sphincter of Oddi, such as the opiates, may cause an elevation in serum amylase. The increase is at a maximum 5 hr after drug administration. So, if possible, the stat amylase should be drawn before the use of opiate drugs. Thiazide diuretics and diagnostic dyes may cause false elevations.

The client does not need to be fasting. Hemolysis does not affect the results of this test. The laboratory needs 0.5 mL of serum.

REFERENCE VALUES FOR AMYLASE

Adult	53–123 U/L
Pregnancy	Pregnancy causes moderate increases. Women taking oral contraceptives have slightly increased amylase levels
Newborn	5–65 U/L or may be undetectable (Hay et al., 1995).
Child	25–125 U/L
Aged	May have higher values (Lawson et al., 1986)

Increased Serum Amylase Level

Clinical Significance. Pancreatitis is the most common reason for marked elevations in serum amylase, which begins to increase about 3–6 hr after an attack of this disease. (See Table 12–3 for a comparison with serum lipase, the other pancreatic enzyme.) The severity of the disease is not always directly related to the levels of the enzyme. In fact, about 10% of patients with fatal pancreatitis have normal serum amylase levels. High levels in alcoholism, pregnancy, and in diabetic ketoacidosis are of salivary rather than pancreatic origin. Renal failure may also cause abnormal elevations not related to pancreatic disease.

In the adult, the two most common reasons for pancreatitis are alcohol abuse and gallstones. Evidently, the obstruction of the pancreatic ducts or pancreatic ischemia triggers an acute inflammatory response, and autodigestion of the pancreas

TABLE 12–3. PANCREATIC ENZYMES USED TO DIAGNOSE ACUTE PANCREATITIS

	Begins Elevation[a]	Peaks[a]	Duration[a]
Serum amylase	3–6 hr	20–30 hr	2–3 days
Urine amylase	6–10 hr after serum levels	Varies	1–2 weeks
Serum lipase	Increases after amylase	Varies	Up to 14 days longer than amylase

[a]Time frames are *general* approximations based on several references. See Lawson et al. (1986); Ravel (1995).

begins. Oral contraceptives, hyperlipidemia, and hyperthyroidism are less common reasons for such response. Ruptured ectopic pregnancies, perforated ulcers, and other acute abdominal conditions may cause some elevation of the serum amylase level due to trauma to the pancreas. In children, pancreatitis is rare and often of an unknown cause. Sometimes it appears to have a hereditary base (Hay et al., 1995). Obesity and the beginning of puberty have been related to the incidence of pancreatitis in girls.

▼ POSSIBLE NURSING DIAGNOSES RELATED TO INCREASED SERUM AMYLASE LEVEL

Risk for Fluid Volume Deficit

Among clients with massive hemorrhagic necrosis, the mortality may be as high as 50–80%. If the pancreatitis is not hemorrhagic, the prognosis is much better, but fluid loss can still lead to shock. Thus one key nursing implication for a client with an elevated serum amylase level is to observe for any change in vital signs that may indicate hypovolemia from the loss of pancreatic fluids or blood.

Pain Related to an Acute Inflammatory Process

Clients with pancreatitis usually have severe abdominal pain. Comfort measures and pain relief are important. Often meperidine (Demerol) is used to relieve pain rather than morphine because opiates may cause spasms of the sphincter of Oddi (Lawson et al., 1986). (Recall that the potential effect of opiates on the sphincter of Oddi can cause the elevation of the pancreatic enzymes as well as of liver enzymes such as the transaminases and ALP.)

Altered Nutrition Related to Measures to Decrease Pancreatic Stimulation

Stimulation of the pancreas needs to be minimized as much as possible. The client must take nothing by mouth and continue to receive intravenous fluids. Total parenteral nutrition may be needed (Bongard and Sue, 1994). A nasogastric (NG) tube may be used to decompress the intestine until the acute inflammation has subsided, although Loiudice et al., (1984) found a NG tube was needed only if ileus or emesis was present and atropine and cimetidine were of little help in resolving the disease. Bowel sounds may be hypoactive or absent if the inflammation is severe.

Risk for Infection

Antibiotics may be used to prevent a secondary infection of the necrotic tissue in the pancreas. (See Chapter 2 on white blood cell (WBC) differentials to assess infections.) The temperature should be assessed every 4 hr.

Risk for Injury Related to Possible Hypocalcemia, Hypokalemia, Hyperglycemia, and Jaundice

When a client has pancreatitis, laboratory tests and diagnostic procedures often influence nursing care:

1. Calcium levels: Serum calcium may be lowered because calcium is deposited in the pancreas because of fat necrosis. The hypocalcemia may be severe enough to cause tetany. (See Chapter 7 for possible nursing diagnoses for clients with a deceased serum calcium level.)
2. Potassium levels: Hypokalemia may result from a lack of intake and a loss of body fluids. (See Chapter 5 for the implications of a lowered potassium level.)
3. Glucose levels: Hyperglycemia may be brought about because the damaged pancreatic cells may not be able to produce sufficient insulin. (See Chapter 8 for serum glucose levels.)
4. Bilirubin levels: Conjugated bilirubin may increase if the pancreatic inflammation is due to obstruction of the common bile duct. (See Chapter 11 for the implications when the client has obstructive jaundice.)
5. Triglyceride levels: Triglyceride levels may be high, particularly if alcohol was a triggering event (see Chapter 9).
6. Blood urea nitrogen (BUN) and creatinine levels: Impaired renal function may occur (see Chapter 4).
7. Assessing for chronic complications: Once the client is over the acute stage of pancreatitis, the most common complications are abscess formation in the pancreas or pseudocysts, which are collections of fluids in sacs outside the pancreas. Gallium scans (Chapter 22) may be used to detect abscesses, whereas sonograms (Chapter 23) may show the presence of the pseudocysts.

Knowledge Deficit Related to Measures to Prevent Recurrent Attacks

Clients who have had an elevated serum amylase level benefit from discharge planning that focuses on the ways that recurrent attacks can be reduced. Alcohol in all forms should be avoided for several months. If alcohol abuse was the precipitating factor, the client may need to seek professional help to deal with a chronic problem. If gallstones are present and a cholecystectomy is to be performed later, dietary modifications may be needed.

▼ URINARY AMYLASE

Amylase, the enzyme elevated in the serum in acute pancreatitis, can also be measured in the urine. The amylase may be elevated in the urine for as long as 2 weeks after an acute episode of pancreatitis. Monitoring amylase levels in urine may be useful after the acute peak in the serum has diminished. (See Table 12–3 for a comparison of the time frames for serum and urine amylases.)

Preparation of Client and Collection of Sample

Usually the test is completed on a collection of urine for a 2-hr period, but sometimes a 24-hr specimen is used. (See Chapter 3 for tips on collecting 24-hr urine specimens.)

REFERENCE VALUES FOR URINARY AMYLASE
0–375 U/L

▼ SERUM LIPASE

Lipase is a pancreatic enzyme that breaks down fat into glycerol and fatty acids. In acute pancreatitis (see Table 12–3), lipase rises later in the serum than does amylase. So lipase may be used as a secondary test for pancreatitis when the diagnosis is questionable. Other types of pancreatic disease, such as carcinoma or traumatic injury, cause some release of the enzyme into the serum. (See the discussion of amylase for nursing diagnoses related to acute pancreatitis.)

Preparation of Client and Collection of Sample

The precautions are the same as those for amylase, except there is no concern about contamination from saliva. The laboratory needs 1 mL of serum.

REFERENCE VALUES FOR LIPASE	
All groups	0–160 U/L or 4–24 U/dL

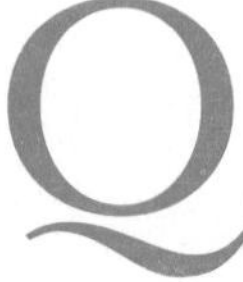

1. Which one of the following factors is the *least* likely to cause elevations in the common serum enzymes such as LDH and CK?

   a. Eating food 4-hr before the test

   b. Vigorous physical activity

c. Administration of intramuscular injections of morphine sulfate
d. Hemolysis of the serum sample

2. A markedly elevated alkaline phosphatase level is a general warning of either

a. Increased bone formation *or* obstruction to bile flow
b. Myocardial infarction *or* angina
c. Cancer of the prostate *or* of the liver
d. Increased bone destruction *or* liver dysfunction

3. Intravenous administration of albumin solutions may cause an elevated serum alkaline phosphatase level for which of the following reasons?

a. Albumin obtained from placentas is rich in this enzyme
b. Alkaline phosphatase is transported by albumin
c. Oncotic pressure is increased in the serum
d. The method used to purify albumin causes the release of the enzyme

4. John Gringo has a history of alcohol abuse but is now in a rehabilitation program. Which of the following tests is used to assess for hepatic injury caused by alcohol abuse?

a. ALP b. LDH
c. Amylase d. GGT

5. When a client has a marked elevation of the transaminases ALT (formerly SGPT) and AST (formerly SGOT), a priority nursing diagnosis is

a. Activity intolerance b. Fluid volume deficit
c. Fluid volume overload d. Impaired gas exchange

6. In myocardial damage, which of the following enzymes is most useful for detecting myocardial damage in the first 24 hr after an episode of chest pain?

a. CK b. AST (SGOT) c. LDH d. ALT (SGPT)

7. A flipped LDH is one of the characteristic signs of an acute myocardial infarction. A flipped LDH means that LDH_1 is which of the following?

a. Greater than LDH_2 b. Less than LDH_2
c. In an abnormal form d. Greater than LDH_4 and LDH_5

8. Mr. Marx is a 50-year-old businessman who was admitted to the coronary care unit with severe chest pain yesterday. His enzyme levels were normal at admission. Because he wants to make several business calls, Mr. Marx has asked where he can find a phone. Which nursing action is appropriate?

a. Allow him to go to a phone via wheelchair, because his enzyme levels are normal
b. Tell him he has most likely had a heart attack, so he must stay on complete bed rest

c. Make sure that Mr. Marx understands the need for further assessment of ECG readings, serial enzyme levels, and a medical exam to rule out a possible myocardial infarction
d. Tell Mr. Marx that phone calls are not allowed and continue to observe him for arrhythmias, hypotension, or distended neck veins

9. Mrs. Jackson is a 44-year-old mother with two teen-aged girls. She has increased CK and aldolase levels caused by a still-undiagnosed muscular disease. Which advice by a home health nurse would be the most appropriate?

a. "Schedule most of your activities for the morning when you have the most strength."
b. "Ask your teenagers to take care of your personal needs such as baths and shampoos."
c. "Why not hire someone to do all your housework?"
d. "Try to alternate each small activity with a short period of rest."

10. Mr. Bigelow is a 35-year-old artist who has been admitted with recurring pancreatitis. Both his serum and urine levels of amylase are markedly increased. The nurse should assess for any signs of which of the following?

a. Hypocalcemia b. Hypoglycemia
c. Hypernatremia d. Hyperkalemia

11. Mr. Bigelow's amylase levels have returned to normal, and he is being discharged. When he returns to the clinic next week, it would be *most important* to reemphasize a diet plan that includes which of the following?

a. Decreased intake of starches and other carbohydrates
b. Total restriction of alcoholic beverages
c. Foods high in fat-soluble vitamins
d. Frequent small feedings with an emphasis on high-calorie foods

▼ REFERENCES

Apple, F., and McGue, M. (1983). Serum enzyme changes during marathon training. *American Journal of Clinical Pathology, 79* (6), 716–718.

Bongard, F.S., and Sue, D.Y. (1994). *Current critical care: Diagnosis & treatment.* Norwalk, CT: Appleton & Lange.

Garty, B.Z., and Nitzan, M. (1994). Benign transient hyperphosphatasemia. *Israel Journal of Medical Science, 30* (1), 66–69.

Hay, W.W., Groothuis, J.R., Hayward, A.R., and Levin, M.J. (1995). *Current pediatric diagnosis & treatment.* (12th ed.). Norwalk, CT: Appleton & Lange.

Kaplan, A., Jack, R., Opheim, K.E., et al. (1995). *Clinical chemistry interpretation and techniques.* (4th ed.). Baltimore: Williams & Wilkins.

Lavie, C., and Gersh, M. (1990). Acute myocardial infarction: Initial manifestations, management and prognosis. *Mayo Clinic Proceedings, 65,* 531–548.

Lawson, T., McCarthy, D., and Rogers, A. (1986). Tracking and treating acute pancreatitis. *Patient Care, 20* (1), 76–109.

Loiudice, T., et al. (1984). Treatment of acute alcoholic pancreatitis: The role of cimetidine and nasogastric suction. *American Journal of Gastroenterology, 79* (7), 553–558.

National Heart Attack Alert Program Coordinating Committee. 60 Minutes to Treatment Working Group (1993). *Emergency Department: Rapid identification and treatment of patients with acute myocardial infarction.* Publication No. 93-3278. Bethesda: National Institutes of Health.

Olbrych, D.D. (1993). Interpreting CPK and LDH results. *Nursing 93, 23* (1), 48–49.

Orebaugh, S.L. (1994). Normal amylase levels in the presentation of acute pancreatitis. *American Journal of Emergency Medicine, 12* (1), 21–24.

Ostcheya, Y., and Culnane, M. (1985). Tumor markers. *Nursing 85,* 15 (9), 49–51.

Ravel, R. (1995). *Clinical laboratory medicine: Clinical application of laboratory data* (6th ed.). St. Louis: Mosby–Year Book.

Reis, G.J., Kaufman, H., Horowitz, G., et al. (1988). Usefulness of lactate dehydrogenase and lactate dehydrogenase isoenzymes for diagnosis of acute myocardial infarction. *American Journal of Cardiology, 61,* 754–758.

Simon, H.K., Muehlberg, A., and Linakis, J.G. (1994). Serum amylase determinations in pediatric patients presenting to the ED with acute abdominal pain or trauma. *American Journal of Emergency Medicine, 12* (3), 292–295.

Statland, B. (1979). Strenuous activity and serum enzyme values. *JAMA, 241,* 404.

Zaman, M.K., and White, D.A. (1988). Serum lactate dehydrogenase levels and *Pneumocystis carinii* pneumonia. *American Review Respiratory Diseases, 137,* 796–800.

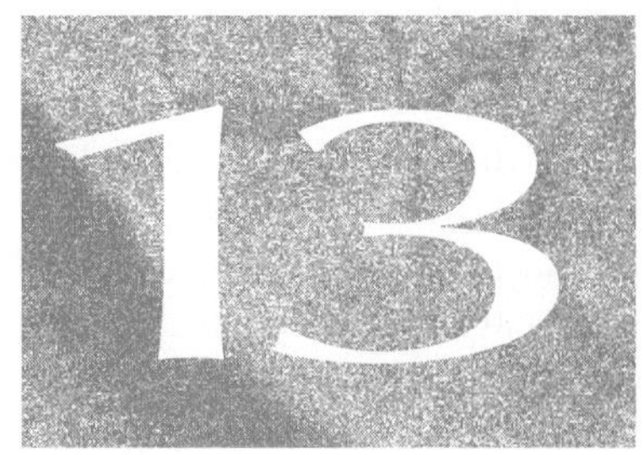

COAGULATION TESTS AND TESTS TO DETECT OCCULT BLOOD

- Prothrombin Time
- Partial Thromboplastin Time
- Activated Clotting Time
- Tests for Low-molecular-weight Heparin
- Hemophilia Tests: Factors VIII and IX
- Platelet Count and Mean Platelet Volume
- Bleeding Time: Modified Ivy, Simplate, Duke Method, Aspirin Tolerance Test
- Clot Retraction Test
- Fibrinogen
- Fibrinogen Degradation Products or Fibrin Split Products
- D-dimer Screen: ELISA and Latex Agglutination Slide Test
- Thrombin Time: Fibrinogen Screen, Thrombin Clotting Time with Reptilase
- Plasminogen Assay
- Protein C and S Anticoagulant System
- Occult Blood: Hematest, Hemoccult, and Other Guaiac Tests

OBJECTIVES

1. Describe the four main stages of the coagulation process, and the difference between the intrinsic and extrinsic systems of clotting as a basis for laboratory tests.
2. Describe clinical situations in which vitamin K is useful for returning the prothrombin time (PT or Pro Time) to normal.

3. Identify important nursing diagnoses for a client who has a bleeding tendency caused by a lack of clotting factors.
4. Devise a teaching plan for a client who is discharged to undergo long-term coumarin therapy.
5. Compare and contrast the two most common coagulation tests, PT and partial thromboplastin time.
6. Describe possible nursing interventions when a client has an abnormally decreased PT or PTT or other signs of hypercoagulability.
7. Explain the screening tests and confirmatory tests for classic hemophilia (hemophilia A).
8. Identify possible nursing diagnoses for clients with increased and decreased platelet counts.
9. Identify the changes in fibrinogen levels, along with the changes in other laboratory tests, that are clues that disseminated intravascular coagulation (DIC) or consumption coagulopathy may be occurring.
10. Describe the important facts a nurse should know about tests used to detect occult blood in the feces or other specimens.

The delicate balance of the coagulation process makes it possible for a healthy person to experience neither hemorrhage nor thrombus formation. Tests such as the PT, PTT, and platelet counts are routine tests for the clotting ability of the blood. Tests of individual factors are needed to detect specific diseases, such as hemophilia A (test for factor VIII). Other tests, such as fibrinogen assays, help in the assessment of severe coagulation problems, such as DIC.

Besides the common tests for clotting ability, this chapter includes information on guaiac and other tests used to detect hidden or occult blood. Occult blood tests are used not only to detect bleeding tendencies but also to screen for rectal cancer.

Coagulation tests are of use to the nurse in three primary ways. First, these tests may alert the nurse to the possibility that the client is vulnerable because of an increased bleeding tendency. Second, some of these tests may indicate that the client is vulnerable because of an increased risk of thrombus formation. Third, three of these tests are specifically used to monitor the effects of anticoagulant drugs. The role of the nurse in anticoagulant therapy is emphasized. No "magic number" determines when a client will bleed or experience thrombus formation. At the very best, these laboratory tests are only guidelines for helping the nurse assess the potential problems.

COAGULATION PROCESS

Twelve factors are involved in the clotting process. Remembering all the factors is not necessary, but knowing which test measures which factors is useful. A list of the 12 factors, along with the tests that show the deficiencies and the relation of vitamin K, is presented in Table 13–1. Vitamin K was named K because it is the "koagulation" factor. If the liver cannot obtain vitamin K, four coagulation factors cannot be manufactured: factors II, VII, IX, and X. Note that the table contains

TABLE 13–1. COAGULATION FACTORS TESTED BY SPECIFIC TESTS AND RELATION TO VITAMIN K

Name of Factor	Test of Deficiency	Vitamin K Needed for Production By Liver
I (fibrinogen)	Fibrinogen level[a] PT, PTT	
I (prothrombin)	PT, PTT	Yes
III (thromboplastin)		
IV (calcium)		
V (labile or proaccelerin)	PT, PTT	
VI (unassigned at present time)		
VII (stable factor or proconvertin)	PT	Yes
VIII (antihemophilic globulin)	PTT	
IX (partial thromboplastin component [PTC], Christmas factor)	PTT	Yes
X (Stuart-Prower factor)	PT, PTT	Yes
XI (plasma thromboplastin antecedent)	PTT	
XII (Hageman factor)	PTT	
XIII (fibrin-stabilizing factor)		

[a]Specific assays can be performed to test for each factor (see the reference values in Appendix A, Table 4).

13 numbers, because one factor (VI) was found to be part of another factor. The factors were numbered, instead of named, in the order of their discovery, so there could be a universal understanding of which factor was being discussed.

Table 13–1 illustrates that both the PT and PTT are used to test several factors but not always the same ones. Although the PTT is a broader screening test, certain deficiencies can be assessed by using both the PT and PTT. Also the laboratory can add one factor at a time to see which factor is missing.

The coagulation process can be initiated two ways. With the *extrinsic system,* the clotting is triggered by the release of tissue thromboplastin. With the *intrinsic system,* the coagulation process requires only the factors that are present in the plasma.

Regardless of how the process is initiated, the coagulation process occurs in four stages. Stage I involves the release of platelet factors that begin the clotting process. Stage II is the generation of thromboplastin as calcium and other factors interact. Stage III is the conversion of prothrombin to thrombin, and stage IV is the formation of fibrin from fibrinogen. Some sources list three stages of coagulation because stages I and II are combined as stage I. Table 13–2 outlines the stages of clotting.

The importance of calcium in the clotting process should be noted. Usually a lack in calcium is not a problem because of the tremendous reservoir of calcium in the bones and teeth (see Chapter 7 on calcium). About 90% of all clotting defects occur in stage II, the thromboplastin generation stage. Thus the PTT is a useful screening tool for many bleeding disorders.

After the factors are used in the coagulation process, fibrin inhibitors, such as antiplasmin, protein C, and antithrombin III, inactivate excess amounts of certain clotting factors so that clotting does not occur inappropriately. Pathologic defects or decreases in these factors may be responsible for thrombotic episodes, so these fibrin inhibitors may sometimes be measured to help determine a coagulation prob-

TABLE 13–2. STAGES OF CLOTTING AND COMMON LABORATORY TESTS

Time of Stage	Stage	Factors Involved[a]	Tests for Stage
	I	Platelets initiate clotting	Platelets, clot retraction
Takes 3–5 min	II	Thromboplastin (factor III) is generated by reaction of factors VIII, IX, X, XI, and XII. Factor IV, CA^{2+} also needed	PTT very sensitive
Takes 8–16 min	III	Factor II (prothrombin) is converted to thrombin. Accelerator factors V, VII, and X are involved	PT very sensitive
Almost instantly	IV	Factor I (fibrinogen) is converted to fibrin. Factor XIII, the fibrin-stabilizing factor, is needed	Fibrinogen levels

Some references combine Stages I and II so that

Stage I: Formation of thromboplastin or activation of factor X

Stage II: Prothrombin to thrombin

Stage III: Fibrinogen to fibrin

[a]Moderate reductions in multiple factors prolong PT and PTT, but this synergistic action usually imposes little clinical risk of hemorrhage (Burns et al., 1993).

lem. Inactive plasminogen is converted to plasmin by a tissue plasmin activating factor (TPA). Plasmin is useful as a fibrinolytic agent. TPA derived from human cells and synthesized by recombinant DNA technology is used to dissolve clots.

▼ PROTHROMBIN TIME

Prothrombin, or factor II, is a plasma protein produced by the liver. The confusing thing about the test is that although it is called *prothrombin time,* it does not measure just prothrombin but also several other factors (see Table 13–1.) The point to remember is that a change in all, or any, of these factors causes an abnormal PT. Just like prothrombin, these other factors are manufactured in the liver, and most of the factors require vitamin K for their manufacture.

The PT is the specific, and the only, laboratory test used to measure the effectiveness of the coumarin type of anticoagulant drugs, such as warfarin sodium (Coumadin). Although heparin, a different type of anticoagulant, in large doses may change the PT, two other tests are used to monitor heparin therapy. These are the PTT and the activated clotting time (ACT), both of which are discussed later in this chapter. Although the abbreviations PT and PTT are very similar and thus often confusing to the novice, the tests are very different and used for two very different anticoagulants (Table 13–3).

Measurement in Seconds, Percentages, and International Normalized Ratio

Prothrombin results may be reported (1) as time in seconds, (2) as a percentage of normal activity, and (3) if used to monitor the coumarin-type drugs, as an Interna-

TABLE 13–3. COMPARISONS OF PT AND PTT

	PT	PTT (Activated)
Drugs monitored	Coumarin-type drugs, e.g., bishydroxycoumarin (Dicumarol), warfarin sodium (Coumadin, Panwarfin)	Heparin
Reference values (control)	60–140% activity 12–15 sec	Not reported in percentage 25–37 sec
Desirable therapeutic levels	INR usually 2.5–3.5[a]	1.5–2.5 times control
Time of drug to affect laboratory test	Oral coumarin takes several *days* to achieve therapeutic level.	Intravenous heparin acts immediately (subcutaneous not usually used except for prophylaxis)
Usual timing of laboratory test	On daily basis until stabilized. Then once every 4–6 weeks for long-term control	Once a day if continuous intravenous infusion or more often if unstable
Measures used to return laboratory test to normal	1. Reduction of dosage 2. Fresh frozen plasma 3. Vitamin K_1 parenterally (Aqua Mephyton)	1. Reduction of dosage 2. Fresh frozen plasma 3. Protamine sulfate parenterally
Time of reversibility	1. Varies with dosage reduction 2. Immediate with transfusion 3. Several hours for vitamin K	1. Varies with dosage reduction 2. Immediate with transfusion 3. Immediate with protamine
Examples of common drugs affecting results of test[b]	Increase PT Antibiotics Cimetidine (Tagamet) Salicylates Sulfonamides Decrease PT Barbiturates Oral contraceptives Vitamin K in nutritional supplements, such as Ensure	Increase PTT Salicylates Dipyridamole (Persantine) May decrease PTT Digitalis Tetracyclines Antihistamines Nicotine

[a]See text on INR—some conditions require slightly higher INR.
[b]Many other drugs may affect test results, so consult a pharmacology text.

tional Normalized Ratio (INR). The seconds reflect how long the blood sample takes to clot when certain chemicals are added. To obtain a control value, the laboratory also tests a known "normal" sample of blood with the same technique. It is important for each laboratory to establish control values because many environmental variables may change the PT by several seconds. If the client's blood sample is deficient either in prothrombin or in one of the other clotting factors that affect the test, the client's PT in seconds will be higher than the control PT in seconds.

Although many laboratories report the PT only in seconds, others also report the percentage. The percentage is more difficult to understand than the time. The percentage is a way of expressing the client's clotting ability as compared with the normal or control activity. In other words, the activity of the factors being tested is considered to be 100% in a control or normal blood sample. With no straight-line relation between time and percentage, a graph has to be plotted to convert seconds to a percentage. The laboratory dilutes the normal sample to various concentrations. These various dilutions, or percentages of concentrations, are then measured to see how long each takes to clot. A graph is made that plots how percentage equals time. If a client's blood sample clots in, for example, 19 sec, the laboratory can look at the curve and see where 19 sec intersects with a certain percentage. The time of 19 sec may reflect 50% of normal clotting ability.

Percentages may vary somewhat because each laboratory must make its own graph for correlating times and percentages. Because the percentages must be based on dilution curves, their use may lead to inaccuracy. It is important to realize that 19 sec may be translated into two different percentages by two different laboratories. In a general sense, the percentage is useful in illustrating how the client's clotting ability compares with the control. For example, a client with a PT of only 20% has only about one-fifth of the clotting ability of the "normal" person used as the control. One might suppose that the greatest clotting factor ability that a client could have would be 100%. Yet remember that for a percentage of normal activity there is a range in "normal." So a figure greater than 100% can result for a client who has a clotting time faster than the control picked by the laboratory. Thus percentages of 60–140% are considered normal individual variations. (See Appendix A for percentage values for all the other factors that may be measured. Note that some have as wide a variation as 50–200%.)

Relation of Time to Percentage

An increase in time always means a decrease in percentage of activity, and vice versa, because as the clotting activity of the blood decreases, the blood takes longer to clot. If the percentage of activity is less than 60%, the client's PT in seconds is increased to more than the control time. However, if the client's PT in seconds decreases from, for example, 20 to 12 sec, the percentage of clotting activity has increased or risen to near the 100% normal activity. PT results in textbooks or on charts are sometimes reported only as "increased PT." This notation means an increase in *time,* not in activity. An increase in PT means the percentage of activity is less than normal.

Use of International Normalized Ratio

The reporting of the PT in seconds or prothrombin activity in a percentage can be problematic in determining the therapeutic range for anticoagulation because the PT in seconds varies depending on the type of reagent used. In the past, only the ratio of the PT to the control was used as a standard. The United States Food and Drug Administration (FDA) recommended that the PT be 1.2–1.5 times control for basic anticoagulation needs and 1.5–2.0 times control for more sustained risks of thromboembolism (Krokosky and Vanscoy, 1989). In the early 1990s, laboratories began converting the PT ratio to the INR, so results were standardized (Corbett, 1990).

The INR, first used in European laboratories and now common in North America, adjusts for the variability in the type of tissue thromboplastin used for the PT. In the 1980s, the World Health Organization developed a plan to standardize the

PT by comparing various commercial preparations of rabbit brain thromboplastin with the more sensitive human brain tissue thromboplastin (Katzung, 1995). This comparison of the thromboplastin from the animal source to the purer human source gives the International Sensitivity Index (ISI). The ISI, obtained from the manufacturers of the thromboplastin reagents, is used with the PT ratio to obtain the INR. The laboratory uses a table like Table 13–4 to match the PT ratio with the ISI for the reagent used. For example, if the control is 12 sec and a patient has a PT of 24 sec, the PT ratio is 2.0. If the reagent used is 1.6, the corresponding INR is 3.0 based on Table 13–4. However, if the ISI were 1.8, the INR would be 3.5. Laboratories report both the PT ratio and the INR for decision making about anticoagulation. For most clinical conditions that necessitate anticoagulation, the recommended INR is 2.5–3.5 (Eckman et al., 1993). Clients with mechanical prosthetic valves or recurrent systemic embolism need a higher level (Nichols and Bowie, 1993).

Preparation of Client and Collection of Sample

Many drugs can affect the PT (see Table 13–3). Record on the laboratory slip any heparin dosage, because the PT may be affected at the peak of heparin activity. Venous blood (1.8 mL) is collected in plastic tubes with 3.8% sodium citrate (blue top). For point-of-care testing, a portable laser photodetector measures the PT in 2 min. Only a finger stick is needed. Results are apparently as reliable as the traditional plasma method (Vanscoy and Gyi, 1988).

REFERENCE VALUES FOR PT	
Adult	Control 8.8–11.6 sec (±2 sec). Percentage of normal activity should be close to 100, but most sources consider a range of 60–140% to be a normal variation.
Newborn	Some clotting factors are lower than in adults, so reference values may be about 12–21 sec. Premature infants may have even higher reference values in seconds.
Pregnancy	In late pregnancy, some clotting factors are increased, so reference values may be slightly decreased for time in seconds.

See text for explanation of INR.

Increased PT (Increase in Time and Consequent Decrease in Percentage) or Hypoprothrombinemia

Clinical Significance. A variety of pathologic conditions cause an increased PT. (Remember that an "increased" PT means an *increase* in the seconds and a *decrease* in the percentage. It is easier to speak of an increased PT, rather than spelling it out.)

A client may have an increased PT because the liver is unable to make prothrombin and the other factors measured with the PT test. An increased PT is characteristic of advanced cirrhosis of the liver because a large amount of scar tissue

TABLE 13–4. TABLE FOR CONVERSION OF PROTHROMBIN TIME RATIO TO INTERNATIONAL NORMALIZED RATIO

Prothrombin Time Ratio	International Sensitivity Index (ISI)																				
	1.0	1.1	1.2	1.3	1.4	1.5	1.6	1.7	1.8	1.9	2.0	2.1	2.2	2.3	2.4	2.5	2.6	2.7	2.8	2.9	3.0
1.0	1.0	1.0	1.0	1.0	1.0	1.0	1.0	1.0	1.0	1.0	1.0	1.0	1.0	1.0	1.0	1.0	1.0	1.0	1.0	1.0	1.0
1.1	1.1	1.1	1.1	1.1	1.1	1.2	1.2	1.2	1.2	1.2	1.2	1.2	1.2	1.2	1.3	1.3	1.3	1.3	1.3	1.3	1.3
1.2	1.2	1.2	1.2	1.3	1.3	1.3	1.3	1.4	1.4	1.4	1.4	1.5	1.5	1.5	1.5	1.6	1.6	1.6	1.7	1.7	1.7
1.3	1.3	1.3	1.4	1.4	1.4	1.5	1.5	1.6	1.6	1.6	1.7	1.7	1.8	1.8	1.9	1.9	2.0	2.0	2.1	2.1	2.2
1.4	1.4	1.4	1.5	1.5	1.6	1.7	1.7	1.8	1.8	1.9	2.0	2.0	2.1	2.2	2.2	2.3	2.4	2.5	2.6	2.7	2.7
1.5	1.5	1.6	1.6	1.7	1.8	1.8	1.9	2.0	2.1	2.2	2.3	2.3	2.4	2.5	2.6	2.8	2.9	3.0	3.1	3.2	3.4
1.6	1.6	1.7	1.8	1.8	1.9	2.0	2.1	2.2	2.3	2.4	2.6	2.7	2.8	2.9	3.1	3.2	3.4	3.6	3.7	3.9	4.1
1.7	1.7	1.8	1.9	2.0	2.1	2.2	2.3	2.5	2.6	2.7	2.9	3.0	3.2	3.4	3.6	3.8	4.0	4.2	4.4	4.7	4.9
1.8	1.8	1.9	2.0	2.1	2.3	2.4	2.6	2.7	2.9	3.1	3.2	3.4	3.6	3.9	4.1	4.3	4.6	4.9	5.2	5.5	5.8
1.9	1.9	2.0	2.2	2.3	2.5	2.6	2.8	3.0	3.2	3.4	3.6	3.8	4.1	4.4	4.7	5.0	5.3	5.7	6.0		
2.0	2.0	2.1	2.3	2.5	2.6	2.8	3.0	3.2	3.5	3.7	4.0	4.3	4.6	4.9	5.3	5.7					
2.1	2.1	2.3	2.4	2.6	2.8	3.0	3.3	3.5	3.8	4.1	4.4	4.7	5.1	5.5	5.9						
2.2	2.2	2.4	2.6	2.8	3.0	3.3	3.5	3.8	4.1	4.5	4.8	5.2	5.7								
2.3	2.3	2.5	2.7	3.0	3.2	3.5	3.8	4.1	4.5	4.9	5.3	5.7									
2.4	2.4	2.6	2.9	3.1	3.4	3.7	4.1	4.4	4.8	5.3	5.8										
2.5	2.5	2.7	3.0	3.3	3.6	4.0	4.3	4.7	5.2	5.7											
2.6	2.6	2.9	3.1	3.5	3.8	4.2	4.6	5.1	5.6												
2.7	2.7	3.0	3.3	3.6	4.0	4.4	4.9	5.4	6.0												
2.8	2.8	3.1	3.4	3.8	4.2	4.7	5.2	5.8													
2.9	2.9	3.2	3.6	4.0	4.4	4.9	5.5														
3.0	3.0	3.3	3.7	4.2	4.7	5.2	5.8														
3.1	3.1	3.5	3.9	4.4	4.9	5.5															
3.2	3.2	3.6	4.0	4.5	5.1	5.7															
3.3	3.3	3.7	4.2	4.7	5.3	6.0															
3.4	3.4	3.8	4.3	4.9	5.5																
3.5	3.5	4.0	4.5	5.1	5.8																
3.6	3.6	4.1	4.7	5.3	6.0																
3.7	3.7	4.2	4.8	5.5																	
3.8	3.8	4.3	5.0	5.7																	
3.9	3.9	4.5	5.1	5.9																	
4.0	4.0	4.6	5.3																		
4.1	4.1	4.7	5.4																		
4.2	4.2	4.8	5.6																		
4.3	4.3	5.0	5.8																		
4.4	4.4	5.1	5.9																		
4.5	4.5	5.2																			
4.6	4.6	5.4																			
4.7	4.7	5.5																			

See text for prothrombin time ratio determination. The ISI is supplied by the manufacturer.

takes the place of functioning liver cells, and these nonfunctioning liver cells can no longer make prothrombin. PT is a valuable tool in assessing the amount of liver damage in a client with liver disease. Unlike other situations in which the PT is increased, vitamin K injections usually do not help much with advanced liver disease. The inability of the liver to respond to vitamin K, as evidenced by little change in the PT after vitamin K injection, demonstrates that the liver is so damaged that it cannot produce more prothrombin and other factors, even with abundant vitamin K.

Another clinical reason for an increased PT is the inability of the body to absorb vitamin K from the gastrointestinal (GI) tract. Because vitamin K is a fat-soluble vitamin, absorption depends on the presence of bile salts. With an obstruction of the common bile duct, bile salts cannot be released into the duodenum. So a client who has obstructive jaundice, which is caused by an obstruction in the common bile duct, has an increased PT because the liver cannot get vitamin K.

Much rarer is a true deficiency of vitamin K in the body, because humans do not depend much on dietary sources for vitamin K. This vitamin is manufactured by the bacteria that normally reside in the intestinal tract. So if a client is undergoing long-term antibiotic therapy that depletes the normal bacteria in the GI tract, the client may have an increased PT caused by a deficiency of vitamin K. Unlike a client with a failing liver, a client with a vitamin K deficiency or malabsorption problem has an increased PT that can be returned to normal by the administration of vitamin K. When the vitamin is given parenterally, it is absorbed into the bloodstream and bypasses the digestive step that requires bile salts. (See Chapter 11 for more discussion on obstructive jaundice and hypoprothrombinemia in relation to the test of direct bilirubin.)

A newborn's PT is slightly prolonged because infants do not have the same quantity of some of the clotting factors as adults. Newborns also do not have a store of vitamin K, and they have not yet acquired the normal intestinal bacteria to produce the vitamin. Newborn infants of mothers who are deficient in vitamin K are thus susceptible to a disease called *hemorrhagic disease of the newborn.* A dose of vitamin K, given prophylactically to all newborns, guards against the possibility of hemorrhage in the first few days.

Another hemorrhagic situation with an increased PT is in the complex bleeding disorder called *DIC*. This clinical situation is discussed in detail at the end of this chapter, as are fibrinogen levels.

Effect of Coumarin on PT. In all the situations discussed thus far, an increased PT of 24 sec, with a corresponding percentage of normal activity of about 20–25%, would be indicative of a severe pathologic state. For a client who is undergoing anticoagulation with one of the coumarin-type drugs, such as warfarin sodium (Coumadin), the therapeutic goal is usually to have only about 25% of normal activity (Katzung, 1995). Coumarin-type drugs cause a decrease in the production of prothrombin and of other factors because these drugs interfere with the use of vitamin K by the liver. Because the coumarin-type drugs work in this indirect way, by depressing liver function, the change in the PT does not occur for a day or longer. It usually takes several days for the PT to reach the desired INR. Vitamin K, taken orally or parenterally, reverses the effects of these drugs, returning the PT to normal within several hours. A PT in the normal range may be dangerous for a client who needs to undergo anticoagulation in the first place. (Refer to Table 13–3 for a summary of information about coumarin drugs and PT monitoring.)

▼ POSSIBLE NURSING DIAGNOSES RELATED TO INCREASED PT

Risk for Bleeding Related to Hypoprothrombinemia

A nurse caring for a client with an increased PT needs a clear understanding of whether this client is likely to be vulnerable to bleeding for a long time or if this abnormal PT is of short duration. For example, if the client has an increased PT as a result of obstructive jaundice, vitamin K brings the PT back to normal within a few hours or at most within a day or so. In this case, one should not need to burden the client and family with a long list of all the possible ways to protect the client from bleeding. However, a client who is being discharged to take a coumarin-type drug needs to know that a PT that represents 20–25% normal clotting activity makes a client vulnerable to bleeding. These clients and their families need detailed instructions on how to treat bleeding episodes. Vitamin K is one antidote for coumarin overdosage (frozen plasma is the other), but many physicians do not want clients to carry this drug if they are close to a medical facility. Clients with severe liver disease may also be functioning with an increased PT that is of a chronic nature. They need to be taught how to protect themselves from bleeding. As mentioned earlier, vitamin K probably does not help this PT very much. Clients with liver disease are very likely eventually to have severe bleeding episodes.

Assessing and Preventing Bleeding Episodes. Nurses must always be looking for symptoms that could indicate a client might be bleeding, because a bleeding episode is the possible consequence in any client with an increased PT. Nurses must also be aware of the ways to prevent bleeding. They must use their own judgment about which parts of the following assessment and interventions are needed for an individual client. The degree of client involvement in protecting him- or herself from bleeding depends on the level of illness and the setting of home or hospital. Nurses must assess the client's level of understanding, readiness for information about the condition or treatment, and willingness and ability to participate in health care.

When caring for a client who has a bleeding tendency because of an abnormal PT and other factors, nurses need to be aware of all the subtle clues that can be a symptom of bleeding. As the professionals who probably spend the most time with the client, nurses have the opportunity and responsibility to detect these subtle changes before a bleeding episode becomes a catastrophe. So a complete assessment and prevention of bleeding includes the following:

1. Headaches or changes in neurologic status could indicate bleeding into the cranium. A headache is of particular concern for a client who has sustained a head injury.
2. Clients with an increased PT must be protected from falls. Sports or other activities that could lead to head blows are risky.

3. Clients who shave should do so with an electric razor to prevent bleeding from accidental cuts.
4. Epistaxis (nose bleeding) and gum bleeding may occur. So too vigorous tooth brushing, hard coughing, or blowing the nose may trigger bleeding. Nose bleeding in these clients can be a serious matter.
5. Nurses must be particularly careful when suctioning a client who has a bleeding tendency.
6. Vomiting or coughing blood can be quite serious. The physician should be notified immediately, even if the vomitus contains only a small amount of blood. Often the small amount of blood that is vomited first is only the first indication. Fresh blood looks like blood. Older blood, which has been acted on by the gastric juices, has a characteristic dark brown color that is called *coffee-ground.*
7. In a client with a nasogastric (NG) tube, the drainage may be coffee-ground color rather than the yellowish to pale green of normal stomach contents. Not all coffee-ground drainage from NG tubes means the client is experiencing a large amount of bleeding. Sometimes simply the presence of the NG tube causes enough irritation to produce minimal and clinically insignificant bleeding. Yet for a client with an increased PT, any bleeding may be serious.

   Tests can be performed to detect occult bleeding in gastric secretions. Yet, obviously, if there is frank blood, a guaiac test is a waste of time and effort. The nurse must also be very careful about irrigation of a NG tube for a client with bleeding tendencies. Iced saline lavage may be used to control gastric bleeding. Antacids and histamine-2 blockers such as cimetidine (Tagamet) may be ordered to decrease gastric hyperacidity. (See the section on guaiac and other tests at the end of this chapter.)
8. A client with severe liver disease may also have esophageal varices (varicosities) that can be the source of massive bleeding. A client with suspected varices may have dietary restrictions so that only soft foods are served.
9. Abdominal or flank pain may indicate slow internal bleeding. Internal bleeding can be very subtle in the beginning, with few symptoms, because the bleeding usually is slow. A client may describe a backache that cannot be relieved with back rubs, a change of position, or the administration of a mild analgesic. No one may consider a possible connection to the anticoagulant the client is receiving until the client faints when he or she tries to get out of bed. Then it is discovered that the client has been slowly bleeding into the retroperitoneal area.

(*continued*)

▼ POSSIBLE NURSING DIAGNOSES RELATED TO INCREASED PT (*continued*)

Internal bleeding can cause pain because of the increasing pressure as blood collects. If the bleeding is into the GI tract, however, there probably is not any associated pain because the blood does not cause undue pressure, and if the client has an ulcer, the blood acts as a buffer. The blood eventually passes into the stool, but it may be occult, or hidden.

Clients with a bleeding tendency should periodically test the stools for occult blood. Hematocrits (hcts) are useful to assess the exact amount of blood loss (see Chapter 2). The tests for occult blood, described at the end of this chapter, are simple enough that clients can be taught to conduct a test at home if the situation warrants doing so. If the bleeding is fairly copious and high enough in the GI tract to be in contact with the digestive juices, the stools take on a dark black color that is described as "tarry." Straining at stool may cause bleeding, especially if the client has hemorrhoids, so the nurse needs to help the client find ways to avoid constipation.

10. Dark or smokey-looking urine may indicate blood in the urine. Hematuria is often the first indication of overdosage with anticoagulants. Sometimes the blood is bright red if it is fresh. Urine tests to check for the presence of red blood cells (RBCs) in the urine should be routine (Schuster and Lewis, 1987). Although the laboratory can check for red cells by means of microscopic examination, which is more sensitive for intact erythrocytes, nurses may conduct dipstick tests for blood in the urine (see Chapter 3 on hematuria). Clients who have catheters may bleed because of irritation caused by the catheter. Nurses should make sure the catheter is securely anchored with tape so it does not slide up and down the meatus.
11. Women with bleeding tendencies caused by an abnormal PT probably have heavy menses, and they should be aware of this possibility.
12. Pain in or immobility of a joint can indicate bleeding into the joint. Nurses must consider all precautions necessary to protect the client from falls and trauma. When active children are clients, doing so may be a real challenge to the parents and to the nurse. Specific points about bleeding caused by classic hemophilia (hemophilia A) are discussed with the test for factor VIII.
13. Taking blood pressure and pulse are two other ways to detect bleeding. A slight but steady increase in pulse may be a subtle sign of bleeding, long before the blood pressure drops.
14. It is wise to have a policy of avoiding intramuscular injections, if at all possible, for clients with bleeding tendencies. If an intra-

muscular injection must be given, choose the smallest-gauge needle possible and apply pressure for 10 min after the injection.

When laboratory personnel come to draw blood, a nurse needs to remind them of the potential bleeding problem. The finger stick method to obtain blood should be used whenever possible if the bleeding tendency is severe (see Chapter 1 for the finger stick procedure). Some hospitals put a sign on the client's door to alert all personnel to the bleeding tendency. The nurse can be inventive in particular settings to make sure everyone caring for the client knows about the bleeding tendency.

Special Needs for a Client Receiving Surgical Care. If a client with an increased PT must undergo an operation, it is imperative that the PT be medically corrected before the operation. To get the PT back to a safe level for the operation, vitamin K injections may be ordered. For example, clients who have undergone valve replacements are usually receiving long-term anticoagulation therapy to prevent thrombus formation around the valve. If the client needs an emergency appendectomy, the conversion to a normal PT is done in conjunction with heparin replacement for anticoagulation. When anticoagulant therapy is necessary during a surgical procedure, the client's drug is switched to heparin because this short-term anticoagulant can be more easily controlled (see PTT) and quickly reversed with protamine. Whole blood or fresh frozen plasma should always be available for a client with an abnormal PT who must undergo an operation. A type and cross match are performed as part of the preoperative preparation (see Chapter 14 on type and cross match).

Impaired Home Management Related to Need for Frequent PT

Dosages of long-term anticoagulant must be adjusted frequently until the PT reaches the desired INR for the client. The PT may be drawn daily during the adjustment phase. Once the client knows the maintenance dose, the PT can be measured about once a month or as little as every 6 weeks. On discharge, clients need written instructions about the anticoagulant and the time for the next PT. In the past, clients would be kept in the hospital until dosages were stabilized. Because hospital stays are short now, a steady anticoagulation state may not be reached before discharge, so the problem of home management of the anticoagulant is intensified. Krokosky and Vanscoy (1989) found that an anticoagulation clinic run by nurses and a pharmacist has decreased the problems associated with long-term anticoagulation therapy.

Knowledge Deficit Related to Long-term Anticoagulation and Other Medications

When the client is taking coumarin-type drugs, a wide variety of other drugs may interact with them to cause changes in the PT, either to increase or to decrease the PT. Aspirin and other salicylates potentiate the effect of coumarin,

(continued)

▼ POSSIBLE NURSING DIAGNOSES RELATED TO INCREASED PT (*continued*)

thus increasing the PT time. Often the client is not aware that many pain medications, such as cold remedies, contain aspirin. Brand drugs, such as Percodan, Empirin, or Darvon Compound, all contain aspirin. In fact, more than 500 aspirin-containing compounds are available. Certainly the client needs to be instructed not to take any medication without consulting the physician who is prescribing the anticoagulant. The coumarin-type drugs are responsible for more adverse drug reactions than any other group (see Table 13–3 for some common interactions).

Knowledge Deficit Related to Effects of Anticoagulation During Pregnancy

Women undergoing anticoagulation therapy need information on birth control and the risks of anticoagulation in pregnancy. Oral anticoagulants may cause nasal hypoplasia, neurologic deficits, and other malformations known as the fetal warfarin syndrome (Wong et al., 1993). Women who need anticoagulants during pregnancy usually take maintenance doses of heparin, although warfarin may be used except between 6–12 weeks gestation and 2–3 weeks before delivery (Greaves, 1993). With both warfarin and heparin, nurses must monitor laboratory tests and assess the pregnant woman for bleeding and other complications (Cosico and Rothlauf, 1992; Corbett and Kenney, 1994).

Decreased Prothrombin Time

Clinical Significance. Sometimes clients may have a PT of 8 or 9 sec, compared with a control of 11 or 12 sec. It may reflect a pathologic condition, such as thrombophlebitis or a malignant tumor. The reduced PT, however, is not of clinical significance as a diagnostic tool.

▼ POSSIBLE NURSING DIAGNOSIS RELATED TO REDUCED PT

Risk for Injury Related to Formation of Venous Thrombi

A reduced PT may indicate hypercoagulability of the blood. Hypercoagulability of the blood, venous stasis, and injury to the venous wall are the three conditions that contribute to the formation of *venous* thrombi. (Note that the condition associated with *arterial* thrombosis is atherosclerosis. See Chapter 9 on lipid metabolism.) It is thought that at least two of the three conditions (Virchow's triad) must be present to have thrombosis formation in the veins. Venous thrombi are found most often in the deep veins of the legs or in pelvic veins.

When a client has known hypercoagulability of the blood, the primary goal of the nurse is to decrease the possibility of venous thrombus formation by such measures as leg exercises, adequate hydration, and no venous constrictions, such as crossing the legs. (See the discussion in the section on PTT on the effectiveness of low doses of heparin to prevent deep venous thrombosis [DVT].) Hickey (1994) described a tool to assess 20 risk factors for DVT. Prophylactic treatments are based on whether the client is at low, moderate, or high risk.

▼ PARTIAL THROMBOPLASTIN TIME

The PTT, a nonspecific test, can demonstrate a lack of any of the various clotting factors, except factor VII (stable factor), that function in the intrinsic clotting system (see Table 13–1). Because some clotting tests, such as PT, bypass the intrinsic clotting system, they are not useful to screen for general plasma deficiencies. The PTT, on the contrary, is useful in detecting the presence of many types of bleeding disorders caused by defective or deficient circulating factors that compose the intrinsic system. If the PTT is abnormal, further tests are needed to pinpoint exactly which factor is defective or deficient.

The other purpose of the PTT is to monitor heparin therapy because heparin, a short-acting anticoagulant that circulates in the plasma, increases the PTT. Table 13–3 summarizes the use of the PTT for monitoring heparin.

Essentially, the laboratory technique for measuring PTT involves adding chemicals to the client's blood sample and timing, in seconds, the formation of a clot. If chemicals are also added to accelerate the clotting time, the result is reported as an activated PTT. The client's results in seconds are compared with a control that was tested using the same method. Like the PT, a control is conducted on "normal" blood because so many environmental variables can affect each individual situation. Unlike the PT, there is no percentage report.

Preparation of Client and Collection of Sample

Venous blood is collected (1.8 or 4.5 mL) in tubes containing 3.8% sodium citrate (blue vacuum tube). If the client is undergoing anticoagulation therapy, record the time, dosage, and route of administration of the heparin.

REFERENCE VALUES FOR PTT	
Adult	24–37 sec for activated PTT, 60–90 sec if not activated
Pregnancy	May be normally decreased by a few seconds Also may be decreased with oral contraceptives
Newborn	Range is increased above adult level for about 3 months

Increased PTT

Clinical Significance. An increased PTT, when the client is not taking heparin, signifies a bleeding disorder. Further tests must be performed to determine which factor is deficient. Also, the client may have abnormal factors such as the lupus anticoagulant factor (Samuel et al., 1989). The abnormality, or the lack of a factor, may be either acquired or hereditary.

The most common hereditary disorder is lack of factor VIII (antihemophilic globulin), which results in the classic hemophilia, or hemophilia A. An inherited deficiency in factor IX (plasma thromboplastin component or Christmas factor) results in the condition known as *Christmas disease,* or hemophilia B. Often the client's history gives clues that the increased PTT is due to a familial condition (see the tests for factors VIII and IX). Specific assays for different factors in the plasma definitively establish the diagnosis.

Acquired deficiencies may be more subtle and difficult to connect to any specific cause. The PTT becomes elevated in a complex bleeding disorder in which the clotting factors are used up at an abnormal rate. This disorder, DIC, is discussed in detail at the end of this chapter, along with fibrinogen levels. Autologous blood transfusions may cause an elevated PTT (Gillott and Thomas, 1984).

If the client is taking heparin, an increase in the PTT is the result of the effects of the circulating anticoagulant in the plasma. Usually the PTT is kept about 1.5–2.5 times the control value. So if the control is 36 sec, a report greater than 90 sec indicates more-than-adequate anticoagulation for the moment the blood is drawn. A report of less than 53 sec indicates inadequate anticoagulation for the moment the blood is drawn. (At the very best, the PTT reflects only heparin activity at the moment the sample is taken, because heparin activity in the blood varies from moment to moment.)

▼ POSSIBLE NURSING DIAGNOSES RELATED TO ELEVATED PTT

Risk for Injury Related to Bleeding

An abnormal PTT necessitates postponement of an operation unless it is an emergency. If the PTT is being used as a routine check before an operation such as a tonsillectomy, the test must be completed early enough so that the reports are on the chart before the client goes to the operating room. Easy bruisability does not always mean a bleeding disorder, but any evidence of past bleeding difficulties needs to be assessed medically before operative or other invasive procedures, such as an arteriogram, are performed. (See Chapter 25 for the risk of bleeding with invasive procedures.)

Anxiety Related to Bleeding Disorder

If the PTT is elevated, several tests may be needed to evaluate the client's clotting ability. Nurses may be helpful in allowing the client and the family to express their concerns and anxieties about an unknown medical diagnosis. Any client with an elevated PTT has an increased tendency to bleed, and thus client teaching for preventing bleeding, discussed earlier, is appropriate. Griffin (1986) noted that stress may activate the bleeding process, so biofeedback and imagery may be useful tools to decrease the client's stress.

Risk for Injury Related to Heparin Therapy

Before assuming responsibility for heparin administration, the nurse should check to see the results of the latest PTT. An abnormally high PTT should always be reported immediately. Failure to report an increased PTT has led to a law suit (Northrop, 1986). The nurse must also record if the PTT is *below* the therapeutic range. It can be as dangerous for the client to remain *under*anticoagulated as *over*anticoagulated.

Because heparin activity may vary from moment to moment, it would be a mistake to believe that all one needs to adjust the dosage is one PTT. Seeing the range of the PTT gives guidelines to the physician in adjusting the dosage for each client. Some hospitals use flow sheets, so the PTT can be charted with the dosage of heparin and compared over an extended period. This chart makes it easier to get a clear idea of the ongoing status of the anticoagulant therapy. Heparin-associated thrombocytopenia can develop, so platelet counts should be ordered (Rizzoni et al., 1988) (see the discussion later in this chapter).

Checking for Drug Interferences. Drugs that interfere with the action of heparin are not as numerous as those that interfere with the coumarin-type drugs, but some drugs do affect the PTT (see Table 13–3). The potential interaction of these drugs may be important if the drugs are added or deleted during the time the client is undergoing heparin therapy. Because drugs containing aspirin increase the bleeding time, they should be avoided when the client is taking heparin. Platelet aggregation is the main defense against bleeding, and aspirin decreases the adhesiveness of platelets, potentiating the bleeding tendency from any type of anticoagulation.

Use of Heparin in Minidoses. There is one type of clinical situation in which the PTT need not be checked, even though the client is taking heparin. This is when heparin is given in low doses of usually about 5,000 units subcutaneously every 8–12 hr. The purpose of the minidose is to prevent the possible occurrence of thromboembolic episodes in clients who are at high risk because of a surgical procedure or prolonged bed rest. More than 70 randomized studies have shown that the prophylactic use of heparin in small doses can de-

(*continued*)

▼ POSSIBLE NURSING DIAGNOSES RELATED TO ELEVATED PTT (*continued*)

crease the risk of pulmonary embolus in high-risk clients (Collins et al., 1988). These doses of heparin are small enough so that they do not affect the PTT. A baseline PTT may be ordered, but nurses do not need to check PTT results before giving each small prophylactic dose of heparin.

Knowledge Deficit Related to Possible Need for Long-term Anticoagulation

If long-term use of anticoagulants is necessary to prevent other thromboembolic episodes, the usual pattern is to begin with a coumarin-type drug after a few days of heparin therapy and continue both types of anticoagulants until the PT is within the desired range. For example, long-term anticoagulation might be needed for a client who has had a pulmonary embolus. During this switch from heparin to long-term oral anticoagulants, both the PT and PTT need to be monitored, and clients need the instructions about coumarin described earlier. (Also see the section on tests for low-molecular-weight heparin.)

Decreased PTT

Clinical Significance. A PTT lower than the control sample is not diagnostically significant, but it may be a clue reflecting hypercoagulability (see the discussion of PT for nursing interventions to help prevent venous thrombus formation). Some degree of hypercoagulability is normal in pregnancy.

▼ ACTIVATED CLOTTING TIME

Although the PTT is usually used to monitor heparin therapy, the ACT also can be used. The ACT, measured at the bedside, is commonly used during cardiovascular operations and in intensive care units. The ACT may also be used to screen for some coagulation deficiencies and is needed for regulation of heparin dosages in clients with the lupus anticoagulant factor.

As with the PTT, the results are not clinically significant unless the timing is correlated with heparin administration. For a clear representation of the true anticoagulated state of the client, clinicians need to use a flow sheet that lists all the test results with the time and route of administration. If the clotting time is not in the desired therapeutic range, the nurse has the responsibility to notify the physician. The nursing implications for a client with bleeding tendencies are covered in the discussion of PT and PTT. The nurse must always keep in mind that a client undergoing any anticoagulation therapy can bleed, even if laboratory results indicate a satisfactory condition.

Preparation of Client and Collection of Sample

The test is performed at bedside by a technologist or other clinician. Whole blood is drawn into special tubes that contain an activator such as siliceous earth (tubes and syringes should be warmed to 37°C). Time to clot is observed immediately. If the client is receiving a continuous heparin drip, the venous sample is obtained from the arm without the intravenous catheter.

REFERENCE VALUES FOR ACT

70–120 sec (depends on type of activator used)
Desirable range for anticoagulation may be 150–190 sec

▼ TESTS FOR LOW-MOLECULAR-WEIGHT HEPARIN

The introduction of low-molecular-weight (LMW) heparin, enoxaparin (Lovenox), has made it much easier to care for clients with thromboembolism at home. Administration of LMW heparin is less time-consuming and does not require as much laboratory monitoring as conventional heparin (unfractionated heparin) (Simonneau et al., 1993). Unlike conventional heparin, LMW heparin is not monitored with PTT. An automated test, called the Heptest has been developed to assess the presence of several LMW heparins (Ozawa et al., 1993). Check with the laboratory for reference values.

In addition to some screening tests for antiplatelet antibodies, the manufacturer of enoxaparin also recommends periodic monitoring of complete blood count, platelet count, and stool for occult blood (Wilson, 1994).

▼ HEMOPHILIA TESTS: FACTORS VIII AND IX

The two main types of hemophilia are called *A (classic hemophilia)* and *B (Christmas disease)*. Classic hemophilia has affected several royal families in Europe. Christmas disease was named for the family who was studied with the genetic defect of factor IX. The specific diagnosis of classic hemophilia is made by means of assay of factor VIII and of Christmas disease by means of assay of factor IX. The cause of more than 80% of all hemophilias is a deficiency of factor VIII. Because the PTT is prolonged in hemophilia, it is a screening test for bleeding disorders. The client has a normal PT and platelet counts.

Preparation of Client and Collection of Sample

Venous blood (4.5 mL) is collected in plastic tubes with 3.8% sodium citrate (blue vacuum tube).

REFERENCE VALUES FOR FACTORS VIII AND IX	
Factor VIII (antihemophilic globulin)	50–200%
Factor IX (plasma thromboplastic cofactor)	60–140%
See Appendix A, Table 4, for reference values for other factors	

▼ POSSIBLE NURSING DIAGNOSES RELATED TO DEFICIENCY IN COAGULATION FACTORS

Impaired Home Maintenance Management Related to Risk for Bleeding

The general nursing implications for a client with bleeding tendencies are discussed in the section on PT. Because factor replacement therapy can be provided, many bleeding episodes can be prevented or treated before damage occurs to joints or to other vital areas. Older children and their parents are taught to mix the factor concentrate and to administer the intravenous infusion. Home therapy for children with hemophilia has been successful, and research (McGuire, 1985) has shown children treated at home display improved social adaptive skills as well as improved physical capabilities.

Anxiety Related to Transmitting a Genetic Disease

See Chapter 18 for a discussion of genetic counseling. Both hemophilia A and B are inherited as X-linked recessive traits. Females who receive the defective gene do not have the disease because they also have another "healthy" X chromosome. On the contrary, any male who receives the defective X shows symptoms because he does not have a healthy X chromosome to balance the effect. Hemophilia may be mild, moderate, or severe, depending on how much of the factor is produced. Hemophilia can also result from spontaneous mutations, since some affected males do not demonstrate the disease in the family tree.

Anxiety Related to Safety of Factor Transfusions

The contamination of pooled factors with the human immunodeficiency virus (HIV) was possible until 1985, when viral inactive clotting factor concentrates were introduced. See Chapter 14 on the current status of testing for HIV. More than 7,000 people with hemophilia were infected with HIV, and some clients may fear that such a catastrophe could occur again if the blood supply is contaminated (Pierce, 1994). The National Hemophilia Foundation may be contacted for the latest information on this subject.

▼ PLATELET COUNT AND MEAN PLATELET VOLUME

Sometimes platelets are considered as a third type of blood cell in the plasma (see Chapter 2 for RBCs and white blood cells [WBCs]). Actually, platelets are not intact cells but only fragments of cytoplasm that function in blood coagulation. As platelets adhere to the wall of an injured vessel, they clump together (or aggregate) and release a substance that begins coagulation. Platelets are formed by the bone marrow and removed by the spleen when they are old or damaged.

Preparation of Client and Collection of Sample

The laboratory uses 0.5 mL of blood. EDTA is used as the anticoagulant (lavender-topped tube). If platelets clump with EDTA, a blue-topped tube may be used. The count is usually performed with a machine, but if the count is low, it is confirmed by means of microscopic examination. Smears can also be performed to estimate the number of platelets.

REFERENCE VALUES FOR PLATELETS AND MPV[a]

Adult 150,000–350,000/mm^3

Women have a greatly decreased platelet count for the first few days of menses

Platelets are increased after labor and delivery

Newborns have lower values

[a]Mean platelet volume (MPV) can be measured. Reference values are 6.6–11.0 µm^3. Larger platelets apparently have better hemostatic function.

Increased Platelet Count (Thrombocytosis)

Clinical Significance. Malignant tumors, especially advanced or metastatic lesions, may cause an elevated platelet count, or thrombocytosis. Many clients with an "unexpected" high platelet count are found to have a malignant neoplasm. Clients with polycythemia vera often have high platelet counts. (Polycythemia vera is discussed in Chapter 2 in the section on RBCs.) Another reason for an increased platelet count is the splenectomy, which causes a temporary increase in the platelet count.

▼ POSSIBLE NURSING DIAGNOSES RELATED TO ELEVATED PLATELET COUNTS

Risk for Injury Related to Thromboembolic Episodes

A logical assumption is that an increased amount of platelets tends to make the blood more coagulable. As discussed in the section on decreased PT and

(*continued*)

▼ POSSIBLE NURSING DIAGNOSES RELATED TO ELEVATED PLATELET COUNTS (*continued*)

hypercoagulability, dehydration could be dangerous for a client with a high platelet count. Venous stasis may be of particular concern. Depending on the reason for the thrombocytosis, thrombus formation may or may not be a possibility. For example, the increased platelet count after a splenectomy does not seem to cause any problems.

If thrombus formation is considered a possibility, aspirin, which is used as a mild anticoagulant in some situations, is sometimes ordered to decrease the adhesiveness of platelets. To prevent gastric irritation, the client needs to be taught either to take aspirin with milk or to dilute it with water.

Risk for Injury Related to Bleeding

Surprisingly, an increased number of platelets does not always mean an increased tendency to clot. In fact, it may mean an increased tendency to bleed. This paradox can be partially explained by the fact that sometimes the increased number of platelets are abnormal ones that cannot function properly in the coagulation process. Thus a client with thrombocytosis may need to be watched for bleeding tendencies. (See the detailed assessment guide in the section on PT.)

Low Platelet Count (Thrombocytopenia)

Clinical Significance. If the cause of the low platelet count, or thrombocytopenia, is unknown, the condition is called *idiopathic* (unknown cause) thrombocytopenic purpura. *Purpura* refers to bruising. Children who have idiopathic thrombocytopenic purpura often have spontaneous remissions. Chronic idiopathic thrombocytopenia in adults, an autoimmune disease, is more difficult to treat (Schwartz, 1994). Low platelet counts may occur after viral infections and are common with acquired immunodeficiency syndrome (AIDS). Thrombocytopenia is also common in clients with systemic lupus erythematous. A low count can be associated with some types of anemias or other hemolytic disorders. Entities that depress bone marrow function, such as chemotherapeutic drugs or radiation, also depress the platelet count. An overactive spleen (hypersplenism) or an enlarged spleen (splenomegaly) destroys platelets at too fast a rate. Severe thrombocytopenia often follows any type of extracorporeal bypass or autotransfusion (Gillott and Thomas, 1984). Because heparin can cause thrombocytopenia, platelet counts must be monitored while a client is taking heparin (Rizzoni et al., 1988). The LMW heparins have less effect on platelets than does conventional heparin (Wilson, 1994).

▼ POSSIBLE NURSING DIAGNOSES RELATED TO THROMBOCYTOPENIA

Risk for Injury Related to Bleeding

When a client has a low platelet count, the most important nursing concern is protecting the client from bruising and bleeding. Petechiae are the most common manifestations of thrombocytopenia because the many microscopic injuries that occur continuously in the capillaries are not immediately sealed off because of the lack of platelets. Invasive procedures may be withheld if platelet counts are as low as 50,000/mm.^{3} The risk of spontaneous hemorrhage is about 50% if the level drops to 20,000/mm^3 (Weber, 1994). Some activities may need to be curtailed until the platelet count returns to normal. In the case of an active child, protection from trauma requires a great deal of ingenuity on the part of the nurse and the parents. Symptoms that indicate bleeding are described in detail in the section on nursing implications for an increased PT. Clients may be embarrassed by the bruises on their arms and legs, and so they appreciate clothing that conceals the bruises from curious onlookers.

Risk for Infection Related to Leukopenia, Anemia, or Drug Therapy

If the thrombocytopenia is a result of general bone marrow depression, the implications about leukopenia (low WBC) and anemia (low RBC) must also be considered. (Related nursing diagnoses are discussed in Chapter 2.) Adult clients, and sometimes children, with a low platelet count may undergo corticosteroid therapy, which is given to raise the platelet count to normal. The risk for infection is due to the use of the cortisone-type drugs. (See Chapter 15 on cortisone therapy and other nursing diagnoses.)

In idiopathic thrombocytopenia purpura, sometimes the removal of the spleen is necessary to return the platelet count to normal (Berchtold and McMillan, 1989). If such an operation is scheduled, the nurse can help prepare the client for the surgical experience. Adult clients usually have few problems after the spleen is removed because the role of the spleen can be taken over by other parts of the reticuloendothelial system. For children, a splenectomy is usually not performed because the spleen is important for antibody production.

Risk for Injury Related to Platelet Transfusions

If thrombocytopenia results from a malignant tumor or from treatment with chemotherapeutic drugs, platelet transfusions may be given. One unit of platelet concentrate increases the platelet count by at least 5,000 (National Heart, Lung and Blood Institute, 1989). Clients with counts less than 10,000–20,000/mm^3 usually require platelet transfusions, whereas those with more may receive transfusions only if hemorrhage begins. Because patients may become sensitized to the platelet concentrates, transfusions are reserved for those who are at great risk. Three of the most important problems in platelet transfusions are allergic reactions, hypervolemia, and bacterial sepsis.

▼ BLEEDING TIME: MODIFIED IVY, SIMPLATE, DUKE METHOD, ASPIRIN TOLERANCE TEST

Bleeding time is a screening test for disorders of platelets or for vascular defects in the clotting process. The laboratory technologist performs the test at the bedside. For the modified Ivy method, a commercial device (Simplate Bleeding Time Device; General Diagnostics) is used to make two small puncture wounds in the forearm. (The Ivy method is performed freehand.) If the arm cannot be used, the ear lobe is used (Duke method).

Preparation of Client and Collection of Sample

The technologist places a blood pressure cuff on the client's arm. The pressure is kept at 40 mmHg. After two small puncture wounds are made on the forearm, the bleeding time is measured with a stopwatch. The bleeding area is blotted with filter paper every 30 sec. There is a small possibility of scar formation from the wound punctures, so some laboratories have the client or guardian sign a consent form. A small dressing is placed over the site. The client should not have had any aspirin or anticoagulants for at least 1 week before the test. Sometimes the test is performed before and after aspirin dosage to assess the effect of the aspirin on the bleeding time (aspirin tolerance test).

REFERENCE VALUES FOR BLEEDING TIMES	
Duke Method (ear lobe)	1–4 min
Modified Ivy	2–9 min
Simplate	3–9.5 min

▼ CLOT RETRACTION TEST

Platelets have an important role in clot formation and in making the clot firm by causing retraction. If platelets are lacking or defective, the clot does not shrink or retract but stays soft and watery. Also, if fibrinolysins are present in the serum, no clot retraction takes place. Fibrinolysis is discussed in the section on decreased levels of fibrinogen.

REFERENCE VALUES FOR CLOT RETRACTION
50–100% in 2 hr

▼ FIBRINOGEN

Fibrinogen (factor I) is a plasma protein manufactured by the liver. Vitamin K is *not* necessary for the formation of this factor, as it is for many of the others manufactured by the liver (see Table 13–1). The sole purpose of fibrinogen seems to be the formation of fibrin as the end product (stage IV) of blood coagulation (see Table 13–2).

Preparation of Client and Collection of Sample

Venous blood (4.5 mL of plasma) is collected in a tube with sodium citrate (blue-topped tube).

REFERENCE VALUES FOR FIBRINOGEN	
Adult	0.15–0.35 g/dL Women tend to have slightly higher levels
Pregnancy	Values may be as high as 0.06 g/dL

Decreased Levels of Fibrinogen

Clinical Significance. Low fibrinogen levels can result from rare genetic disorders or from severe liver disease, either of which might first be detected with the PTT.

More commonly, however, the decrease of fibrinogen is due to DIC. DIC is a pathologic overstimulation of the coagulation process. It is also called *consumption coagulopathy* or the *defibrination syndrome.*

Not a primary disorder, DIC is secondary to other severe illnesses. The theory is that widespread tissue injury somehow triggers the clotting mechanism so that a pathologic formation of small thrombi occurs in the microcirculation. Paradoxically, the client begins to bleed because the clotting factors are eventually depleted. Besides the low fibrinogen level, the PT is increased, the PTT is increased, and the platelet count is lowered. Thrombocytopenia is a cardinal diagnostic finding (Griffin, 1986). Because the placenta is a rich source of tissue thromboplastin, abnormalities such as abruptio placentae and fetal death can trigger massive clotting problems. Pregnant women have a reduced activity of the fibrolytic system. The increase of clotting factors and the decrease in fibrolysis protect against severe hemorrhage, but these changes can also contribute to coagulation problems in pregnancy (DeCherney and Pernoll, 1994). Other clients most likely to experience this abnormal clotting process are clients with toxemia of pregnancy, metastatic cancer, shock, sepsis, or burns. Respiratory distress syndrome, malaria, snake bite, and extracorporeal bypass also may contribute to DIC.

If the PT, PTT, platelet count, and fibrinogen levels are positive for DIC, additional tests to check for fibrinolysis and fibrin degradation products may be ordered. (See the following section for values for these tests.)

▼ POSSIBLE NURSING DIAGNOSES RELATED TO DECREASED FIBRINOGEN LEVELS

Risk for Injury Related to Bleeding and Clotting in the Microcirculation

Because a low fibrinogen level is often part of a complex pathologic situation, clients most likely to experience DIC are usually those who are already in an intensive care unit with a primary illness. (See the tests for FDP and D-dimer.) Shock is often present. In the obstetric area, women with toxemia or with any abnormality of the placenta should be observed for DIC. The nurse giving direct care may be first to notice signs of bleeding, such as bruise marks or the appearance of blood in drainage tubes or on dressings. (Refer to the section on PT to review the ways a nurse can make objective assessments for occult or hidden bleeding.) If thrombi have developed in the microcirculation, the client may have unexplained pain or symptoms of poor circulation to specific areas, such as cyanosis of the fingers or toes.

Assisting with Medical Interventions. Whole blood or blood components may be given intravenously to replace the clotting factors. Nurses must understand the correct rate of flow for the particular blood component used as well as the complications that may occur. Because blood components are obtained from a pool of donors, hepatitis may occur later. (See Chapter 14 for tests used to screen blood products.) Not only is bleeding occurring but also thrombus formation may be taking place. So heparin may be part of the therapy for this complex situation if there is a large thrombus (DeCherney and Pernoll, 1994).

▼ FIBRINOGEN DEGRADATION PRODUCTS OR FIBRIN SPLIT PRODUCTS

The fibrinogen degradation products (FDP) test measures the products that result from the breakdown of fibrin clots by the action of the enzyme plasmin. Fibrin degradation products are found in DIC. In addition to being useful in diagnosing the presence of DIC, the FDP may also be used to monitor fibrinolytic therapy. Tests of fibrin metabolism may also be used to evaluate the clot formation that occurs after pulmonary embolism. Hypofibrinogenemia and fibrin split products (FSP) occur after autologous transfusions (Gillott and Thomas, 1984).

Preparation of Client and Collection of Sample

Venous blood (4.5 mL) is collected in a special tube that contains thrombin and an antifibrinolytic agent. Blood should be drawn before heparin therapy is begun.

REFERENCE VALUES FOR FSP

For screening tests, no agglutinations at 1:4 dilution
Quantitative tests <10 μg

▼ D-DIMER SCREEN: ELISA AND LATEX AGGLUTINATION SLIDE TEST

D-Dimer refers to the degradation products of cross-linked fibrin. This byproduct of clot lysis may be measured by enzyme-linked immunosorbent assay (ELISA) or a slide test. ELISA is time-consuming and expensive but may be needed to confirm a screening test for FSP. A more rapid screening test is the latex agglutination slide test. Sensitivity and negative predictive values were similar for both types of tests when used to evaluate for venous thrombosis in an emergency unit (Hansson et al., 1994). The D-dimer slide test also has proved useful for screening for abruptio placentae (Nolan et al., 1993). D-dimer testing is also important to confirm DIC (DeCherney and Pernoll, 1994).

Preparation of Patient and Collection of Sample

Current PT, PTT, platelet count, and fibrinogen are obtained for baseline values. The blood sample is collected in a blue topped tube, 1.8 mL in a 2-mL tube or 4.5 mL in a 5-mL tube.

REFERENCE VALUE FOR D-DIMER SCREEN

Less than 0.5 μg/mL

▼ THROMBIN TIME: FIBRINOGEN SCREEN, THROMBIN CLOTTING TIME WITH REPTILASE

The thrombin time measures the time it takes blood to clot when thrombin is added to the sample. If a clot does not form immediately, a fibrinogen deficiency is present. Heparin therapy also keeps the blood sample from clotting. A reagent called *reptilase* (derived from snake venom) has an action similar to thrombin as it clots fibrinogen. However, reptilase is not inhibited by heparin, so it can be substituted for the conventional thrombin time test when the client is receiving heparin. In addition to assessing for some bleeding disorders, the thrombin time is also used to monitor clients receiving fibrinolytic therapy.

Preparation of Client and Collection of Sample

Whole blood, 4.5 mL, is collected in a plastic tube with sodium citrate (blue top). For the reptilase test, a special tube is obtained from the hematology laboratory.

REFERENCE VALUES FOR THROMBIN TIME AND REPTILASE TIME	
Thrombin time	14–16 sec or within 5 sec of control
Reptilase time	18–22 sec

▼ PLASMINOGEN ASSAY

Plasminogen is the inactive precursor of plasmin, an enzyme that has the ability to dissolve clots. The amount of this substance is useful information when the client is taking thrombolytic agents. The test also may be used to evaluate a client who has DIC. A decrease in plasminogen activity may be associated with the tendency for thrombosis.

Preparation of Client and Collection of Sample

Venous blood is collected in a special tube with a plasmin inhibitor.

REFERENCE VALUE FOR PLASMINOGEN ACTIVITY
73–122%

▼ PROTEINS C AND S ANTICOAGULANT SYSTEM

Protein S is a naturally occurring anticoagulant and protein C is necessary for its action. Congenital or acquired decreases or a defect in either of these proteins increases the risk for vascular thrombosis (Ravel, 1995). Thrombotic episodes often occur in high-risk situations such as pregnancy, a surgical procedure, or trauma. Tests for the protein C and protein S antigens and a functional assay of each are conducted.

Preparation of Client and Collection of Sample

The coumarin drugs alter the results, so blood is drawn before administration of oral anticoagulants or after a stable therapeutic level is established. Whole blood, 4.5 mL, is collected in a blue topped vacuum tube. This procedure may require approval from the laboratory. The turn-about time for results may be 2–4 weeks.

REFERENCE VALUES FOR PROTEIN C AND S
Protein C (immunoassay for antigen and functional clotting assay) 70–140%
Protein S (immunoassay for antigen and functional clotting assay) 70–140%

▼ OCCULT BLOOD: HEMATEST, HEMOCCULT, AND OTHER GUAIAC TESTS

Occult (hidden) blood can be detected by simple tests that cause color changes in the presence of blood. Although all tests for blood in stool, urine, or other secretions are sometimes called *guaiac tests,* not all of them use the chemical guaiac. Some tests, Hematest (Ames) being the common one, use another chemical, orthotolidine. Although tests such as Hematest and Hemostix (Ames) can be used to detect occult blood in urine, a microscopic examination is needed to detect intact erythrocytes. (See Chapter 3 on tests for hematuria.) The various tests for occult blood can also be performed on emesis, but note that a histamine-2 blocker may make the test falsely positive and a low pH falsely negative. Gastroccult (Smith Kline Diagnostics) is specifically designed to test for occult blood and the pH of gastric secretions. Nurses may use Gastroccult for on-the-spot assessment of occult blood in emesis or NG drainage. Only a drop of gastric juices is needed.

Nurses can also perform point-of-care assessments for blood in the stool by obtaining a small amount of feces by means of digital examination if necessary and using one of the commercial preparations discussed later. The most important use of such tests is to screen clients for cancer of the colon, because bleeding is one of the early symptoms. A screening for blood in the stool is much easier and less expensive than sigmoidoscopy (Ahlguist et al., 1985). The emphasis on early diagnosis of colorectal cancer has increased the overall 5-year survival rate to nearly 50% (Mehler, 1994).

Preparation of Client and Collection of Sample

The client may be instructed to avoid meat and to eat a high-fiber diet for 1–3 days before a screening test of the feces. Meat, especially red meat, may cause a false-positive result, and a high-fiber diet increases the chances of finding occult blood if a lesion is present in the GI tract. Some places may restrict a client's diet only after an initial screening test is positive. More than one stool specimen may be needed to detect intermittent bleeding. At least three are recommended. Stool specimens do not have to be tested immediately but must be protected from sunlight.

Nurses should be aware of influences on these tests. Vitamin C (>250 mg) may produce false-negative results, whereas iron pills may give false-positive results. Turnips and horseradish, which contain peroxidase, may also cause a false-positive result; aspirin and anti-inflammatory drugs, which tend to cause slight GI bleeding, should be avoided 2 days before the test. Long-distance runners may have occult blood in the feces after a vigorous run.

The client can collect stool at home with a commercially prepared filter paper in a protective cover, such as Hemoccult by Smith Kline Diagnostics. The written instructions tell the client to collect a small specimen of stool on an applicator and smear the stool on Part A of the paper. A second specimen from a different part of the stool is put on Part B of the paper. After three samples are collected and brought to the clinic or laboratory, two drops of a commercially prepared developing solution are placed on each smear, and the color change is noted after 30 sec.

Newer techniques for assessing for occult blood have been developed so that initial screenings do not require the handling of fecal samples. Compliance with return of three sets of guaiac-impregnated cards had been noted to be low (Rodney and Ruggiero, 1985). One type of screening uses a pad that is placed into the toilet after a bowel movement. The pad does not have to actually touch the stool. It simply floats in the toilet. The pad contains a performance monitor that changes color as long as the pad is not outdated. Another spot on the pad changes color if there is blood in the stool. Another method uses filter paper as toilet paper. The stool is then tested for blood by spraying the paper in the toilet. The reader is encouraged to investigate the range of commercial products available for home use.

REFERENCE VALUES FOR OCCULT BLOOD IN STOOL

Blue indicates the presence of blood. A second test may be completed to confirm a positive report.

▼ POSSIBLE NURSING DIAGNOSIS RELATED TO OCCULT BLOOD

Knowledge Deficit Related to Health Maintenance by Checking for Occult Blood

Nurses may be involved in instructing clients on how to test stools for blood as a screening measure at home. Nurses can educate the public about the importance of the resources available in their communities. The tests discussed above can be bought without prescriptions and are advertised in publications for the general public. As discussed in Chapter 1, screening for occult blood in the feces is one of only a few tests that are generally recommended routinely for even apparently healthy people older than 40 years of age. The community health nurse or the family nurse practitioner can offer this screening test to clients. (See Chapter 27 for information on sigmoidoscopy, which may be needed as a follow-up to the screening test for occult blood in the feces.)

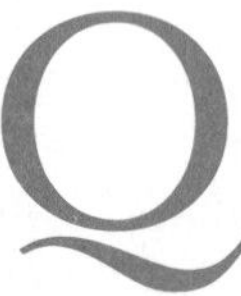

1. Mrs. Rodriguez has just begun hyperalimentation therapy because she is severely malnourished. The hyperalimentation therapy consists of amino acids, a concen-

trated glucose solution, minerals, and water-soluble vitamins. How could this situation affect the PT drawn today? It is likely the

a. Percentage and seconds will both be increased
b. Percentage will be increased and seconds decreased
c. Percentage and seconds will both be decreased
d. Percentage will be decreased and seconds increased

2. The case manager is scanning the laboratory reports that were just sent to the unit. A PT reported as an INR of 2.5 would be evidence of an appropriate therapeutic outcome for

a. Mr. Ramos, who is undergoing coumarin therapy
b. Mr. Wong, who is undergoing heparin therapy
c. Mrs. Saxon, who is scheduled for a liver biopsy
d. Mrs. Java, who had an injection of vitamin K_1 yesterday

3. A prophylactic injection of vitamin K_1 is given to newborns because the

a. PT of newborns is increased in seconds
b. Fibrinogen level of newborns is decreased
c. Platelet count may be lowered in some instances
d. Intestinal bacteria may destroy the vitamin K

4. Vitamin K injections are the least likely to return the PT to normal for which client?

a. Mr. Richards, who is suffering from malnutrition
b. Mr. Ringer, who has liver dysfunction
c. Mrs. Saxon, who is undergoing long-term coumarin therapy
d. Mrs. Java, who has obstructive jaundice caused by a pancreatic tumor

5. Mr. Ringer, a patient with cirrhosis, has had two episodes of gastrointestinal bleeding but seems stabilized now. His PT is 20 sec (control, 13 sec), and his platelet count is 100,000/mm^3 (reference value 150,000–350,000/mm^3). He eats a conventional diet but has little appetite. The *most important* instruction for the nurse to give Mr. Ringer when he goes home is for him to

a. Maintain a balanced diet with emphasis on foods containing vitamin K
b. Check his pulse regularly and report a rate greater than 100 beats per minute
c. Always drink a glass of milk when he takes aspirin
d. Report any dark-colored or black stools to his physician immediately

6. Mrs. Bender is being discharged to undergo long-term coumarin therapy. When the nurse formulates a discharge teaching plan, the *least important* topic to include is the necessity of

a. Carrying identification that she is undergoing long-term anticoagulant therapy
b. Having periodic PTs drawn

c. Not taking nonprescription drugs that contain aspirin
d. Assessing the amount of potassium (K^+) in her diet

7. Mrs. Jones has a PTT of 130 sec (control is 35 sec). She is receiving an intravenous heparin drip at a rate of 700 U/hr. Which action by the nurse is most appropriate after the physician is notified of the laboratory result?

   a. Prepare an injection of vitamin K for emergency use by the physician
   b. Increase the heparin rate, as ordered, because this will decrease the PTT time
   c. Encourage walking to increase circulation
   d. Keep the client on bed rest and assess the client often for any symptoms of bleeding

8. Mr. Jacobs, 66 years of age, is a postoperative client who had deep venous thrombosis (DVT) after a previous operation. His PTT is slightly lower than the normal control value. He takes a "minidose" of heparin as a preventive measure. Thus, the nursing action that has the highest priority is to

   a. Assess frequently for bleeding
   b. Encourage as much walking as possible
   c. Ascertain if protamine, the antidote for heparin, is readily available
   d. Monitor fluids to prevent circulatory overload

9. If a client has a low platelet count, the initial physical assessment is most likely to reveal

   a. Large hematomas on abdomen and back
   b. Delayed capillary filling when the skin is blanched
   c. Evidence of gastrointestinal bleeding such as a positive test for blood in the feces
   d. Petechiae on the legs

10. Which of the following nursing actions is the *most appropriate* for Sally, who reports a headache and is asking if she may take an over-the-counter medication for pain. Her platelet count today is 20,000/mm^3 (reference value is 150,000–350,000/mm^3).

   a. Allow her to take her usual over-the-counter medication for headache because it is usually very effective
   b. Offer her fluids to decrease the viscosity of her blood
   c. Obtain an order for aspirin for her headache
   d. Assess her for any changes in level of consciousness (LOC)

11. Sally has a platelet count of 10,000/mm^3 caused by idiopathic thrombocytopenia; John has a platelet count of 780,000/mm^3 caused by a malignant tumor (reference values 150,000–350,000 mm^3). Because of these laboratory reports, *both* these clients should be assessed for

   a. Bone marrow depression and polycythemia
   b. Thrombus formation in lower extremities

c. Bleeding episodes from minor trauma
d. Infection of mucous membranes

12. Which of the following changes in laboratory tests are most indicative of the complex bleeding disorder that is called disseminated intravascular coagulation (DIC) or consumption coagulopathy?

    a. Increased PT, increased PTT, and increased platelet count
    b. Decreased PT, decreased PTT, and decreased fibrinogen levels
    c. Increased PT, decreased platelet count, and increased fibrinogen levels
    d. Increased PT, decreased platelet count, and decreased fibrinogen levels

13. Johnny, 8 years of age, is scheduled for a tonsillectomy and adenoidectomy (T and A) tomorrow. The test that will most clearly demonstrate that he has an intact intrinsic clotting system is the

    a. Fibrinogen level
    b. PTT
    c. Platelet count
    d. PT

14. Mr. Ringer is scheduled for a liver biopsy tomorrow. He has a tentative diagnosis of cirrhosis caused by alcohol abuse. Which two of these laboratory tests are used in assessing adequate liver function before the invasive procedure of a liver biopsy?

    a. PTT and fibrinogen levels
    b. PT and platelet counts
    c. Fibrinogen levels and platelet counts
    d. PT and antihemophilic factor (factor VIII)

15. Linda Everett, 32 years of age, delivered a premature infant yesterday. Because of massive blood loss, she received three units of blood. Today she is having only slight vaginal bleeding. The laboratory data to best substantiate the need for continued close observation of vital signs would be

    a. PT, 11 sec (control, 12 sec)
    b. Fibrinogen, 0.10 g/dL (reference value 0.15–0.60 g/dL)
    c. PTT, 37 sec (control, 35 sec)
    d. Platelet count, 400,000/mm^3 (reference value 150,000–350,000/mm^3)

16. Two days ago, Mr. Frank, 58 years of age, underwent a complex abdominal operation for cancer of the colon. He has a nasogastric tube, which is draining greenish drainage. He can walk with help. Today's laboratory reports show a PT of 9 sec (control, 12 sec), a PTT of 30 sec (control, 34 sec), and a platelet count of 350,000/mm^3 (reference value 150,000–350,000/mm^3). *Based on this laboratory data,* a priority nursing action is to

    a. Encourage the client to walk
    b. Check the nasogastric drainage for occult (hidden) bleeding
    c. Check stools for occult (hidden) bleeding
    d. Monitor for infection or other signs of bone marrow depression

17. Which of the following statements is accurate about testing for occult blood in the feces?

   a. Red meat may cause false-negative results in the feces
   b. The test is useful as a screening test for cancer of the colon
   c. The stool specimen must be tested within 2–4 hr after collection
   d. Blue indicates a negative reaction for the presence of blood

▼ REFERENCES

Alhquist, D., et al. (1985). Fecal blood levels in health and disease: A study using Hemo-Quant. *New England Journal of Medicine, 312,* 1422–1428.

Berchtold, P., and McMillan, R. (1989). Therapy of chronic idiopathic thrombocytopenia in adults. *Blood, 74* (7), 2309–2315.

Burns, E.R., Goldberg, S.N., and Wenz, B. (1993). Paradoxic effect of multiple mild coagulation factor deficiencies on the prothrombin time and activated partial thromboplastin time. *American Journal of Clinical Pathology, 100 (2), 94–98.*

Collins, R., Scrimgeaur, A., Yusus, S., et al. (1988). Reduction in fatal pulmonary embolism and venous thrombosis by perioperative administration of subcutaneous heparin. *New England Journal of Medicine, 318* (1), 1162–1172.

Corbett, J.V. (1990). Monitoring anticoagulants: Use of INR and other tests. *California Nursing Review, 12* (2), 30.

Corbett, J.V., and Kenney, C. (1994). Anticoagulants during pregnancy. *MCN American Journal of Maternal Child Health Nursing, 20* (6), 56.

Cosico, J.N., and Rothlauf, E.B. (1992). Indications, management and patient education: Anticoagulant therapy during pregnancy. *MCN American Journal of Maternal Child Health Nursing, 17* (3), 130–135.

DeCherney, A.H., and Pernoll, M.L. (1994). *Current obstetric & gynecologic diagnosis & treatment* (8th ed.). Norwalk, CT: Appleton & Lange.

Eckman, M.H., Levine, H.J., and Pauker, S.G. (1993). Effect of laboratory variations in the prothrombin-time ratio on the results of anticoagulant therapy. *New England Journal of Medicine, 329,* 696–702.

Gillott, A., and Thomas, J. (1984). Clinical investigation involving the use of the haemonetic cell saver in elective and emergency vascular operations. *American Surgeon, 50* (11), 609–612.

Greaves, M. (1993). Anticoagulants in pregnancy. *Pharmacology Therapeutics*, 59, 311–327.

Griffin, J. (1986). The bleeding patient. *Nursing 86, 16* (6), 34–40.

Hansson, P.O., Eriksson, H., Eriksson, E., et al. (1994). Can laboratory testing improve screening strategies for deep vein thrombosis at an emergency unit? *Journal of Internal Medicine, 235,* 143–151.

Hickey, A. (1994). Catching deep vein thrombosis in time. *Nursing 94, 24* (10), 34–42.

Katzung, B. (1995). Basic and clinical pharmacology (6th ed.). Norwalk, CT: Appleton & Lange.

Krokosky, N., and Vanscoy, G. (1989). Running an anticoagulation clinic. *American Journal of Nursing, 89* (10), 1304–1306.

McGuire, P. (1985). Home therapy for children with hemophilia: Development, implementation and evaluation. *Syllabus of Abstracts for National Symposium on Nursing Research.* Stanford, CA: Department of Nursing, Stanford Hospital.

Mehler, E. (1994). Preparing your patient to use a fecal occult blood test. *Nursing 94, 24* (5), 32R.

National Heart, Lung and Blood Institute. (1989). *Indications for the use of red blood cells, platelets, and fresh frozen plasma.* Publ. No. 89–2974A. Bethesda: National Institutes of Health.

Nichols, W.L., and Bowie, E.J. (1993). Standardization of the prothrombin time for monitoring orally administered anticoagulant therapy with use of the international normalized ratio system. *Mayo Clinical Proceedings, 68,* 897–898.

Nolan, T.E., Smith, R.P., Devoe L.D. (1993). A rapid test for abruptio placentae: Evaluation of a d-dimer latex agglutination slide test. *American Journal of Obstetrics and Gynecology, 169,* 265–269.

Northrop, C. (1986). Look and look again. *Nursing 86, 16* (1), 43.

Ozawa, T., Domagalski, J., and Mammen, E. F. (1993). Determination of low-molecular-weight heparin by Heptest on the automated coagulation laboratory system. *American Journal of Clinical Pathology, 99,* 157–162.

Pierce, G.F. (1994). Hemophila A (Letter to editor). *New England Journal of Medicine, 350* (22), 1617.

Ravel, R. (1995). *Clinical laboratory medicine: Clinical application of laboratory data* (6th ed.). St. Louis: Mosby–Year Book.

Rizzoni, W., et al. (1988). Heparin-induced thrombocytopenia and thromboembolism in the postoperative period. *Surgery 103* (4), 470–476.

Rodney, W., and Ruggiero, C. (1985). The Coloscreen self-test for detection of fecal occult blood. *Journal of Family Practice, 21* (3), 200–204.

Samuel C., et al. (1989). Comparison of laboratory tests used for identification of the lupus anticoagulant. *American Journal of Hematology, 30* (4), 213–220.

Schuster, G., and Lewis, G. (1987). Clinical significance of hematuria in patients on anticoagulant therapy. *Journal of Urology, 137* (5), 923–925.

Schwartz, R.S. (1994). Treating chronic idiopathic thrombocytopenic purpura: A new application of an old treatment. *New England Journal of Medicine, 330* (22), 1609–1610.

Simonneau, G., Charbonnier, B., Decousus, H., et al. (1993). Subcutaneous low-molecular-weight heparin compared with continuous intravenous unfractionated heparin in the treatment of proximal deep vein thrombosis. *Archives of Internal Medicine, 153,* 1541–1546.

Vanscoy, G., and Gyi, F. (1988). A new era in warfarin therapy. *U.S.Pharmacist, 13* (4), H-24–H-30.

Weber, M.S. (1994). Thrombocytopenia. *American Journal of Nursing, 94* (11), 46.

Wilson, B. (1994). Enoxaparin and a new look at clot prevention. *MEDSURG Nursing, 3* (1), 66–67.

Wong, V., Cheng, C.H., and Chan, K.C. (1993). Fetal and neonatal outcome of exposure to anticoagulants during pregnancy. *American Journal of Medical Genetics, 45,* 17–21.

SEROLOGIC TESTS

- ABO Grouping
- Rh Factor
- Rh Antibody Titer Test
- Direct Antiglobulin (Coombs' Test) or RBC Antibody Screen
- Antibody Screening Test (Indirect Coombs)
- Hepatitis B Surface and e Antigens and Antibodies Against Hepatitis B Antigens and the Delta Agent
- Hepatitis A Tests: Anti-HAV, IgM, IgG
- Antibodies to Hepatitis C Virus
- Acquired Immunodeficiency Syndrome Tests: Antibodies for HIV
- Human T-Cell Lymphotropic Virus Types I and II
- Serologic Tests for Syphilis: VDRL and RPR, FTA-ABS and MHA-TP
- Infectious Mononucleosis
- Streptococcal Infections
- Rubella
- Toxoplasmosis
- Amebiasis
- Herpesvirus Family
- Cytomegalovirus Titers
- TORCH Screen
- Varicella-zoster Antibody Titer
- Fungal Antibodies: Histoplasmosis and Coccidioidomycosis
- Fungal Antigens
- Rickettsial Disease: Proteus OX-19, Proteus OX-2, and Proteus OX-K (Weil–Felix Reaction)

- C-Reactive Protein
- Complement Activity: C_3, C_4, and C_1 Esterase Inhibitor
- Antinuclear Antibodies
- Tests for Systemic Lupus Erythematosus
- Rheumatoid Factor
- Thyroid Antibodies

OBJECTIVES

1. Explain the basic procedures for serologic tests for blood bank, microbiologic, and immunologic procedures.
2. Describe the role of the nurse in the prevention and assessment of transfusion reactions due to ABO incompatibility.
3. Explain the rationale for the administration of Rh immunoglobulins.
4. Identify the most important nursing diagnoses when a client has a positive report for hepatitis B surface antigen (HBsAg) or for hepatitis A.
5. Describe the usefulness of the test for antibodies against human immunodeficiency virus (HIV) in prevention of the spread of acquired immunodeficiency syndrome (AIDS).
6. Describe what a client should be taught about the various serologic tests for syphilis (STS).
7. Describe the clinical usefulness of serologic tests for common bacterial, viral, fungal, and rickettsial diseases.
8. Describe the information that should be given to a woman of childbearing age who has a negative titer of rubella antibodies.
9. Explain why positive serologic tests or skin tests may not be indicative of an active infection.
10. Describe how C3 and C4, two components of the complement system, are altered by antigen–antibody reactions.
11. Describe how humoral antibodies, such as rheumatoid factor (RF) and antinuclear antibodies (ANA), are useful in assessing autoimmune disease.

The category of serologic tests is broad. It includes blood bank procedures (immunohematology), identification of antibodies against infectious diseases (microbiology), and studies of immune diseases (immunology). The basic principle underlying serologic tests is that a reaction between an antibody and antigen results in a recordable event. In some tests, the client's blood sample is mixed with an antigen to see if there are antibodies in the serum. In other tests, antibodies may be added to the blood sample to see if the antigen exists.

Serologic tests alone, however, are usually not specific enough to establish a diagnosis. For example, clients may have antibodies against an infectious agent, such as a fungus, but they may not have the disease when the test is administered. As another example, two clients may both have a high level of RF, which is a type of immunoglobulin. Yet one client has all the symptoms of rheumatoid arthritis, and the other has no symptoms. Likewise, some clients with syphilis may have what is termed a *seronegative* result, and some who do not have the disease have a *seropositive* result. This lack of total specificity is a common problem of older serologic tests because drugs, infections, and diseases such as carcinoma often cause unpredictable changes in immunologic response.

The first part of this chapter describes the techniques used in blood banking procedures. The blood types ABO demonstrate in a dramatic way the antigen–antibody basis for tests.

The second part of the chapter discusses the common serologic tests used in microbiology. (Specific microbiologic tests, such as cultures and microscopic examinations, are described in Chapter 16). Some serologic tests are only indirect tests for the presence of an organism, such as a virus, which may have many different antigens. Other tests can detect specific antibodies to a bacterial, viral, fungal, protozoan, or rickettsial antigen or antigens.

The last part of the chapter contains a discussion on the common serologic tests used to assess immunologic diseases such as systemic lupus erythematosus (SLE). Serologic testing in autoimmune diseases is rapidly becoming more common as researchers discover more about the antigen–antibody reactions that occur in these baffling diseases.

COMMON TECHNIQUES IN SEROLOGIC TESTING

Serologic testing is based on the fact that antigen–antibody reaction causes an observable event. From a nursing point of view, the exact testing technique is not of primary interest. Nonetheless, to understand the description of the test, nurses do need to be familiar with the general meaning of these techniques:

1. Agglutinations and titer levels
2. Complement fixation (CF)
3. Immunofluorescence antibody test (IFA)
4. Radioimmunoassay (RIA)
5. Enzyme immunoassay (EIA) and enzyme-linked immunosorbent assay (ELISA)
6. Immunoglobulin electrophoresis

Agglutination and Titer Levels

Agglutination, or clumping, which often occurs when antibodies attach to an antigen, is the most basic type of serologic testing. Cold agglutins and the Coombs' test are examples of an observable clumping of cells in the blood sample when there is a certain ratio of antibodies to antigens.

The serum is diluted with normal saline solution in graduated amounts. For many serologic tests, rather than reporting only agglutination (positive) or no agglutination (negative), the laboratory represents the results as a *titer,* which is the last dilution at which a reaction occurred. For example, the laboratory uses the standard dilutions in Table 14–1 to test for antibodies against streptolysin-O (ASO) that is produced by group A β-hemolytic streptococci. In the example in the table, the last dilution to cause a reaction was 1:170, which would be the titer reported. In essence, this finding means that the client's serum contained enough antibodies still to cause a reaction with the antigenic material when the serum was diluted 1:170.

One titer does not give as much information as do two titers separated by a time interval, because a *rise* in titer is more significant than any one high number. So, to catch a rise or fall, the timing of titers is very important. A fourfold increase in titer between an acute and a convalescent sample is usually necessary to confirm the presence of an infection. The time interval between acute and convalescent phase depends on the organism causing the disease.

Complement Fixation

Complement factors are a group of proteins in the bloodstream that enter into some antigen–antibody reactions. One or more of the constituents of complement (see the test for C3 and C4) can be consumed during an antibody–antigen reaction. Because the complement used in the reaction is fixed, it cannot be used again. The tests using complement fixation are hard to standardize, so the newer techniques IFA, RIA, and ELISA have become common. The now-outdated Wasserman test for syphilis is an example of a test using CF.

Immunofluorescence Antibody Tests

The IFA test can be direct or indirect. In the direct method, an antibody labeled with a fluorescent dye (fluorescein) is mixed with a sample of blood from the client. If an antigen is present, the antigen–antibody complex can be seen under a microscope with an ultraviolet light source. With the indirect method, the known antigen is

TABLE 14–1. TITER DILUTION CHART FOR ASO

1:60	Positive
1:85	Positive
1:120	Positive
1:170	Positive
1:240	Negative
1:340	
1:480	
1:680	
1:960	
1:1360	
1:2720	

ASO, anti-streptolysin O antibodies.

An antibody titer is reported as the last dilution that causes an antigen–antibody reaction, or agglutinization. Thus, in this example, the laboratory report would read "ASO titer 1:170." See text for further explanation.

mixed with the serum and any antigen–antibody complex is then mixed with fluorescein-labeled anti-immunoglobulin antibodies.

An example of a fluorescent type of test is the FTA-ABS for syphilis. *FTA* stands for *fluorescent treponemal antibody,* and *ABS* stands for a special absorption technique that helps eliminate some of the nonspecific antibodies that may also be stained with the fluorescent dye. Another example of an IFA discussed in this chapter is the IFA for toxoplasmosis. The IFA test can be falsely positive if the serum contains ANA. (See the ANA test at end of the chapter.)

Radioimmunoassay and Enzyme Immunoassay

The use of radioactive-tagged and enzyme-tagged substances is discussed in Chapter 1.

Immunoglobulin Electrophoresis

See Chapter 10 for a discussion of how γ-globulins can be separated into patterns on a graph. The specific identification of immunoglobulins supplements the information gained from serologic testing. IgM antibodies are indicative of an acute infection, and IgG antibodies are indicative of past exposure and probable immunity. (For examples, see the discussion on tests for rubella and hepatitis.)

IMMUNOHEMATOLOGIC TESTS

The tests performed on blood used for transfusions are often called *immunohematologic* rather than *serologic,* which is a broader term.

Screening Blood for Transfusions

Several routine laboratory tests are performed on a unit of donor blood (see Table 14–2). Nurses need to be up to date about these tests because clients are concerned about the safety of blood (Corbett, 1991). An alternative to transfusions with blood bank

TABLE 14–2 ROUTINE TESTS ON DONOR BLOOD

1. ABO typing
2. Rh factor and variations
3. Syphilis (VDRL)
4. Red cell antibody screen (Coombs' or direct antiglobulin)
5. Hepatitis B surface antigen (HBsAG)
6. Antibody to hepatitis B core antigen (anti-ABcAg)
7. Hepatitis C antibody (anti-HCV)
8. HIV antibody (AIDS tests by ELISA and Western blot)
9. HTLV-I (T-cell leukemia)
10. ALT (alanine aminotransferase, an enzyme for hepatitis)[a]

[a]See Chapter 12 for documentation for ALT.
Consult local blood banks for the most current information on screening tests.

blood is the use of an autologous blood recovery unit that recycles the client's blood lost in the surgical field. Disposable collection units are available to collect chest drainage for autotransfusion (Smith et al., 1995).

Blood banks take precautions to ensure that donor blood is as safe as possible to administer to a client and also that it is safe for the person to donate blood. For example, the donor must weigh at least 110 lb (50 kg) and have a hemoglobin (hgb) level of 13.5 g for men and 12.5 g for women. (See Chapter 2 on the measurement of hgb levels.) The donor must have a temperature no higher than 98.6°F (37°C), a heart rate of 50–100 beats per minute with no irregularities, and a blood pressure between 200/100 and 100/50 mm Hg. The blood bank physician may modify these guidelines depending on the individual situation. Overall, the donor must be in generally good health with no upper respiratory infections or allergies. Blood donations are not taken from people who have ever had hepatitis, malaria, jaundice, or a sexually transmitted disease. Pregnancy or a blood transfusion excludes donors for 6 months. Travel to other countries also excludes donors for 6 months. (Note that the incubation period for hepatitis B is 6 months.) Dental operations or tooth extraction in the 72 hr before the donation excludes a donor. (See Chapter 16 on how even minimal dental work can cause transient bacteria in the bloodstream [bacteremia].) Vaccines and some immunizations are other reasons for deferral (Kotwas et al., 1990).

Typing and Cross Matching of Blood

To type and cross match (T&C) blood, the laboratory needs at least 15–30 min to make sure that the donor unit of blood is compatible with the blood of the recipient. The client's blood type and Rh factor are determined so that a matching unit of blood can be taken from the blood bank. It is never safe to assume that any unit of A-positive blood can be given to any client with A-positive blood. So the cross match mixes a small sample of the two bloods to see if any clumping occurs. The full range of tests for a T&C are listed in Table 14–2.

Typing and Screening

If there is only a faint possibility that blood will be needed, the physician may order typing and screening (T&S) rather than cross matching. In a screening, the client's blood is tested, so that if blood is needed, the actual cross matching can be performed in a few minutes. The advantage of screening is that it does not tie up a unit of blood when the need is slight. For example, if two units of blood are typed and cross matched for a surgical client, those two units of blood cannot be used for another client until the operation is over and the blood is released for re–cross matching for another client.

Typing for Packed Cells

If a client needs red blood cells (RBCs) but not serum, the physician orders a unit of packed cells. A unit of packed RBCs contains only about one-fourth the amount of plasma as a unit of blood. T&C is as necessary for packed cells as it is for whole blood. Packed cells are now much more commonly used for blood transfusions than is whole blood. In this discussion, *blood transfusion* refers to either whole blood or packed cells.

Preparation of Client

There is no special preparation of a client for T&C or for T&S. For either procedure, the laboratory needs 10 mL of whole blood. Dextran, a plasma expander, should not be started before a T&C because it interferes with cross matching.

▼ ABO GROUPING

All humans have one of four blood types—A, B, AB, and O—which are genetically determined. Even though type A has subgroups, one generally speaks of only four types, the frequency of which is shown in Table 14–3 along with a description of the antigens and antibodies in each type. Besides the ABO grouping, which is the most important variable, the matching of donor and recipient must take into account many other factors.

Understanding the concept of the universal donor and recipient may help the nurse visualize, in a simple way, the importance of antibody–antigen response in immunologic testing. Type O blood is theoretically the universal donor because none of the principal antigens occur on the RBCs of people with type O blood. Type O blood does have antibodies against A and B, but in one unit of donor blood, the donor antibodies become so diluted in the plasma of the recipient that the antibodies are of minimal importance. In fact, in an emergency situation such as a disaster, health care personnel ask the blood bank to send O-negative packed cells so they are ready even before victims arrive at the hospital (McCormac, 1990). A person with AB blood has both A and B antigens on the RBCs, so the plasma contains no antibodies against A or B antigens. Thus people with AB blood are sometimes called universal recipients. It is interesting to note that a person born with one type of ABO antigens has the antibodies against the other antigens, even though the person has never had contact with the other types of blood. In contrast, a person with Rh negative blood does not have antibodies against the Rh factor until there is sensitization. (The Rh factor, which, like ABO types, is genetically determined, is discussed later in this chapter.)

TABLE 14–3. ABO BLOOD TYPING

Estimated Percentage of Population	Type	Description
46	O	No A or B antigens on RBCs. Antibodies against A and B antigens[a]
41	A	Antigen A on RBCs. Antibodies against B antigens
9	B	Antigen B on RBCs. Antibodies against A antigen
4	AB	Antigens A and B on RBCs. No antibodies against A or B antigens

[a]From birth, the person has the antibodies, even with no exposure to the antigens. In contrast, a person with Rh-negative blood does not have antibodies against the Rh factor until exposed to the factor.

Clients must *never* be given a type of blood that contains foreign A or B antigens. For example, a client with type A blood who is given a unit of type B blood would undergo a severe hemolytic reaction. The antibodies against the B antigen, which are present in the A client, attack the RBCs of the type B donor blood. The hemolysis of the RBCs causes the release, directly into the bloodstream, of free hemoglobin, which can be damaging to the renal tubules. The end result of a transfusion of incompatible blood may be renal failure and death.

▼ POSSIBLE NURSING DIAGNOSIS RELATED TO BLOOD TRANSFUSION

Risk for Injury Related to Complications of Blood Transfusion

In most institutions, at least two clinicians must check the client's nameband against the unit of blood to be administered. T&C is of no value if the blood is given to the wrong client. Not only the client's name but also the medical record number must match the identification number of the unit of blood. After the unit of blood is hung, the nurse's responsibility is to see that the blood is given correctly. Ravel (1995) noted that most transfusion-related problems are due to human error. (See Chapter 13 for a discussion of platelet transfusion and Chapter 2 for leukocyte replacement.) Special programs including on-line recording of transfusion history, have been designed to facilitate the administration, tracking, and documentation of blood products (Gonterman et al., 1994).

Assessing for Complications. The nurse must also be aware of the signs and symptoms of an adverse reaction to a blood transfusion. The most severe hemolytic reaction is due to donor-recipient ABO incompatibilities. Rh and other factors may also cause some hemolysis, but usually the reaction is not as pronounced as with ABO incompatibility. (See the next section on laboratory tests done after a hemolytic transfusion reaction.) Checking of vital signs before and during the blood transfusion is the basic nursing action. Also, running the blood slowly for the first 15 min minimizes the severity of a reaction, should it occur. Freedman et al. (1990) described the nurse's role in the detection and treatment of hemolytic transfusion reactions, as well as of other transfusion reactions, such as allergic reactions, febrile reactions, circulatory overload, and air embolism.

If a client begins to exhibit symptoms such as fever, chills, and low back pain, it is essential that the nurse not let the transfusion continue. Normal saline solution can be infused to keep the intravenous line patent when the unit of blood is discontinued.

The unfinished unit of blood must be sent back to the laboratory with a specimen of the client's blood for the laboratory to try to determine what caused the reaction. The client's blood and the donor's blood are re–cross matched to see if they are truly incompatible.

Because one of the dreaded complications of an incompatible blood transfusion is renal failure, the laboratory may want a urine specimen to check for the presence of hgb in the urine. Intake and output should be meticulously recorded, and all urine should be saved for laboratory examination for at least 24 hr.

The laboratory checks for free hgb in the plasma and, if needed, indirect bilirubin and haptoglobin, the presence of which helps confirm hemolysis. (See Chapter 11 for an explanation of why unconjugated bilirubin is elevated with hemolysis.) Haptoglobin is a serum glycoprotein the role of which is to bind free hgb released from destroyed RBCs. Evidently, haptoglobin is diminished in severe hemolysis because it cannot be replaced quickly enough. Reference values for haptoglobin vary considerably, depending on the methods of evaluation used. A 2-min slide test is available.

Assessing for and Preventing Bacterial Contamination. In addition to the tests for hemolysis, the laboratory may also perform a blood culture from the donor bag of blood. (See Chapter 16 on culture reports from blood specimens.) Blood at room temperature becomes an attractive culture medium for bacteria. Nursing actions to prevent sepsis from blood transfusions include the aseptic technique for starting the transfusion, hanging the blood within 30 min after it is taken from the blood bank, and ensuring that the entire unit is transfused within 2–4 hr.

▼ RH FACTOR

The Rh factor is named after the rhesus monkey used in the original research on this factor. Actually, several different Rh factors have been identified, but usually only the main factor is clinically significant. The Rh factor, like the ABO types, is genetically determined.

There are two different nomenclatures for the Rh factors. In the Weiner system the main Rh factor is Rh0. In the Fisher–Rose system, the main Rh factor is *D*. In the literature, Rh0 or *D* is often called the *Rh factor*. In this discussion, the term *Rh factor* specifies the main factor involved when one speaks of Rh positive or Rh negative blood. Table 14–4 provides a description of Rh positive and Rh negative.

Normally, a person with Rh negative blood does not have any antibodies against the Rh factor. An Rh negative male can become sensitized (i.e., antibodies develop against the Rh factor) by transfusion with Rh positive blood. In an Rh negative female antibodies can develop against the Rh factor not only through blood transfusions with Rh positive factors but also through a pregnancy in which the fetus is Rh positive. Once an Rh negative person has antibodies against the Rh factor, another transfusion with Rh positive blood, or another pregnancy with an Rh positive fetus, can have serious consequences.

TABLE 14–4. Rh FACTOR

Estimated Percentage of Population	Type	Description
85–90	Rh+	Rh antigen on RBCs. No antibodies against Rh factor
10–15	Rh−	No Rh antigen on RBCs. Develops antibodies against Rh factor if sensitized by transfusion of Rh positive blood. Also, the pregnant woman can be sensitized by an Rh positive infant.

Some sources note up to 20% of population may be Rh negative (Ravel, 1995).

Rh Factor in Blood Transfusions

To keep antibodies against the Rh factor from developing in a person with Rh negative blood, the Rh negative person is given only Rh negative blood. Hence, Rh typing is one of the components of cross matching. The administration of Rh positive blood to an Rh negative person who has antibodies against the Rh factor (i.e., who is sensitized) causes a hemolytic reaction because the person's antibodies attack the RBCs that contain the Rh factor. The severity of this hemolytic reaction is usually not as great as it is in ABO incompatibility, but it is nevertheless to be avoided. (See the nursing implications for when a client has any kind of transfusion reaction.)

Rh Factor in Pregnancy

An Rh negative mother and an Rh positive father can produce either an Rh negative or an Rh positive baby, depending on the gene passed from the father. Laboratory tests can be performed to determine if the Rh positive father has either two positive genes for Rh or one positive and one negative. (Note that an Rh positive mother can carry an Rh negative fetus without any Rh-related problem.)

A problem occurs when an Rh negative mother is carrying an Rh positive child. Hemolytic disease of the newborn, formerly called *erythroblastosis fetalis,* occurs when an Rh negative mother produces antibodies against the Rh positive RBCs of her fetus. With the first pregnancy, the fetus is usually not affected because the mother has not had time to build antibodies against the Rh factor. However, at the time of the infant's separation from the placenta (a full-term birth or an abortion), some of the RBCs from the fetus enter the mother's general circulation and trigger the production of antibodies against the Rh factor. Subsequent pregnancies with another Rh positive fetus may present problems because the woman's serum is now sensitized against Rh positive antigens.

▼ POSSIBLE NURSING DIAGNOSIS RELATED TO THE Rh FACTOR

Knowledge Deficit Related to the Use of Rh Immunoglobulins

About 13% of all Rh negative mothers become sensitized (i.e., antibodies develop against the Rh factor) by their first pregnancy with an Rh positive fetus. If the woman is not immunized by the administration of Rh immunoglobulins, each subsequent pregnancy with an Rh positive fetus incurs a further 13% risk of starting antibody production. The use of Rh immunoglobulins is based on the principle of passive immunity. Because the mother has been given antibodies against the Rh factor, her body is not stimulated to begin active production of antibodies against the Rh factor.

Nurses who work with women in the childbearing years should have a good understanding of the Rh factor so that they can help these women understand the possible implications in relation to pregnancy. The laws of some states make it mandatory that any woman whose blood is typed must be told the results of the Rh factor.

▼ Rh ANTIBODY TITER TEST

The Rh antibody titer test is used to monitor the course of an Rh negative woman who is carrying an Rh positive fetus. If the mother is in a second pregnancy and did not receive Rh0 (D) immunoglobulin (RhoGAM) after a first pregnancy or abortion, the rise of the titer helps determine the need for medical intervention, such as exchange transfusions or an early delivery.

Preparation of Client and Collection of Sample

The laboratory needs 10 mL of blood. This test may also be performed on a sample of cord blood.

REFERENCE VALUES FOR RH TITER

A normal Rh antibody titer is negative. A rising titer may indicate the need for immediate medical intervention to prevent serious damage to the fetus or newborn. (See Chapter 28 on amniocentesis for titers of 1:16 or greater.)

▼ DIRECT ANTIGLOBULIN (COOMBS' TEST) OR RBC ANTIBODY SCREEN

In certain types of sensitization, such as to the Rh factor, the erythrocytes become coated with antibodies or immunoglobulins. The Coombs' test is used as a screening test to detect whether immunoglobulins have become attached to the RBCs.

The test is referred to as a direct antiglobulin test (as opposed to the indirect or antibody screening test discussed next), because the RBCs are tested without any intervening manipulations. A sample of the client's blood is mixed with Coombs' serum, which is a rabbit serum that has antibodies against human globulins. If the client's RBCs are coated with immunoglobulins, agglutination occurs. The Coombs' test is performed for the following reasons:

1. To screen blood for cross matching. If a client's erythrocytes have been exposed to incompatible blood, the erythrocytes are coated with an antibody or globulin complex.
2. To check for hemolytic transfusion reactions.
3. To assess hemolytic disease of the newborn. In hemolytic disease of the newborn, the antibodies from a sensitized Rh negative mother cross the placenta and coat the fetal red cells. (See Chapter 28 on amniocentesis.)

Other factors may also cause the client's RBCs to be coated with immunoglobulins. For example, many drugs, as well as autoimmune diseases that cause hemolytic anemia, may cause a positive Coombs' reaction. If necessary, further testing can be completed to identify the specific immunoglobulins present. (See Chapter 10 on immunoglobulin testing.)

Preparation of Client and Collection of Sample

In the newborn, the blood sample is taken directly from the umbilical cord. In children and adults, a venous sample is used. This test is routine for one aspect of T&C, which requires 10 mL.

REFERENCE VALUES FOR COOMBS' TEST

The Coombs' test should be negative. A positive test indicates that some type of globulin is coating the RBCs.

▼ ANTIBODY SCREENING TEST (INDIRECT COOMBS')

An antibody screen is used to detect Rh antibodies in maternal serum. This test used to be called the *indirect* Coombs' because the serum is subjected to several different conditions to detect various antibodies. The indirect Coombs' should be thought of as a laboratory technique rather than an actual test (Ravel, 1995). If there is a positive result from the antibody screening, the laboratory performs more tests to identify the specific antibodies. This test is also performed as part of a cross match.

Preparation of Client and Collection of Sample

The laboratory should be consulted for specific instructions.

REFERENCE VALUE FOR ANTIBODY SCREEN

The antibody screening test should be negative.

MICROBIOLOGIC SEROLOGIC TESTS

The tests in this section are used for various types of diseases with infectious agents. Table 14–5 provides an overview.

Serologic Tests for Hepatitis

The several different forms of viral hepatitis are designated as hepatitis A (formerly called *infectious hepatitis*), hepatitis B (formerly called *serum hepatitis*), and hepatitis C (formerly called *non-A non-B hepatitis*). Hepatitis D, caused by the delta virus,

TABLE 14–5. COMMON SEROLOGIC TESTS USED IN MICROBIOLOGY

Test	Organism	Remarks
VDRL RPR FTA-ABS MHA-TP	*Treponema pallidum,* which causes syphilis	Confirming tests are performed if screening tests are positive
HBsAg	Hepatitis B virus (formerly called serum hepatitis)	Can also measure antibodies against HBsAg and other antigens
Anti-HAV	Hepatitis A virus (formerly called infectious hepatitis)	See Table 14–6 for all tests for hepatitis A and B
Anti-HCV	Hepatitis C virus	Useful in blood screening
HIV antibodies and antigen	Virus associated with AIDS	See text and current literature for update
Cold agglutinins	Eaton agent of pleuropneumonia-like organism (PPLO) may cause atypical pneumonia	Positive in some cases, not all
HSV	Herpes simplex virus	Not used routinely. See Chapter 16 for other tests
CMV	Cytomegalovirus	Problematic in pregnancy and for immuno-suppressed clients
HAT Monospot	Epstein-Barr virus of infectious mononucleosis	Also see WBC with differential in Chapter 2
ASO Anti-DNase-B Streptozyme test	Group A β-hemolytic streptococci	Measures antibodies *after* an acute infection with streptococci. Not useful during initial infectious stage
Rubella titer	Rubella virus (3-day measles)	Even a low antibody titer probably indicates immunity
TPM or Toxo	*Toxoplasma gondii,* a protozoan that causes toxoplasmosis	Most tests are indirect measurements of the protozoan
Hemagglutination for amebiasis	*Entamoeba histolytica* (causes amebic dysentery and hepatic abscess)	Stool cultures also performed (see Chapter 16)
Fungus antibody tests	Histoplasmosis Coccidioidomycosis	Cultures also performed (see Chapter 16)

Note: A TORCH screen includes *t*oxoplasmosis, others such as syphilis or hepatitis, *r*ubella, *c*ytomegalovirus, and *h*erpes.

appears as a coinfection with hepatitis B. Hepatitis E, a type of enteric hepatitis, has only been recently identified and is more common in countries with poor sanitation (Gurevich, 1993a). Clinical laboratory tests for hepatitis E and other forms of non A-non B hepatitis are not yet available but are being developed (Ravel, 1995). Table 14–6 describes a wide array of tests used to detect hepatitis.

▼ HEPATITIS B SURFACE AND e ANTIGENS AND ANTIBODIES AGAINST HEPATITIS B ANTIGENS AND THE DELTA AGENT

The virus that causes hepatitis B was discovered in 1965 in an Australian man. It was originally named the *Australian antigen,* and early laboratory tests were called HAA, for hepatitis Australian antigen. The commonly used test now is called *hepatitis B surface antigen* (HBsAg). Because a typical virus has many different antigens, a surface antigen is but one component of the hepatitis B virus (HBV). Numerous tests are now available to identify the hepatitis B antigens and antibodies (Table 14–6).

TABLE 14–6. TESTS USED TO DIAGNOSE HEPATITIS A, HEPATITIS B, AND HEPATITIS C

Name of Test	Explanation
Anti-hepatitis A virus (anti-HAV) IgM IgG	Measures antibodies to the hepatitis A virus. Antibodies of IgM type indicate *current* infection, whereas IgG antibodies represent past infection and probable immunity. Used to diagnose or rule out hepatitis A in a suspected case of hepatitis.
Hepatitis B surface antigen (HBsAg)	Measures surface antigen of hepatitis B virus. Indicates infection with hepatitis B and carrier state if it persists. Used to screen potential blood donors and to diagnose or rule out hepatitis B in suspected cases of hepatitis.
Hepatitis B core antigen (HBcAg)	Measures a core antigen of hepatitis B virus in liver cells, not serum. Used only for research.
Hepatitis B e antigen (HBeAg)	Measures the e antigen of the hepatitis B virus. Correlates well with high titers of the virus, so used to evaluate infectiousness, particularly in chronic states.
Anti-HbsAg	Measures antibodies to hepatitis B surface antigen. Demonstrates immunity to hepatitis B virus, except for a few unusual subtypes. Used to demonstrate if vaccine is needed for person at risk for hepatitis B.
Anti-HBcAg IgM IgG	Measures antibodies to the core antigen of hepatitis B. Appears in the serum earlier than anti-HBsAg, so may be used to diagnose hepatitis B in the "window" or convalescent state. IgM indicates *current* infection. IgG indicates past infection and probably immunity. Also can demonstrate if vaccine is needed for person in high-risk group.
Anti-HBeAg	Measures antibodies to the e antigen of hepatitis B virus. Appears late in infection and may be an index of infectivity. May be too weak to be detected.
Antibody to delta antigen (anti-delta) (Delta antibody)	Suggests recent infection or carrier for a defective virus active only in the presence of hepatitis B.
Hepatitis C antibodies (Anti-HCV)	Measures antibodies to the hepatitis C virus, which was formerly known as one type of non-A non-B hepatitis.

Note: See Chapter 10 for discussion on IgM antibodies, which indicate active infection, and IgG antibodies, which indicate prior infections.

The detection of HBsAg in a client's serum means either that the client is ill with the disease or is a carrier. In either case, the blood is a possible source of infection for other people. Most people do not carry the virus after the disease is over, but 5–15% do become carriers (Ravel, 1995). Hepatitis B is spread primarily by blood and body secretions. Because the incubation period is 50–180 days, a client who gets hepatitis B from a blood transfusion may not show symptoms for as long as 6 months. Thus no one who has undergone a blood transfusion is permitted to donate blood for 6 months. Tests of HBsAg have become very useful in screening blood donors, many of whom are not aware they are carriers.

In addition to testing for the presence of HBsAg, the laboratory can also test for antibodies against the hepatitis B antigens. A person who has antibodies against HBsAg is presumed to be immune to hepatitis B, but not necessarily to other types of hepatitis. Table 14–6 summarizes information about the usefulness of three different antibody tests, including antibodies to the delta agent, a defective RNA virus that seems to infect only people who already have HBV infection.

Preparation of Client and Collection of Sample

The laboratory uses venous blood to test for hepatitis B. The exact amount needed depends on the test used.

REFERENCE VALUES FOR HEPATITIS B

A positive HBsAg test indicates either active hepatitis or a carrier state. In either case, the client's blood may be a source of infection.

A positive antibody titer to HBsAg presumably indicates immunity to hepatitis B

Negative antigen and antibody tests for HBsAg indicate the client is susceptible to hepatitis B.

▼ POSSIBLE NURSING DIAGNOSES RELATED TO POSITIVE TEST FOR HEPATITIS B

Knowledge Deficit Related to Spread of Infection

Clients who are carriers of HBV must be informed of their risk to others through blood or contact with body secretions such as semen. Printed information on safe sexual practices should be made available. Information about safe sex has become readily available since the AIDS epidemic began (Barrick, 1990). Although universal precautions are standard practice in all clinical settings and dental offices, clients should be told to notify health care workers

(*continued*)

▼ POSSIBLE NURSING DIAGNOSES RELATED TO POSITIVE TEST FOR HEPATITIS B (*continued*)

about the positive test for hepatitis B if these workers will be handling the client's blood.

Of particular concern is the spread of hepatitis B to newborns, which usually occurs on entry into the birth canal. The use of hepatitis B immune globulin (HBIG), which gives immediate passive immunity, and hepatitis B vaccine, which promotes active immunity, is usually effective in protecting the babies of mothers who are carriers of HBV.

Knowledge Deficit Related to Prevention of Disease

γ-Globulin may lessen the severity of hepatitis, but only a vaccine totally prevents the disease. The first vaccine for hepatitis B, made from pooled donors, was marketed in 1981. Now the vaccine is produced by DNA recombinant technology and is about 90% effective (Katzung, 1995). After completion of the three injections, antibody titers may be performed to validate the effectiveness of the vaccine. The vaccine was first used for groups at high risk such as homosexuals, abusers of intravenous drugs and their sexual partners, and health care workers who might be contaminated with blood. One of the most effective provisions of the 1992 regulations on protecting health care workers from blood-borne pathogens was the requirement that free HBV vaccine be made available to all health care employees who are at risk for exposure to hepatitis B (Kolodner, 1993).

Immunization of all newborns is now recommended because the estimated cost of universal use of the vaccine is less than 5% lifetime risk of infection (Gurevich, 1993b). Health care practitioners are also urging all adolescents to have vaccinations before beginning sexual activity. Widespread use of the vaccine can considerably reduce or even eliminate the transmission of hepatitis B, so nurses need to help educate the public on this issue.

Activity Intolerance Related to Extreme Fatigue

See the sections on hepatitis A and on bilirubin levels (Chapter 11) and transaminase levels (Chapter 12) for more information on other nursing diagnoses for clients with hepatitis. Hepatitis B tends to be more severe than hepatitis A, and chronic hepatitis does occur. Interferon treatment may be used if the elevated liver enzymes persist for more than 6 months.

▼ HEPATITIS A TESTS: ANTI-HAV, IgM, IgG

Hepatitis A is spread primarily by the oral–fecal route. It is often spread by food handlers or by means of sexual contact. The incubation period is about 15–45 days, which is much shorter than the 50–180 days for hepatitis B. There is no evidence of progression to chronic liver disease. Clinical features cannot be used to differentiate hepatitis A from other types of hepatitis. As noted in Table 14–6, there are two tests for hepatitis A and many more for hepatitis B, as well as one for hepatitis C.

Preparation of Client and Collection of Sample

The laboratory needs 2 mL of serum in a serum separator tube (SST).

REFERENCE VALUES FOR HEPATITIS A

A positive test for hepatitis A antibodies of the IgM type is strong evidence of acute infection with the virus. Antibodies of the IgG type are indicative of past exposure to hepatitis A. About 40–50% of adults have IgG antibodies against hepatitis A (Ravel, 1995).

▼ POSSIBLE NURSING DIAGNOSES RELATED TO POSITIVE HEPATITIS A TEST

Knowledge Deficit Related to Spread of Disease

If the test indicates acute infection, the most important nursing implication is to initiate enteric precautions so that feces-to-mouth transmission of the virus does not occur. The person should not be allowed to handle or prepare any food for others. The disease can also be transmitted by means of sexual contact. In a hospital, a patient with poor hygiene may need a private room (Marx, 1993).

Risk for Injury Related to γ-Globulin Injections

If there is a possibility that a client with an infection may have infected others by food handling or by intimate contact, the contacts may be offered γ-globulin. γ-Globulin (Gamastan) is also recommended for people who plan to travel in areas where hepatitis A is common. γ-Globulin, which can be given up to 2 weeks after exposure, does not prevent the disease, but it may lessen the severity. The immune serum globulin against hepatitis A comes from human sources. The product information sheet gives the recommended dosages based on weight. Note that anaphylactic reactions, although very rare, can occur. Vaccines for hepatitis A are not yet available.

Activity Intolerance Related to Extreme Fatigue

There is no drug to cure hepatitis; the mainstays of treatment are rest and a diet that promotes liver regeneration. (For other nursing diagnoses, see bilirubin levels (Chapter 11) and transaminase levels (Chapter 12), which are used to monitor the progress of the client.)

▼ ANTIBODIES TO HEPATITIS C VIRUS

In the late 1980s, researchers cloned a protein associated with the hepatitis C virus (HCV). This protein was used to develop a test to detect antibodies to HCV (anti-HCV) in the blood. This was the first time a viral genome was used to develop a serologic assay without actually first isolating the agent. Studies revealed that the predominant virus for non-A non-B transfusion hepatitis was this C virus, which could be detected with the antibody test (Alter et al., 1989). By May 1990, the United States Food and Drug Administration (FDA) approved the use of test kits to detect anti-HVC, and the test became part of the routine screen of donor blood (see Table 14–2). The technique for the test was improved in 1992, so fewer false-negative results are obtained. Hepatitis C was found in some immune globulin products, but since May, 1994, all these products should not pose a risk for HCV infection (FDA, 1994).

Some clients with HCV infection may have an elevated alanine aminotransferase (ALT) but a negative test for anti-HCV. In these clients a diagnosis of hepatitis C is possible with the use of the nucleic probe and the polymerase chain reaction (see Chapter 1 on this technique).

Preparation of Patient and Collection of Sample

The laboratory needs 1 mL of serum.

REFERENCE VALUES FOR ANTI-HVC
Negative titer

Clinical Significance. Many clients with hepatitis C do not have jaundice so the clue to diagnosis may be an elevated ALT level. The clinical signs and symptoms of hepatitis C are similar to those of hepatitis B but less severe. However, progression to chronic hepatitis and cirrhosis is more frequent with hepatitis C (Ravel, 1995). Hepatitis C, like hepatitis B, is associated with the development of liver cancer. Clients with chronic hepatitis C may benefit from interferon treatment (Gurevich, 1993b).

▼ POSSIBLE NURSING DIAGNOSES RELATED TO POSITIVE ANTI-HCV TEST

Knowledge Deficit Related to Prevention of Disease

At present, the most commonly recognized risk factors for HCV infection are use of contaminated needles, history of blood transfusions, hemodialysis, and health care employment. Sexual spread of the disease and transmission to the newborn are relatively uncommon. No vaccine is available, so prevention involves avoiding contaminated blood and blood products. The American Liver Foundation, at 1-(800)223-0179, has excellent information for patient education about hepatitis C and for other types of hepatitis.

▼ ACQUIRED IMMUNODEFICIENCY SYNDROME TESTS: ANTIBODIES FOR HIV

Since the beginning of the AIDS epidemic, much research has been centered on studying the effects of HIV-1, which used to be called a lymphadenopathy-associated virus (LAV) or a human T-cell lymphotropic virus (HTLV type III).

Until 1988 only two types of tests were used to detect HIV-1 antibodies: a screening test performed with ELISA, and confirmation by the Western blot test, which uses electrophoresis, a process discussed in Chapter 10, to separate out component proteins of the virus. These proteins are transferred or blotted to a support medium. If antibodies to these specific viral proteins are present in the client's serum, mixing the medium with a sample of the client's serum causes a reaction. In 1989, the FDA licensed a latex agglutination test for HIV-1 antibodies that can give results in 5 min. This was the first test to use a protein engineered by DNA technology. The test does not replace the ELISA, but it can be used in situations in which there is not full laboratory support. Although not originally approved for home use, the test may soon be purchased for use by the general public. The reader is encouraged to talk with laboratory personnel and to consult the most current literature to determine the validity and reliability of various tests for HIV-1 and for other possible types of HIV. At present, a version of the Western blot remains the standard as the confirming test for HIV. The time between exposure to HIV and the appearance of antibodies is probably quite variable; a range of 12 days to 5 years is reported in the literature. Ravel (1995) noted that seroconversion usually occurs 6–10 weeks after exposure.

Other tests for HIV identify specific proteins or antigens such as P24, a core protein, or GP 41, a glycoprotein on the envelope of the virus. Viral antigens may also be identified by nucleic acid probes and polymerase chain reaction (PCR) amplification. The sensitivity of PCR for HIV-1 appears to be about 40–60% in the first 1 to 2 weeks of life and up to 98% by 3 months of age (Ravel, 1995).

Cultures of HIV-1 may be the only method to confirm infection in the first 2–3 weeks after exposure. These tests are available in only a few laboratories at research institutions. (See Chapter 2 on CD4 lymphocyte counts, which are used to monitor HIV progression.)

Blood banks began using the test for antibodies against HTLV-III or HIV in 1985. The use of this screening test dramatically reduced the risk of transmission of AIDS by means of blood transfusions. Also in 1985, the U.S. Public Health Service announced establishment of alternative sites for antibody testing so clients at high risk for AIDS could undergo the test without going to a blood bank (Mason, 1985). Groups at high risk included male homosexuals, users of intravenous drugs, and people with hemophilia. The risk for people with hemophilia is reduced now because of the screening test, but an estimated 20,000 people with hemophilia already had positive serologic results (Helquist, 1986). The sexual contacts of people with hemophilia with the antibodies are also likely to develop antibodies (Jason, 1986). Although heterosexual transmission is less likely than transmission through male homosexual activity, transmission of the AIDS virus is possible from men to women and vice versa (Lederman, 1986). Although male-to-female transmission has been known for many years, many women with HIV do not receive an early diagnosis because they do not consider themselves at risk. Specific guidelines (Sipes, 1995) are available to assess for HIV in women. Besides targeting groups of people at high risk, prevention must target *high-risk behaviors,* because adolescents are being affected by the epidemic (Nelson, 1995).

The establishment of test centers raised many legal and ethical issues, which are still being debated. Counseling after an HIV test is recommended by the Centers for Disease Control (CDC) and is mandated by law in some states. Killian (1990) noted that more and more nurses are becoming involved in posttest counseling, and therefore to reduce the risk of liability, nurses must keep in mind the three basic principles of *completeness, consistency,* and *confidentiality.* Nurses must constantly read current literature to provide clients with information in accord with the prevailing standards of care. For example, studies are ongoing regarding the benefits of zidovudine during pregnancy and delivery (Boyer et al., 1994). Nurses need to keep up to date about the use of this drug and other antiviral agents used in pregnancy so that they can help explain the choices to pregnant women. The hope remains that it is possible to slow the spread of a deadly epidemic to the next generation (Corbett and Kenney, 1995).

Preparation of Client and Collection of Sample

A test for HIV antibodies requires 5 mL of clotted blood. Clients may refuse HIV tests (Kirton, 1994). The client must give written consent for the test, and the clinician providing the pretest counseling must sign the form. All results are confidential. Check for specific laboratory procedures and the latest legal requirements.

REFERENCE VALUES FOR HIV ANTIBODIES
Negative for antibodies to HIV

▼ POSSIBLE NURSING DIAGNOSIS RELATED TO POSITIVE HIV TEST

Altered Health Maintenance Related to a Positive HIV Test

In addition to psychological counseling, clients who have positive HIV tests need the most current information on drug therapy available to them, including participation in clinical trials for new promising drug therapy. Studies continue on subjects who, without treatment, have no symptoms for many years after documented HIV-1 infection (Cao et al., 1995). To maintain health, clients also need concrete information on the importance of good nutrition and control of stress. Information about ways to express sexual needs without endangering others is important in helping the client maintain a balanced life.

Morrison (1986) noted that the care of clients with AIDS is nursing's special challenge, and hence the *California Nurse* devoted an entire issue to this challenge at a time when some were unaware of the magnitude of the epidemic. Nurses continue to be on the forefront helping both clients with positive HIV tests and those with AIDS lead lives as fulfilling and productive as possible. Maybe what is needed most when a client has a positive HIV test are positive-thinking nurses who are unsurpassed in giving compassionate and competent care to all.

▼ HUMAN T-CELL LYMPHOTROPIC VIRUS TYPES I AND II

HTLV-I is a distinct retrovirus associated with adult T-cell leukemia. It has also been associated with tropical spastic paraparesis. Although distantly related to HIV, which used to be called HTLV-III, HTLV-I does not cause immunodeficiency syndrome. In 1989, the FDA approved three EIA test kits for use in screening blood supplies for HTLV-I. The tests for HTLV-I may also detect HTLV-II, a closely related retrovirus. However, some HTLV-II is missed, so several new ELISA tests can be used. A nucleic probe with PCR is the best way to differentiate the two types (Ravel, 1995).

▼ SEROLOGIC TESTS FOR SYPHILIS

Except for the common cold and flu, sexually transmitted diseases are the most common infectious diseases in the United States. Although chlamydia and herpes infections and gonorrhea are more common than syphilis, syphilis is the more dangerous if left undetected and thus untreated. (See Chapter 16 for the tests for gonorrhea and chlamydia and herpes infections.)

Although the spirochete, *Treponema pallidum,* that causes syphilis may occasionally be identified from a syphilitic sore, or chancre, syphilis is more commonly diagnosed with a serologic test. Testing for syphilis may be divided into tests for screening and those for a confirmation of a positive screening test. The Venereal Disease Research Laboratories (VDRL) or rapid plasma reagin (RPR) are screening tests, whereas the FTA-ABS and the microhemagglutination (MHA) are confirmatory tests for syphilis. The Wassermann test, which used a complement fixation technique, was the first serologic test for syphilis, but it is no longer used.

Dark-field Examination

A small amount of serum expressed from the base of a lesion is examined under a microscope. A dose of penicillin renders the dark-field useless.

VDRL and RPR

The VDRL is named for the research laboratory that perfected this flocculation test for syphilis. The test measures a globulin complex called *reagin* that appears early in the course of syphilis. If the globulin complex reagin is present, an aggregation occurs that can be reported as either negative, weakly reactive, or reactive. The RPR uses the VDRL antigen, but it adds some carbon particles so that the flocculation can be seen on a plastic card.

The VDRL and variations of it are indirect tests for syphilis because they are tests for a reaction to a globulin, not to the spirochete itself. A person who has just contracted syphilis may not have had time to build up antibodies against *T pallidum,* so these tests usually become positive 3–4 weeks after exposure. Because the screening tests react to abnormal globulins, other diseases, such as malaria, other infections, malignant tumors, and some connective tissue disorders, may cause false-positive reactions.

FTA-ABS and MHA-TP

The FTA-ABS may be used to confirm an infection with the spirochete that causes syphilis. It tests for the specific antibodies against *T pallidum.* The laboratory prepares a slide and stains it to make the antibodies appear yellow-green under an ultraviolet microscope. Technical difficulties are involved in the test, and false positives can occur. Another confirming test is the MHA for *T pallidum* (MHA-TP) test. The MHA-TP may be substituted for the FTA-ABS in some situations to confirm the diagnosis of syphilis. The MHA-TP is easier to perform and costs less than the FTA-ABS.

Preparation of Client and Collection of Sample

The laboratory uses 4 mL of venous blood for STS. Alcohol may interfere with some tests. Fasting is usually not required but is preferred by some laboratories. A premarital test for syphilis may be required by state law if the woman is younger than 50 years or has not had a hysterectomy. However, many states no longer mandate premarital testing.

REFERENCE VALUES FOR STS

These tests should be negative.

Note that various conditions may cause false-positives, as explained in the text. Also note that the tests are most strongly positive 4–6 weeks after exposure.

▼ POSSIBLE NURSING DIAGNOSIS RELATED TO POSITIVE SEROLOGIC TEST FOR SYPHILIS

Knowledge Deficit Related to Need for Screening and Follow-up with Sexual Contacts

If not detected in the early stages, syphilis may eventually spread, causing severe neurologic problems, blindness, and even death. The treatment of syphilis is extremely easy: penicillin by means of injection. Other antibiotics are used if the client is allergic to penicillin.

As a communicable disease, syphilis must be reported to the public health department either by the physician or through the laboratory (Nettina, 1990). Public health departments have staffs who follow up with the sexual contacts of the client who has a positive STS. Clinicians unsure of local reporting requirements should seek advice from local health departments or state sexually transmitted disease programs (Pigg, 1994). Nurses may take an active role in educating the public about the importance of screening people who may have been exposed to the disease. Nurses working with clients who have a positive STS can help impress on them the importance of early detection and early treatment of their sexual partners and the need for safe sex. Nurses must be nonjudgmental in their approach.

Because syphilis can be passed to a fetus, it is extremely important that a pregnant woman be treated for syphilis. (See Chapter 16 for information about other sexually transmitted diseases and pregnancy.) A nurse working in a prenatal clinic can explain to clients why an STS is done in early pregnancy. Screening maternal blood at delivery is also important and may be more effective than screening cord serum (Stepanuk, 1994).

▼ INFECTIOUS MONONUCLEOSIS

Heterophil Antibody Titer

The heterophil antibody titer (HAT) is a test for infectious mononucleosis, a viral disease. The word *heterophil* refers to an affinity for more than one group or species. Normally humans do not have antibodies against the RBCs of sheep, but clients with infectious mononucleosis do develop antibodies that agglutinate the RBCs of sheep.

The test, however, is not specifically diagnostic, because other factors may also cause an increase in heterophil antibodies. For example, allergic reactions, such as serum sickness, cause an increased HAT. Tests to confirm infectious mononucleosis include testing for the Epstein-Barr nuclear antigen (EBNA) as well as for antibodies to the viral capsid antigen (VCA). These antibodies can be identified as either IgG or IgM (see Chapter 10).

Diagnostic Kits for Infectious Mononucleosis

Spot tests for infectious mononucleosis use a saline suspension of antigen derived from RBCs of horses. The mixture of the test material with a drop of the client's serum causes a coarse granulation if the client has infectious mononucleosis. The spot tests are rapid, specific, and sensitive as screening tests, and they are valuable in supporting a clinical diagnosis of infectious mononucleosis. Yet they do not positively identify the Epstein-Barr virus of infectious mononucleosis, and titers may be needed, as discussed earlier. Other criteria for diagnosing infectious mononucleosis include lymphocytosis and the presence of atypical lymphocytes in the serum (see Chapter 2 for a discussion of lymphocytes as part of a differential white blood cell (WBC) count).

Preparation of Client and Collection of Sample

The screening tests require 1–2 mL of blood. A WBC count with differential is also ordered.

▼ NURSING DIAGNOSIS FOR A POSITIVE HAT OR SPOT TEST

Activity Intolerance Related to Fatigue

Nursing care for clients with infectious mononucleosis includes providing rest and other general measures to help them overcome a viral infection. There is no drug therapy for the disease. Although infectious mononucleosis is sometimes called the *kissing disease,* the exact mode of transmission is unknown. Isolation is not necessary. Many people have antibody titers against the Epstein–Barr virus. Transaminase levels (Chapter 12) and bilirubin levels (Chapter 11) are used to assess the degree of liver dysfunction.

▼ STREPTOCOCCAL INFECTIONS

Definition and Purpose

Three tests are used to identify a recent infection with group A β-hemolytic streptococci:

1. Anti-streptolysin-O (ASO)
2. Anti-streptodornase-B or anti-deoxyribonuclease-B (anti-DNase-B)
3. Streptozyme test

Group A β-hemolytic streptococci produce several substances (antigens) that induce the formation of measurable antibodies in the serum. Because the aftermath of group A streptococci infections may be diseases such as rheumatic fever or glomerulonephritis, one or more of these three streptococcal antigen tests is used to help in confirming that the client did have a streptococcal infection in the recent past. Rheumatic fever is becoming rarer because of early recognition and treatment of streptococcal infections such as strep throat. (See Chapter 16 on the importance of throat cultures to identify strep throat.)

Anti-streptolysin-O. The antibodies to streptolysin-O appear about 7–10 days after an acute streptococcal infection. The antibodies peak 2–4 weeks later, remaining high for weeks to months. The test may not always be elevated with streptococcal infections, and other disease conditions, such as liver disease, may make the test falsely positive.

Anti-streptodornase-B. Anti-DNase-B measures the antibodies formed against another of the streptococcal enzymes called *deoxyribonuclease-B.* It may be used in conjunction with the test for streptococcal antigens.

Streptozyme Test. This test, a commercial product, is more general than the ASO or anti-DNase-B. It measures antibodies against five different streptococcal enzymes: (1) streptolysin-O, (2) deoxyribonuclease-B, (3) hyaluronidase, (4) streptokinase, and (5) nicotinamide adenine dinucleotidase. False-positive results can occur.

Preparation of Client and Collection of Sample

These tests require venous blood. Record on the laboratory slip if the client is taking antibiotics, because titers may not increase if the client has been taking antibiotics.

REFERENCE VALUES FOR TESTS FOR STREPTOCOCCAL INFECTIONS

ASO titers:	
Preschool	1:85
Age 5–18 y	1:170
Adults	1:85
Anti-DNase-B titers:	
Preschool	1:60
Age 5–18 y	1:170
Adults	1:85
Streptozyme titers	<100 Streptozyme units

Ravel (1995) noted there is considerable debate over which of these tests is most useful.

▼ RUBELLA

Rubella (also called *3-day measles* or *German measles*) is usually of no clinical significance unless it occurs in a pregnant woman. Rubella may cause a miscarriage, or it may bring about congenital heart disease, cataracts, deafness, and brain damage in the fetus. Thus, it is important to assess whether women who are to become pregnant have an immunity against rubella. In the past, rubella tests were often mandated for women of childbearing age obtaining a marriage license. Many states no longer require premarital tests.

Preparation of Client and Collection of Sample

The test requires venous blood, 0.5 mL in a SST vacuum tube.

REFERENCE VALUES FOR RUBELLA

Titers of 1:32 or more indicate immunity
If tested by EIA, IgG: index greater than 1.2 shows immunity
IgM: index greater than 1.09 is positive for acute infection

Once a person has had rubella, an elevated titer of antibodies persists for many years or perhaps for life. Even a small number of antibodies indicates some immunity from the disease. Women who are not immune to rubella (i.e., who have no antibody titer) should be vaccinated before becoming pregnant. The rubella test for antibodies is one of the blood tests that may be necessary to obtain a marriage license in some states.

▼ POSSIBLE NURSING DIAGNOSES RELATED TO NEGATIVE RUBELLA TITER

Knowledge Deficit Related to Need for Vaccine

The lack of a titer to rubella is clinically significant in women who may become pregnant. Since 1969, when the first rubella vaccine was licensed in the United States, there has been a mass immunization program for school-aged children. However, there are still women in their childbearing years who are susceptible to rubella. A single dose of rubella vaccine is recommended not only for children more than 12 months old but also for any woman who has no antibody titer for rubella and who may become pregnant.

Whether some action should be taken may be a disturbing question for a woman who contacts rubella during her pregnancy. If a pregnant woman is believed to have rubella, a rise in maternal rubella IgM is evidence of recent infection. The client needs to confer with the physician about possible damage to the fetus.

Health care workers must take all measures necessary to prevent susceptible pregnant women from contracting rubella. All health workers who might transmit rubella to pregnant women should be immunized against the disease.

Risk for Injury Related to Vaccine

Nurses should be aware that adult women who are given the vaccine should avoid pregnancy for 3 months. Giving the client information about reliable birth control may be necessary. Also, because the vaccine can cause some joint symptoms, particularly in adults, the possible side effects of the vaccine need to be explained (Katzung, 1995). Women may need to sign an informed consent noting the risks inherent in becoming pregnant within 3 months of the injection.

▼ TOXOPLASMOSIS

Toxoplasmosis (TPM or Toxo) is caused by infestation with the protozoan *Toxoplasma gondii,* which is found in raw or poorly cooked meat and in the feces of cats. The disease causes fatigue, fever, and lymph gland swelling. TPM can be treated with drugs, so usually the disease is not serious in an adult unless the host is immunocompromised, as in AIDS. TPM can be passed to a fetus and cause neurologic damage and eye problems.

Preparation of Client and Collection of Sample

Check with the laboratory for the specific type of serologic test being used. Most tests for toxoplasmosis require about 4 mL of whole blood. Pertinent history includes whether the client has been exposed to cats, may be pregnant, or is immunosuppressed.

REFERENCE VALUES FOR TPM

IgM antibody titer is negative if <8 for an adult and <2 for an infant.

Infants may have an increased titer because of the transfer of antibodies from the mother. Infants need to be retested later.

▼ POSSIBLE NURSING DIAGNOSES RELATED TO POSITIVE TITER

Knowledge Deficit Related to Danger for Pregnant Women

People should be aware that poorly cooked or raw meat can introduce organisms into the human body. Also the importance of avoiding hand contamination from the feces of cats should be made common knowledge. Because cats are the host, the pregnant woman needs to be careful about handling the feces of a cat and certainly to avoid strange cats. A veterinarian can be contacted about the health status of a house cat. About 90% of mothers with acute TPM during pregnancy have no symptoms. Because systemic serologic screening is cost effective, some authorities recommend screening for TPM in pregnancy to reduce the risk of congenital TPM (Lappalainen et al., 1994).

(*continued*)

▼ POSSIBLE NURSING DIAGNOSES RELATED TO POSITIVE TITER (*continued*)

Anxiety Related to Unknown Diagnosis

The presence of lymphadenopathy (enlarged lymph glands) and vague symptoms in an otherwise healthy person may suggest a viral infection. A client with suspected TPM may also undergo tests done for infectious mononucleosis. In contrast to infectious mononucleosis, there is no elevated HAT in TPM. (See earlier in this chapter for the discussion of the HAT.) Until the diagnosis is made by the physician, the client may be afraid that the lymph gland swelling is due to a malignant tumor and is likely to be very relieved to find out that the problem is an infection with a protozoan. In an immunosuppressed client, TPM may be a serious or even fatal disease unless treated early (Scherer, 1990).

▼ AMEBIASIS

Entamoeba histolytica is an ameba that causes amebic dysentery and hepatic abscesses. The ameba can be identified by means of microscopic examination. (See Chapter 16 for the technique used to obtain a stool culture for ameba.) The stool examination is the most definitive test for ameba, but it is technically difficult to obtain live ameba for direct examination. Serologic tests can identify antibodies to *E histolytica,* which are present in 90–95% of clients with a hepatic abscess caused by the ameba and in 85–90% of clients with an intestinal infestation with *E histolytica* (Ravel, 1995).

Preparation of Client and Collection of Sample

The test requires venous blood. Check with the laboratory for the exact amount.

REFERENCE VALUES FOR AMEBA

Fourfold titer increase indicates infestation with the ameba. Antibody levels persist for several years after an active infestation.

▼ POSSIBLE NURSING DIAGNOSIS RELATED TO INCREASING TITER

Knowledge Deficit Related to Spread of Disease

See Chapter 16 for the client teaching needed when a client must follow enteric precautions.

▼ HERPESVIRUS FAMILY

A primary infection with herpes simplex virus (HSV) (either HSV 1 for oral herpes or HSV 2 for genital herpes) may produce rising antibody titers. Because exposure to one of the herpesviruses is almost universal in the population, the serologic test for herpes is usually not useful for clinical management. However, the titers of HSV are useful in epidemiologic studies or for research. Clinical diagnosis of genital herpes is usually made on the basis of history and symptoms. The two specific tests to confirm HSV 2, the Tzanck test and viral cultures, are discussed in Chapter 16. Diagnosis is particularly important in pregnant women. Epstein–Barr virus, CMV, and the varicella virus are also in the herpesvirus family and are discussed in this chapter. In 1986, human herpesvirus 6 (HHV 6) was isolated and in 1990, HHV 7 was isolated. Serologic testing is being developed, as is a nucleic acid probe with PCR amplification (Ravel, 1995).

▼ CYTOMEGALOVIRUS TITERS

Cytomegalovirus (CMV), a type of herpesvirus found in almost all body secretions, can cross the placenta and be transferred in blood. Many adults have been exposed to the virus and thus have immunity. The virus may be dangerous for pregnant women because of damage to the fetus. The virus can cause cerebral malformation and necrosis of brain tissue (Bullock and Rosendahl, 1988). Immunosuppressed clients are highly susceptible to CMV infection. Clients with AIDS usually have high titers for CMV. Acute infection with the virus in the client with AIDS often leads to eye damage and blindness as well as cerebral damage.

The risk to health workers is low because healthy people have adequate immune systems. Young et al. (1983) conducted a study to see if CMV was a serious hazard to female staff caring for newborns infected with CMV. The precaution of screening the antibody status of employees, tried for 18 months, did not prove necessary because CMV was not a substantial risk to staff. Standard techniques to avoid contamination with body secretions, including the admonition that babies should not be kissed by nursery personnel, are adequate to protect the staff, including those who are pregnant (Jacobson, 1990).

REFERENCE VALUES FOR CMV

A fourfold or greater rise in titer between acute and convalescent samples is evidence of infection. A single IgM-specific titer of more than 1:8 is evidence of an acute infection.

The CMV antigen can be detected with a DNA probe and electron microscopy, but both methods are expensive.

▼ TORCH SCREEN

The TORCH screen includes testing for *t*oxoplasmosis, *o*ther (usually hepatitis or syphilis), *r*ubella, *c*ytomegalovirus, and *h*erpes simplex. The TORCH screen is performed in newborn infants to evaluate possible congenital infection with one of these viruses. By evaluating the type of antibody present in umbilical cord blood, the laboratory may be able to determine if there is passive transfer from the mother (IgG antibodies) or actual congenital infection (IgM antibodies). Because antibody production may not occur early enough in the infection, the TORCH screen is not always useful and is being replaced with more specific tests for the suspected organism.

▼ VARICELLA-ZOSTER ANTIBODY TITER

A varicella-zoster antibody screen is performed to see if the client has immunity to the herpes zoster virus that can cause both chickenpox (varicella) and shingles (herpes zoster). Titers are not as useful for determining acute infections. Vesicle scrapings can be used for viral culture (Chapter 16).

Preparation of Client and Collection of Sample

The laboratory needs 0.5 mL of serum.

REFERENCE VALUE FOR VARICELLA-ZOSTER ANTIBODY TITER
Negative finding means the client is susceptible to infections with the herpes zoster virus.

Clinical Significance. To curtail an epidemic of chickenpox in the clinical setting, it is useful to know which staff do not have an immunity to the herpes zoster virus, because they should not take care of patients who are believed to have shingles or chickenpox. The incubation period is 10–20 days after the initial exposure. However, the disease is infectious for 5 days before the rash and continues to be so until all the lesions have crusted over (Krause and Straus, 1990). Clients who are immunosuppressed should be protected from patients or staff who have negative titers and hence could become carriers of the virus if exposed. Disseminated chickenpox can be fatal to an immunosuppressed person.

▼ FUNGAL ANTIBODIES: HISTOPLASMOSIS AND COCCIDIOIDOMYCOSIS

By use of the CF or immunodiffusion techniques, the laboratory can identify antibodies that occur in response to fungal diseases, such as histoplasmosis or coccidioidomycosis. Histoplasmosis is found particularly in the Ohio Valley area, and coccidioidomycosis (valley fever or desert fever) is prominent in the San Joaquin Valley of California. Because many people who live in an area where a fungus is endemic may have positive serologic tests from past exposures, one titer is not enough to be diagnostic. A fourfold rise in titer is evidence of current infection. Although some types of fungus are endemic in certain areas, clients with the disease may be far from the origin. A travel history is mandatory when a fungal disease is suspected (Wheat et al., 1986).

Skin testing and cultures may also be used to identify the particular fungus causing the systemic infection. (See Chapter 16 for some tips on cultures for fungus.) A positive skin test does not indicate that an infection is currently present, because the antibodies may be from past exposure. More diagnostically significant is conversion of a negative skin test to a positive one. Because skin tests can also cause a serologic test to become positive, they should be started after the blood is drawn for serologic tests for fungal antibodies.

▼ FUNGAL ANTIGENS

Tests to identify antigens (rather than antibodies) for various fungi continue to be developed. Antigen tests are used for cryptococcosis and candidiasis, two fungi often found in immunocompromised clients.

Preparation of Client and Collection of Sample

These tests require venous blood. Antibody tests should be drawn before any skin testing is done.

REFERENCE VALUES FOR FUNGAL ANTIBODIES AND ANTIGENS
Fourfold rise in antibody titer is evidence of infection. Specific antigens may be found in blood, urine, or cerebrospinal fluid.

▼ NURSING IMPLICATIONS

The nurse should confer with the physician to see if the client presents any danger to other clients or to the staff. Refer to a nursing text for detailed information on the care of clients with fungal disease. Nurses may administer ordered skin tests for fungus. The technique for intradermal injection, the diluent strength of the antigen, and the times to read the results are clearly explained with the product information that accompanies the test material.

▼ RICKETTSIAL DISEASE: *PROTEUS* OX-19, *PROTEUS* OX-2, AND *PROTEUS* OX-K (WEIL-FELIX REACTION)

The nonpathogenic organism, *Proteus* OX-19, is agglutinated by the serum of clients with certain rickettsial diseases, such as Rocky Mountain spotted fever and typhus. This reaction is called the Weil-Felix reaction. Other types of *Proteus,* such as OX-K (Ravel, 1995) may be used to determine other specific types of infection with rickettsiae. Culturing the rickettsiae is possible, but it must be completed in a special laboratory. So the *Proteus* test may be performed when a rickettsial disease is suspected.

Preparation of Client and Collection of Sample

The test requires 6 mL of venous blood. Because the Weil-Felix reaction involves a reaction to the *Proteus* antigen, the test is not indicative of rickettsial disease if the client has an infection with certain pathogenic strains of *Proteus.* Note the possibility of any *Proteus* infections. (See Chapter 16 for a discussion of *Proteus* infections of the urinary tract, respiratory tract, and wounds.) Other diseases, such as typhus, may occasionally cause agglutinations of *Proteus* OX-19, and conditions such as liver disease may cause false-positive results. Antibody titers for specific rickettsiae are sent to specialized laboratories. Two titers about 3 weeks apart are needed.

REFERENCE VALUES FOR WEIL-FELIX REACTION

A titer of 1:40 or 1:80 is considered possible evidence of rickettsial disease.

A titer of 1:160 or greater is presumptive evidence of infection with one of the Rickettsia species.

Antibody tests for rickettsial disease, sent to a public health laboratory are more specific. A negative titer would be <8.

All rickettsiae are spread by vectors. For example, epidemic typhus is spread by body lice, and Rocky Mountain spotted fever is spread by ticks. The laboratory needs to know of possible exposure to these vectors. Because transmission requires a vector, the client does not pass the infection to others.

IMMUNOLOGIC TESTS

The few tests discussed in this section are used primarily to assess for diseases such as SLE, rheumatoid arthritis, or other autoimmune reactions. See Table 14–7 for a list of the common serologic tests used in immunology and Appendix A, Table 3, for less common ones.

TABLE 14–7. COMMON SEROLOGIC TESTS USED IN IMMUNOLOGY

Test	Description
C-reactive protein	Measures an abnormal protein found in the serum in certain inflammations. Compare with ESR in Chapter 2
Complement activity	Measures activity of the complement system
C3 and C4	Specific measurements of the amount of two of the complement factors
ANA	Measures antinuclear antibodies, which are sometimes increased in SLE
Anti-DNA	Other humoral antibodies, which are sometimes elevated in SLE
RF	Measurement of antibodies, which may be elevated in rheumatoid arthritis
Thyroglobulin and microsomal antibodies	Measurement of antibodies, which may be elevated in some types of thyroiditis

ANA, antinuclear antibodies; ESR, erythrocyte sedimentation rate; RF, rheumatoid factor; SLE, systemic lupus erythematosus.

▼ C-REACTIVE PROTEIN

The C-reactive protein (CRP), not normally present in the blood, appears with inflammatory processes or with tissue destruction. Sometimes this test is used to monitor rheumatic fever or rheumatoid arthritis. Like the erythrocyte sedimentation rate (ESR), the CRP is a nonspecific test that indicates only an inflammation. New methods, such as fluorescent immunoassay, have made it possible to quantify the CRP. Quantitative CRP measurements are useful to monitor acute inflammations, but ESR is still the preferred test for chronic inflammation (Ravel, 1995). (See Chapter 2 for the discussion of ESR as the more common test used to monitor rheumatoid arthritis.

Preparation of Client and Collection of Sample

The test requires 3 mL of venous blood.

REFERENCE VALUE FOR C-REACTIVE PROTEIN

0–8 mg/dL

▼ COMPLEMENT ACTIVITY: C3, C4, AND C1 ESTERASE INHIBITOR

The complement system consists of several proteins that are active in producing the inflammatory response that sometimes occurs after an antigen–antibody reaction. In the classic pathway, the complement is activated by an antigen–antibody response. In the alternate pathway, polysaccharides, endotoxins, or immunoglobulins activate the complement cascade. The final reaction of the complement system produces a complex protein capable of lysing cell membranes.

The total amount of complement activity may be measured with a hemolytic assay and expressed in units as compared with a normal standard. The test of total complement activity is difficult to perform and to standardize because it must use fresh human or guinea pig complement. A simpler test involves measuring two of the components of the complement system. These two components, C3 and C4, as well as the other components of the complement system, are used up in the complicated series of reactions that follow some antibody–antigen reactions.

C3 is the preferred test in most clinical situations. C3 composes about 70% of the total protein in the complement system and is central to activation of both the classic and alternate pathways. C4 is used only in the classic pathway. Diseases such as hereditary angioedema (HAE) can be screened with C4. HAE is an autosomal dominant trait that causes a lack of C1 esterase inhibitor, a serum protein that regulates activation of the first component of the complement cascade (Huber and Calliari, 1985).

Preparation of Client and Collection of Sample

Tests for C3 and C4 require 2 mL of serum collected without additives. The C1 esterase inhibitor test and the test for total hemolytic activity require 5–10 mL of blood sent on ice.

REFERENCE VALUES FOR TOTAL COMPLEMENT, C3, C4, AND C1 ESTERASE INHIBITOR

Complement, total hemolytic activity	150–250 U/mL
C3	83–177 mg/dL
C4	15–45 mg/dL
C1 esterase inhibitor	13.2–24 mg/dL

Values are lower at birth and slightly higher in the aged.

Clinical Significance. An increase in the total complement activity occurs in some acute inflammatory diseases, but depressed levels have more clinical significance. Decreased serum levels of C3 and C4 indicate the presence of immune complexes that have used up the complement factors (assuming no inherited complement deficiencies). Complement deficiencies can be genetic, but acquired ones are most common. Studies have shown that newborns and preterm infants have impaired complement activity as compared with adults. The lack of complement may help explain why newborns, particularly premature infants, are prone to life-threatening pyogenic infections (Wolach et al., 1994).

Although an increase in the amount of complement activity and a decrease in serum C3 and C4 indicate that immune complexes are being formed, the actual diagnosis may be very difficult to establish. These tests are likely to be only part of the assessment needed to help the physician establish a diagnosis of autoimmune disease.

A normal level of serum complement does not rule out the possibility of an immune reaction, because some antigen–antibody responses do not cause an activation and depletion of the complement factors. Much research is being carried out on the complicated immune response.

▼ ANTINUCLEAR ANTIBODIES

ANA are γ-globulins found in clients with certain types of autoimmune diseases. ANAs are directed against components within the nucleus of the cell. Although they may be of various classes, most of the antibodies are of the IgA class (see Chapter 10). The test is typically used to rule out SLE because most clients with SLE have a positive ANA. However, the test is not specific for SLE because the test may also be positive in rheumatoid arthritis, scleroderma, carcinoma, tuberculosis, and hepatitis. Various drugs may also cause an increased ANA titer.

Identification of the various staining patterns for ANA such as a rim (peripheral), solid, or speckled pattern can also give important information. However, not all investigators agree on which pattern is found most often in various diseases (Ravel, 1995).

Preparation of Client and Collection of Sample

The test requires 2 mL of serum, which should be sent to the laboratory immediately.

REFERENCE VALUES FOR ANA	
Test is considered positive if detected with serum diluted 1:8 or titer >40	
Aged	ANA levels seem to increase with age even in people without immune diseases

▼ OTHER TESTS FOR SYSTEMIC LUPUS ERYTHEMATOSUS

In addition to the more general ANA test, tests of individual antigen–antibody reactions have been developed to help with the diagnosis of SLE. The four common tests are: anti-DNA, anti-Sm, anti-RNP, and anti-Ro. (See Kuper and Failla [1994] for the criteria for classifying lupus or call the Lupus Foundation of America, 1(800)558-0121 for the most current information on the use of these tests.)

▼ RHEUMATOID FACTOR

The RF is a test of abnormal proteins found in the serum of many clients with rheumatoid arthritis. Evidently the RF really consists of different types of IgM antibodies. (See Chapter 10 for the measurement of IgM.) Although the RF is present with other diseases, the highest levels are found in clients with rheumatoid arthritis, but the levels do not always correlate with the severity of the disease activity. Some "normal" people, particularly the elderly, may have the factor. Clients with tuberculosis, bacterial endocarditis, syphilis, and collagen diseases may have the RF.

Preparation of Client and Collection of Sample

The test requires 10 mL of clotted blood. A fasting sample is preferred.

REFERENCE VALUE FOR RF
<30 IU/mL

▼ POSSIBLE NURSING DIAGNOSIS RELATED TO RF

Altered Health Maintenance

A client with rheumatoid arthritis needs nursing care both during the acute stages and during remissions. Fatigue is common and affects many activities of daily living (Belza et al., 1993). Nurse practitioners may manage clients with this chronic disease. The basic triad of treatment includes (1) physical therapy and exercises, (2) emotional and psychological support, and (3) monitoring of anti-inflammatory drug therapy. The ESR (Chapter 2) is used to follow the disease process.

▼ THYROID ANTIBODIES

In some types of thyroid disorders, the body produces antibodies against certain thyroid constituents. The end result is inflammation and destruction of the thyroid gland. Although the level of antibodies does not exactly correlate with the severity of the symptoms, identifying the probable cause of thyroid dysfunction is a help. (See Chapter 15 for a complete discussion on hypo- and hyperthyroidism, along with the tests used.) Relatives of clients with thyroid autoimmunity problems may also have high titers of thyroid antibodies. Because other diseases, such as the collagen diseases, may cause increased titers, the client may also undergo other types of antibody tests (see Appendix A, Table 3).

Preparation of Client and Collection of Sample

The test requires 1 mL of serum. Because oral contraceptives may cause titers to become detectable, record whether the client is taking birth control pills.

REFERENCE VALUES FOR THYROID ANTIBODIES

Microsomal antibodies	titer <100
Thyroglobulin antibodies	titer <10

Titers increase with age, particularly in some elderly, healthy women

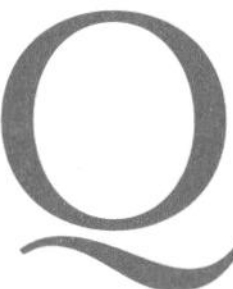

1. Which one of the following tests is routinely performed on a unit of donated blood?

   a. HAA (hepatitis A antigen)
   b. ANA (antinuclear antibodies)
   c. ASO titer (anti-streptolysin titer)
   d. ALT (alanine transferase)

2. Mr. Royal has type AB blood. Theoretically, based on the ABO typing, Mr. Royal could receive any type of blood because he has which of the following?

   a. No A or B antigens
   b. No antibodies against A and B antigens
   c. Only antibodies against O
   d. Only AB antibodies

3. Mrs. Tudor had a hemolytic transfusion reaction, possibly caused by incompatible blood. She had fever, chills, and low back pain. The transfusion was stopped, and the unit of blood was returned to the laboratory. The nurse should save a urine specimen for which reason?

   a. The urine may need to be checked for free hemoglobin
   b. Dehydration must be prevented
   c. A bilirubin test should be performed stat
   d. Circulatory overload may require use of a diuretic

4. Mrs. Sanchez, who is Rh negative, just delivered a healthy 8-lb (3.6 kg) baby boy who is Rh positive. She was given an injection of RhoGAM. She asks the nurse why she had the shot. Which of the following explanations by the nurse is accurate? "This shot

   a. Prevents you from having any problems with any other pregnancies because it eliminates the Rh factor."
   b. Gives you temporary antibodies against the Rh factor so that your body won't make any on your own, which could still be present if you have another Rh positive pregnancy."

c. Helps to eliminate any antibodies that you might have gotten from this pregnancy so that the next pregnancy will be normal."

d. Helps your body to manufacture antibodies, so that if you have another pregnancy with an Rh baby there won't be any problems."

5. A positive Coombs' test indicates coating of erythrocytes by some type of globulin. Which of the following clinical situations is assessed with a Coombs' test?

   a. Hemolytic disease of the newborn
   b. Autoimmune thyroid disorders
   c. Systemic lupus erythematous (SLE)
   d. Fungal infections

6. Mr. Wayler is a client receiving renal dialysis three times a week. His laboratory test shows a positive report for HBsAg (hepatitis B surface antigen). Mr. Wayler does not have any symptoms of hepatitis. Based on these data, which precaution should be instituted?

   a. None, because he has no evidence of clinical disease
   b. Administration of hepatitis B vaccine to Mr. Wayler
   c. Use of gloves when any blood-contaminated articles must be handled
   d. Administration of γ-globulin to staff who must work directly with Mr. Wayler

7. The school nurse has been asked to provide some information about syphilis to a group of adolescent girls. Which of the following statements is inaccurate?

   a. A blood test for syphilis should be performed on anyone who had sexual contact with a person who has syphilis
   b. Syphilis is treated with a penicillin injection or with other antibiotics if the person is allergic to penicillin
   c. Syphilis is a communicable disease that must be reported to the health department
   d. A positive laboratory test for syphilis is always indicative of active infection

8. A nurse in advanced practice is seeing many women who may have been exposed to HIV. In setting up a testing protocol for the clinic, the nurse must follow a procedure that provides for

   a. Oral consent to a blood test and documentation of pretest counseling
   b. Written consent to HIV testing and the name of person drawing the blood
   c. Oral consent for HIV testing and a signed form detailing the extent of the pretest counseling session
   d. Written consent to HIV testing and the signature of the person who provided pretest counseling

9. Shirley Bowden is a college freshman who has had considerable lower abdominal discomfort and a low-grade fever. She is believed to have a repeat episode of pelvic inflammatory disease (PID). Which of the following may be used to assess for an acute inflammatory response?

   a. Heterophil antibody test and Mono spot test
   b. Anti-DNA, anti-Sm, anti-RNP, and anti-Ro
   c. Total complement activity
   d. C-reactive protein (qualitative)

10. ASO, anti-DNase-B, and Streptozyme (the serologic tests for antibodies against group A β-hemolytic streptococci) would be the *least* useful for

   a. Carolyn, 10 years of age, who has just been told she has "strep" throat
   b. Billy, 8 years of age, who has symptoms of possible rheumatic fever
   c. Tommy, 14 years of age, who has acute glomerulonephritis
   d. Barbara, 9 years of age, who has a history of repeated sore throats and joint pain

11. Martha Leahy, 25 years of age, who wants to get pregnant, has a negative titer of rubella antibodies. What should Martha do before she becomes pregnant?

   a. Nothing, because a negative titer shows immunity to rubella
   b. Try to catch rubella by means of exposure to young children with measles
   c. Consult her physician about receiving the rubella vaccine if she becomes pregnant
   d. Ask her physician to give her the rubella vaccine now and practice birth control for at least 3 months

12. Ginny Jasper is to undergo a serologic test for toxoplasmosis. Which of the following is a significant factor in her health history in relation to the test for TPM?

   a. Has had a tick bite
   b. Just moved from the San Joaquin Valley
   c. Has a cat
   d. Likes raw fruits and vegetables

13. In the Ohio Valley area, where the fungus *Histoplasma capsulatum* is endemic, people who have positive skin and serologic tests for histoplasmosis are

   a. Highly susceptible to the fungus
   b. Always carriers of the fungal disease
   c. Always infected with the fungus
   d. Showing evidence of exposure to the fungus

14. The laboratory test, *Proteus* OX-19, is an indirect test for
    - a. *Proteus* infection
    - b. Rickettsial disease
    - c. Protozoan infestation
    - d. *Entamoeba histolytica* infestation

▼ REFERENCES

Alter, H., et al. (1989). Detection of antibody to hepatitis C virus in prospectively followed transfusion recipients with acute and chronic non-A, non-B hepatitis. *New England Journal of Medicine, 321* (22), 1494–1500.

Barrick, B. (1990). Light at the end of a decade. *American Journal of Nursing, 90* (11), 37–40.

Belza, B.L., Henke, C.J., Yelin, E.H., et al. (1993). Correlates of fatigue in older adults with rheumatoid arthritis. *Nursing Research, 42* (2), 93–99.

Boyer, P.J., Dillon, M., Navaie, M., et al. (1994). Factors predictive of maternal-fetal transmission of HIV-1. *JAMA, 271* (24), 1925–1930.

Bullock, B., and Rosendahl, P. (1988). *Pathophysiology: Adaptations and alterations in function* (2nd ed.). Boston: Scott, Foresman.

Cao, Y. Qin, L., Zhang, L., et al. (1995). Virologic and immunologic characterization of long-term survivors of human immunodeficiency virus type 1 infection. *New England Journal of Medicine, 332* (4), 201–208.

Corbett, J.V. (1991). Screening donor blood grows complicated. *California Nursing, 13* (1), 44.

Corbett, J.V., and Kenney, C. (1995). Zidovudine in pregnancy. *MCN American Journal of Maternal Child Nursing, 20* (2), 122.

Food and Drug Administration. (1994). Immune globulin-associated hepatitis C transmission. *FDA Medical Bulletin, 24* (2), 2–3.

Freedman, M., et al. (1990). Nursing considerations in the administration of blood component therapy. *Seminars in Oncology Nursing, 6* (20), 155–162.

Gonterman, R., Kiracofe, S., and Owens, P. (1994). Administering, documenting, and tracking blood products and volume expanders. *MEDSURG Nursing, 3* (4), 269–276.

Gurevich, I. (1993a). Hepatitis Part I. Enterically transmitted viral hepatitis: Etiology, epidemiology, and prevention. *Heart and Lung, 22* (4), 370–372.

Gurevich, I. (1993b). Hepatitis Part II. Viral hepatitis B, C, and D. *Heart and Lung, 22* (5), 450–456.

Helquist, M. (1986). Hemophilia and AIDS. *Focus: A Review of AIDS Research, 1* (6), 3–4.

Huber, M., and Calliari, D. (1985). Hereditary angioedema, the swelling disorder. *American Journal of Nursing, 85* (10), 1090–1092.

Jacobson, E. (1990). Hospital hazards: How to protect yourself. *American Journal of Nursing, 90,* 48–53.

Jason, J., et al. (1986). HTLV-III/LAV antibody and immune status of household contacts and sexual partners of persons with hemophilia. *JAMA, 255* (2), 212–215.

Katzung, B. (1995). *Basic & clinical pharmacology.* (6th ed.). Norwalk, CT: Appleton & Lange.

Killian, W. (1990). HIV counseling: Know the risks. *American Nurse, 22* (8), 28.

Kirton, C.A. (1994). AIDS: When your patient refuses HIV testing. *American Journal of Nursing, 94* (11), 48–53.

Kolodner, D.E. (1993). The new federal bloodborne pathogens standard: Significance to the health care worker. *MEDSURG Nursing, 2* (1), 59–61.

Kotwas, L., et al. (1990). Blood collection techniques. *Seminars in Oncology Nursing, 6* (2), 109–116.

Krause, P., and Straus, S. (1990). Zoster and its complications. *Hospital Practice, 25,* 61–76.

Kuper, B.C., and Failla, S. (1994). Shedding new light on lupus. *American Journal of Nursing, 94* (11), 26–32.

Lappalainen, M., Koskela, P., Hedman, K., et al. (1994). Screening of toxoplasmosis during pregnancy. *Israel Journal of Medical Science, 30,* 362–363.

Lederman, M. (1986). Transmission of the acquired immune deficiency syndrome through heterosexual activity. *Annals of Internal Medicine, 104,* 115–117.

Marx, J. (1993). Viral hepatitis. *Nursing 93, 23,* (1), 35–41.

Mason, J. (1985). Alternative sites for screening blood for antibodies to AIDS virus. *New England Journal of Medicine, 313* (18), 1157–1158.

McCormac, M. (1990). Managing hemorrhagic shock. *American Journal of Nursing, 90* (9), 22–28.

Morrison, C. (1986). Nursing's special challenge. *California Nurse, 82* (4), 1–16.

Nelson, J.A. (1995). HIV in adolescents. *MCN American Journal of Maternal Child Health Nursing, 20* (1), 34–37.

Nettina, S. (1990). Syphilis: A new look at an old killer. *American Journal of Nursing, 90* (4), 68–70.

Pigg, R.M. (1994). 1993 sexually transmitted diseases treatment guidelines. *Journal of School Health, 64* (4), 156–159.

Ravel, R. (1995). *Clinical laboratory medicine.* (6th ed.). Chicago: Mosby–Year Book.

Scherer, P. (1990). How AIDS attacks the brain. *American Journal of Nursing, 90* (1), 44–53.

Sipes, C. (1995). Guidelines for assessing HIV in women. *MCN: American Journal of Maternal Child Nursing 20* (1), 29–33.

Smith, R.N., Fallentine, J., Kessel, S., et al. (1995). Instilling the facts about autotransfusion. *Nursing 95, 25* (3), 52–54.

Stepanuk, K.M. (1994). Congenital syphilis: Are we missing infected newborns? *MCN: American Journal of Maternal Child Health Nursing, 19* (5), 272–274.

Wheat, L., et al. (1986). Diagnosis of disseminated histoplasmosis capsulatum in serum and urine specimens. *New England Journal of Medicine, 314* (2), 83–88.

Wolach, B., Carmi, D., Gilboa, S., et al. (1994). Some aspects of the humoral immunity and the phagocytic function in newborn infants. *Israel Journal of Medical Science, 30,* 331–335.

Young, A., et al. (1983). Is cytomegalovirus a serious hazard to female hospital staff? *Lancet, 1,* 975–976.

ENDOCRINE TESTS

- Growth Hormone or Somatotropin
- Prolactin
- Adrenocorticotropic Hormone
- Cortisol Plasma Levels
- Urinary Cortisol Levels
- 17-Hydroxycorticosteroids (Porter–Silber Test)
- 17-Ketosteroids
- Urinary Pregnanetriol
- Aldosterone
- Renin
- Catecholamines, Vanillylmandelic Acid, and Metanephrines
- Parathormone or Parathyroid Hormone
- Thyrotropin or Thyroid-stimulating Hormone
- L-Thyroxine Serum Concentration (Total T_4)
- Triiodothyronine Serum Concentration (T_3)
- Free T_4 and Free Thyroxine Index
- Follicle-stimulating Hormone
- Luteinizing Hormone
- Estradiol and Other Forms of Estrogen
- Progesterone
- Pregnanediol (Progesterone Metabolite)
- Estrogen and Progesterone Receptors
- Testosterone and Other Androgens

OBJECTIVES

1. Explain the concepts of negative feedback, circadian rhythms, and ectopic hormone production.
2. Give examples of how laboratory tests are used to assess the relation between the anterior pituitary gland and other endocrine glands.
3. Determine the appropriate nursing diagnoses for a client with increased or decreased serum cortisol levels.
4. Devise a teaching plan for parents who have a child with adrenogenital syndrome.
5. Identify the characteristic clinical manifestations of increased and decreased levels of serum aldosterone, including changes in renin activity.
6. Explain the purpose of 24-hr urine specimens for vanillylmandelic acid (VMA) and metanephrines.
7. Describe the clinical effect of an increased level of parathyroid hormone (PTH) and the most important nursing intervention needed.
8. Explain the usefulness of thyroid-stimulating hormone (TSH) and free thyroxine (T_4) index in evaluating clients with hyper- or hypothyroidism.
9. Determine the appropriate nursing diagnoses for clients with increased or decreased serum thyroid hormones.
10. Explain why infants who may have hypothyroidism (cretinism) need immediate medical evaluation and treatment.
11. Identify the key nursing diagnoses when a client has altered levels of the sex hormones.

The brief discussions of the negative feedback system, circadian rhythms, ectopic hormone production, and other physiologic information in this chapter should help the reader understand the tests performed to measure hormone levels.

Except for ectopic hormone production (discussed later), each hormone is produced by a specific endocrine gland, and each has a specific function or functions. These functions are briefly discussed in relation to the tests for each hormone.

Table 15–1 gives an overview of the endocrine glands, the hormones produced by each gland, and how the hormones are tested with specific laboratory tests of blood and urine samples. The releasing factors (discussed in the following section) are not included in this table because they are not usually measured.

BACKGROUND INFORMATION

Releasing Factors That Stimulate Anterior Pituitary Gland

The central nervous system is closely connected to the endocrine system because some releasing factors from the hypothalamus are carried to the pituitary gland through the venous system that connects the hypothalamus and the pituitary gland. Because *hypophysis* is another name for the pituitary gland, this venous system is called the *hypophyseal portal system.* These releasing factors from the

TABLE 15–1. COMMONLY MEASURED HORMONES

Source of Hormone	Name of Hormone	Tests Used to Assess Hormone Levels
Anterior pituitary gland	Growth hormone (GH) or somatotropin (STH)	Serum GH levels
	Adrenocorticotropin (ACTH)	Serum ACTH levels; see section on adrenal gland for ACTH suppression and stimulation tests
	Thyroid-stimulating hormone	Serum TSH levels; see section on tests of thyroid gland
	Follicle-stimulating hormone (FSH) (one of the gonadotropins)	Serum and urine FSH levels; see section on sex hormones
	Luteinizing hormone (LH), sometimes called interstitial-cell-stimulating hormone (ICSH) in male (the other gonadotropin)	Serum and urine levels; see section on sex hormones
	Prolactin (PRL)	Serum prolactin
	Melanocyte-stimulating hormone (MSH)	Serum MSH not usually measured directly; see discussion about increase of MSH with cortisol lack
Posterior pituitary gland	Antidiuretic hormone (ADH) or arginine vasopressin (AVP) (Pitressin)	Not commonly measured; see Chapter 4 on serum and urine osmolality
	Oxytocin (Pitocin)	Not measured as diagnostic test; oxytocin is used in obstetrics as drug to induce labor
Adrenal cortex	Glucocorticoids (cortisol as principal one)	Plasma and urine cortisol; 17-hydroxycorticosteroids (17-OHCS) or Porter–Silber test; 17-KGS; see also ACTH tests
	Mineralocorticoids (aldosterone as principal one)	Serum and urine aldosterone levels; tests for renin activity; see Chapter 5 for serum levels of sodium and potassium
	Sex hormones (androgens, progesterone, and estrogen)	Pregnanetriol in urine; 17-ketosteroids (17-KS) in urine
Adrenal medulla	Norepinephrine Epinephrine	Catecholamines in urine; metanephrines in urine; vanillylmandelic acid (VMA) in urine; norepinephrine and epinephrine are not commonly measured in serum; pharmacologic tests not commonly performed
Parathyroid	Parathyroid hormone (PTH)	Serum PTH; serum and urine calcium and phosphate levels; see Chapter 7
Thyroid	Calcitonin	Calcitonin not commonly measured; see Chapter 7 on serum calcium
	L-thyroxine (T_4) and triiodothyronine (T_3)	Free T_4; free T_4 index; total T_4; T_3; TSH levels
Pancreas	Insulin Glucogen	See Chapter 8 for tests of glucose metabolism
Testes	Androgens	Serum testosterone; see 17-KS urine test for androgens

(*continued*)

TABLE 15–1. *(Continued)*

Source of Hormone	Name of Hormone	Tests Used to Assess Hormone Levels
Testes *(continued)*		
	Estrogen and progesterone in minute amounts	Serum estradiol; see also tests for FSH and LH
Ovaries	Estrogens	Serum estradiol; serum and urine estradiol in pregnancy (see Chapter 18) Serum progesterone
	Progesterone	Pregnanediol in urine
	Androgens in minute amounts	17-KS for androgens; see also tests for FSH and LH

hypothalamus stimulate the pituitary gland to release certain hormones. For example, thyrotropin-releasing factor (TRF) is sent from the hypothalamus to the pituitary gland. The pituitary gland is thus stimulated to release TSH, which in turn acts on the thyroid gland to produce T_4.

Currently, several releasing factors from the hypothalamus are being extensively studied in relation to the effect of various drugs. The susceptibility to drugs of the hypothalamus–anterior pituitary system is taking on considerable clinical importance as more is being learned about the interaction between drugs and hormone levels.

Negative Feedback System for Endocrine Functioning

The anterior pituitary gland secretes hormones that act on specific target organs to cause the release of other hormones. For example, the pituitary gland releases adrenocorticotropic hormone (ACTH), which then stimulates the adrenal gland to produce cortisol. When the cortisol reaches a certain level in the bloodstream, continued secretion of ACTH from the pituitary gland is suppressed. In other words, a high level of cortisol turns off the secretion of ACTH. Conversely, a low level of serum cortisol is a stimulus for the increased production of ACTH. This interplay, in which the increased level of one hormone causes a decrease in the level of the other hormone, is called *negative feedback*. The hormones from the adrenal cortex, thyroid gland, ovaries, and testes all have negative feedback systems with hormones from the anterior pituitary gland. Understanding negative feedback is important because tests for the suppression or stimulation of hormones are based on the physiologic principle that levels of one hormone should change the level of another hormone.

Other Methods to Control Hormone Production

Not all hormones are controlled with a negative feedback system through the pituitary gland. For example, PTH is regulated by the serum calcium and phosphorous levels (see Chapter 7). A high level of serum calcium causes a suppression of PTH from the parathyroid gland. A decrease in the serum calcium level causes an increased production of PTH.

The intricate balance between too much and too little of a hormone is one of the wonders of the human body. In a healthy state, all hormones are kept within a precise range that can fluctuate as body needs change. All hormones are interrelated to some degree, so changes in the one hormone may affect the level of others, although not in as direct a manner as in negative feedback.

Circadian Rhythms and Other Rhythms

A change in the levels of a hormone every 24 hr is called a *circadian* (around the day) *rhythm*. For example, cortisol is higher in the morning than in the evening. Although cortisol seems to be relatively independent of the sleep pattern, growth hormone is strongly bound to the sleep pattern. Much research is being conducted to investigate which factors, other than activity patterns and sleep, regulate the normal variations every 24 hr. In addition to cortisol and growth hormone, aldosterone, prolactin, TSH, testosterone, luteinizing hormone (LH), and follicle-stimulating hormone (FSH) all vary considerably during each 24-hr period. Because the hormones do fluctuate, more than one blood sample or one urine specimen may be needed for an accurate reflection of an individual client's hormone level.

The female hormones, estrogen and progesterone, are, of course, on another rhythm that must also be taken into account in comparing reference values. Rhythms that are longer than circadian (24-hr) rhythms are termed *infradian rhythms*. In adult women, the menstrual cycle is an infradian rhythm, because the variations in FSH and LH are on a monthly, not a daily, cycle. Besides the sex hormones, other hormones may fluctuate with menstrual cycles. In women, therefore, various hormones must be considered in relation to the menstrual cycle.

Ectopic Hormone Production

Most elevations of serum hormone levels are due to an overproduction by the specific endocrine gland. They can also occur if there is production of the hormone from a nonendocrine source. Hormones from nonendocrine sources are called *ectopic hormones* because they come from the wrong place or originate outside the normal pathway. For example, some benign and malignant tumors manufacture hormones similar to the hormone produced by the endocrine gland. ACTH, melanocyte-stimulating hormone (MSH), gonadotropins, antidiuretic hormone (ADH), and PTH are common ectopic hormones.

In some malignant conditions, hormone tests may be performed to see if some of the symptoms are due to ectopic hormone production. For example, a tumor that produces PTH may cause symptoms of hypercalcemia. (See Chapter 7 for a discussion of hypercalcemia.) The physician may order a variety of tests to determine whether the symptoms of a hormone imbalance are due to a malignant tumor or to primary dysfunction of the endocrine gland.

Screening Tests and Definitive Tests for Primary and Secondary Imbalances

In general, screening tests for hormone imbalances are performed by measuring the concentration of the hormone in the serum. If the serum level is greater or lesser than the reference values, more definitive tests are completed to find out if the prob-

TABLE 15–2. SCREENING AND DEFINITIVE TESTS OF HORMONE FUNCTION

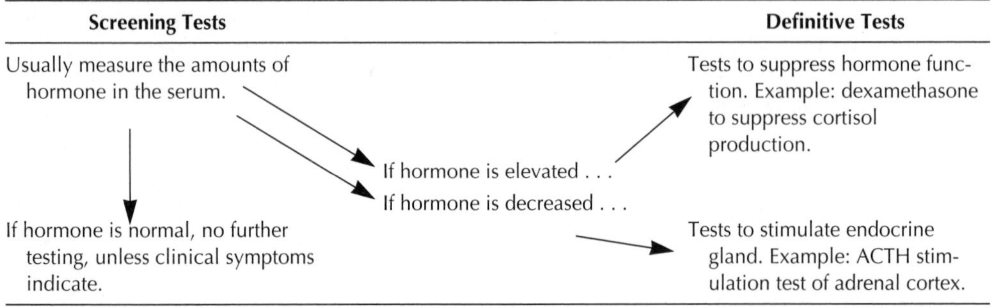

lem is in the gland itself. If the disorder is due to a problem in the gland itself, the disorder is called *primary*. If the endocrine imbalance is due to other causes, such as pituitary dysfunction, the endocrine disorder is termed *secondary*. For example, if hypothyroidism is due to malfunction of the thyroid gland, the disorder is called *primary hypothyroidism*. If the hypothyroidism is due to pituitary insufficiency, the disorder is called *secondary hypothyroidism*. Laboratory tests that use drugs to stimulate or to suppress hormone production are useful in determining if the disorder is primary or secondary (Table 15–2).

PITUITARY TUMORS

Pituitary tumors are classified as either hyperfunctional or nonfunctional on the basis of their effects on hormone production. The most common symptom of nonfunctional pituitary tumors is bitemporal hemianopsia caused by pressure on the optic nerve. The client has impaired vision in either the right or left side of both eyes. Symptoms of hyperfunctional tumors vary greatly depending on the type or types of hormones released. The most common syndrome is due to overproduction of prolactin, which can cause galactorrhea and changes in menses. A transphenoidal approach is often used for resection of these tumors (Smith-Rooker et al., 1993).

▼ POSSIBLE NURSING DIAGNOSES RELATED TO PITUITARY DISORDERS

Anxiety Related to the Disease

Emotional problems with mood changes are likely to be a part of most disorders of the pituitary gland. Some of the symptoms are directly related to the hormonal imbalance, whereas others may be brought on by the delay before an accurate diagnosis is made. Cowan (1984) noted that if the client is a woman, the symptoms may be labeled "hysteria." Because it is not unusual for the condition to be misdiagnosed for several years, a sense of bitterness and anger may complicate the efforts to help the client deal with the problems of the disease. After the diagnosis is established, clients and their significant others may need help to deal with surgical or other planned treatment.

Disturbances of Self-concept Related to Change in Body Image

Various pituitary disorders cause physical changes such as acromegaly, dwarfism, or obesity. Clients may need help accepting the physical changes that may or may not be remedied with therapy. For example, acromegaly may necessitate reconstruction of the bones of the face. The physical changes may also affect sexual functioning, an issue often overlooked.

▼ GROWTH HORMONE OR SOMATOTROPIN

Growth hormone (GH), produced by the anterior pituitary gland, stimulates the growth of bone and other tissue. GH affects metabolism by increasing protein synthesis, decreasing carbohydrate utilization, and increasing fat mobilization. GH is higher in children, but it is present in small amounts all through life. GH levels are performed to evaluate lack of growth of a child. For adults, GH is measured as one assessment of pituitary function. Researchers noted (Press et al., 1984) the importance of GH in mediating the metabolic derangements of diabetes.

Several factors influence the production of GH. Diets low in protein cause an increased production of the hormone. Hypoglycemia also causes an increased surge of GH in the serum, and hyperglycemia causes a decreased production of it. Because GH production is suppressed by hyperglycemia and stimulated by hypoglycemia, tests for GH may involve the administration of a glucose load or an insulin injection. Because exercise and sleep also cause variations in plasma GH levels, the activity of the client and the timing of specimen collection are important to note. (For reasons that are still unknown, GH levels increase during sleep.)

Preparation of Client and Collection of Sample

The laboratory needs 1 mL of serum. The activity of the client, including sleep patterns, needs to be normal. A baseline level is performed with the client fasting and at rest, although the client should have been eating a conventional diet before the fasting period.

GH levels may also be drawn after the client has been given drugs such as L-dopa (Ravel, 1995). Several serum blood samples are drawn after the administration of a drug to see how much the GH increases.

In clients with GH excess, a glucose load may be given to demonstrate that the GH cannot be suppressed. The procedure may consist of a glucose tolerance test (GTT) with simultaneous glucose and GH measurement. (See Chapter 8 for the procedure for GTT.)

REFERENCE VALUES FOR GH

Adult (fasting and at rest)	2–6 ng/mL
Newborn	10–40 ng/mL
Children	<10 ng/mL

In adults, the usual values may be so low that the hormone cannot be detected. Stimulation with L-dopa may increase GH to measurable levels

With sample drawn at 8 AM after normal sleep.

Increased GH Serum Level

Clinical Significance. Severe malnutritional states cause a prolonged elevation of GH. Various types of tumors, either benign or malignant, can cause excess secretion of GH. In children, an abnormal increase of GH causes *gigantism.* Increased GH after puberty brings about a distortion of bony structures because the bones are stimulated to grow after closure of the epiphyses. Growth hormone excess in the adult creates *acromegaly.*

▼ POSSIBLE NURSING DIAGNOSIS RELATED TO INCREASED GH

A client with a pituitary tumor may undergo radiation or surgical therapy to remove the tumor. (See earlier discussion of general nursing diagnoses.) An important point to remember in relation to increased GH levels is that hyperglycemia may be a clinical problem. An increased level of GH decreases the body's ability to handle glucose. (See Chapter 8 for more discussion of hyperglycemia and appropriate nursing diagnoses.)

Decreased GH Serum Level

Clinical Significance. Lack of GH is due to hypofunction of the pituitary gland, which can result from a tumor, from trauma, or from an unknown cause. In children, a lack of GH causes *dwarfism.* In adults, although the lack of GH does not cause clinical symptoms, it may be associated with deficiencies of other pituitary hormones, so symptoms are related to the other deficiencies. Hence a measurement of GH may be used to help in assessing the presence of hypopituitarism in the adult.

Sheehan's syndrome is a type of hypopituitarism that sometimes occurs after a complicated delivery with bleeding and shock. During the postpartum period, a thrombus may occur in the hypophyseal vessels, which causes destruction of the pituitary gland. Symptoms of a deficiency may occur months or years later.

▼ POSSIBLE NURSING DIAGNOSIS RELATED TO DECREASED GH

Knowledge Deficit Related to Replacement Therapy

In a child, a lack of GH is treated medically with injections of GH so that the child develops normally. In 1985, the United States Food and Drug Administration (FDA) approved the manufacture of GH by means of gene splicing. (This was the second product of recombinant DNA technology to be approved for human use. The first was insulin, approved in 1982.) Human GH-releasing factor is also available for experimental use (Katzung, 1995). Parents need detailed instructions about the injections and follow-up care. In infants, a lack of GH may cause an immediate problem by causing hypoglycemia. Older clients with a lack of GH may show symptoms of hypoglycemia only if they are fasting. Adults are not usually given injections of GH, but they may need replacement of other pituitary hormones, all of which can be replaced by means of parenteral injection. Also, hormones from specific glands, such as thyroid, may be given. The nursing implications for specific hormone therapy are briefly covered in the discussion of each hormone. (See also the two general nursing diagnoses discussed earlier.)

▼ PROLACTIN

Prolactin (PRL), a hormone from the anterior pituitary gland, is normally increased during pregnancy and the subsequent lactation period. Tumors of the pituitary gland, drugs, or other variables can result in increased PRL secretion. Women have an abnormal secretion of breast milk and suppression of menstruation (amenorrhea-galactorrhea syndrome). Some women may not realize they have galactorrhea until a milking pressure is applied to the breast. Other symptoms, such as headaches and weight gain from sodium retention, may occur. Men may experience impotence because excess PRL has a negative feedback to the pituitary gland, suppressing gonad function.

An enlarging tumor can cause visual problems because of pressure on the optic chiasm. The impairment of vision is particularly noted in pregnant women who have a pituitary tumor because the pituitary gland increases in pregnancy.

If the increased secretion is a result of a tumor, the lesion is usually benign and can be removed surgically. Bromocriptine (Parlodel) is a drug used for short-term therapy. Some drugs, such as tranquilizers, can mimic the PRL tumor syndrome, and thus treatment is elimination of the causative factor. Magnetic resonance imaging (MRI) (see Chapter 21) can be used to evaluate the effect of drug treatment on the size of the tumor (Glaser et al., 1986).

Preparation of Client and Collection of Sample

Test requires 2 mL of serum.

REFERENCE VALUES FOR PROLACTIN	
Adult: Men	0–10 ng/mL
Women	0–15 ng/mL Increases up to 40 ng/mL in luteal phase
Pregnancy	1st trimester: <80 ng/mL 2nd trimester: <160 ng/mL 3rd trimester: <400 ng/mL
Newborn	<500 ng/mL

▼ NURSING DIAGNOSES RELATED TO INCREASE OR DECREASE OF PROLACTIN LEVELS

See the general nursing diagnoses for pituitary disorders discussed earlier.

ADRENAL CORTEX

The adrenal cortex secretes three types of hormones (Table 15–3):

1. The glucocorticoids. The glucocorticoid usually measured in the plasma is cortisol. Free cortisol can also be measured in the urine. Various metabolites of the glucocorticoids can be measured in the urine as 17-hydroxycorticosteroid (17-OHCS).
2. The mineralocorticoids. The mineralocorticoid measured in the serum is aldosterone.

TABLE 15–3. EFFECTS OF THREE TYPES OF HORMONES FROM ADRENAL CORTEX

Hormone	Effect
Glucocorticoids (cortisol)	Effects on metabolism of carbohydrates, fats, and proteins. Suppresses immune responses.
Mineralocorticoids (aldosterone)	Effect on fluid and electrolyte balance. Increased retention of sodium and water. Decreased retention of potassium.
Sex hormones (androgens, progesterone, and estrogen)	Affect secondary sex characteristics but not as substantially as hormones from ovaries and testes.

3. The sex hormones. The sex hormones produced by the adrenal cortex include the androgens, progesterone, and estrogen. Both males and females have the male hormones (androgens, such as testosterone) and the female hormones (progesterone and estrogen). Measurement of androgens becomes important when there is hyperplasia of the adrenal gland, which increases the production of the sex hormones. A urine test, 17-ketosteroid (17-KS), is one way to determine an increase of sex hormones from the adrenal gland.

ACTH–ADRENAL AXIS

Production of cortisol by the adrenal cortex is controlled by the ACTH–adrenal axis. Because ACTH and cortisol are related by a negative feedback system, the pituitary is stimulated to produce ACTH when the plasma cortisol level is low. ACTH then increases production of cortisol by the adrenal cortex. The increasing plasma cortisol level becomes the stimulus for the pituitary gland to discontinue the high levels of ACTH production. Homeostasis is maintained by the increases and decreases of ACTH, which balance cortisol in the serum. ACTH also increases production of the sex hormones by the adrenal cortex, but this effect is usually not clinically significant except in some adrenogenital syndromes. (Androgen excess is discussed in the section on the clinical significance of decreased cortisol levels.) ACTH has little or no effect on the serum levels of the third type of adrenal cortex hormones, the mineralocorticosteroids, or aldosterone. Aldosterone is controlled by the renin–angiotensin system, which is explained in the section on aldosterone.

▼ ADRENOCORTICOTROPIC HORMONE

A measurement of ACTH helps determine whether the lack of serum cortisol is due to hypofunction either of the adrenal cortex or of the pituitary gland. The administration of drugs such as dexamethasone (Decadron) or metyrapone is used to stimulate or to suppress the production of ACTH. Each of these tests is discussed briefly with a summary of the clinical significance of the findings.

Preparation of Client and Collection of Sample

The baseline specimen, for which the laboratory needs 5 mL of plasma, is usually collected in the morning. The specimen should be put on ice and sent to the laboratory immediately. The blood should not come in contact with glass. The collection tube may contain EDTA or heparin.

REFERENCE VALUE FOR ACTH
6–76 pg/mL

ACTH Stimulation Test with Metyrapone

Metyrapone interferes with the normal production of cortisol by blocking some enzymatic actions so compound S is not converted to cortisol. Because of negative feedback, a fall in plasma cortisol level should cause an increase in the level of circulating ACTH. If clients have pituitary insufficiency, however, ACTH level is *not* increased, even with the blockage of cortisol production by metyrapone. Because several ACTH levels may be drawn after the administration of metyrapone, nurses must check with the individual laboratory for the exact timing of the specimens. Phenytoin (Dilantin) interferes with the test because the drug has a variety of endocrine effects. Estrogen compounds also interfere with the test.

ACTH Suppression Test: Dexamethasone Suppression Test

Normally, high plasma corticosteroid levels suppress the formation of ACTH (the negative feedback concept again). Dexamethasone (Decadron), which is a potent corticosteroid that suppresses the formation of ACTH, is given as a test to determine whether the client continues to produce large amounts of cortisol after ACTH is suppressed. Clients with a hyperactive adrenal cortex (Cushing's syndrome) do continue to have high serum cortisol levels because the suppression of pituitary ACTH does not affect the hyperactive adrenal gland.

For screening purposes, 1 mg of dexamethasone is given orally at 11 PM (a client who weighs more than 200 lb (90 kg) takes a larger dose) to suppress ACTH formation. A sample for serum cortisol measurement is drawn the next morning at 8 AM. The plasma levels of cortisol should drop below 5 μg/100 mL. Urine levels of cortisol and other metabolites also may be measured. (These tests are discussed later.) For confirmation of the results, the dexamethasone dosage may be increased and given for several days.

Modified Dexamethasone Suppression Test for Depression

The dexamethasone suppression test (DST) is used to screen for depression. Some clients with clinical depression show elevated cortisol levels even after the dexamethasone is given. Those who show no suppression, a positive test, are believed to be more responsive to pharmacologic intervention (Harris, 1982). If the DST is used to evaluate a depressive state, blood levels are drawn at 4 PM and 11 PM rather than 8 AM. Controversy continues over the use of the DST for depression because the sensitivity may be no greater than 50% (Ravel, 1995).

Use of ACTH (Cosyntropin) to Stimulate Cortisol Production

Clients with suspected diseases of the adrenal cortex can be given a test dose of ACTH to determine whether ACTH causes an increased production of cortisol in the serum. A synthetic type of ACTH, called *cosyntropin,* may be given intravenously or intramuscularly as a diagnostic test. The administration of 0.25 mg of cosyntropin should stimulate the adrenal cortex to increase the plasma cortisol level by at least 18 μg/dL (Katzung, 1995). A lack of response to cosyntropin indicates primary hypofunctioning of the adrenal cortex.

▼ CORTISOL PLASMA LEVELS

Cortisol, the glucocorticoid found in the largest concentration in the serum, is the one usually measured to gain information about the functioning of the adrenal cortex. Plasma cortisol has a diurnal variation, its levels being higher in the morning than in the evening. Baseline readings are taken in the morning with the client at rest. The timing of the cortisol levels with suppression and stimulation are determined by the procedure of the particular laboratory.

Preparation of Client and Collection of Sample

The laboratory needs 1 mL of plasma. The specimen is usually drawn in the morning after the client has been fasting. Evening samples may also require about 3 hr of fasting. Water is allowed. Because activity increases the level, the client needs to be supine for 2 hr before the test.

Salivary Cortisol

For research studies, salivary cortisol is a simple noninvasive way to obtain a physiologic index of stress. (See Chang et al. [1995] for details on this procedure.)

REFERENCE VALUES FOR SERUM CORTISOL

8 AM (client at rest) 5–25 μg/dL

8 PM <10 μg/dL

1. There are no age or sex differences, but pregnancy causes an increase. Obese people do have higher levels. Activity also increases levels
2. Dexamethasone suppression should decrease cortisol levels to <5 μg/100 mL
3. Cosyntropin stimulation should increase 8 AM cortisol levels at least 18 μg/100 mL

Increased Serum Cortisol Level

Clinical Significance. An increase in cortisol can be either ACTH-dependent or ACTH-independent. A pituitary tumor can cause an increase of ACTH, which causes an increased cortisol level. This type of cortisol increase is ACTH-dependent, and it is sometimes called *Cushing's disease.* Increases of serum cortisol from other causes are called *Cushing's syndrome.* (Cushing was an American endocrinologist who first described the characteristic signs and symptoms of cortisol excess.)

Plasma cortisol levels increase independently of the pituitary gland when there is hyperplasia of the adrenal cortex. Hypersecreting tumors of the adrenal cortex may be malignant or benign.

Some nonendocrine malignant tumors can secrete ACTH, which can result in increased serum cortisol levels (see earlier discussion on ectopic hormones). Cushing's syndrome, or high plasma cortisol levels, can be caused by the administration of corticosteroids over a long period of time.

The specific medical treatment of elevated cortisol levels depends on the cause. The client may undergo a battery of tests to determine whether there is a tumor of the pituitary gland or of the adrenal gland. If Cushing's syndrome is due to exogenous cortisol administration, the dosage of cortisone may be decreased. Sometimes difficult medical decisions must be made regarding the continuation of cortisone therapy. The problems caused by the disease must be weighed against the untoward effects of the therapy.

▼ POSSIBLE NURSING DIAGNOSES RELATED TO INCREASED SERUM CORTISOL LEVEL

Risk for Infection

Nurses must recognize that clients with cortisol elevations do not have a normal response to infections. Cortisol impairs antibody production and cellular immunity, qualities that are beneficial in the treatment of abnormal inflammatory responses but detrimental in the presence of an infection. Such clients may have little elevation of temperature or other responses to a bacterial invasion. So they must be taught to avoid possible sources of infection.

Altered Nutrition

Cortisol stimulates the formation of glucose from other substances, such as protein (gluconeogenesis), and it interferes with the action of insulin. Clients may thus have problems with hyperglycemia. (See Chapter 8 for nursing implications with hyperglycemia.) Obesity is usually a problem, so a typical eating plan for a client with Cushing's syndrome would be a low-sodium, high-protein, low-carbohydrate, and low-calorie diet.

Risk for Injury Related to Poor Wound Healing

Increased levels of cortisol tend to make the skin fragile. Wound healing is delayed. For a postoperative client taking corticosteroids, dehiscence of wounds is a potential problem. Nursing research (Braden, 1988) has suggested that increased serum cortisol levels in elderly people recently located to a nursing home may precipitate pressure sores in susceptible clients. Thus, inspection of the skin and measures to promote skin integrity and wound healing are important when there are known or suspected high cortisol levels.

Risk for Injury Related to Loss of Calcium from Bone

High levels of cortisol cause a reduction in protein stores. If cortisol levels are elevated for more than 6 months, the matrix of the bone may be damaged and calcium may be released, leading to osteoporosis. The bones are easily fractured, so clients must be protected from falls. Any reports of leg or hip pain necessitate a medical evaluation. Sometimes clients undergo total hip replacements because of erosion of joints.

Risk for Bleeding Related to Development of Gastric Ulcers

Increased cortisol levels cause an increased secretion of hydrochloric acid (HCl) and pepsinogen. There is also an inhibition of collagen formation and of other protective proteins in the gastric mucosa. The exact cause of gastric ulcers is not known, but ulcers are a risk when cortisol levels are high. To protect the gastric mucosa, clients may be given antacids. Any signs of gastrointestinal bleeding should be reported at once. (See Chapter 13 for guaiac tests for occult gastrointestinal bleeding.)

Risk for Fluid Volume Excess

Depending on the level of cortisol increase, clients may have sodium retention and potassium excretion. (See the discussion on the effects of aldosterone.) The increased sodium and water retention may lead to elevated blood pressure, weight gain, and edema. (See Chapter 5 for the nursing implications for clients with hypernatremia or hypokalemia.)

Poor Self-esteem Related to Changes in Body Image

Elevated cortisol levels cause a round, full face ("moon face") and a redistribution of fat deposits. Clients may have a "buffalo hump" on the back. Their trunks are obese, and their wasted muscles make the extremities thin. Females may become masculinized with unwanted hair because of some androgenic effects. Acne may occur. Treatment helps correct most of these body changes, but clients need help to cope with their altered body images.

Ineffective Coping of Family Related to Changes in Mood

Increased cortisol levels tend to cause hyperactivity. Clients may need to be cautioned about too much activity. The client may have dramatic mood changes. Euphoria is often present, and psychotic behavior may occur. The family may need help in learning to deal with such wide mood changes. Perez (1984) noted many clients with Cushing's disease have undergone marital disruption, which they attribute to the fatigue and depression of the disease.

Decreased Serum Cortisol Level

Clinical Significance. A subnormal level of cortisol in the plasma is known as *Addison's disease.* (One way to remember that Addison's disease involves a lack of cortisol is to remember that in Addison's disease, one must *add* some cortisone.) The lack of cortisol in the serum may be due to primary hypofunction of the adrenal cortex, or it may be secondary to hypofunctioning of the pituitary gland. Infections may invade the adrenal cortex. Once the most common cause of adrenal insufficiency was tuberculosis, but now it is idiopathic autoimmune adrenalitis. Adrenal insufficiency can be a complication of acquired immunodeficiency syndrome (AIDS) (Greene et al., 1984).

Long-term administration of high doses of corticosteroids causes suppression of ACTH production and a resulting inactivity of these clients' own adrenal glands. There is some atrophy of the adrenal cortex, so the glands do not respond normally to the need for more cortisone in stress. The inability of the adrenal cortex to increase production of cortisol during stress may cause a collection of symptoms known as an *Addisonian crisis.* If cortisol drugs are not withdrawn gradually (tapered off), the client may have a lowered cortisol level before the adrenal glands can begin to function normally again. (See the section on congenital adrenocortical hyperplasia for an explanation of cortisol lack in newborns and young children.)

Clients with borderline adrenal cortex functioning may not have problems until they are faced with a stressful situation, such as a surgical procedure or some other physical or psychological trauma. Insufficiency occurs when at least 90% of the adrenal glands are destroyed. Once the symptoms of a lack of cortisol and aldosterone are recognized and confirmed, replacement therapy is started. Until the hormones are replaced, or when the need is greater than the supply, these clients may have problems related to the lack of cortisol and aldosterone.

▼ POSSIBLE NURSING DIAGNOSES RELATED TO DECREASED SERUM CORTISOL LEVEL

Fluid Volume Deficit Related to Lack of Retention of Sodium and Water

A lack of cortisol and of the mineralocorticoid aldosterone causes low serum sodium levels, which may lead to hypovolemia. Thus clients with a lack of cortisol tend to become dizzy, and they may faint if they leave bed rapidly (postural hypotension). In more advanced cases, the lack of sodium retention can lead to hypovolemia severe enough to cause shock. (See Chapter 5 for the nursing implications for clients with hyponatremia.)

Risk for Altered Cardiac Output Related to Retention of Potassium

Cortisol and, even more so, aldosterone cause sodium retention and potassium excretion. So in Addison's disease, when cortisol is low, not only is the serum sodium low, but the serum potassium rises. The serum potassium may or may not be high enough to cause symptoms. Certainly the client should not be given additional potassium. (See Chapter 5 for the nursing implications for hyperkalemia.)

Risk for Injury Related to Hypoglycemia with Fasting States

Clients with a lack of cortisol are less able to maintain a normal blood sugar when there is no continual replacement of glucose. Thus clients with suspected cortisol deficiency may have symptoms of hypoglycemia if they fast. (See Chapter 8 for the signs, symptoms, and treatment of hypoglycemic episodes.)

Ineffective Coping Related to Inability to Handle Stress (Addisonian Crisis)

Clients with slightly low cortisol levels may have no symptoms until faced with stress: They cannot cope with a crisis. The client needs to be protected not only from physical stress, such as infections, but also from psychological stress, such as high levels of anxiety. In either case, because the adrenal cortex cannot produce enough cortisol and aldosterone, the person has an addisonian crisis. The symptoms of an addisonian crisis are the extreme of the problems already described. Clients experience shock due to the lack of sodium and water in the plasma, and their serum potassium levels increase. They have pain, nausea, and vomiting. Circulatory collapse and death can occur. Treatment of an addisonian crisis includes the intravenous administration of cortisol and a mineralocorticoid along with the replacement of sodium, chloride, and water.

Altered Self-concept Related to Changes in Body Image

On the whole, a lack of cortisol does not cause as many changes in body image as does an excess of cortisol. One characteristic of a lack of cortisol is pigmentation of the skin, because the lack triggers the release of MSH. The exact reasons for the increase in MSH are not well understood. It is hypothesized that the lowered cortisol triggers the pituitary gland to produce not only more ACTH but also MSH. Clients can be told that the darkening of the skin fades when the cortisol level is brought back to normal.

If the cortisol lack is associated with a lack of androgens, there may not be many changes because most sex hormones are produced by the gonads.

(*continued*)

▼ POSSIBLE NURSING DIAGNOSES RELATED TO DECREASED SERUM CORTISOL LEVEL (*continued*)

However, if only cortisol is lacking, the adrenal cortex may be stimulated to increase the production of androgens. This increase causes a collection of symptoms known as *adrenogenital syndrome,* which causes the masculinization of females. (See the section on androgen levels.) In infants and children, congenital hyperplasia of the adrenal glands caused by cortisol lack causes many body changes, as described in the section on adrenogenital syndrome.

Knowledge Deficit Related to the Need for Lifelong Replacement Therapy

Clients with a lack of cortisol take cortisone supplements. Most of the dose is usually given in the morning because this is in keeping with the normal rhythm of the hormone. Clients should be taught to take the cortisone replacement with food or antacid.

A mineralocorticoid may also be needed; fludrocortisone (Florinef) is one that is taken orally, and desoxycorticosterone (DOCA) is given parenterally. Mineralocorticoid replacement is needed only when clients are deficient in aldosterone as well as in cortisol.

These clients need to carry identification that notes the need for extra cortisone in times of stress. They may also keep parenteral hydrocortisone (Solu-Cortef) for emergency replacement. They may be taught to double their doses for minimal stress and triple them for great stress, such as a surgical procedure (Burnett, 1980). The adult client needs to know exactly how to recognize the need for more cortisone. Also parents need to know when to give extra medication to children. (See the discussion on congenital adrenal hyperplasia.)

ADRENOGENITAL SYNDROME ASSOCIATED WITH CONGENITAL ADRENOCORTICAL HYPERPLASIA

A congenital lack of certain enzymes can decrease production of cortisol and sometimes of mineralocorticoids. At least six different inherited genetic defects cause decreased synthesis of cortisol, and some of these defects also cause a lack of mineralocorticoids.

The lack of cortisol causes an increased production of ACTH and hyperplasia of the adrenal glands. Even when the adrenal glands enlarge, they do not produce more cortisol, because of the genetic defect in manufacturing cortisol. However, the adrenal cortex is stimulated to produce more androgens and the precursors of hydrocortisone. In an infant or young child, although the increase in estrogens is not apparent, the increase in androgens causes masculinization of girls and signs of early puberty in boys. In addition to the genetic defect that causes a lack of manufacture of cortisol, there may be an associated inability to produce aldosterone. Children who also lack aldosterone are called *salt losers* because they are unable to retain sodium and water.

Nursery nurses need to examine each newborn's genitalia for any abnormalities. Sometimes girls are incorrectly assumed to be boys. Infants may experience failure to thrive and milk intolerances. Salt losers may have a very poor appetite, frequent vomiting, and other symptoms of severe fluid and electrolyte imbalance.

Some children may seem normal at birth but show symptoms of very early puberty. In these children, diagnosing the lack of cortisol is important so that the increased androgen level does not create secondary sex characteristics. Girls may need surgical treatment to repair an enlarged clitoris or fused vagina. The parents need reassurance that normal sexual function can be expected later. The child's serum cortisol levels are tested, which are low. Urine tests are also conducted to evaluate the presence of metabolites of the glucocorticoids and the androgens in the urine. (These urine tests are covered next.) Treatment with cortisol and, if necessary, with a mineralocorticoid, reduces the level of ACTH and thus the hyperplasia of the adrenal cortex causing the excess of androgens.

▼ POSSIBLE NURSING DIAGNOSIS RELATED TO CONGENITAL ADRENOCORTICAL HYPERPLASIA

Knowledge Deficit Related to Emergency Replacement Therapy

Children with a cortisol lack and their parents need careful instruction on how to manage the replacement of cortisol. It is recommended that families always keep a plastic syringe, two needles, and an ampule of hydrocortisone (Solu-Cortef) in their automobiles and homes for emergency injections. Parents are told that a dose of Solu-Cortef given unnecessarily does not harm the child, but a delay in giving a dose could be fatal. Older children can be taught to recognize symptoms that indicate a need for more hydrocortisone.

URINARY MEASUREMENT OF THE ADRENAL CORTEX STEROIDS

Free urinary cortisol, as well as various metabolites of the adrenal cortex hormones, can be measured in 24/hr urine specimens. In general, the urinary excretion of steroids increases when the serum levels of the steroids increase and decrease when steroids are low in the serum. Sometimes creatinine in the urine sample is measured to ensure that the volume of urine is normal.

See Chapter 3 for details on urine collection. The nurse should check with the laboratory to see if any preservative is needed. The urine specimens are kept cold to decrease bacterial growth. These urine specimens may be ordered as part of tests of ACTH suppression or ACTH stimulation.

▼ URINARY CORTISOL LEVELS

This test, which measures cortisol itself rather than the metabolites, has become the usual test for evaluating adrenal hyperfunction, or Cushing's syndrome. Some drugs, such as spironolactone (Aldactone) or quinacrine (Atabrine), interfere with the results. Low values do not necessarily mean adrenal hypofunction.

REFERENCE VALUE FOR URINARY CORTISOL
20–70 µg/24 hr or 25–95 ng/mg of creatinine

Increased in pregnancy and with oral contraceptives.

▼ 17-HYDROXYCORTICOSTEROIDS (PORTER–SILBER TEST)

This urine test, sometimes called the *Porter–Silber test,* measures several of the metabolites of both the glucocorticoids and aldosterone. These metabolites are increased in Cushing's syndrome. The administration of ACTH should cause an increase also. These metabolites are decreased in Addison's disease and in the adrenogenital syndrome of lack of cortisol. Abnormal values can be caused by hepatic or renal dysfunctions. Chlorpromazine and related drugs interfere with the assay. The specimen should be kept cold. This test is being replaced with urinary cortisol levels.

REFERENCE VALUES FOR 17-OHCS	
Male	3–10 mg/24-hr urine specimen
Female	2–6 mg/24-hr urine specimen

▼ 17-KETOSTEROIDS

17-KS are metabolites of the steroids from both the adrenal cortex and the testes except for the androgen testosterone. The values for men are considerably higher after puberty. The values are increased in tumors when production of hormones from the adrenal cortex or the testes is increased. These metabolites are also increased in the adrenogenital syndrome. Hypofunctioning of the adrenal gland and certain adrenal adenomas cause a decrease. Meprobamate and many other drugs may make the test invalid. Check for possible drug interferences if the client is receiving any drugs. The urine should be kept cold and may need a preservative such as HCl.

REFERENCE VALUES FOR 17-KS

	Male	Female
Age 10	1–4	1–4
20	6–21	4–16
30	8–26	4–14
50	5–18	3–9
70	2–10	1–7

mg/24-hr urine specimen.

▼ URINARY PREGNANETRIOL

Because pregnanetriol is a precursor in adrenal corticoid synthesis, this test is useful in confirming the presence of the adrenogenital syndrome caused by a lack of an enzyme to make cortisol. (Pregnanediol is a test of progesterone. See the section on gonadotropins.) Pregnanetriol is also increased with some tumors of the ovary or adrenal cortex. The urine specimen may need a preservative such as 33% acetic acid.

REFERENCE VALUES FOR URINARY PREGNANETRIOL

Adult	0.5–2.0 mg/24-hr urine specimen
Children:	
2 weeks–2 years	0–0.2 mg/24-hr specimen
2–16 years	0.3–1.1 mg/24-hr specimen

▼ ALDOSTERONE

Aldosterone, a hormone produced by the adrenal cortex, is a mineralocorticoid. Increases in aldosterone cause an increase in the extracellular fluid (ECF) volume because aldosterone increases the reabsorption of sodium and chloride while increasing the excretion of potassium and hydrogen ions.

A decrease in ECF causes increased production of aldosterone through stimulation of the renin–angiotensin system. A decreased flow of blood through the kidney is a stimulus for the production of renin, a hormone secreted by the kidney. Renin, when secreted into the bloodstream, acts on angiotensinogen to form angiotensin. (Angiotensinogen is formed in the liver and circulates in the plasma.) Angiotensin then stimulates the adrenal cortex to increase production of aldosterone. Thus a drop in ECF volume is corrected by the final action of retaining more sodium and water in the plasma. Conversely, an increased ECF volume is a signal for less production of renin. Without renin, angiotensinogen is not converted to the active form of angiotensin, so the adrenal cortex decreases production of aldosterone. Less aldosterone means less sodium (and water) retention, so the ECF volume is decreased to normal again. (See Table 15–4 for a simple diagram of the regulation of aldosterone and the related laboratory tests.)

Preparation of Client and Collection of Sample

The client needs to eat a conventional diet with the usual intake of sodium and potassium. The client may be instructed to eat a specific sodium diet of 10 or 100–200 mEq (mmol). With more sodium in the diet, the reference values are lower. The dietician must plan the diet if a specific sodium intake is to be followed before the urine and plasma samples are collected.

The laboratory needs 3 mL of plasma or serum for the specimen. The plasma specimen is taken after the client has been resting in the supine position for at least 2 hr. Samples may also be obtained in an upright position for comparison. The peak concentration of aldosterone is in the early morning sample. A 24-hr urine specimen may also be collected, and it needs to be kept cold. (See Chapter 3 on 24-hr urine collection.)

REFERENCE VALUES FOR ALDOSTERONE

Plasma levels	With normal sodium intake	
	7 AM recumbent	<16 ng/dL
	9 AM upright	4–31 ng/dL
Urinary excretion for 24 hr	6–25 µg/24 h	
Pregnancy levels are 3–4-fold higher		

In addition to direct measure of aldosterone levels, serum and urine levels of sodium and potassium are measured. (See Chapter 5 on electrolyte measurements in serum and urine.)

TABLE 15–4. RENIN–ANGIOTENSIN CONTROL OF ALDOSTERONE AND TESTS THAT MEASURE ALDOSTERONE-PRODUCING ABILITY OF ADRENAL CORTEX

Decrease of Na in plasma. (Measurement of Na levels.)		
↓		Aldosterone causes increase of Na in plasma and decrease in K. (Measurement of K levels, aldosterone levels in serum and urine, saralasin test.)
Increased production of renin by kidney. (Measurement of renin activity.)		
↓		↑
Renin converts angiotensinogen into angiotensin I, which through enzyme action becomes angiotensin II.	→	Angiotensin II stimulates production of aldosterone by adrenal cortex.

K, potassium; Na, sodium.

See Larrabee and Hanna (1983) and Groër and Shekleton (1989) for more detail.

Increased Aldosterone Levels in Serum and Urine (Hyperaldosteronism)

Clinical Significance. Increased levels of aldosterone can be either primary or secondary. In primary hyperaldosteronism, a tumor of the adrenal cortex or adrenal hyperplasia (Conn's syndrome) causes increased secretion of aldosterone. The renin level in the serum is low because the increased production of the hormone is not caused by the renin–angiotensin mechanism. (The test for renin is discussed next.)

Secondary hyperaldosteronism is a much more common clinical problem than the primary condition. In secondary hyperaldosteronism, the oversecretion of aldosterone is due to continuous activity of the renin–angiotensin system. This constant stimulation of the system occurs when perfusion to the kidneys is not adequate. For example, clients with congestive heart failure (CHF) often have poor renal perfusion. A lack of pressure in the juxtaglomerular apparatus causes the kidney to secrete more renin because the kidneys interpret the lack of perfusion as a lack of ECF. Renin activates angiotensin, which stimulates aldosterone production. Unfortunately, in CHF, the ECF is already in abundance. So the increased aldosterone level, as a response to poor renal perfusion, does not correct the underlying problem. With secondary hyperaldosteronism, the renin level is therefore high.

Not all cases of increased aldosterone are so simple. Sometimes drugs, such as oral contraceptives, cause an increase in aldosterone levels, although the exact mechanism is not well understood. Clients with severe liver dysfunction, such as cirrhosis, tend to have elevated aldosterone levels, which are partly related to poor renal perfusion. Also, if a failing liver can no longer detoxify aldosterone, levels of serum aldosterone remain higher for longer periods.

▼ POSSIBLE NURSING DIAGNOSIS RELATED TO INCREASED ALDOSTERONE LEVELS

Risk for Injury Related to Hypertension and Hypokalemia

Increased aldosterone levels tend to cause an elevation of serum sodium levels and a decrease of serum potassium levels. In primary aldosteronism many clients do not have edema even though a sodium excess occurs. This lack of edema is probably because ECF volume is controlled by several factors. Hypertension and hypokalemia are the two most outstanding characteristics of primary aldosteronism (Giefer and Cassmeyer, 1994). Monitoring the blood pressure and electrolytes is important. (See Chapter 5 on the nursing implications of hypokalemia.)

(*continued*)

▼ POSSIBLE NURSING DIAGNOSIS RELATED TO INCREASED ALDOSTERONE LEVELS (*continued*)

Risk for Fluid Volume Excess Related to Retention of Sodium

If the increased aldosterone level is due to secondary causes, edema is usually a clinical problem. (See Chapter 5 for a discussion of the nursing implications when a client has edema and needs to follow a restricted sodium diet.) Diuretics may be particularly useful for secondary hyperaldosteronism. The type of diuretic often used is spironolactone because this drug is an aldosterone-blocking agent. Spironolactone (Aldactone) is a steroid compound that presumably acts by competing with aldosterone for cellular receptor sites in the tubules. Thus it promotes sodium and water excretion without a loss of potassium.

Decreased Aldosterone Levels

Clinical Significance. The decrease in aldosterone is often part of a generalized hypofunctioning of the adrenal gland. The causes of Addison's disease are discussed in the section on cortisol deficiencies. In congenital adrenal hyperplasia, the infant lacks an enzyme needed to manufacture cortisol from cholesterol, and this deficiency may or may not be associated with a deficiency of aldosterone. In the most common type of genetic defect that causes a lack of cortisol, about one-third of clients are also deficient in a mineralocorticoid or aldosterone (Burnett, 1980). The lack of aldosterone gives the symptoms of "salt wasting" seen in some genetic defects and in Addison's disease.

▼ POSSIBLE NURSING DIAGNOSIS FOR DECREASED ALDOSTERONE LEVELS

Fluid Volume Deficit Related to Hyponatremia

Clients with decreased aldosterone levels are unable to maintain normal serum sodium and potassium levels and thus can experience hypovolemic shock and hyperkalemia. (See the discussion on addisonian crisis in the section on low cortisol levels.) They must therefore have salt, water, and mineralocorticoid replacement. If they lack aldosterone, clients take fludrocortisone (Florinef) orally or DOCA parenterally to ensure mineralocorticoid activity. These medications are continued for life. Because a lack of mineralocorticoid activity also may be part of the adrenogenital syndrome, children who experience salt wasting as part of their congenital problem must undergo mineralocorticoid replacement. Children born with a severe lack of mineralocorticoids may die, however, before the defect is recognized.

▼ RENIN

Renin is an enzyme produced by the juxtaglomerular apparatus in response to decreased blood flow through the kidneys. A change from the recumbent position to upright also causes an increased production. A high-sodium diet causes a decrease in renin. Thus diet and the position of the client must be taken into account when using reference values for renin activity. The test for renin is used in the differential diagnosis of hypertension.

Preparation of Client and Collection of Sample

Because the values of renin are normally higher in the morning, the test is performed early in the day. The client is usually in the supine position when the blood is drawn, but blood also may be drawn with the patient upright for comparison. The laboratory needs 4 mL of plasma, which is put into a tube with EDTA as an anticoagulant (lavender vacuum tube). The specimen should be iced. Also note the sodium content of the diet, which should be controlled for several days. Diuretics, estrogens, oral contraceptives, and antihypertensive drugs should be withheld for several days before the test.

REFERENCE VALUES FOR SERUM RENIN

Supine	0.5–1.6 ng/mL per hr
Upright	1.9–3.6 ng/mL per hr

▼ CATECHOLAMINES, VANILLYLMANDELIC ACID, AND METANEPHRINES

The adrenal medulla secretes epinephrine and norepinephrine, both of which are essential in assisting the body for the "fight-or-flight" response to stress. These two hormones, called the *catecholamines,* are usually measured in 24-hr urine samples but plasma samples also can be tested. Dopamine, also a catecholamine and the precursor of the other two, may be measured in the serum and urine.

Catecholamines are broken down into intermediate metabolites, which are called *normetanephrine* and *metanephrines.* Laboratories may also measure these intermediate metabolites in the urine. The main product of catecholamine breakdown is an acid called VMA. Because the VMA test is easier to perform than the other urine tests for catecholamines, the laboratory may use the VMA as the screening procedure. Some laboratories prefer to use the metanephrines as the screening test for hypertension (Camuñas, 1983). Although the metanephrine test is slowly gaining preference, VMA and catecholamine assays are still widely used (Ravel, 1995). In some types of neuroblastomas, dopamine and the metabolite homovanillic acid may be more prominent than the other two catecholamines and the metabolites (Kaplan et al., 1995).

Preparation of Client and Collection of Specimen

All the tests for the metabolites of the catecholamines require that the urine remain acid with a pH of 3 or less. Usually 12 mL of HCl is added to the 24-hr specimen bottle. Clients should be warned about the strong acid in the bottle. The usual procedure for collecting urine for 24 hr is followed (see Chapter 3).

The client needs to be relatively free of stress. Vigorous exercise causes an elevation of catecholamines. Blood pressure, height, and weight should be recorded on the laboratory slip.

Nurses must validate the need for restriction of certain foods by checking with the laboratory conducting the test. The client should eat a conventional diet because fasting increases catecholamines. Depending on the procedure used by the laboratory, some foods must be restricted in the diet. For example, coffee, tea, chocolate, bananas, avocados, and anything with vanilla used to interfere with the VMA results. Newer laboratory methods may not be affected by food intake.

A multitude of drugs can lead to confusing results. Drugs that act via the sympathetic nervous system, such as some antihypertensives, and antidepressants, make the test invalid. Ideally, the client should not take any drugs for 3–7 days before the test. Nurses must check with the individual physician to see which drugs can be given.

REFERENCE VALUES FOR CATECHOLAMINES AND METABOLITES IN URINE

Dopamine	65–400
Epinephrine	1.7–22.4
Norepinephrine	12.1–85.5
Metanephrines	0.0–0.9
Vanillylmandelic acid (VMA)	1.4–6.5
Homovanillic acid (HVA)	0.0–15.0

All results are μg/24-hr urine specimen.

Increased Catecholamines in Urine

Clinical Significance. Mild elevations of the catecholamines and of their metabolites can be caused by stress such as operations, burns, or childbirth. (No endocrine response can be effectively evaluated during stress.) A marked increase in the catecholamines has two main causes: The first, a tumor of the adrenal medulla, called a *pheochromocytoma,* causes a marked elevation in catecholamines. The second comes from certain types of malignant tumors, called *neuroblastomas,* which arise from primitive sympathetic tissue. Other tests, such as scans, help pinpoint the presence of a tumor.

▼ POSSIBLE NURSING DIAGNOSES RELATED TO ELEVATED CATECHOLAMINES

Anxiety and Altered Cardiac Output Related to the Effects of Increased Catecholamines

Clients with elevated catecholamines have symptoms reflective of the stimulating effects of epinephrine and norepinephrine. Often their symptoms are attributed to other causes. Some of the outstanding symptoms are increased blood pressure and pulse. Because clients may feel jittery and notice heart palpitations, their symptoms may be wrongly ascribed to an anxiety attack. The surge of catecholamines may be intermittent, so that during an attack the blood pressure may become high and the client can have pounding headaches, nausea, and vomiting. The high levels of epinephrine can cause hyperglycemia and glycosuria, and the client may be believed to have diabetes. (See Chapter 8 on symptoms of hyperglycemia.)

Nurses should carefully monitor the blood pressure and pulse of any client with suspected catecholamine increase caused by pheochromocytoma or a childhood neuroblastoma. A blood or urine sample taken during or soon after an attack may demonstrate the presence of high levels of catecholamines.

Knowledge Deficit Related to Drug Therapy and an Impending Surgical Procedure

Symptoms can be controlled with α-adrenergic blocking drugs, but the definitive treatment is an operation. Some clients are treated with drugs for weeks before the operation, whereas other clients undergo surgical treatment soon after the diagnosis is made (Katzung, 1995).

Catecholamine Deficiency

Clinical Significance. Even when the adrenal medulla is hypofunctional or destroyed by disease or surgical intervention, the client does not have any symptoms of catecholamine deficiency because catecholamines are also produced by the autonomic nerve endings.

▼ PARATHORMONE OR PARATHYROID HORMONE

Parathormone is produced by the parathyroid glands—the only hormone secreted by these glands. The parathyroid glands, usually four in number, are located in the vicinity of the thyroid gland. Unlike that of many of the other hormones, the level of PTH is not under the influence of the pituitary gland.

The function of PTH is to control serum calcium and phosphorus levels (Table 15–5). A lowered serum calcium level is a stimulus for the release of more PTH to keep the serum calcium level normal. PTH works in various ways to keep a constant serum calcium level and a correspondingly normal phosphorus level:

1. It works in concert with vitamin D to stimulate calcium and phosphorus absorption via the intestinal mucosa.
2. It causes mobilization of calcium from the bone.
3. It causes increased excretion of phosphorus in the urine.

An abnormal elevation or decrease in PTH always changes serum calcium and phosphorus levels. (See Chapter 7 for a detailed discussion of the effects of PTH on serum calcium and phosphorus levels. Note that phosphorus is measured as phosphate in the serum.)

Preparation of Client and Collection of Sample

The client does not have to be fasting. Collect a morning sample. The laboratory needs 1 mL of serum, which should be kept on ice in all cases or, if it must be sent a distance, frozen. (Samples are often shipped because the test is difficult to conduct in most laboratories.) PTH is stable for only 2 hr at room temperature. Note that laboratories can measure the intact molecule or several of the fragments (Ravel, 1995). PTH assays should always be performed in conjunction with a measurement of serum calcium. A PTH-Ca normogram may be used to report the results (Kaplan et al., 1995).

REFERENCE VALUE FOR SERUM PTH (INTACT MOLECULE)
10–60 pg/mL

Increased PTH Serum Level

Clinical Significance. Increased PTH levels may indicate primary hyperparathyroidism. Tumors of a parathyroid gland, which are usually benign, cause increased secretion of PTH. Clients have symptoms of high serum calcium levels and low phosphate levels (as discussed in Chapter 7). A persistently low serum calcium level or a high phosphate level causes a secondary rise in PTH. Also, malignant tumors from nonendocrine sources can secrete PTH. (See the discussion on ectopic hormones.)

Because an elevated PTH causes an increased serum calcium level and a decreased serum phosphate level, the nursing diagnoses are based on these imbalances. (See Chapter 7 for the nursing implications when a client has hypercalcemia.) If the client has an adenoma, surgical intervention can restore the balance.

TABLE 15–5. EFFECTS OF PARATHORMONE (PTH) ON SERUM CALCIUM AND SERUM PHOSPHORUS

↑ PTH causes ↑ Ca ↓ P
↓ PTH causes ↓ Ca ↑ P

Decreased PTH Serum Level

Clinical Significance. Decreased levels of PTH can be due to trauma to the parathyroid glands during a thyroidectomy. Infections or other trauma may affect the parathyroid gland. Tumors of the gland usually cause an increase in hormone production, but some tumors may cause decreased function of the gland. Because the levels of PTH are normally low in the serum, a low level may not be helpful in diagnosis.

The symptoms and clinical manifestations of a lack of PTH are reflected in low serum calcium levels and in high phosphate levels. Severe hypocalcemia causes tetany. (See Chapter 7 for a detailed description of tetany and nursing diagnoses for hypocalcemia.)

A lack of PTH is treated with administration of vitamin D and calcium salts. (See Chapter 7 on the treatment of low serum calcium levels and possible client teaching.)

THYROID GLAND

The thyroid gland secretes three hormones: triiodothyronine (T_3), L-thyroxine (T_4), and calcitonin. Calcitonin lowers the plasma calcium level by inhibiting mobilization of calcium from the bone. (See Chapter 7 on the role of calcitonin in the regulation of calcium levels.) Calcitonin levels are measured only for known or suspected cases of medullary carcinoma of the thyroid. (See Appendix A, Table 2 for reference values.) The other two of these hormones, T_3 and T_4, are forms of thyroxine, and they are usually called the *thyroid hormones*. (T_3 contains *three* iodine atoms and T_4 contains *four* iodine atoms in a molecule.) An adequate intake of iodine is necessary for the continual formation of T_3 and T_4. As with the other hormones, protein intake also must be normal. In many countries, table salt has been iodized so that people have an adequate intake of iodine.

Most of the output of the thyroid is in the form of T_4; only a small amount is in the form of T_3, but T_3 is much more potent than T_4. Both T_4 and T_3 can be measured directly. Also, the amount of T_4 can be calculated with other tests, such as the T_3 resin uptake. Each of these tests is discussed individually later in this section. The thyroid hormones, T_4 and T_3, have several functions:

1. They potentiate the effects of epinephrine and decrease the serum cholesterol level.
2. They are necessary for normal development of the central nervous system.
3. They stimulate growth and normal metabolism in all cells.

Tests to Diagnose Thyroid Disease

Although there are several different tests for diagnosing hyper- and hypothyroidism, estimation of the free thyroxine (free T_4) and the newer, more sensitive thyrotropin or TSH are the two principal laboratory tests recommended by the American Thyroid Association (Surks et al., 1990). In some cases, the patient may also have radioactive iodine (RAI) uptakes or thyroid scans, both of which are discussed in Chapter 22.

Cancer of the thyroid is suggested by cold nodules on a thyroid scan not by serum laboratory tests. Some types of thyroid inflammation are associated with increased amounts of antibodies. Chapter 14 discusses the test for thyroid antibodies that are subdivided into microsomal antibodies and thyroglobulin antibodies.

Because the thyroid hormones increase the metabolism of cholesterol, clients with hyperthyroidism tend to have low serum cholesterol levels, and clients with hypothyroidism tend to have high serum cholesterol levels. (See Chapter 9 on cholesterol tests.) Yet the cholesterol level is not particularly helpful in confirming the presence of a thyroid disorder.

▼ THYROTROPIN OR THYROID-STIMULATING HORMONE

The production of T_4 and T_3 is controlled by TSH from the anterior pituitary gland. TSH is released from the pituitary in response to the thyrotropin-releasing hormone (TRH) in the hypothalamus. Thus, like most of the other anterior pituitary hormones, TSH is sensitive to nervous response from the hypothalamus. Measurement of TSH is useful in determining whether hypothyroidism is due to primary hypofunction of the thyroid gland or to secondary hypofunction of the anterior pituitary gland. In sophisticated endocrine evaluations, TRH from the hypothalamus can be measured. High doses of corticosteroids and dopamine infusions can suppress TSH levels.

Preparation of Client and Collection of Sample

The laboratory requires 2 mL of serum. The client does not need to be fasting.

REFERENCE VALUES FOR TSH
0.5–5.0 µU/mL

Thyrotropin has a diurnal variation with the lowest levels about 10 AM and the highest levels at about 10–11 PM (Ravel, 1995). Acutely ill clients may have different patterns.

Increased or Decreased TSH

Clinical Significance. One purpose of measuring TSH is to evaluate the possibility of pituitary failure as the cause of hypothyroidism. A low TSH is an indication for further investigation of pituitary disorders. Primary hypothyroidism, caused by insufficiency of the thyroid gland itself, is a much more common cause of hypothyroidism. In primary hypothyroidism, the TSH level becomes greatly elevated in an attempt to stimulate the failing thyroid gland. For many years, TSH has been used to confirm primary hypothyroidism in newborns (Fisher et al., 1979). In the past, TSH was not useful in the diagnosis of hyperthyroidism because some people with normal thyroid function (euthyroid) had such low levels of TSH that the levels were barely detected if at all. A newer assay, which is very sensitive and is sometimes noted as s-TSH, can clearly define a lower limit of normal range. For clients with hyperthyroidism, the level may be as low as 0.1 mU/L. The very sensitive TSH is also used to monitor the treatment of hypothyroidism. A lower than normal level occurs with overdosage of T_4 (Surks et al., 1990). This is another example of the negative feedback concept discussed at the beginning of this chapter.

▼ L-THYROXINE SERUM CONCENTRATION (TOTAL T_4)

T_4, the thyroxine with four iodine atoms, is the most abundant of the thyroid hormones. The test of total T_4 measures both free thyroxine and the portion carried by the thyroid-binding plasma proteins. Laboratories may also have techniques for controlling the effect of proteins to make a "normalized" T_4 (Ravel, 1995).

Preparation of Client and Collection of Sample

The laboratory requires 1 mL of plasma. Fasting is recommended. If the client is taking a thyroid preparation, this should be recorded on the requisition slip. Many drugs (e.g., propranolol and phenytoin) may interfere with the test results.

REFERENCE VALUES FOR L-THYROXINE (TOTAL T_4)

Adult	4–12 μg/dL Values vary according to different laboratory methods[a]
Pregnancy	Causes an increase, as do oral contraceptives
Infants	Up to 16.5 μg/dL
Children	Up to 15.0 μg/dL (declines with age)
Aged	Values maintained, but decrease in plasma protein lowers values

[a]See free T_4 test.

Decreases and Increases in T_4

Clinical Significance. The hormone is increased in hyperthyroidism and decreased in hypothyroidism. The nursing diagnoses for these two conditions are summarized later in this chapter. In clients with a hydatidiform mole, T_4 may be very elevated. Evidently, there is an increase of some TSH activity from the molar tissue. Another nonthyroid cause of an elevation is liver disease.

▼ TRIIODOTHYRONINE SERUM CONCENTRATION (T_3)

Some resources may list this test as a T_3 RIA to denote that the hormone is measured with a radioimmunoassay. However most laboratories now use immunoassay rather than radioimmunossay, as discussed in Chapter 1. T_3 is more biologically active than T_4, but both hormones have similar actions in the body. T_3 is not usually used in confirming the diagnosis of suspected hypothyroidism because other tests can demonstrate hypofunction of the thyroid gland. Sometimes, however, a client may have clinical signs of thyrotoxicosis with a normal T_4. Measurement of the T_3 is then needed, because T_3 may be elevated in thyrotoxicosis while other thyroid tests are still in the normal range (Ravel, 1995).

Preparation of Client and Collection of Sample

The preparation and collection instructions are the same as those for the T_4 test.

REFERENCE VALUES FOR TOTAL TRIIODOTHYRONINE (T_3)	
Adult	75–195 ng/dL
Pregnancy and oral contraceptives	Tend to increase the values
Infants and children have higher values	

A decrease in plasma proteins causes lowered values.

▼ FREE T_4 AND FREE THYROXINE INDEX

The free part of T_4, the part not bound to the globulins, can be measured by means of direct assay or with indirect measurement, which may be recorded as a free T_4 index or as a free thyroxine index (FTI). Except in rare situations, such as acute nonthyroid disease, the indirect measurement of free T_4 is as useful as and is less expensive than a direct assay of free T_4. A number of different methods are available for estimation of the free T_4, which takes into account the total serum T_4 and the thyroid hormone binding ratio, which is an indirect measurement of the thyroid-binding globulins. The index is reported as a range of numerical values. Surks et al. (1990) noted that the estimation of free T_4 is more useful than the total T_4 for diagnosing hyper- and hypothyroidism.

REFERENCE VALUE FOR FREE T_4 (ACTUAL ASSAY)
0.8–2.7 ng/mL

REFERENCE VALUE FOR FREE T_4 INDEX (CALCULATED)
4.6–11.2

TABLE 15–6. TESTS OF THYROID FUNCTION

Test	Hypothyroidism	Hyperthyroidism
TSH (thyroid-stimulating hormone)	↓ or ↑ (see text)	↑ or ↓ (see text)
T_4 (L-thyroxine) total and free	↓	↑
T_3 (triiodothyronine)	Not usually performed	↑
Free T_4 Index	↓	↑
RAI (radioactive iodine uptake)	↓	↑
Thyroid scans (see Chapter 22)	Used to identify nodules not hypo or hyper states *per se.*	

See text and the work of Surks et al. (1990) for American Thyroid Association Guidelines for use of laboratory tests in thyroid disorders. See Ravel (1995) for the complexity of interpreting these tests when they do not follow an expected pattern.

Elevated Serum Thyroid Levels

Clinical Significance. A diagnosis of hyperthyroidism is made when the client has an elevation of several of the tests discussed in this chapter. (One test alone may not always be diagnostic.) Table 15–6 shows which of the common tests of thyroid function are usually elevated in hyperthyroidism. An excess of thyroid hormone can result from inflammation, tumors, or autoimmune disorders of the thyroid gland. Often the cause of the hyperthyroidism is unknown (i.e., it is idiopathic). A hyperthyroid state associated with goiter and a bulging of the eyes (exophthalmos) is called *Graves' disease,* which is considered the most fully developed hyperthyroid state and is also called *thyrotoxicosus.* It sometimes follows an infection, physical stress, or emotional crisis. Hyperthyroidism is rare in infants, but it does occur in children and particularly in adolescents. Hyperthyroidism is much more common in girls than in boys. Once hyperthyroidism is definitely diagnosed, treatment may include the use of antithyroid drugs, therapy with RAI, or surgical intervention. The goal of treatment is to bring the client back to a euthyroid, or normal thyroid, balance. The client needs help from the nurse and from others in learning to cope with the manifestations of hyperthyroidism.

▼ POSSIBLE NURSING DIAGNOSES RELATED TO ELEVATED SERUM THYROID LEVELS

Risk for Altered Cardiac Output Related to Tachyarrhythmias

In general, most of the symptoms of hyperthyroidism are due to the accelerated metabolism that results from an excess of circulating thyroid hormones. These clients have tachycardia and often arrhythmias, such as atrial fibrillation. Even their resting pulses may be more than 90 beats per minute. Extreme thyrotoxicosis can even cause high-output cardiac failure. The high pulse

(continued)

▼ POSSIBLE NURSING DIAGNOSES RELATED TO ELEVATED SERUM THYROID LEVELS (*continued*)

decreases as the thyroid gland is brought under control. However, the pulse should be monitored to gauge how well clients can tolerate activity so they are not overtaxed. β-Blockers, such as propranolol (Inderal), may be ordered to decrease symptoms until the hyperthyroidism is controlled.

Altered Nutrition: Less than Body Requirements Related to Increased Metabolism

These clients' increased metabolism make them hungry most of the time. They need a well-balanced diet with extra calories, as well as between-meal snacks. Extra fluids are needed because of the diaphoresis. Stimulants, such as caffeine, should be avoided. The client should be weighed periodically to see that weight loss is not continuing. If diarrhea is a problem, the diet should avoid foods that tend to aggravate the hyperactive bowel.

Risk for Hyperthermia Related to Ineffective Thermoregulation

Clients with hyperthyroidism have heat intolerance, so they should be protected from high environmental temperatures. The room should be kept cool, and additional fluids should be offered to prevent hyperthermia. A thyroid storm can occur after an operation if the thyroid hormones are released in increased amounts. Antipyretics are not as helpful as they are with fevers related to hypothalamic control. Measures such as a cooling blanket are useful. Abrupt withdrawal of antithyroid medication can also lead to thyroid storm, so clients need to know the importance of complying with a medication regimen (Corsetti and Buhl, 1994).

Sleep Pattern Disturbance Related to Hyperactivity and Increased Metabolic Rate

Clients with hyperthyroidism often have insomnia. They need a quiet, relaxing environment and perhaps sedatives to sleep. (Sedatives are contraindicated for clients with hypothyroidism.)

Altered Self-concept Related to Exophthalmos

Exophthalmos is an abnormal protrusion of the eye that sometimes occurs with hyperthyroidism when lymphocytes and mucopolysaccharides collect behind the eyeball. This collection may be unilateral or bilateral. The treatment of hyperthyroidism does not seem to have an appreciable influence on the progression or regression of the exophthalmos. The key is to prevent trauma to the eyes and to help clients adjust to the altered body image (Groër and Shekleton, 1989).

Ineffective Coping

Family, co-workers, and friends may find it difficult to understand the actions of a client who has symptoms of hyperthyroidism. Nurses may be helpful by explaining in simple terms why these clients fuss about heat, noise, or what may seem like small irritations. Jenkins (1980) described a personal account of the frustrations of learning to live with thyrotoxicosis and how this affected her jobs in nursing. Control of a hormone imbalance is not always achieved in a short time. It may take months to years to gain adequate balance.

Decreased Serum Thyroid Levels

Clinical Significance. The findings of the several tests to confirm the diagnosis of hypothyroidism are summarized in Table 15–6. In adults, the presence of hypothyroidism is called *myxedema.* The failure of the thyroid gland to produce thyroid hormones is usually a primary dysfunction of the gland itself. However, hypothyroidism can also result from a lack of TSH (as discussed in the section on TSH). Diets deficient in iodine also cause a lack of thyroid hormone and an enlargement of the thyroid gland (goiter). Inflammations and autoimmune responses may cause insufficiency of the gland, but often the hypofunctioning cannot be linked to a causative factor.

Many clients in an intensive care unit have low serum T_4 levels but no symptoms of hypothyroidism, so this is called the *sick low T_4 euthyroid syndrome* (Kaplan et al., 1995). The T_4 returns to normal after recovery from the illness.

In congenital hypothyroidism, the lack of the thyroid hormone can cause cretinism. Lack of thyroid in newborns causes growth failure and mental retardation. The symptoms of hypothyroidism may not be present at birth because the fetus has some thyroid hormones from the mother. Studies (Fisher et al., 1979) have concluded that T_4 should be a screening device for all newborns, so that congenital hypothyroidism can be detected. (See Chapter 18 on newborn screening.) In addition to newborns, other populations particularly susceptible to hypothyroidism are elderly people, postpartum women, people with autoimmune diseases such as Type I diabetes mellitus or Addison's disease, and those who have had treatment for hyperthyroidism in the past.

▼ POSSIBLE NURSING DIAGNOSES RELATED TO DECREASED SERUM THYROID LEVELS

Altered Health Maintenance Related to Need for Lifelong Replacement Therapy

Hypothyroidism in Infants. Nurses must be aware of the symptoms of hypothyroidism in newborns and in adults, because nurses may be involved in case

(*continued*)

▼ POSSIBLE NURSING DIAGNOSES RELATED TO DECREASED SERUM THYROID LEVELS (*continued*)

finding. Case finding in infants is important because mental retardation occurs if the infant is not treated within 2–3 months after birth, and sometimes the effects of lack of thyroid may not be prominent at birth because the fetus has some thyroid hormones from the mother. Some of the outstanding characteristics of a lack of thyroid in a newborn are protruding tongue, a broad, flattened nose, a protruding abdomen with an umbilical hernia, and a generalized muscle hypotonia. The baby has a hoarse cry and may be a poor feeder. The heart rate is slow.

Once hypothyroidism is diagnosed, treatment is begun with thyroid replacement. The medication helps the infant grow and develop normally. The parents need careful teaching about the importance of lifelong administration of the hormone and normal patterns of growth and development.

Older Children and Adults. Symptoms of hypothyroidism, or myxedema, in clients beyond infancy are due to the slowing of metabolism that occurs with insufficient thyroid hormone. These clients may have only slight symptoms, so the disease may be overlooked. They typically have fatigue, lethargy, and an intolerance to cold. Their hair is coarse and their skin is very dry. They gain weight on a limited diet. Constipation may be a problem. Blood pressure and pulse are low. Clients may have memory impairment or a definite slowness in mental ability. Thyroid replacement eradicates these symptoms. The client needs to know the signs of overdosage of the drugs. (See the discussion on the symptoms of hyperthyroidism.) A resting pulse greater than 90 beats per minute is an indicator of possibly too much thyroid replacement. Clients should be taught to check their own pulses. Any improvement in the way thyroid is commercially prepared can cause a need for less medication as the drugs become more potent (Stoffer and Szpunar, 1984).

Altered Comfort Related to Cold Intolerance and Slowness of Thought

Clients with hypothyroidism have a cold intolerance, so the environment needs to be warm. The nurse can provide extra clothing, such as heavy socks. The environment must also be warm in the psychological sense. These clients may be slower in activity so others must let them proceed at their own pace. The clients may need help to adjust to fast-moving situations. Because inactivity may produce more lethargy and dullness, sensory stimulation is needed. In the home setting, the family may need help making the environment warm, relaxed, and relatively quiet for the client.

Altered Nutrition: More than Body Requirements

Clients may need to follow a diet that is low in calories to prevent weight gain. The nurse should see that the diet contains all the essential nutrients and vitamins. Clients can be assured that when their thyroid level is returned to normal, their excess poundage should be easier to lose. (In fact, thyroid pills have been used as a type of diet pill. Thyroid intake by a client who is euthyroid is not a physiologically sound way to lose weight.) Plenty of fluids and fiber in the diet help to decrease the problem of constipation.

Risk for Injury Related to Intolerance for Sedatives and Narcotics

Because these clients have a slower-than-normal metabolism, sedatives and narcotics may have a profound effect. These types of drugs should be used with caution, if at all.

Altered Body Image

Clients may be distressed by their rough skin and coarse hair. They may need to use hair conditioners and plenty of skin lotion to keep their skin and hair attractive looking. These skin and hair problems fade as the hormonal balance is restored.

GONADOTROPINS AND THE SEX-RELATED HORMONES

The sex-related hormones include the gonadotropins from the anterior pituitary gland (FSH and LH) and estrogen, progesterone, and the androgens from the ovaries, testes, and adrenal cortex. Both the ovaries and testes produce progesterone, estrogen, and the androgens but in markedly different proportions in males and females. The sex hormones from the adrenal cortex occur in minute amounts in both sexes.

Infertility, the lack of development of secondary sex characteristics, and changes in sexual characteristics or sexual functioning are common reasons for measuring the sex hormones.

▼ FOLLICLE-STIMULATING HORMONE

FSH from the anterior pituitary gland controls the growth and maturation of the ovarian follicles in women for ovulation. FSH also controls the secretion of estrogen in women. In women, a high FSH is the most reliable indicator of the ovarian failure of menopause. In men, FSH stimulates the testes to produce sperm.

Preparation of Client and Collection of Sample

There is no special preparation of the client. The laboratory needs 5 mL of serum or plasma for the blood test. The same sample can be used for LH.

REFERENCE VALUES FOR FSH	
Adult: Men	4–15 mU/mL
Women	4.6–22.4 mU/mL pre- or postovulatory; 13–41 mU/mL midcycle peak
Prepubertal: Boys	2–10 mU/mL
Girls	3–7 mU/mL
Postmenopausal women	30–170 mU/mL

▼ LUTEINIZING HORMONE

LH is the second gonadotropic hormone secreted by the anterior pituitary gland. In women, LH, along with FSH, is necessary for ovulation to take place. Various test kits are available to measure the surge of LH in the urine as a signal of ovulation. (See Chapter 28 on tests for fertility.) After ovulation, LH stimulates the ruptured follicle to secrete increasing amounts of progesterone. In men, LH stimulates the production of androgens, which are important in determining the secondary sex characteristics. LH in men is sometimes referred to as the interstitial cell-stimulating hormone (ICSH). In men, LH may be measured if serum testosterone levels are low.

REFERENCE VALUES FOR LH	
Adult: Men	3–18 mU/mL
Women	2.4–34.5 mU/mL pre- and postovulation 43–187 mU/mL, midcycle peaks
Children	2–12 mU/mL
Postmenopausal women	30–150 mU/mL

Preparation of Client and Collection of Sample

The requirement of 3 mL of blood or plasma for LH is the same as for FSH, and both tests can be performed on the same specimen.

Changes in FSH and LH Serum Levels

Clinical Significance. FSH and LH levels are measured to see whether clients with hypogonadism have a primary gonad problem or a secondary problem of pituitary insufficiency. Pituitary insufficiency may be first manifested by a lack of function of the testes or ovaries. LH and FSH are low if the failure of the gonads is due to pituitary insufficiency (secondary hypogonadism). The levels of FSH and LH in serum and urine are high if the failure of the gonads is primary failure of the ovaries or testes. Drugs, such as clomiphene (Clomid) or gonadotropin-releasing factor (GRH), may be given to see if the level of gonadotropins increases. Increased levels of FSH are also used to verify that a woman is undergoing menopause.

▼ ESTRADIOL AND OTHER FORMS OF ESTROGEN

Different forms of the estrogens, including estradiol, estrone, and estriol, can be measured. Estriol is the estrogen present in largest amounts at pregnancy. (See Chapter 18 for the use of estriol as a test of fetal well-being during pregnancy.) Because estrogens are produced not only by the ovaries but also by the adrenal cortex and testes, estradiol levels may be useful to assess pathologic conditions in all three glands.

The level of estradiol is increased in men who have testicular or adrenal tumors. In women, the increased estradiol arises from estrogen-secreting ovarian tumors. Decreases of estradiol in women, or a lack of increase during a menstrual cycle, can be due either to ovarian failure or to pituitary insufficiency. Other factors, such as anorexia nervosa, may also cause decreases in estradiol. Hepatic and renal failure can cause abnormal increases of estrogens in the serum. Women may show no symptoms when estrogens are increased. Men may exhibit feminizing signs, such as enlarged breasts, when any of the estrogens is increased.

Preparation of Client and Collection of Sample

For estradiol, collect 5 mL in a red-topped tube. Include date of LMP. Values vary considerably as to ranges considered normal (see Appendix A, Table 2 for other values).

REFERENCE VALUES FOR SERUM ESTRADIOL	
Men	20–90 pg/mL
Women	
Follicular phase	20–120 pg/mL
Midcycle	80–300 pg/mL
Luteal phase	60–170 pg/mL
Menopause	<20 pg/mL

▼ PROGESTERONE

In women of childbearing age, progesterone is low during the first part of the menstrual cycle (follicular phase). When LH is increased at the time of ovulation (luteal phase), there is a resulting surge of progesterone for several days. Progesterone remains elevated in early pregnancy. Progesterone levels are used to document the occurrence of ovulation. Progesterone is also secreted by the adrenal glands, so progesterone levels may be elevated in neoplasms of either the ovaries or the adrenal glands.

Preparation of Client and Collection of Sample

The laboratory needs 2 mL of serum in a red-topped tube. Include date of LMP and trimester of pregnancy. Reference values vary (see Appendix A, Table 2 for other ranges).

REFERENCE VALUES FOR SERUM PROGESTERONE	
Men	0–1.0 ng/mL
Women	
Follicular phase	0–1.5 ng/mL
Luteal phase	2–30 ng/mL
Postmenopausal	0–1.5 ng/mL
Pregnancy	Peaks in third trimester to as high as 200 ng/mL

▼ PREGNANEDIOL (PROGESTERONE METABOLITE)

Pregnanediol is the principal form of progesterone in the urine. (Pregnane*tri*ol is another urine test performed to evaluate adrenocortical function. See the discussion earlier in this chapter.) In women the level of pregnanediol in the urine rises rapidly after ovulation and steadily during pregnancy. The 24-hr urine specimen may be performed to evaluate the need for progesterone replacement.

REFERENCE VALUES FOR URINARY PREGNANEDIOL	
Children	0.4–1.0 mg/24-hr specimen
Men	0.5–1.5 mg/24-hr specimen
Women	
Pregnancy, 28–32 weeks	27–47 mg/24-hr specimen
Nonpregnant	0.5–7.0 mg/24-hr specimen
Luteal phase	2.0–7.0 mg/24-hr specimen
Postmenopausal	0.3–1.5 mg/24-hr specimen

▼ ESTROGEN AND PROGESTERONE RECEPTORS

Estrogen and progesterone receptors are measured routinely in biopsy specimens of tumors because they have important prognostic implications. The positive or negative results for these receptor sites also help the clinician plan chemotherapy (Allred, 1993). A newer type of immunohistochemical determination is easier to perform and less expensive than the older biochemical assays (Tesch et al., 1993). Clinicians and clients can call 1 (800) 4-CANCER to obtain up-to-date information about clinical trials for breast cancer and other information about cancer and diagnostic testing.

▼ TESTOSTERONE AND OTHER ANDROGENS

The male sex hormones, the androgens, are produced by the adrenal cortex, the testes, and the ovaries. The most powerful of the androgens, testosterone, comes mainly from the testes. Men with increased testosterone levels do not have any symptoms. In boys before puberty, there is precocious development of secondary sex characteristics. In women and girls there is masculinization. The adrenogenital syndrome, which occurs because of a lack of cortisol and an abundance of androgens, is discussed earlier in this chapter. In men a lack of testosterone, which can be due to primary failure of the testes or secondary to pituitary insufficiency, causes feminization. To evaluate impotence, serum testosterone is ordered before the gonadotropins.

Preparation of Client and Collection of Sample

The laboratory needs 4 mL of serum.

REFERENCE VALUES FOR SERUM TESTOSTERONE	
Men	300–1,100 ng/dL
Women	20–90 ng/dL
Adolescent males	>100 ng/dL
Some laboratories use 250 ng as the lower limit in men	

▼ POSSIBLE NURSING DIAGNOSES RELATED TO IMBALANCES IN SEX HORMONES

Disturbance in Self-concept Related to Changes in Body Image

Hormones are potent in shaping and altering secondary sex characteristics. For example, a woman who has an increase of testosterone has more facial hair, more muscle mass, and a deeper voice. One of the key nursing implications for clients undergoing sex hormone changes caused by pathologic conditions is to help them cope with the disturbance in their body images. Alterations in sexual characteristics are corrected if the hormone balance can be established. The mood changes and depression may be due to both hormonal influences and the effect of the physical changes. Nurses can help these clients reduce the effect of the unwanted characteristics. Even details,

(continued)

▼ POSSIBLE NURSING DIAGNOSES RELATED TO IMBALANCES IN SEX HORMONES (*continued*)

such as helping a woman find a place to have unwanted hair removed, can mean a great deal.

Specific Interventions for Malignant Tumors. Several of the tumors that cause masculinizing features in women or feminizing features in men are malignant. Nurses must be aware of the specific nursing care guidelines related to the pathophysiologic features of the tumor. Some types of cancer are treated with hormone therapy, which causes an imbalance of sex hormones and permanent changes in body image.

Sexual Dysfunction Related to Hormonal Changes

A client may need professional counseling to deal with problems related to sexual functioning. The emphasis for any sex-hormonal change is to help the client deal with a decreased sexual self-concept. If hormone tests are being performed as part of an infertility evaluation, the nurse needs to be sensitive to the anxiety of the couple who have not been able to conceive a child. (See Chapter 28 for diagnoses related to infertility.)

Ineffective Family Coping Related to Precocious Puberty in Children

The problem of mistaken sexual identity in newborns is discussed in the section on adrenogenital syndrome. (See the section on cortisol.) Masculinization of a girl or precocious puberty in either sex is disturbing for the child and probably much more so for the parents. Endocrine problems in children are usually treated by specialists who can also help parents, who may be alarmed by the changes in their child. A visiting nurse may be helpful in assessing the adjustment of child and family to these changes. School nurses can be instrumental, too, in recognizing children who may need counseling to deal with the physical and psychological problems of early maturity. Sexual precocity is three times more prevalent in girls than in boys. Some girls are capable of reproduction at 8 or 9 years of age.

Altered Health Maintenance Related to Use of Anabolic Steroids for "Sports Doping"

Anabolic steroids are sometimes abused by athletes to enhance athletic performances. Therefore, laboratory studies may be ordered to evaluate the possible presence of these drugs. Duncan and Shaw (1985) discussed the implications for the nurse practitioner who may be involved in identifying the effect of these drugs on the health of a client.

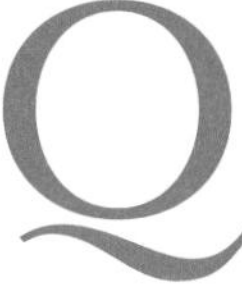

1. Which of the following illustrates the concept of a negative feedback system for control of serum cortisol?

   a. An increase of serum cortisol when ACTH secretion is increased
   b. A decreased level of serum cortisol when ACTH secretion is decreased
   c. A decreased secretion of ACTH when serum cortisol is increased
   d. An increased secretion of ACTH when serum cortisol is increased

2. Mrs. Wu has an elevated serum cortisol level with a tentative diagnosis of Cushing's syndrome caused by an adrenal cortex tumor. Which nursing action would be most needed?

   a. Observing and reporting any gastric distress, because gastric ulcers may develop
   b. Assessing for fluid deficit and high serum potassium levels (hyperkalemia)
   c. Taking the temperature every 4 hr to assess for infection
   d. Encouraging physical activity to counteract lethargy and boredom

3. Mr. Lee has a lower-than-normal serum cortisol level. Which nursing action would be appropriate for this client with a diagnosis of Addison's disease?

   a. Informing the client that his increased skin pigmentation will not fade even though cortisol hormone replacement is adequate
   b. Checking the urine for sugar because hyperglycemia is a potential problem
   c. Helping Mr. Lee prevent postural hypotension by teaching him to get out of bed slowly
   d. Encouraging compliance with a restricted sodium diet

4. Bobby, 5 years of age, has been referred to an endocrinologist because he has an enlarged penis and secondary sex characteristics. His serum sodium was low, and his serum potassium was elevated. A 24-hr urine for 17-ketosteroids (17-KS) was elevated. The increased elevation of serum androgens in adrenogenital syndrome is due to a basic lack of which of the following?

   a. ACTH production   b. Cortisol production
   c. Gonadotropic hormones   d. Testosterone

5. Mrs. Rodriguez has congestive heart failure with secondary aldosteronism. An elevation of the mineralocorticoid aldosterone would cause which of the following symptoms?

   a. BP of 90/60 mm Hg
   b. Serum potassium of 5.8 mEq/L

c. Pitting edema of the ankles
d. Polyuria (urine output of 2,500 mL in 24 hr)

6. Urine testing for metanephrine and for vanillylmandelic acid (VMA) are two of the screening tests for tumors of the

a. Adrenal cortex b. Adrenal medulla
c. Pituitary gland d. Parathyroid gland

7. An increased level of parathormone (PTH) causes an increased serum level of which?

a. Sodium b. Potassium

c. Phosphorus d. Calcium

8. The test least often used to follow clients with hyper- or hypothyroidism is which of the following?

a. TSH (thyroid-stimulating hormone test)
b. Free T_4 (L-thyroxine)
c. T_3 (triiodothyronine)
d. Free T_4 index

9. Mrs. Graves has been admitted to the hospital because of suspected hyperthyroidism. Which of the following nursing actions would be appropriate in caring for Mrs. Graves?

a. Seeing that she has a low-calorie diet
b. Keeping her room slightly warmer than usual
c. Encouraging her to increase her activity level
d. Checking an apical pulse when vital signs are taken

10. Mr. Lane has come to the clinic to begin tests for hypothyroidism because symptoms were noted by a home care nurse who was visiting the Lane family. Which of the following symptoms is characteristic of a client with suspected hypothyroidism?

a. Agitation b. Diarrhea
c. Intolerance to cold d. Weight loss

11. Baby Finley, diagnosed as having congenital hypothyroidism, has been started on a thyroid preparation. If hypothyroidism is not detected in early infancy (2–3 months), the infant will experience which of the following?

a. Mental retardation b. Cardiovascular problems
c. Generalized muscle hypertrophy d. Vision abnormalities

12. The most important nursing implication for clients with alterations in sex hormones is to be aware that they often need help in coping with which of the following?

a. Decreased appetite and weight loss
b. Changes in secondary sex characteristics
c. Changes in energy level
d. Physical stress, such as an infection

▼ REFERENCES

Allred, D.C. (1993). Should immunohistochemical examination replace biochemical hormone receptor assays in breast cancer? (Editorial.) *American Journal of Clinical Pathology, 99,* 1–2.

Braden, B. (1988). The relationship between serum cortisol and pressure sore formation among the elderly recently located to a nursing home. *Reflections, 14* (4), 11.

Burnett, J. (1980). Congenital adrenocortical hyperplasia: The syndrome and nursing interventions. *American Journal of Nursing, 80,* 1306–1311.

Camuñas, C. (1983). Pheochromocytoma. *American Journal of Nursing,* 83 (6), 887–891.

Chang, H., Anderson, G.C., and Wood, C.E. (1995). Feasible and valid saliva collection for cortisol in transitional newborn infants. *Nursing Research, 44* (2), 117–119.

Corsetti, A., and Buhl, B. (1994). Managing thyroid storm. *American Journal of Nursing, 94* (11), 39.

Cowan, D. (1984). Prejudices toward pituitary disorders. *Newsletter of Brain and Pituitary Foundation (Western Chapter), 1* (2), 8.

Duncan, D., and Shaw, E. (1985). Anabolic steroids: Implications for the nurse practitioner. *Nurse Practitioner, 10* (12), 8, 13–15.

Fisher, D., et al. (1979). Screening for congenital hypothyroidism: Result of screening one million North American infants. *Journal of Pediatrics, 94* (5), 700–705.

Giefer, C.K., and Cassmeyer, V.C. (1994). The syndrome of primary aldosteronism: A case study. *MEDSURG Nursing, 3* (4), 277–284.

Glaser, B., et al. (1986). Magnetic resonance imaging of the pituitary gland. *Clinical Radiology, 37* (1), 9–14.

Greene, L., Cole, W., Greene, J., et. al. (1984). Adrenal insufficiency as a complication of acquired immunodeficiency syndrome. *Annals of International Medicine, 101* (4), 497–498.

Groër, M., and Shekleton, M. (1989). *Basic pathophysiology: A holistic approach. St. Louis:* Mosby.

Harris, E. (1982). The dexamethasone suppression test. *American Journal of Nursing, 82* (5), 784–785.

Jenkins, E. (1980). Living with thyrotoxicosis. *American Journal of Nursing, 80* (5), 956–958.

Kaplan, A., Jack, R., Opheim, K.E., et al. (1995). *Clinical chemistry interpretation and techniques.* (4th ed.). Baltimore: Williams & Wilkins.

Katzung, B. (1995). *Basic and clinical pharmacology.* (6th ed.). Norwalk, CT: Appleton & Lange.

Larrabee, P., and Hanna, N. (1983). Saralasin infusion test. *American Journal of Nursing, 83* (12), 1958.

Perez, C. (1984). Up and coming research. *Newsletter of Brain and Pituitary Foundation (Western Chapter),* 1 (3), 7.

Press, M., et al. (1984). Importance of raised growth hormone in mediating the metabolic derangements of diabetes. *New England Journal of Medicine, 310* (13), 810–815.

Ravel, R. (1995). *Clinical laboratory medicine: Clinical application of laboratory data.* (6th ed.). St. Louis: Mosby–Year Book.

Smith-Rooker, J.L., Garrett, A., and Hodges, L.C. (1993). Case management of the patient with pituitary tumor. *MEDSURG Nursing, 2* (4), 265–274.

Stoffer, S., and Szpunar, W. (1984). Potency of levothyroxine products. *JAMA, 251* (5), 635–636.

Surks, M., Chopra, I.J., Mariash, C.N., et al. (1990). American Thyroid Association guidelines for use of laboratory tests in thyroid disorders. *JAMA, 263* (11), 1529–1532.

Tesch, J., Shawwa, A., and Henderson, R. (1993). Immunohistochemical determination of estrogen and progesterone status in breast cancer. *American Journal of Clinical Pathology, 99,* 8–12.

CULTURE AND SENSITIVITY TESTS

- β-Lactamase Assay
- Minimal Inhibitory Concentration
- Minimum Bactericidal Content or Minimum Lethal Concentration
- Urine Cultures
- Blood Cultures
- Sputum Cultures and Acid-fast Bacillus
- Throat Cultures
- Nasal and Nasopharyngeal Cultures
- Wound Cultures
- Eye Cultures
- Vaginal and Urethral Smears
- Stool Cultures
- Cultures of Cerebrospinal Fluid and Other Fluids

OBJECTIVES

1. Describe the classification system used by the laboratory to identify bacteria.
2. Interpret the clinical significance of culture and sensitivity (C&S) and minimal inhibitory concentration (MIC) reports.
3. Identify the general nursing implications when a client has cultures ordered for a possible bacterial infection.
4. Describe in detail the various ways urine is collected for urine cultures.

5. Explain the procedures used to obtain blood cultures, as well as the timing of preliminary and final reports.
6. Describe what the nurse should teach the client to obtain a useful sputum specimen.
7. Explain why it may be important to perform throat cultures for children with sore throats.
8. Describe the correct procedure to obtain a wound culture and what should be taught to the client.
9. Describe how gonorrhea and other sexually transmitted diseases (STDs) are detected by smears and cultures.
10. Describe the proper procedure for collecting a stool specimen for laboratory examination.

The first part of this chapter provides background information about the classification of bacteria and about how the laboratory performs cultures and sensitivity testing on clinical specimens. Nursing implications for culture collection are outlined. In addition, the nurse's role in caring for clients with infections is reviewed. The last part of the chapter outlines the purpose, procedure, and preparation of the client for each common type of culture.

CLASSIFICATION OF BACTERIA AT MICROSCOPIC EXAMINATION

Bacteria can be classified into groups according to

1. Whether the bacteria take a Gram stain
2. The shape of the bacteria—round (cocci), rod-shaped (bacilli), or spiral-shaped (spirilla)
3. Whether the bacteria thrive with oxygen (aerobic) or without (anaerobic)

The distribution of cocci in pairs (diplococci), in a string (streptococci), or in a cluster (staphylococci) helps the microbiologist classify bacteria. A preliminary stain may not identify the exact bacteria, but it can help with a presumptive diagnosis and help rule out what the bacteria are not. For example, if the Gram stain shows gram-negative diplococci, gonorrhea is most likely the causative organism. If the Gram stain reveals gram-negative rods, the infection may be caused by organisms such as *Escherichia coli* or *Pseudomonas*. Table 16–1 shows the classification of some of the common bacteria identified in laboratory specimens.

The laboratory technician also records other details, such as the number of different bacteria present, to estimate the probability of an infection. Gram stains are scanned for polymorphonuclear lymphocytes (PMNs), which are present in infection, and for squamous epithelial cells, which are present in mucosal contamination. The technician also is able to see that the specimen is grossly contaminated with normal flora.

Gram stains may be useful for the presumptive identification of gonorrhea in endocervical smears in women and urethral smears in men and for meningitis in

TABLE 16–1. EXAMPLES OF COMMON BACTERIA FOUND IN CULTURES

Organism	Culture in Which Commonly Found
Aerobic	
Gram-positive cocci	
Staphylococcus aureus (coagulase-positive)	Blood, wound, sputum
Streptococcus (A β-hemolytic)	Throat, wound, sputum
Streptococcus pneumoniae (pneumococcus)	Sputum, CSF in adult
Gram-negative cocci	
Neisseria meningitidis (meningococcus)	CSF, throat
Neisseria gonorrhoea (gonococcus)	Urethra, endocervix, throat
Gram-negative rods or bacilli	
Escherichia coli (many strains)	Urine, blood, wound
Proteus	Urine, sputum, wound
Enterococcus	Blood, sputum, wound
Pseudomonas	Sputum, urine, wound
Salmonella	Stool
Shigella	Stool
Anaerobic	
Gram-positive cocci	
Anaerobic streptococci	Wound, stool, vagina
Gram-positive bacillus	
Clostridium group	Wound, stool
Gram-negative bacillus	
Bacteroides	Wound, stool
Acid-fast bacillus	
Mycobacterium tuberculosis	Sputum, gastric contents, CSF

CSF, cerebrospinal fluid.
Information compiled from several references.

cerebrospinal fluid (CSF). Gram stains of stool and urine may or may not be helpful. In several specimens, such as sputum smears, the usefulness of a Gram stain is controversial (Ravel, 1995).

CULTURE GROWTHS

A stain is only a presumptive identification of bacteria. A culture allows the bacteria to grow and to multiply so that the exact organism can be identified by various methods of analysis. The laboratory usually takes 2 or more days to make a final identification of the organisms present in a specimen. For some specimens it may take 6–10 days. The growth on the culture takes about 24 hr. The laboratory must then use various tests to determine the species of bacteria present. Various methods, such as the addition of sugars, are used to identify different strains of a species. These tests to identify a type of bacteria may take another 24 hr or more.

The amount of growth on the culture varies with the organism. For example, some bacteria, such as *E coli,* reproduce every 20 min. At the other extreme, the organism that causes tuberculosis, *Mycobacterium tuberculosis,* reproduces only about once a day. Thus a final report of a culture for tuberculosis may take 1–6 weeks. (See the section on sputum collection for acid-fast bacillus [AFB] for a faster way to detect mycobacterium by nucleic acid probe.)

Anaerobic Cultures

Unless there is a specific order to the contrary, bacterial cultures are usually performed under aerobic conditions because most disease-causing organisms require oxygen. However, if the client may have an infection with an anaerobic organism, the specimen must be cultured without oxygen. For an anaerobic specimen, the nurse should call the laboratory to obtain the needed container for anaerobic transport, or a syringe with the needle capped with a cork may be used for transport. The specimen should be sent to the laboratory immediately. With blood cultures, the routine is to put the blood specimens into two different containers so that both an anaerobic culture and an aerobic culture can be performed. Two laboratory requisitions should be sent with the two specimens so the laboratory is aware of the need to perform both types of culture.

Cultures for Fungus

Cultures for fungus require specific preparations with india ink, KOH (potassium hydroxide), or PAS (periodic–acid Schiff stain). With swabs moistened with saline solution small scrapings may be taken from a lesion. The nurse should consult with the laboratory on exactly how to collect the specimen.

The cultures for fungus take a long time to grow, and they must be handled carefully because the spores from the fungus can get into the air. For most of the systemic fungal diseases, such as histoplasmosis, various serologic tests are performed. (See Chapter 14 on serologic tests.) Skin tests are also used to identify clients who have antibodies against certain fungal infections (see Chapter 10 on cellular immunity).

Cultures for Viruses

The laboratory identification of viral diseases is usually performed with serologic tests because a culture of a virus requires a living cell culture, which demands the services of a specialized laboratory. Some viruses have been identified by means of electron microscopy, but the positive identification of certain viruses is still performed only at large medical centers. Specimens for virus isolation should be collected in the first 4 days of illness. Almost all viruses are extremely labile outside the human host, so the specimen should be put in the special viral holding medium supplied by the laboratory. Viral testing is expensive, so the laboratory may require a detailed clinical history of the client for approval of the test. (Serologic titers for some viral diseases are discussed in Chapter 14.)

CULTURE AND SENSITIVITY TESTS

Sometimes, in addition to knowing the exact organism causing the infection, it is necessary to demonstrate if the organism is sensitive to a certain antibiotic. In regard to C&S, *sensitivity* refers to the ability of the antibiotic to inhibit the growth of the bacteria. *Sensitivity* has an entirely different connotation when describing the reaction of a client to an antibiotic. A client who is allergic to a drug is said to be *sensitive* or *hypersensitive* to the drug. Sensitivity of the *client* to the drug is undesirable, whereas sensitivity of the *organism* to the antibiotic is essential. If the antibiotic does not inhibit growth of the bacteria, the organism is said to be *resistant* to the antibiotic.

The most common way that a laboratory checks the sensitivity of organisms to specific antibiotics is to put disks of paper impregnated with antibiotics in a culture. Laboratories may list the test as a Kirby–Bauer susceptibility test. If the growth of an organism is retarded, the report is an *S* for *sensitive* or *susceptible.* If the antibiotic disk does not retard the growth of the specific bacteria in the culture, the report is *R* for *resistant.* An *I* on a report means that the results are in an *intermediate* zone or *inconclusive* of growth retardation. Some laboratories place an intermediate growth into the resistant category. Usually the laboratory uses only one member of an antibiotic family because sensitivity differences are usually minor.

The purpose of conducting C&S is to ensure that the client is receiving the correct antibiotic for the particular organism causing the infection. For example, suppose a client were receiving ampicillin. If a report showed the organisms to be resistant to ampicillin but sensitive to other antibiotics, the physician must change the antibiotic order. (See Table 16–2 for an example of a C&S report that necessitates notification of the physician before the next dose of ampicillin is given.) C&S is particularly useful when a client is not responding to therapeutic dosages of antibiotics. A routine sensitivity for every culture may not be needed and could be an unnecessary health cost to the client. The physician must determine if a culture *and* sensitivity are cost-effective in a particular situation.

TABLE 16–2. EXAMPLE OF SENSITIVITY REPORT (SHORTENED LIST)

Drug	*Escherichia coli*	*Pseudomonas aeruginosa*
Amikacin	S	S
Ampicillin	R	R
Chloramphenicol	S	S
Gentamicin	S	S
Methicillin	R	R
Penicillin G	R	R
Tobramycin	S	S

S, sensitive; R, resistant.

▼ β-LACTAMASE ASSAY

Some bacteria become resistant to some of the penicillins and cephalosporins because the bacteria produce enzymes that make the drugs ineffective. These enzymes, the β-lactamases, affect a certain structure in the antibiotic known as the β-*lactum ring*. The first of these enzymes was called *penicillinase* because it made penicillin ineffective as an antibiotic. Ravel (1995) noted that several types of β-lactamase assays are performed, and most tend to be accurate, particularly when a positive reaction is reported. A positive reaction means that the organism in question is resistant to many of the penicillins and the first and second generation cephalosporins. Like C&S, which takes longer, a β-lactamase assay helps with the choice of the most effective and least expensive drug for a particular infection. For example, if the test shows that the staphylococci do not produce β-lactamase, penicillin G is the most potent and the least expensive drug to use (Katzung, 1995).

▼ MINIMAL INHIBITORY CONCENTRATION

MIC is a report of the concentration of an antibiotic that inhibits the growth of the organism. Venous blood containing the microorganism is put into liquid culture mediums, each containing an antibiotic at a specified concentration. Table 16–3 shows the range of testing for some antibiotics. The concentration of antibiotic that inhibits the growth of the microorganism in vitro is then noted. The MIC helps the physician choose antibiotics that are clinically appropriate and cost-effective. For an organism to be considered sensitive to an antibiotic, attainable blood levels should be at least two to four times the MIC. For urinary tract infections, the dose of antimicrobial agent in the urine needs to be 10 times the MIC.

For example, if for organism X the MIC is reported as 4.0 µg/mL for methicillin, one uses the information in Table 16–3 to determine if methicillin would be effective. If the approximate blood level is only 4.0, the drug would not be effective. For intravenously administered methicillin, the obtainable blood levels are much higher (10–40 µg/mL), and thus it would be considered an appropriate antibiotic. However, the MIC that is effective in vitro (test tube) may not always correlate well with the effectiveness in vivo. Blood levels vary according to body fat and hepatic and renal functioning.

▼ MINIMUM BACTERICIDAL CONTENT OR MINIMUM LETHAL CONCENTRATION

The minimum bactericidal content (MBC) or minimum lethal concentration (MLC) denotes the concentration of antibiotic needed to actually kill an organism. The technique is an in vitro one as described for MIC. End reports for the MBC may note either 99%, 99.9%, or 100% colonies killed. Not a routine test, the MBC may be used

TABLE 16–3. RANGES TESTED FOR MINIMAL INHIBITORY CONCENTRATION (MIC) BY LABORATORY

Antibiotics (Range Tested)	Representative Adult Dose (g)	Approximate Blood Levels (μg/mL)	Approximate Urine Levels (μg/mL)
Clindamycin (0.25–16)	p.o. 0.15–0.3 q6h	2–4	30–90
	IV 0.3–6 q6–8h	4–8	45–240
Erythromycin (0.25–16)	p.o. 0.25–0.5 q6h	1–4	(5%)
	IV 0.3 q4–6h	10–20	
Methicillin (0.25–16)	IV 1–2 q4h	10–40	
Penicillin (0.06–4)	(p.o. 0.25–0.5 q6h)	1.5–4.0	300–450
	IV 1–2 mL q4h	20–40	3,000–5,000
Ampicillin			
(0.12–8, gram-pos.)	p.o. 0.25–1.5 q6h	1.5–4.0	50–100
(0.25–16, gram-neg.)	IV 1–2 q4h	15–30	200–400
Cephalothin (1–64)	p.o. 0.25–0.5 q6h	2–15	300–1,000
	IV 1–2 q4h	25–85	800–2,000
Gentamicin (0.25–16)	IM,IV q8–12h (3–5 mg/kg per day)	5–10	65–300
Tetracycline (0.25–16)	p.o. 0.25–5 q6h	1.5–4.0	200–800
	IV 0.5 q6–12h	10–20	600–1,000
Carbenicillin (8–512)	p.o. 1q6h	5–10	350–14,000
	IV 4 q4h	125–175	2,000–10,000
Chloramphenicol (0.5–32)	p.o. 0.25–0.5 q6h	1.5–4.0	200–700
	IV 0.5–1 q6h	10–20	500–1,400
Kanamycin (1–64)	IV,IV 5 q12h (15 mg/kg per day)	15–20	100–200
Tobramycin (0.25–16)	IM,IV q8-12h (3–5 mg/kg per day)	5–10	65–300
Amikacin (1–64)	IM,IV q8-12h (15 mg/kg per day)	16–21	700–830

Reprinted laboratory report courtesy of Kaiser Hospital, San Francisco, Calif.

for debilitated clients with leukopenia or subacute bacterial endocarditis. (See Chapter 2 for decreased white blood cell [WBC] count.)

COLLECTING SPECIMENS FOR CULTURE

General Nursing Implications

Specific information about each common type of culture is covered in the second half of this chapter. This section presents general guidelines for the collection of all specimens for bacterial culture.

Collect Specimens Before Giving Antibiotics. If possible, cultures should be collected before administration of the antibiotic is begun. If the client is already taking antibiotics, the laboratory should be notified, because techniques to counteract the effect of the antibiotic, such as adding enzymes, may be performed, or special collection tubes are used.

Use the Correct Specimen Container. All specimens, except stool, must be collected in a sterile container, and anaerobic specimens must be collected in oxygen-free containers. Some cultures, such as throat cultures, may be transferred to the culture medium immediately. The nurse should call the laboratory if there is any doubt about the type of culture medium to be used. For example, the laboratory has specific cultures for blood, and it may be desirable to have the blood transferred to the culture medium as soon as it is drawn. In other settings, the laboratory may prefer to receive blood in tubes and make the transfer to the culture medium in the laboratory. If the specimen is not placed in the correct medium, it is useless.

Know How Much of the Specimen Is Needed. For example, the laboratory can perform a culture on only a few milliliters of sputum, so it is useless to keep the container longer to try to obtain a larger amount. Table 16–4 lists the amounts needed for each type of specimen. Information on the amount needed for each type of specimen is also covered with the discussion on the specific test.

Do Not Expose Others to the Infectious Material. Meticulous handwashing before and after obtaining a culture is essential. The nurse must make sure that the outside of the specimen container does not become contaminated with the contents inside it.

TABLE 16–4. AMOUNTS NEEDED FOR CULTURE AND TIPS FOR COLLECTION

Type of Culture	Amount Needed	Special Notes
Urine	2–3 mL in sterile container (if also for urinalysis, send 15–30 mL)	Must be clean-catch or catheterized specimen so not contaminated by perineal flora
Blood	10 mL by venipuncture. Keep in syringe or put into culture at bedside—5 mL aerobic, 5 mL anaerobic	Be sure not contaminated with skin flora. Special skin cleansing needed.
Sputum	2–3 mL in sterile container	Sputum, *not* saliva
Throat	One swab put in prepared culture (Culpak)	Touch back of throat only
Nasopharyngeal	One swab in test tube	Swab gently
Wound	One swab in test tube. May use syringe for anaerobic specimens.	Clean skin around wound first—see text on chronic wounds
Eye	One swab	Be careful not to touch cornea
Vaginal	One swab. If anaerobic, need special container	Need cervical specimen for gonorrhea
Urethral	One swab	See text for other ways to detect gonorrhea in men
Stool	1-inch lump (walnut size) or 20 mL if diarrhea	See text for special techniques
CSF; (pleural fluid; peritoneal fluid)	1 mL—aerobic and anaerobic	Need to notify lab that CSF is coming. CSF, pleural, or peritoneal fluid is collected in other tubes for other types of analysis.

CSF, cerebrospinal fluid.
Information compiled from several references.

Because the contents are potentially infectious, the personnel handling the container must be protected. If the outside of the container does become contaminated, the nurse can use gloves to transfer the contents to another container. As an alternative, the nurse may also put the container into a bag and note that the outside of the container has been contaminated. Thus laboratory personnel will not touch the outside of the container with their bare hands.

Make Sure that the Specimen Is Properly Labeled. The laboratory requisition must be filled out correctly. A specimen that is not properly identified is useless. If the specimen is for an outpatient, making sure that the home phone number of the client is available is important. Information required on the laboratory slip includes the client's name and other identification, such as medical record number, hospital room number, or clinic site. The type and *source* of the specimen, as well as the date and time collected, are essential. Sometimes laboratories receive yellow liquid marked for C&S. The laboratory cannot assume that this is urine. Even if it is marked urine, the technicians have no idea if it is from a Foley catheter or is a clean catch. Other details, such as the need for an anaerobic report or whether the client is on antibiotics, should be recorded.

Send the Culture to the Laboratory as Soon as Possible. All cultures should be sent to the laboratory immediately, but some specimens, such as urine, can be refrigerated if there is a delay in transporting the specimen. Some commercial kits contain an ampule of transport medium that keeps samples moist for as long as 72 hr. For some specimens, such as a culture of CSF, the laboratory needs to be called before the culture is sent, so that the personnel are available to begin immediate examination of the fluid when it arrives at the laboratory. In the hospital setting, cultures are not usually collected on the evening or night shift unless the laboratory provides 24-hr service. If specimens are collected in a home, the nurse must check with the laboratory to see how the specimen can be transported without causing the death of the organism to be cultured.

▼ GENERAL NURSING DIAGNOSIS WHEN CULTURES ARE ORDERED

Risk for Injury Related to Transmission of Infectious Material

Universal precautions, first introduced in 1987 and modified in 1988 (Centers for Disease Control [CDC], 1988), heightened the awareness of the risks to health care workers who are careless with body secretions. Much attention is paid to avoiding blood and blood-containing secretions. In addition to universal precautions, specific precautions and hospital protocols are needed that are category- or disease-specific (Jackson and Lynch, 1990). Staff may need to be reminded that the spread of bacteria is best controlled by handwashing after

(continued)

▼ GENERAL NURSING DIAGNOSIS WHEN CULTURES ARE ORDERED (*continued*)

every physical contact with every client. Some staph infections are staff induced. Mayer et al. (1986) found that feedback about handwashing did increase compliance. Thus, when clients are known to have a positive bacterial culture, it behooves the nurse to see if proper handwashing and isolation procedures are being carried out and to give feedback to those who are breaking technique. Consultation with an infection control nurse may be needed. In the home setting, family members need to be taught how to protect themselves from the spread of infection.

Assessing for Signs and Symptoms of Infection. Often the nurse may be the first one to detect that the client may be getting an infection. For example, a nurse in a nursing home may notice that the urine in a drainage bag has a foul odor. A pediatric nurse may notice that the lungs of a child have crackles and that the child has a fever. A nurse making a home visit may notice that a wound appears inflamed and sore to the touch.

Although fever is usually present in infections, in some clients, particularly the elderly, fever may be absent and the WBC count and differential normal. (See Chapter 2 for a discussion of the "shift to the left" as a characteristic sign of a developing bacterial infection.) Elderly clients who describe "not feeling good" or who are weak or lethargic may need a complete physical examination to rule out the possibility of an unnoticed infection. In newborns the WBC count may not be elevated, but an increase in the erythrocyte sedimentation rate (ESR) and the bands (see Chapter 2) may be important in screening for newborn sepsis.

Assisting the Client to Combat Infection. Too often health professionals consider that the administration of antibiotics is the *only* way to treat infections, but a holistic approach to the treatment of an infection includes more. Increased fluids, a diet adequate in protein, and plenty of rest are other ways to help the body combat a bacterial invasion. Adults may need antipyretic drugs to reduce the fever, if the fever is high or the client is uncomfortable. Gurevich (1985) noted it is not necessarily desirable to decrease a fever, even up to 105°F (41°C) in adults. Pediatric guidelines are different (Thomas, 1985), so treatment may be administered for a temperature of 101°F (39°C). Griffin (1986) suggested tepid baths for fever in adults. Aspirin or acetaminophen is prescribed to reduce fevers in adults. Aspirin is not used with children because of the association with Reye's syndrome. A moderate increase in temperature is considered useful in helping the body mobilize the defense against bacterial invasion. The natural defenses of the body against infection need to be encouraged along with the proper use of antibiotics and antipyretics. Some studies have supported the health attributes of yogurt in combating diarrhea and vaginal infections that may accompany antibiotic use (Sanders, 1993). Stress reduction should also be employed, so the body is free to mobilize against the infection.

Recognizing Situations that Allow the Growth of Opportunistic Organisms. Poor techniques by health professionals are not always to blame when clients have an infection in the hospital or nursing home. Always present in our environment are opportunistic pathogens, which do not usually cause an infection unless the resistance of the host is low. Reducing all possible pathogens in an environment may be difficult. For example, food is not sterile. Salad is a notorious source of organisms, and even pepper has been shown to carry potential pathogens. Opportunistic organisms such as *Pneumocystis carinii* are commonly present but only cause pneumonia in immunosuppressed clients, such as those with acquired immunodeficiency syndrome (AIDS). Clients who are immunosuppressed need extra careful observation for any signs of infection.

▼ URINE CULTURES

General Indications

For routine microscopic urinalysis, the findings that suggest a urinary tract infection (UTI) are the presence of a large number of WBCs and bacteria in the urine. Two screening tests for a UTI, nitrites and leukocyte esterase (LE), are discussed in Chapter 3. For nonpregnant women, treatment with antibiotics can be given without a culture if there are no signs suggestive of pyelonephritis, vaginitis, or chlamydial urethritis and the client has not had more than one other UTI in the past year (Komaroff, 1984; Leiner, 1995). If the UTI does not respond quickly to medication, the culture may be needed to determine appropriate therapy. The most common organism causing such infections is *E coli*. Other gram-negative rods, such as the *Proteus* or *Pseudomonas* groups, are occasionally present in UTIs.

Female clients are particularly susceptible to UTI because of the short length of the urethra and the possible contamination from perineal organisms. ("Honeymoon" cystitis often occurs when sexual activity introduces organisms into the urinary tract). Girls are also much more likely to have UTIs than are boys. Catheterization procedures for either sex increase the risk for UTI.

Preparation of Client and Collection of Sample

Ideally, urine for cultures should be the early morning specimen because the urine is concentrated. However, urine can be collected at any time for the culture. Most laboratories consider a clean-catch, midstream urine the best for a culture. The laboratory needs only 1 mL to grow the culture, so the urine can be transmitted in a syringe if the specimen is removed from a Foley catheter. (See discussion on Foley specimens.) If a routine urinalysis is to be performed before a C&S, the laboratory needs at least 15 mL of urine.

There are various diagnostic kits for urine cultures. Clients may be taught to use these at home. (See Chapter 1 for a discussion of diagnostic kits.)

Clean-Catch or Midstream Specimens. The problem in collecting urine for C&S is that the urine may be contaminated with the bacteria normally present in the perineal area. Thus the perineal area must be cleansed thoroughly before the urine is collected. In one study, client instruction with diagrams on how to use iodophor-soaked tissues as a cleanser did reduce the number of nonpathogenic organisms that often contaminate a urine specimen (McGuckin, 1981). Current practice is to use simple soap and water to clean the perineal area. Women should use a tampon to prevent menstrual fluid or vaginal secretions from contaminating the urine specimen.

The urine is collected midstream so it contains fewer of the bacteria that reside on the perineal surfaces near the urinary meatus. To collect a midstream specimen, the client must be able to stop the urine flow after it is begun and then urinate into a sterile cup or directly onto a dipstick for culture. Women hold the labia apart so that the urinary meatus is clear. If the client is unable to clean the area, the nurse can clean around the meatus. (A nonsterile glove can be used to protect the nurse who washes the perineal area.) In an uncircumsized male client, the foreskin must stay retracted during the procedure.

Collecting Urine by Direct Catheterization. In the past, urine specimens for culture were often collected by means of direct catheterization to make sure that the specimen did not become contaminated from perineal secretions. For example, if a woman had a heavy menstrual flow, the urine would be contaminated with blood. However, the danger of infection as a result of catheterization is a reason to try to obtain urine by means of clean-catch whenever possible. During the menstrual flow, or when there are vaginal secretions, the client can clean the perineal area, insert a tampon, and then clean around the meatus again before urinating. If catheterization is necessary to collect a urine specimen, sterile technique must be followed. Faller and Lawrence (1994) described how to catheterize a urinary stoma using a large (16 Fr) catheter to avoid blockage with mucus.

Collecting Urine from a Foley Catheter. If the client has an indwelling (Foley) catheter, urine can be collected from it. The Foley catheter must be clamped so that urine can accumulate in the bladder. (Urine taken from a drainage bag is never suitable for a culture because the urine is not fresh.) Foley catheter drainage tubes have a special sample port for inserting a needle and a syringe to remove a few milliliters of urine for tests. The tube below the area may be bent back on itself so that urine collects near the port. Some tubes have a special clamp. The sample port should be cleaned with alcohol before the needle is inserted. It is important for microscopic urinalysis to remove the needle from the syringe before emptying the urine from the syringe into the specimen cup. Forcing urine through the needle breaks up cells.

Collecting Urine in Children. A sterile cotton ball can be placed in the diaper of an infant. Another technique is to clean the perineal area and attach a sterile collection bag around the meatus. This procedure is easier with male infants. For older children, meatal cleaning and midstream collection may be no more effective than simply having the child void into a sterile container (Wong, 1990).

REFERENCE VALUES FOR URINE CULTURES

Urine is sterile in the bladder, but it becomes contaminated with organisms normally present in the perineal area. The amount of organisms is counted and usually interpreted as follows:

<10,000 organisms/mL	Unlikely UTI, probable contamination
10,000–100,000 organisms/mL	Probable UTI, particularly if urine specimen is from a catheter
>100,000 organisms/mL	Definite UTI

These numbers exclude the presence of normal genital flora such as lactobacilli.

In low-grade pyelonephritis, the urine culture may be negative even though bacteria are present in the pelvis of the kidney.

Screening Tests for UTI: Slide Centrifuge Gram Stain, LE, and Nitrite Dipsticks

Gram staining of a slide centrifuge of urine (Cytospin) is a reliable screening test for the presence or absence of bacteria. In addition, this technique provides information on the morphology of the bacteria, which may help in precise selection of an antibiotic (Goswitz et al., 1993). An even more common screening test for UTI is the nitrite and LE dipstick test discussed in Chapter 3 as part of a routine urinalysis.

▼ POSSIBLE NURSING DIAGNOSIS RELATED TO POSITIVE URINE CULTURE

Knowledge Deficit Related to Preventive and Therapeutic Measures for Urinary Tract Infection

The key measure to assist a client in overcoming a UTI is to keep the urine as dilute as possible so that bacteria cannot multiply rapidly. Keeping the urine acidic may also be helpful for some bacterial infections. (See Chapter 3 on the use of cranberry juice to make the urine more acidic.) The client needs to know exactly how much fluid should be consumed each day. Caffeine may irritate the bladder. The physician may prescribe sulfa drugs or antibiotics, such as

(continued)

▼ POSSIBLE NURSING DIAGNOSIS RELATED TO POSITIVE URINE CULTURE (*continued*)

ampicillin, depending on the causitive organism for the UTI, and the client should know the possible side effects of the drugs. In addition, the nurse should make sure that the client knows ways to prevent infections in the future by continuing adequate fluid intake. Also, some women are not aware that wiping the perineal area should be front to back so that intestinal bacteria are not transmitted to the meatus. Avoiding bubble baths and nylon pants are other preventive measures often suggested. However, sexual intercourse and use of a diaphragm and spermicide are the two behavioral factors most consistently associated with UTIs in otherwise healthy adult women (Leiner, 1995).

Conti and Eutropius (1987) noted that virtually all clients with long-term use of catheters do have bacteriuria, but cultures are not routinely performed unless the client has symptoms. Proper catheter care is a concern in extended care facilities. Nurses have an important role in reducing the risk of infection of indwelling catheters by promoting excellent catheter care. New devices, such as silver-impregnated or coated catheters, have been shown to postpone bacteriuria and prevent urethral entry of microorganisms (Pinkerman, 1994).

▼ BLOOD CULTURES

General Indications

Blood cultures are ordered when a client is believed to have septicemia. In many localized infections, a few bacteria may enter the bloodstream (bacteremia), but they are usually not sufficient to cause symptoms of sepsis (septicemia). A client with septicemia is usually severely ill with fever, chills, and other signs of serious infection. Newborns may have no symptoms. The spikes of fever may be related to the release into the bloodstream of more bacteria. So sometimes blood cultures are ordered to be performed when the client has another spike in temperature.

Bacteria can enter the bloodstream from infections in soft tissues, from contaminated intravenous lines, such as those used for hyperalimentation, or even from simple surgical procedures, such as a tooth extraction or instrumentation with endoscopes, particularly cystoscopes. Bacteremia in elderly clients can result from pneumococcal pneumonia. In adults the most common organisms causing septicemia are gram-negative rods, such as *E coli* or *Aerobacter* species, which can enter the bloodstream because of UTI or instrumentation of the urinary tract. *Staphylococcus aureus* may also cause septicemia. In newborns, *E coli* and β-hemolytic streptococci are the two most frequent causes of septicemia. In newborns, sepsis is often a result of prolonged labor and early rupture of the membranes (more than 24 hr before delivery), maternal infection (proved or suspected), and neonatal aspiration.

The early and efficient diagnosis of neonatal bacterial sepsis is difficult because blood cultures have low sensitivity and must be combined with other tests (Gerdes, 1994).

Preparation of Client and Collection of Sample

Usually blood samples for blood culture are drawn at least two different times and in both arms to increase the chance of detection of any organisms. For example, the order may read, "Blood cultures now and in 3 hr. If the client has another temperature spike, draw blood cultures immediately." The physician, nurse, or laboratory technician may draw the blood for the cultures. Solitary venipunctures are preferred, but if the client has poor veins, blood cultures can be obtained from an arterial line (Pryor, 1984).

Usually 10 mL is obtained from one venipuncture. Half the specimen (5 mL) is put into a culture for anaerobic bacteria and 5 mL into a culture for aerobic bacteria. Pediatric specimens may require only 3–5 mL and newborns even less. For infants, a heel stick may be performed to obtain blood for a culture. Some laboratories have the person who draws the blood add the blood directly to the culture media. Other laboratories prefer that the blood sample be sent directly to the laboratory and that the transfer to culture be made by the bacteriologic technician. Blood culture bottles also come with an antibiotic adsorbing resin that is useful for clients who have received antibiotics before the cultures were drawn.

The main problem with blood cultures is that the specimen is often contaminated with bacteria from the environment. The skin is specially prepared before the venipuncture is performed. The preparation, much like a surgical preparation, consists of thorough cleansing with iodine and alcohol solutions. The skin over the vein must not be touched after preparation is completed. If the skin over the vein is probed, the person drawing the blood uses a sterile glove. The transfer of the blood sample to the culture medium must also be a sterile procedure. Leisure et al. (1990) noted it is not of benefit and is a high risk to change the needle before inoculating blood cultures.

REFERENCE VALUES FOR BLOOD CULTURES

Any bacteria in the blood are clinically significant. Yet, because there is always the possibility of contamination from the skin, the bacteriologist may make an interpretation of possible contaminants if certain skin bacteria are present in small amounts. At least three cultures in 24 hr may be ordered to determine if bacteria are actually in the blood. A final diagnosis from a blood culture may take several days. However, if the laboratory identifies the presence of certain pathogens, even in small amounts, it issues a preliminary positive report so that the physician can order appropriate antibiotics. *E coli* is a common pathogen in both adults and children. Other pathogens may be *S aureus* and various streptococci. Some fungi, such as *Candida* and *Cryptococcus,* grow in routine blood culture medium.

Culturing of Catheter Tip. Septicemia can result from use of an indwelling intravenous catheter, particularly a central venous catheter used to deliver hyperalimentation fluids. The high glucose content of hyperalimentation fluids supports bacterial growth. Sometimes when the intravenous catheter is removed, the tip is cut off with sterile scissors and sent to the laboratory for culturing. The tip should not be allowed to touch the client's skin or the bedclothes. A sterile towel can be used to catch the catheter when it is removed.

REFERENCE VALUES FOR CULTURING TIP OF CATHETER

If an intravenous catheter tip is cultured, a count of 15 or fewer colonies is usually not significant. A count of more than 15 colonies on the culture suggests the catheter as the source of septicemia.

▼ POSSIBLE NURSING DIAGNOSIS RELATED TO POSITIVE BLOOD CULTURE

Risk for Injury Related to Septic State

Clients with septicemia often have low resistance to infection because they are already critically ill from other causes. Most of the appropriate nursing care is that given to acutely ill clients. Septic shock may occur and be fatal. Usually clients with septicemia are not a source of infection for others, but this possibility should be carefully assessed. Sepsis has become a greater threat as microorganisms are becoming more virulent and resistant to drug therapy. In addition, some microorganisms now identified as neonatal pathogens were not a problem in the past. Lott and Kenner (1994a,b) discussed these new infections and the role of the nurse in preventive and therapeutic measures. In the infant, hypoglycemia (Chapter 8) and hyperbilirubinemia (Chapter 11) are often concurrent problems with septicemia.

▼ SPUTUM CULTURES AND ACID-FAST BACILLUS

General Indications

Sputum cultures are often ordered when a client has lung congestion (crackles), elevated temperature, and other signs of a probable respiratory infection. Respiratory infections cause an increased secretion of respiratory secretions or sputum. Sputum originates in the bronchi, not in the upper respiratory tract. Different bacteria cause the sputum to be greenish, yellowish, or rust-colored. The sputum may have a foul smell.

Almost all the bacteria that cause respiratory infections are normally present in the upper respiratory tract in small amounts. In healthy people, these organisms, such as *Klebsiella* or *Staphylococcus,* do not cause disease because they are present in small amounts. Yet when an organism has a chance to grow quickly because of stagnant respiratory secretions, the client can experience pneumonia. Postoperative clients and those who are immunosuppressed are at high risk for pneumonia. Caruthers (1990) noted that infectious pneumonia is a problem among elderly clients who have both acute and chronic illnesses. Sputum cultures can identify which organism is in abundance and thus the cause of the respiratory problem. If tuberculosis is suspected, a special type of culture for AFB is done. Parasites such as *P carinii* are not easily found in routine sputum. Also, sputum culture is not reliable for *Legionella* infection, so pleural fluid or lung tissue may be needed if either type of pneumonia is suspected. (See Chapter 27 on bronchoscopy.)

Preparation of Client and Collection of Sample

The laboratory needs only a few milliliters of sputum for a culture. Sputum, however, is not the same thing as saliva. The sputum specimen must be from the bronchial tree, not simply saliva from the mouth. Having clients rinse out their mouths before the sputum is obtained is a good idea, so that the sputum is not contaminated with saliva and mouth bacteria. An early morning specimen is ideal because the sputum is concentrated then. Early morning sputum also tends to be plentiful if the client has been sleeping through the night and the secretions have pooled.

Sputum from the bronchial tree can be obtained in several ways. If at all possible, the client should be allowed to cough up the sputum. If the client is unable to cough, suctioning can be performed with a special catheter that allows some of the secretions to be caught in a special reservoir. Sputum cultures are also obtained with a bronchoscope.

If the purpose is to determine the presence of the AFB that causes tuberculosis, the culture may be performed on at least three different days. If no sputum can be obtained, the physician may order a gastric analysis, because *M tuberculosis* is acid-resistant and thus not destroyed by gastric acidity. (Urine may be cultured for AFB, too, if tuberculosis of the kidney is suspected.)

Wet Mounts of Sputum Specimens

The first laboratory examination of a sputum specimen is a wet mount. If a large number of epithelial squamous cells are observed, no further testing is conducted, because these cells indicate the specimen is oropharyngeal secretion. Another specimen of sputum, not saliva, must be obtained. A wet mount may also be used to detect a large number of eosinophils. Sputum eosinophilia is associated with asthma and other nonbacterial pulmonary diseases. Baigelman et al. (1993) noted that if as many as one-fourth of the cells are eosinophils, a sputum Gram stain has less than a 1% chance of providing clinically useful bacteriologic information. Not continuing with a Gram stain and culture may be cost-effective.

REFERENCE VALUES FOR SPUTUM CULTURES

Various organisms, if present in large amounts, can cause acute respiratory infections. The laboratory reports the predominant organism or organisms present in the sputum. Common pathogenic organisms include *Streptococcus pneumoniae, Staphylococcus aureus,* and *Haemophilus influenzae.* Various gram-negative bacilli may also cause respiratory infections. The culture for these common bacteria is completed in 24–48 hr.

A culture for tuberculosis (AFB culture) grows very slowly. It may take 1–6 weeks to obtain a final report. The AFB may also be identified with a nucleic probe. See Chapter 1 on this technology. Results are available within 1 day.

▼ POSSIBLE NURSING DIAGNOSES RELATED TO POSITIVE SPUTUM CULTURE

Ineffective Airway Clearance

Clients need encouragement to perform deep breathing and coughing exercises. They may also need intensive respiratory therapy by suctioning or postural drainage. The nurse needs to make sure that hydration is adequate because without adequate fluids the sputum becomes tenacious.

Knowledge Deficit Related to Spread of Disease to Others

Teaching clients to cover their mouths when coughing seems common sense, but the nurse may have to remind clients. The nurse also needs to teach clients how to safely dispose of sputum that is excreted. If clients are coughing up large amounts of sputum, cleaning an emesis basin is easier if the basin is first lined with tissues. Otherwise sputum tends to become encrusted in the basin. As a rule, clients with most types of pneumonia are not isolated. However, depending on the type of organism in the sputum, respiratory isolation might be justified.

Tuberculosis has re-emerged as a public health concern, so aggressive drug treatment that reflects a philosophy of treating all tubercular infections as if they were drug resistant has been instituted (Anastasi and Thomas, 1994). Nurses may contact the CDC for the latest information on prevention and treatment of tuberculosis.

▼ THROAT CULTURES

Throat cultures are the only reliable means of differentiating strep throats from viral sore throats. Most sore throats are caused by viruses; only about 10–15% of them in children are caused by group A β-hemolytic streptococci. Yet identifying whether the patient has group A β-hemolytic streptococci is important because rheumatic fever and glomerulonephritis may follow such infections. Streptococci are classified according to the antigens. Some are not considered particularly pathogenic, whereas group A β-hemolytic strep is. (See Chapter 14 on the streptococcal antigen-antibody tests of anti-streptolysin-O, anti-streptodornase-B, and streptozyme.) Occasionally a throat culture for gonorrhea may be performed if the client has been engaging in oral sex with a partner who has gonorrhea.

Certain clinical signs and symptoms should alert nurses to the possibility that a sore throat is indeed a bacterial infection rather than a viral one. For bacterial infections

1. Temperatures are higher than with viral infections.
2. Symptoms usually occur more abruptly and the client seems more ill.
3. The patches on the throat are often distinctive.
4. The WBC count is characteristically elevated—not so with viral infections. (See Chapter 2 on the significance of the WBC count in bacterial infections.)

Preparation of Client and Collection of Sample

Throat cultures are performed with a swab that is immediately placed into a test tube or kit with a special medium for the growth of bacteria. The client's tongue is depressed with a tongue blade and a flashlight is used to visualize the inflamed area of the throat. The sterile swab is rubbed over each tonsilar area and the posterior pharynx without touching the lips or tongue. Any white patch should be cultured. The results of throat cultures take 24–48 hr. Special test kits for strep throat show a positive reading in 7 min (as a stat test) or 70 min as a batch test. Evaluation of the Directigen Group A strep test kit showed that the kit method is relatively simple to perform, easy to interpret, and provides accurate assessment for the organism with little or no cross reactivity with other β-hemolytic groups (Miller et al., 1984). Many companies now manufacture test kits for group A streptococci (Ravel, 1995).

REFERENCE VALUES FOR THROAT CULTURES

The diagnosis of strep throat is based on finding group A β-hemolytic streptococci. Other possible pathogens, *H influenzae, Corynebacterium diphtheriae,* gonococci, or meningococci, can be identified with culture.

▼ POSSIBLE NURSING DIAGNOSES RELATED TO POSITIVE TEST FOR GROUP A STREPTOCOCCI

Knowledge Deficit Related to Needed Treatment

If streptococci are the cause of the sore throat, penicillin, or erythromycin in the case of penicillin allergy, is prescribed. Clients sometimes stop taking antibiotics after they begin to feel better. Yet antibiotic therapy for strep throat must be con-

(*continued*)

▼ POSSIBLE NURSING DIAGNOSES RELATED TO POSITIVE TEST FOR GROUP A STREPTOCOCCI (*continued*)

tinued for at least 10 days, regardless of how well the client feels. So the nurse may assess to make sure that the parents, or the clients themselves, understand the reason why the antibiotic is to be continued for 10 or more days. Either the physician or the nurse may have to explain to the parents that undertreating strep throat increases the possibility of the later development of rheumatic fever.

Health Maintenance Management to Reduce Community Spread

Clients with strep throat are not isolated because the disease is considered noninfectious a few hours after antibiotic therapy is begun. Other family members should be tested because about half of siblings and nearly one-fourth of parents of a child with strep throat also have the organism. Because streptococci are transmitted in droplets from the respiratory tract, an infected client should not cough or breathe on others. The nurse may become involved with follow-up contacts for other family members. In a school, the nurse or public health nurse can be effective in both detecting and preventing the spread of strep throat in a population. Preventing strep infections helps prevent rheumatic fever. Rheumatic heart disease is the only principal form of cardiovascular disease that is preventable at present. (See Chapter 14 on the streptococci antigen tests used to assess for previous acute infections with streptococci.)

▼ NASAL AND NASOPHARYNGEAL CULTURES

General Indications

Nasopharyngeal cultures are performed to screen for *Bordetella pertussis, Candida albicans, C diphtheriae, Neisseria meningitidis, H influenzae,* and others. Nasal cultures may be performed to identify carriers of organisms, such as *S aureus,* that are also called *coag-positive.* The differentiation between carrier state and infection is often difficult because some pathogens do transiently appear in the normal human pharynx. Health workers in areas such as newborn nurseries or operating rooms may have nasal cultures to screen out potential sources of spread once an outbreak has occurred.

Preparation of Client and Collection of Sample

A flexible swab is inserted gently into the nose and rotated against the anterior nares for a nasal culture. A longer flexible swab makes it possible also to collect a culture specimen from the posterior pharynx (nasopharyngeal). The swab is placed into a tube of transport medium and sent to the laboratory. Identification of particular strains of *Staphylococcus* may require special laboratory resources not found in all institutions.

REFERENCE VALUES FOR NASOPHARYNGEAL CULTURES

Pathogens such as streptococci, pneumonococci, or *N meningitidis* may or may not be clinically significant. Coag-positive staphylococci may be present in 20% of people who undergo nasopharyngeal cultures (Ravel, 1995).

▼ POSSIBLE NURSING IMPLICATIONS RELATED TO POSITIVE NASAL CULTURES

If a health worker has a positive culture, the physician must evaluate the importance of the person as a carrier. A health worker who is a potential source of pathogens may be assigned to areas where the risk of infecting others is minimal. The actual danger to others is somewhat controversial because many pathogens are always present to some degree and become disease-producing only when the opportunity arises. These opportunistic pathogens are probably dangerous for the already ill and immunodeficient person. Many hospitals have an infection control nurse as part of an infection control team. As employees, nurses should seek out information about how their institutions handle the problem of carriers.

▼ WOUND CULTURES

General Indications

Normally wounds should not be infected with any organisms. Yet once the integrity of the skin is broken, there is a direct pathway for skin flora to reach tissue. An infected wound is usually obvious even to the untrained eye. The characteristic signs are redness, heat, and swelling. There may also be drainage that contains pus (purulent) and that may have a foul odor. If the wound cannot drain, the infection can cause pain and swelling, such as in an abscess. The wounds of surgical clients should be inspected daily for any sign of infection. Clients with burns are also susceptible to infections of the open skin areas.

Preparation of Client and Collection of Wound Culture

A specimen for a wound culture may be obtained by swab, aspiration with a needle and syringe, or tissue biopsy. Most experts agree that swab cultures are the least reliable method because of contamination from skin flora. Aspiration of wounds is usually a much better technique. It is important to reach an area of viable tissue because more microorganisms survive there than in the exudate. Cuzzell (1994) suggested irrigation of the wound with normal saline solution to eliminate the exudate.

The saline solution is soaked up with sterile gauze, and the wound is massaged slightly to produce fresh drainage, which is aspirated. Contents from aspiration usually are collected in an anaerobic container. All air must be expressed from the syringe before the specimen is injected into the container. An anaerobic container also can be used for aerobic collection. Tissue biopsy, most often used for clients with burns or long-standing decubitus ulcers, is analyzed for bacterial growth per gram of tissue. Debrided tissue may be used, but it is viable tissue that supports the colonization of pathogens. Included with all specimens should be the location of the wound and the clinical diagnosis, such as cellulitis, furuncle, abscess, or decubitus ulcer.

REFERENCE VALUES FOR WOUND CULTURES

Common organisms found in wounds are *S aureus,* group A streptococci, gram-negative bacilli, and fungi. If the wound is deep and hence not in direct contact with the air, anaerobic bacteria such as clostridia or anaerobic streptococci may also thrive.

▼ POSSIBLE NURSING DIAGNOSIS RELATED TO POSITIVE WOUND CULTURE

Risk for Injury Related to Spread of Infection

If the wound is completely covered and is not draining to the outside, simple wound isolation is needed. In essence, wound isolation means using a gown and gloves when the wound must be dressed. Sometimes staff tend to become careless in using sterile technique when the client has a wound infection. A break in sterile technique is shrugged off as being not important because "the client already has an infected wound." This kind of thinking is not justifiable because, no matter how infected a wound may be, adding other organisms is possible. Dressing changes of an infected wound require the same careful sterile technique as do wounds that are not already infected.

If the wound is draining enough that the dressings become soaked, the client may become a source of infection to others. So more extreme isolation procedures may need to be carried out. Refer to the specific policies of the institution. Many hospitals now have an infection control nurse who can help nursing personnel decide the level of isolation required for a hospitalized client with a wound infection. In the home, the nurse needs to teach the client how to avoid transmitting the infection to others. Because proper wound healing requires good nutrition, the dietary needs of the client should be assessed. (See the ideas discussed earlier in this chapter about ways to increase a person's resistance to infection.)

▼ EYE CULTURES

Although the eye does contain some bacteria, the bathing of the eye with tears usually keeps the actual count of bacteria low. An infected eye is easy to see even by an untrained person. Because of the need to treat most eye infections with topical antimicrobial agents, the laboratory may routinely use a Kirby–Bauer disk to test the organisms found for susceptibility to drugs such as neomycin and chloramphenicol.

Preparation of Client and Collection of Sample

A sterile swab is used to collect some of the purulent matter from the eye. The client should be told to look up while the nurse gently pulls down on the cheek. The swab can be placed on the conjunctiva. *Not touching the cornea with the swab is important.* After the specimen is collected, it is put into a sterile culture tube.

REFERENCE VALUES FOR EYE CULTURES

S aureus and *P aeruginosa* are two bacteria that may cause eye infections. In newborns, infections can be transmitted during passage through the birth canal. To prevent this transmission of gonorrhea or other infections, state laws require delivery room personnel to instill silver nitrate or an antibiotic ointment in every newborn's eyes. Many nurseries now use erythromycin ointment because it prevents chlamydial infections and gonorrhea.

▼ POSSIBLE NURSING DIAGNOSIS RELATED TO POSITIVE EYE CULTURE

Knowledge Deficit Related to Care for Eye Infection

Clients should be taught not to wipe the infected eye. They must also avoid transmitting the infection to the other eye. Dark glasses may offer some comfort to clients if they need to be outdoors. Clients also may need instructions on the proper way to instill eye drops. For example, clients may not know how to put pressure on the lacrimal duct to prevent the drop from entering the nasal cavity.

▼ VAGINAL AND URETHRAL SMEARS

The vagina normally contains bacteria such as *Lactobacillus, Staphylococcus,* and *E coli* and some yeast. Most commonly, vaginal infections are due to *Trichomonas vaginalis* or to the fungus *C albicans*. Smears of the discharge may detect the causative agent. If gonorrhea is suspected in a female client, an endocervical smear is performed. In the male clients, smears or cultures of the drainage from the urethra may be performed for gonorrhea or other organisms. Also in male clients, centrifuged urine may be cultured for gonorrhea. Newer tests for herpes and chlamydia have increased the ability to detect STDs. (See Chapter 14 for serologic tests for syphilis.)

Preparation of Client and Collection of Sample

Vaginal and Endocervical Smears. To obtain a vaginal smear or culture, the swab must be inserted well into the vagina. Check with the laboratory regarding any special techniques needed for smears, such as a wet saline swab for *Trichomonas* or KOH for *Candida.* The client or the nurse needs to hold the labia apart so that the swab does not touch the outer lips. If the nurse must separate the lips of the vagina, a non-sterile glove should be used. An endocervical specimen, necessary for suspected gonorrhea or chlamydia, requires the use of a speculum as for other pelvic examinations. Only water is used to lubricate the speculum. Excess cervical mucus is wiped off with a dry cotton ball, and then a cotton-tipped swab is inserted in the endocervical canal for 30 sec to absorb any organisms. Two specimens are put on one special culture medium. (If an anal specimen is collected, it is put on a separate culture medium.)

Urethral Smears in Male Clients. Collection of urethral smears in male clients is often performed at the time the physician is examining the client because of discharge from the penis. The exudate is collected on a swab, which is rolled, not rubbed, on a slide. A special loop swab can be gently inserted into the urinary meatus to obtain exudate. If the client has no discharge from the penis, a urine specimen may be centrifuged to obtain a smear or culture for possible gonorrhea.

REFERENCE VALUES FOR VAGINAL, ENDOCERVICAL, AND URETHRAL SMEARS

The presence of pathogens on a smear is considered diagnostic. A culture may or may not be needed to confirm the identification of certain organisms, such as fungus (*Candida*) or protozoan *(Trichomonas),* that may be causing vaginitis.

Clinical Significance of Positive Smears or Cultures

Gonorrhea. About half the cases of pelvic inflammatory disease (PID) in women are due to infection with *gonorrhoeae.* Although a smear may be diagnostic for men with gonorrhea, women need a culture because the smear may not allow differentiation between other vaginal flora and gonorrheal organisms. The sample for the culture must be taken from the endocervical canal, not from the vagina. Oropharyngeal and rectal smears and cultures must be performed if the person has had oral or anal sex with an infected person.

Chlamydia. *Chlamydia* is a bacteria-like microbe with some of the characteristics of a virus. The disease may have few symptoms and often is found with other STDs. Unlike syphilis and gonorrhea, chlamydial infection is not eliminated by penicillin. If left untreated, the disease may cause sterility because of chronic inflammation in the urogenital tract. Chlamydia antigen tests are available to screen clients at high risk, but the cell tissue culture is the standard of reference for diagnosis because the rapid tests may often lead to false-positive diagnoses. However, urine testing for chlamydia by means of a nucleic acid amplification technique (see Chapter 1) has been found to be highly effective (Lee et al., 1995).

Herpes Simplex. The genital type of herpes is caused by a virus called herpes simplex virus 2 (HSV 2). (HSV 1 causes cold sores in the mouth.) Exudate from the lesions present during an acute episode of herpes infection can be examined with a microscope. A herpes culture takes several days, but an antibody test can detect active herpes in 4 hr. Nettina (1989) noted that because this test (Herp-Check) can determine whether a pregnant woman has active lesions close to the time of birth, women with genital herpes may be able to avoid unnecessary cesarean deliveries. For the tests for herpes, a specimen can be obtained by scraping the vesicle, but the ideal way is aspiration of fluid from an intact vesicle. A tuberculin syringe with a 28-gauge needle is used.

Herpes is treated with topical acyclovir (Zovirax). Clients should use a finger cot or rubber gloves to reduce the spread to other sites, particularly the eye. After an initial outbreak, stress reduction and general good health habits may keep the virus in remission.

Trichomonas. *T vaginalis* is a protozoan that grows optimally under anaerobic conditions. Sometimes a wet smear may be performed to detect the active protozoa in a drop of vaginal discharge or in a drop of urine from a male client. Culturing of urogenital discharges can reveal protozoa even if direct microscopic examination seems normal.

Moniliasis or Other Yeast Infections. *C albicans* and, less frequently, other species of *Candida* may be normally present in vaginal secretions. These yeast-like fungi may become invasive under conditions that favor their rapid growth. Predisposing factors for rapid growth of fungi include long-term antibiotic therapy, pregnancy, oral contraceptives, diabetes, and wearing nonventilating pants. The vaginal discharge viewed with a microscope on a wet mount using KOH preparation shows many budding yeast cells and may be diagnostic.

Bacterial Vaginosis. Bacterial vaginosis may be caused by *Gardnerella, Corynebacterium,* or *Haemophilus* species. It may be called nonspecific or anaerobic vaginitis. Bacterial vaginosis may be diagnosed after the other pathogens have been ruled out. The pH of secretions helps with ruling out some organisms: *Gardnerella* and *Trichomonas* species occur with a pH above 4.5 and *Candida* with a pH less than 4.5 (Ravel, 1995).

Toxic Shock Syndrome. Toxic shock syndrome (TSS) is a rare disease believed to be caused by toxin-producing strains of the bacterium *S aureus*. Clients believed to have TSS undergo blood and urine cultures as well as a vaginal culture to detect a focal staph infection. The use of high-absorbency tampons may be linked to an increased incidence, but a rise of the syndrome in 1983, after use of high-absorbency tampons declined because of published warnings, has not been explained (Petti, 1986). Because of the possible association with tampon use, manufacturers of tampons now include detailed information about the symptoms of TSS in their product information folders. Early symptoms may be fever and a rash. Abnormal laboratory reports include leukocytosis with pronounced left shift (Chapter 2), elevated BUN and creatinine (Chapter 4), severe acidosis (Chapter 6), hypocalcemia (Chapter 7), hyperbilirubinemia (Chapter 11), elevated CPK (Chapter 12), and thrombocytopenia (Chapter 13). Treatment involves the use of antibiotic therapy and treatment of the circulatory collapse that may occur.

▼ POSSIBLE NURSING DIAGNOSES RELATED TO POSITIVE VAGINAL OR URETHRAL SMEAR OR CULTURE

Knowledge Deficit Related to Sexual Transmission of Disease

Gonorrhea is a communicable disease that must be reported to the health department, which employs people who serve as case finders. Although the sexual contacts of these clients need to be examined for case finding, clients may or may not wish to name their sexual partners. The nurse can be sensitive to their needs and yet also impress on them the importance of the disease as a public health problem.

Other diseases, such as trichomoniasis, do not require reporting, but the spread from person to person is also of concern. Women may be reinfected by a male partner unless he, too, is cultured and treated (the ping-pong effect). Thus treatment of any STD involves not only the client but also the person or persons who have been and who will be sexual partners of the client (Lutz, 1986). At present, herpes infection cannot be cured, but the disease is infectious only when it is active. The nurse can help set a climate that is conducive to assisting these clients help themselves and others by learning about safe sexual practices. Clients need factual information on how to best proceed as a sexual being and how to live with a chronic STD (Swanson et al., 1995).

Learning Needs Related to Treatment

Female clients may need specific instructions on how to insert vaginal suppositories or to administer douches, if medicine is ordered in these forms. Again, the nurse must foster a climate that helps clients feel comfortable about discussing intimate details. Excellent literature and video tapes for patient teaching are available free of charge from the pharmaceutical companies that manufacture vaginal medications.

▼ STOOL CULTURES

Many normal bacteria live in the feces. In fact, a large percentage of the weight of feces is bacteria. Most of the organisms in the intestine are many types of gram-negative bacilli. *Escherichia coli* is a common normal inhabitant in adults, but it can also be a pathogen. For example, *E coli* in poorly cooked meat caused an epidemic of enteric infection in several western states. The molecular studies of the meat strains showed that they were identical to the human isolates (Tarr, 1993). Bacterial cultures of stool are routinely checked for *S aureus, Salmonella, Shigella,* and other enteropathogens. If anaerobic organisms are suspected, such as *Clostridium botulinum,* an anaerobic culture also is performed. A microscopic examination to detect the presence of fecal blood, leukocytes, and organisms called *vibros* can be performed in 30 min. A test for fecal leukocytes differentiates infectious from non-infectious colitis.

In addition to cultures for bacteria, stool specimens may also be collected to identify parasites that can be protozoa or worms (helminths). Protozoa are more common in most areas than are helminths, unless there is a history of travel to the tropics or a heavy influx of immigrants (Most, 1984). If the laboratory is checking for protozoa such as *Entamoeba histolytica,* the nurse must collect several specimens over a period of days. Because protozoan parasites have cyclical life spans, multiple collections increase the chance of spotting a parasite. The use of enzyme immunoassay (EIA) has made it possible to screen for *Giardia* in one stool specimen. If the laboratory is still using the traditional microscopic examination, three specimens are required. (See Chapter 14 for a serologic test performed for amebae.) For helminths, a single stool specimen is usually sufficient.

Infant botulism, first identified in 1976, differs from the food-borne botulism seen in adults and older children because the spores germinate in the infant's intestinal tract (Bechler-Karsch and Berro, 1994). The organism, or more likely the toxin, can be identified in the stool. *Cl difficile* can be identified by the toxin in the stool. *Cl difficile* infection is an important nosocomial disease associated with recent antibiotic use, particularly use of third-generation cephalosporins (Anand et al., 1994).

Two other methods of collecting stool specimens for examination involve cellophane tape and a rectal swab. The cellophane tape may be pressed over the perineal area to pick up pinworms, which are very small intestinal worms. Rectal swabs are sometimes performed for *Shigella* infection and for gonorrhea, if this disease is suspected. Yet few organisms live in the rectal wall; the mass of bacteria or parasites is in the feces.

Preparation of Client and Collection of Sample

For bacterial or protozoan cultures, a walnut-sized piece of feces is all that is needed. Diarrheal stool can also be cultured; only about 15–20 mL is needed, and the rest of the stool is discarded. The specimen should be sent to the laboratory immediately. Check with the laboratory for the time span permissible.

The client must defecate into a clean bedpan. Urine in the bedpan may kill some of the growth. A tongue blade can be used to transfer the small amount of stool to the stool container. Commercial kits contain small spoons inside a specimen container. When handling the bedpan, the nurse should wear disposable, nonsterile gloves. Because parasites or bacteria may often be harbored in mucus or in streaks of blood, some of this material should be included in the sample. The stool specimen is put into a waxed container with a tight-fitting lid. It is important not to contaminate the outside of the specimen container. Clients may collect a stool specimen at home. If so, they need to be taught how to collect the specimen properly and how to wash their hands properly so that the outside of the container is not contaminated. (Enteric diseases are spread by oral–fecal transmission.) A plastic bag or newspaper can be taped under the toilet seat so the client can sit on the toilet.

If a rectal swab or cellophane tape is used to collect material from the rectal area, the nurse should wear a glove when touching the perineal area. A sterile cotton-tipped swab is inserted 1 inch (2.5 cm) into the anal canal. The swab should be moved side to side and left for 30 sec for absorption of organisms. Record on the laboratory slip whether the client is taking antibiotics because these drugs can change the flora in the intestines. Also, the use of antacids may change the pH of the stool and affect bacterial growth.

If the fat content of the stool is to be measured because of malabsorption problems, the *entire* stool for 1–3 days is sent to the laboratory. The client follows a 100-g fat diet.

REFERENCE VALUES FOR STOOL CULTURES

The laboratory may issue a preliminary report of probable findings of *Salmonella* or *Shigella,* so that enteric precautions can be started. Parasites or worms may be immediately identified at examination. The two important protozoan infections in the United States are amebiasis and giardiasis. Immunosuppressed clients may have an infection with *Cryptosporidium* or other uncommon organisms.

▼ POSSIBLE NURSING DIAGNOSES RELATED TO POSITIVE STOOL CULTURE

Knowledge Deficit Related to Spread of Infection to Others

Depending on the type of pathogen in the stool, the nurse must make sure that the client does not spread the pathogens to others. Isolation is usually not required if clients can wash their hands properly and if the feces can quickly be flushed into the sewage system. Stool precautions are not needed for botulism, *Cl perfringens* infection, or staph food poisoning. The nurse should be aware that the collection of stool and the focus on the anal area is often a source of embarrassment for the client. (Saving a stool is frowned on since the age of 2 years and the anal stage.) The client should not be made to feel "unclean" because of the extra precautions needed to protect others. Children are prone to spread disease because of poor hygiene. In fact, giardiasis has been called *daycare diarrhea* (Bonner and Dale, 1986). Positive cultures for *Cl difficile* have been obtained from hospital rooms up to 40 days after a client's discharge (Carpenter and Zielinski, 1992). The organism has been isolated from toilet seats, shelves where bedpans are stored, and numerous other locations. The organism also has been cultured from the hands of personnel caring for clients with *Cl difficile* infection.

Knowledge Deficit Related to Effect of Drugs

Once appropriate therapy has been started, clients need follow-up stool samples to evaluate the effectiveness of the therapy. Some of the drugs used for intestinal pathogens cause gastrointestinal symptoms; so it is important that clients know what may be expected from the drug and what may be an indication that therapy is not being effective. Later stool samples may show a second type of pathogen also is present.

▼ CULTURES OF CEREBROSPINAL FLUID AND OTHER FLUIDS

Specimens of CSF are obtained by means of lumbar puncture. CSF is sterile, and it is collected under sterile conditions. Various organisms may be responsible for meningitis, including *H influenzae, N meningitidis,* and *Strep pneumoniae.* The first is common in infants and the last in adults.

The laboratory performs an immediate smear to see if any organisms exist. The laboratory should be notified that CSF is going to the laboratory so that immediate analysis can begin. Specific identification of the organism may take 48–72 hr. (See Chapter 25 on the procedure for lumbar puncture.)

Cultures of Pleural Fluid, Peritoneal Fluid, and Joint Fluid

Pleural fluid, obtained by means of thoracentesis, can be cultured for possible bacterial growth, as can peritoneal fluid obtained at paracentesis (see Chapter 25). Joint fluid from a joint aspiration may also be cultured. The role of the nurse in carefully marking the specimens and sending them to the laboratory is discussed in the beginning of this chapter. Careful labeling is necessary for *all* specimens. If a urine specimen is not labeled correctly, it is usually possible to obtain another specimen, but it may be much less feasible to obtain a second specimen of any fluid that requires an invasive technique.

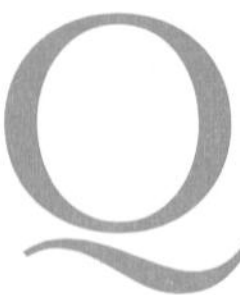

1. The laboratory reports a large number of gram-negative rods *are* present on the preliminary stain of a urine specimen. Which one of the following organisms is thus ruled out?

   a. *Escherichia coli* b. *Proteus species*
   c. *Neisseria gonorrhoeae* d. *Pseudomonas species*

2. Mrs. Siegel's urine was sent to the laboratory for a C&S (culture and sensitivity). The report notes an *S* next to all the listed antibiotics except penicillin, which is marked with an *R*. An *R* next to the penicillin indicates

   a. Penicillin is the right drug for the urine infection
   b. Mrs. Siegel is resistant to penicillin
   c. Penicillin must be increased to obtain a successful urine level
   d. The organisms in the culture were resistant to penicillin

3. Common bacteria that cause nosocomial infections are staphylococci and gram-negative rods. Which nursing action would be the most effective way to prevent these nosocomial infections?

   a. Administering all prescribed antibiotics on time
   b. Emphasizing handwashing before and after caring for every client
   c. Isolating all clients with fevers of undetermined origin (FUO)
   d. Culturing all open wounds

4. Mrs. Mozian, 78 years of age, has undergone cultures of blood, urine, and sputum because of a persistent fever and general malaise. In planning care for Mrs. Mozian, the nurse in the nursing home should

   a. Assess the fluid intake and determine how much fluid by mouth should be taken daily
   b. Move the client to a private room for isolation
   c. Encourage more activity to keep the client stimulated
   d. Use aspirin as needed to keep the temperature normal

5. Which of the following is a correct statement about the collection of urine for urine cultures?

   a. The meatus of a male client requires more cleaning than does the meatus of a female client

b. A disinfectant is always used to clean the genital area before a clean-catch is performed
c. A clean-catch urine specimen requires that the urine be caught in midstream
d. Only a catheterized urine specimen is suitable for urine culture

6. Mr. Edwards has been having fever and chills from an unknown cause. He is to have blood cultures drawn twice. The nurse should be aware of which of the following?

    a. The skin over the venipuncture site must be prepared with an iodine solution to reduce contamination by skin flora
    b. Two blood samples can be drawn at the same time if the specimens are drawn from two different sites
    c. Blood cultures should not be drawn after a spike of fever or a chill
    d. A positive confirmation of a diagnosis can be made in 24 hr

7. Mrs. Solado has had a central venous catheter in place for several days for hyperalimentation. The physician is removing the catheter because of possible sepsis. The catheter is to be cultured. How should the nurse prepare the specimen for the laboratory?

    a. Wrap the entire catheter in a sterile towel and send to the laboratory
    b. Cut off the tip of the catheter with sterile scissors, put the tip into a sterile container, and send it to the laboratory
    c. Cut off the tip of the catheter with bandage scissors, put the tip in a clean test tube, and send it to the laboratory
    d. Put a sterile swab inside the tip of the catheter and then send the swab to the laboratory

8. Mr. McKay is to have a sputum specimen obtained because of lung congestion and fever. Which of the following instructions by the nurse is correct to tell Mr. McKay?

    a. "Save as much sputum as you can in the next 2 hr because the laboratory needs at least an ounce (30 mL) of sputum."
    b. "Discard the first specimen in the morning because the secretions will not be fresh."
    c. "Saliva will be all right for a specimen if it hurts to cough deeply."
    d. "Rinse out your mouth before obtaining the specimen so bacteria from the mouth will be less numerous."

9. Mrs. Gardeni is to provide sputum specimens three times for AFB. If the preliminary report is positive, she will be on respiratory isolation to prevent the spread of

    a. Tuberculosis
    b. *Legionella pneumophila*
    c. Influenza
    d. *Pneumocystis carinii*

10. Timmy, 10 years of age, has come to see the school nurse for a sore throat. The concern for correctly identifying the cause of the sore throat is important because rheumatic fever or glomerulonephritis sometimes occurs after infection with which organism?

    a. Any of the staphylococci **b.** Group A β-hemolytic streptococci
    c. *Staphylococcus aureus* **d.** Any of the streptococci

11. Mr. Ricardo has a Penrose drain inserted into an abdominal stab wound that is inflamed and draining around the drain. Which of the following measures would be the most appropriate for the nurse to obtain a specimen for wound culture?

    a. Swab the end of the Penrose drain
    b. Swab the base of the wound
    c. Use a needle and syringe to aspirate fluid
    d. Obtain a tissue biopsy specimen

12. Mr. Rabinowitz has an infected eye. Which of the following actions by the visiting nurse is inappropriate?

    a. Using a sterile swab to collect some exudate and putting the swab into culture medium supplied by the laboratory
    b. Lightly touching the cornea with the swab to obtain the specimen
    c. Instructing the client not to rub his eye with his fingers
    d. Showing the client how to rinse off the exudate without contaminating the other eye

13. Johnny Phillips, 17 years of age, is concerned that he may have gonorrhea. He asks the nurse in the clinic how gonorrhea can be detected. The nurse should explain to Johnny that the test for gonorrhea involves which of the following?

    a. Drawing blood by venipuncture for a serologic test
    b. Obtaining some secretions from the end of the penis for a microscopic examination
    c. Both urine and blood tests
    d. Only a finger stick for a blood sample

14. Mr. Cohen is to have a stool specimen collected because of a possible *Salmonella* infection. He just had a bowel movement in the bedside commode. Which action by the nurse is appropriate?

    a. Send a small portion of the stool in a waxed container to the laboratory
    b. Discard the stool because it was diarrhea rather than formed stool
    c. Use sterile gloves to transfer all the stool to a sterile container and send it to the laboratory
    d. Send the entire stool in a waxed container to the laboratory

▼ REFERENCES

Anand, A., Bashey, B., Mir, T., et al. (1994). Epidemiology, clinical manifestations and outcome of *clostridium difficile*-associated diarrhea. *American Journal of Gastroenterology, 89* (4), 519–521.

Anastasi, J.K., and Thomas, F. (1994). Dealing with H.I.V. related pulmonary infections. *Nursing 94, 24* (11), 60–64.

Baigelman, W., Chodosh, S., Beiser, A., et al. (1993). Sputum eosinophilia negates need to perform Gram's stain. *Lung, 171,* 15–18.

Bechler-Karsch, A., and Berro, E.A. (1994). Infant botulism. *MCN: American Journal of Maternal Child Health Nursing, 19* (5), 275–280.

Bonner, A., and Dale, R. (1986). Giardia lamblia: Day care diarrhea. *American Journal of Nursing, 86* (7), 818–820.

Carpenter, D.R., and Zielinski, D.A. (1992). How do you treat and control *C difficile* infection? *American Journal of Nursing, 92* (9), 22–24.

Caruthers, D. (1990). Infectious pneumonia in the elderly. *American Journal of Nursing, 90* (2), 56–60.

Centers for Disease Control. (1988). Update: Universal precautions for prevention of transmission of human immunodeficiency virus, hepatitis B virus, and other bloodborne pathogens in health care settings. *Morbidity and Mortality Weekly Report, 37* (24), 376–383.

Conti, M., and Eutropius, L. (1987). Preventing UTI's: What works? *American Journal of Nursing 87* (3), 307–309.

Cuzzell, J.Z. (1993). The right way to culture a wound. *American Journal of Nursing, 93* (5), 48–50.

Faller, N.A., and Lawrence, K.G. (1994). Obtaining a urine specimen from a conduit urostomy. *American Journal of Nursing, 94* (1), 37.

Gerdes, J.S. (1994). Clinical symptoms in neonatal sepsis. *Israel Journal of Medical Science 30* (5), 430–441.

Goswitz, J., Willard, K.E., Eastep, S.J., et al. (1993). Utility of slide centrifuge Gram's stain versus quantitative culture for diagnosis of UTI. *American Journal of Clinical Pathology, 99* (2), 132–136.

Griffin, J. (1986). Fever: When to leave it alone. *Nursing 86, 16* (2), 58–61.

Gurevich, I. (1985). Fever: When to worry about it. *RN, 48* (12), 14–19.

Jackson, M., and Lynch, P. (1990). Infection control: In search of a rational approach. *American Journal of Nursing, 90* (10), 65–74.

Katzung, B. (1995). *Basic and clinical pharmacology.* (6th ed.). Norwalk, CT: Appleton & Lange.

Komaroff, A. (1984). Acute dysuria in women. *New England Journal of Medicine, 310* (6), 368–375.

Lee, H.H., Chernesky, M. A., Schachter, J., et al. (1995). Diagnosis of *Chlamydia trachomatis* genitourinary infection in women by ligase chain reaction assay of urine. *Lancet, 345,* 213–216.

Leiner, S. (1995). Recurrent urinary tract infections in otherwise healthy adult women. *Nurse Practitioner, 20* (2), 48–56.

Leisure, M., et al. (1990). Changing the needle when inoculating blood cultures. *JAMA, 264* (16), 2111–2112.

Lott, J.W., and Kenner, C. (1994a). Keeping up with neonatal infections: Designer bugs, Part I. *MCN: American Journal of Maternal Child Health Nursing, 19* (4), 207–213.

Lott, J.W., and Kenner, C. (1994b). Keeping up with neonatal infection: Designer bugs, Part II. *MCN: American Journal of Maternal Child Health Nursing, 19* (5), 264–271.

Lutz, R. (1986). Stopping the spread of sexually transmitted diseases. *Nursing 86, 16* (3), 47–50.

Mayer, J., Dubbert, P.M., Miller, P.M., et al. (1986). Increasing handwashing in an intensive care unit. *Infection Control, 7* (5), 259–262.

McGuckin, M. (1981). Getting better urine specimens with the clean catch midstream technique. *Nursing 81, 11,* 72–73.

Miller, J.M., Phillips, H.L., Graves, R.K., et al. (1984). Evaluation of the Directigen group A strep test kit. *Journal of Clinical Microbiology, 20* (5), 846–848.

Most, H. (1984). Treatment of parasitic infections of travelers and immigrants. *New England Journal of Medicine, 310,* 298–304.

Nettina, S. (1989). When patients with genital herpes turn to you for answers. *Nursing 89, 19* (8), 61–64.

Petti, D. (1986). The incidence of toxic shock syndrome in northern California. *JAMA, 255* (3), 368–372.

Pinkerman, M.L. (1994). Indwelling urinary catheters: Reducing infection risks. *Nursing 94, 24* (9), 66–68.

Pryor, A. (1984). A comparison of blood cultures withdrawn from the arterial line and by venipuncture. *Heart and Lung, 13* (4), 411–415.

Ravel, R. (1995). *Clinical laboratory medicine: Clinical application of laboratory data.* (6th ed.). St. Louis: Mosby–Year Book.

Sanders, M.E. (1993). Healthful attributes of bacteria in yogurt. *Contemporary Nutrition, 18* (5), 1–2.

Swanson, J.M., Dibble, S.L., and Chenitz, W.C. (1995). Clinical features and psychosocial factors in young adults with genital herpes. *Image: Journal of Nursing Scholarship, 27* (1), 16–22.

Tarr, P.I. (1993). Food safety: What do nutrition professionals need to know about *E coli? Food and Nutrition News, 65* (5), 34–35.

Thomas, D. (1985). Fever in children. *RN, 48* (12), 18–19.

Wong, D. (1990). Clean-catch midstream urine collection may not be necessary in children. *American Journal of Nursing, 90* (1), 43.

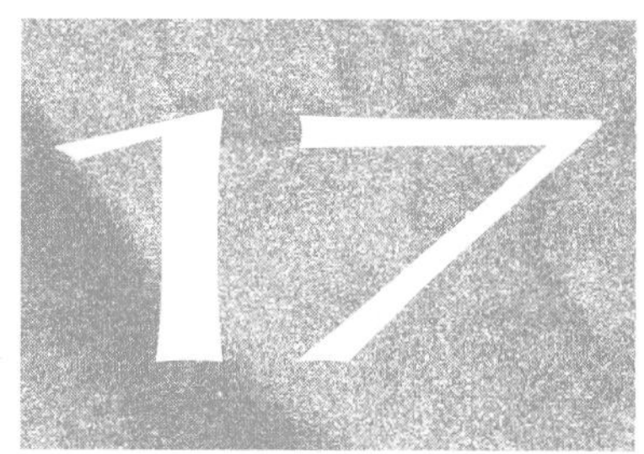

THERAPEUTIC DRUG MONITORING AND TOXICOLOGY SCREENS

- Antibiotics: Aminoglycosides
- Antibiotics: Vancomycin
- Immunosuppressive Agent: Cyclosporine Assay
- Anticonvulsants: Phenytoin, Free Phenytoin, Primidone, Valproic Acid, Phenobarbital, Carbamazepine, and Ethosuximide
- Antipsychotic Agent: Lithium Carbonate
- Tricyclic Antidepressants
- Bronchodilators: Theophylline Products and Caffeine Levels
- Cardiac Drugs: Digoxin and Digitoxin
- Antiarrhythmic Drugs: Quinidine, Procainamide and NAPA, Phenytoin, Lidocaine, and Tocainide
- Salicylates: Acetylsalicylic Acid
- Urine Testing: Phenistix
- Acetaminophen
- Blood Alcohol
- Barbiturates
- Toxicology Screens in Blood and Urine
- Bromide
- Lead

OBJECTIVES

1. Discuss nine reasons for monitoring serum or urine drug levels.
2. Describe how plasma peak and trough levels are used to monitor aminoglycoside levels.
3. Name five anticonvulsants that are sometimes monitored with serum levels and indicate the clinical symptoms of each that may indicate toxicity.
4. Identify the antipsychotic drug that must be monitored with serum drug levels to avoid toxicity.
5. Describe possible nursing diagnoses related to toxicity from antidepressants and other drugs.
6. Identify the two main clinical problems that may develop if a client has a serum theophylline level above the therapeutic range.
7. Identify which cardiac drugs are most commonly monitored with serum drug levels, along with the key nursing implications for each drug.
8. Describe three different clinical situations in which aspirin (acetylsalicylic acid [ASA]) serum levels are useful.
9. Identify the important facts that emergency department nurses should know about blood levels of alcohol and other depressant drugs.
10. Identify the usual medication history of a client with bromide toxicity.
11. Describe current protocols for screening for lead poisoning in young children.

Clinical toxicology is the study of drugs that are therapeutic as well as those that are toxic. In clinical practice, the line between therapeutic effects and toxic effects may be narrow. The cardinal principle of experimental toxicology, first expressed by a 16th-century physician and alchemist, is that only the *dose* differentiates between a poison and a remedy (Scala, 1978). For example, digoxin in the correct dosage for an individual is therapeutic, but if the dose is increased even slightly, the drug may be extremely toxic. Measurements of arsenic, carbon monoxide, or lead (all poisons) are traditional examples of toxicologic tests. Therapeutic drug monitoring, as a type of clinical toxicology, has expanded in the past few years because more and more drugs can be easily measured in the serum. The radioimmunoassay (RIA) and enzyme methods (discussed in Chapter 1) have made it possible for the laboratory to detect even small amounts of a drug or toxic substance in the bloodstream.

Although any drug can be measured in the serum, this chapter focuses on the drugs that are commonly measured and that have clinical significance for the nurse. Some general reasons for monitoring drugs, some of the pitfalls of using drug levels as assessment tools, and the general nursing implications when drug levels are used are discussed at the beginning of the chapter. Tests for specific drugs, along with any needed precautions about collection of the sample and about the specific nursing implications, are listed separately in the second part of this chapter.

PLASMA DRUG LEVELS

Reasons for Monitoring

Richens and Warrington (1979) listed seven reasons why plasma drug levels need to be measured. In addition, two other reasons for monitoring are discussed.

When the Rate of Metabolism of a Drug Has a Wide Interindividual Variation

Many drugs are given at about the same dosage for all people because the rate of metabolism does not vary much from person to person. For other drugs, such as theophylline, the rate of metabolism may vary greatly, depending on metabolic variations in the individual. With regard to theophylline, the United States Food and Drug Administration (FDA) has published specific guidelines for dosage based on weight, age, smoking or nonsmoking, and presence of certain diseases (FDA, 1980). The dosage of theophylline must be tailored to fit the particular individual. For example, if a smoker becomes a nonsmoker, the theophylline dose may have to be decreased. Serum theophylline concentrations can be measured to make sure that the dosage is maintaining the correct serum level.

When Saturation Kinetics Occur

For some drugs, such as phenytoin (Dilantin), an increase in dosage beyond a certain point does not increase the effectiveness of the drug because the body is saturated. The actual pharmacokinetics of a drug may be very complex, and they are used to determine the serum level considered therapeutically effective. However, for some drugs, the serum level is not at all reliable because the main action of the drug may be in tissues.

When the Therapeutic Ratio of the Drug Is Close to the Toxic Level

If a drug leaves considerable leeway between its therapeutic effect and its toxic effect, careful monitoring with serum levels is usually not considered necessary. Lithium, however, is a good example of a drug that has a narrow margin of safety and that must be monitored.

When Signs of Toxicity Are Difficult to Recognize Clinically

Serum levels of certain drugs help detect or prevent toxicity that might otherwise not be noticed because of other clinical problems. An antiarrhythmic drug, such as quinidine, may depress the myocardium and cause symptoms that could be wrongly attributed to a worsening of the underlying cardiac disease rather than to the toxicity of the drug. Longe (1989) found serum drug levels very helpful in monitoring clients in a skilled nursing facility who were undergoing long-term therapy with medications known to cause toxicity in the elderly.

When Gastrointestinal, Hepatic, or Renal Disease Is Present

If gastrointestinal (GI) problems are present, any oral medication may have an erratic drug absorption. (Usually the drug would be ordered for parenteral administration to avoid this problem.) If hepatic disease is present, drugs that are metabolized by the liver—and almost all are—are not cleared from the serum normally. (See Chapter 11 for the role of the liver in conjugating drugs and other substances, such as bilirubin.) Finally, because most drugs are excreted in the urine, renal disease means a problem with excretion. For example, the aminoglycoside antibiotics, if given at all, must be carefully monitored with serum levels when renal disease is present. (See Chapter 4 for assessment of renal function.)

When Drug Interactions Result from the Use of Several Drugs

Clients with epilepsy may take two types of anticonvulsants, both of which can cause central nervous system symptoms, such as lethargy and depression. It may not be at all clear which drug or combination of drugs is causing the toxic effects. A serum level of the drugs helps pinpoint the culprit.

When Noncompliance Is Suspected

Noncompliance means that a client is not taking a drug as ordered. The reasons for not taking a drug can be varied, including simple misunderstanding of the need. Clients for whom certain drugs are prescribed may be overly afraid of side effects, so they reduce the amount of drug prescribed or they "forget" to take the pill at certain times. Squire et al. (1984) found that many clients using antiarrhythmic drugs for a long time had low serum levels, most likely because of noncompliance. Sometimes when clients are admitted to the hospital, they have a toxic reaction to a drug, such as digoxin, because in the hospital they are given it routinely every day as ordered. At home, the administration may not be on schedule. A community health nurse can be of assistance in visiting clients at home to determine whether noncompliance is a reason for erratic serum drug levels.

When an Overdose of an Unknown Substance or Substances Has Occurred

Therapeutic drugs, such as aspirin or barbiturates, are often taken in toxic amounts either accidentally (poisoning) or deliberately as a suicidal gesture. With drug experimentation, the client may have inhaled, ingested, or injected a variety of different drugs. The laboratory can screen serum, urine, and gastric contents to identify the chemicals present. In chronic poisoning with heavy metals, such as lead, the laboratory can identify the toxic substances in both the serum and urine.

To Detect Abuse of Drugs for Legal Prosecution

The legal implications of the blood alcohol test are discussed in the section on alcohol tests. Other legal problems are discussed in the section on opiate abuse.

Reasons for Not Monitoring

Although there are many reasons to monitor drugs, there are also reasons not to monitor them. One good reason is cost. If the drug is not particularly toxic and if the client responds well to the usual prescribed dosage, a serum drug level is unnecessary. The nurse can help explain to clients in simple terms why drug monitoring either is or is not necessary. For some drugs, the effect of the drug on other laboratory tests is more important than the actual serum level of the drug. For example, if the client is taking anticoagulants, either partial thromboplastin time (PTT) (for heparin) or prothrombin time (PT) (for coumarin) is used to monitor the dosage of the respective anticoagulants. (See Chapter 13 on tests for coagulation.) If the client is undergoing insulin therapy, blood glucose levels are used to monitor drug effects, not the insulin level per se. (See Chapter 8 on glucose.)

Caution in Interpretation

Because serum drug levels reflect only the amount of the drug in the plasma at a given time, the level may not reflect the actual physiologic activity of the drug. Laboratory tests of serum drugs measure both the bound and unbound parts of the drug. A client with less albumin in the serum may thus have a larger amount of free drug in the serum. It is the free or unbound drug that is biologically active and thus toxicity is related to the amount of plasma proteins available for binding. (See Chapter 10 on the measurement of albumin.) Also, some drugs affect the serum level of the drug being measured.

Variation in results caused by a lack of standardization in different laboratories may be a problem. McCormick et al. (1978) found a wide range of test results when three different laboratories performed tests on standardized samples of digoxin, phenobarbital, and phenytoin. Therapeutic drug monitoring assays in general have differed more greatly between laboratories than have simple tests such as blood urea nitrogen (BUN) or glucose measurement (Ravel, 1995). Although laboratory error is not a nursing problem, the risk for laboratory error must be kept in mind when serum drug levels do not correlate well with the clinical signs and symptoms.

▼ GENERAL NURSING IMPLICATIONS

Correct Sample Timing: Peaks, Troughs, and Steady States

Serum samples of drug levels may be ordered as peak levels, as trough levels, or after obtaining a steady state. For serum drug levels, *peak* times refer to measurements of the highest level of drug reached in the serum; *trough* times represent the lowest levels. Some laboratories may refer to the trough levels as *residuals*.

(continued)

▼ GENERAL NURSING IMPLICATIONS (*continued*)

The *steady state* of a drug refers to the time when the plasma level has been stabilized with a maintenance dose. For some drugs, a steady state is not obtained for several days. A practical way to estimate the steady state is to multiply the half-life by 5, which gives the approximate time to reach 97% of the steady-state value. Howard (1986) suggested that nurses ask the hospital pharmacist to compile a list of optimal sampling times for all drugs being monitored. Each drug has its own distribution time and volume of distribution (VD) to the tissues. Some drugs have a small VD, which means they remain in the serum. Other drugs have a large VD, which means they are distributed to the tissues.

Controversy exists about whether peak or trough levels are better indicators of toxicity for specific drugs. In general, the peak is a determination of the rate of absorption of the drug, whereas the trough is a measurement of the drug's rate of elimination. A timetable for drawing peak and trough levels for tobramycin is shown in Table 17–1.

Peak and trough levels of serum drug levels are meaningless unless it is known when the drug was given, the amount given, and the route. Knowing what other drugs are being taken by the client is also important, because they may interfere with some tests. If the client is being assessed for a steady state of the drug, make note not only of this information but also of the daily dosage that has been maintained for a certain period. (Also, question the client and make sure that the ordered dosage was, in fact, the dosage being taken at home.) In summary, the laboratory needs the following information:

1. The exact timing of the last dose of the drug
2. The exact amount of the drug given
3. The route of the drug (peak times change dramatically between oral and parenteral administration)
4. How long the client has been taking a certain dosage (if the client is being assessed for a steady-state level)
5. Other medications that may interfere with the specific test (check with the individual laboratory to determine this)

The information gained by serum drug levels is used primarily by the physician, who readjusts the dosages if needed. Nurses need to be aware of the reference values used in a particular setting, so that deviations from normal can be reported before another drug dosage is given. For example, if a trough level shows a range as high, or nearly as high, as the expected peak, continuing with the drug may be dangerous. Contacting the physician before the next dose of the drug is administered would be wise. Unless the information from the laboratory report is used in a timely way, the serum drug levels are only an expensive academic exercise that has no benefit to the client.

TABLE 17–1. PEAK AND TROUGH LEVELS

Timing of Medication	Peak to be Drawn 30 min After IV Infusion Completed	Trough to be Drawn 5 min Before Next Dose
Tobramycin 80 mg in 100 mL of D_5W q8h intravenously over 1 hr 8 AM–9 AM	Draw sample at 9:30 AM	Draw sample at 3:55 PM

Note: Check with indiividual laboratory for peak time for other drugs.
See Chapter 4 on serum creatinine levels also used to monitor drug nephrotoxicity.

▼ ANTIBIOTICS: AMINOGLYCOSIDES

Serum antibiotic levels are not routinely measured if the antibiotic is not usually toxic, if the infection is responding appropriately, and if the client does not have liver or renal dysfunction. For example, because penicillin and the cephalosporins have a much wider range between therapeutic doses and toxic doses than do the antibiotics that are classified as aminoglycosides, clients taking penicillin or the cephalosporins are not routinely monitored with serum antibiotic levels.

All aminoglycosides have a central amino sugar—hence the name *aminoglycoside* (sugar). These antibiotics are used for serious infections with gram-negative bacteria, such as *Escherichia coli* and *Pseudomonas* species. (See Chapter 16 on cultures and sensitivities.) The aminoglycosides that are commonly monitored with serum levels are gentamicin (Garamycin), tobramycin (Nebcin, Tobrex), amikacin (Amikin), and netilmicin (Netromycin) (Deglin and Vallerand, 1995).

Preparation of Client and Collection of Sample

The laboratory needs 1 mL of serum. Usually blood samples for peak levels of antibiotics are drawn 30–60 min after completion of intravenous infusion of an antibiotic. The trough or residual level is measured immediately before the next dose of antibiotic is due. The nurse should check with the laboratory about exact trough and peak times. Table 17–1 gives an example of the timing of levels for tobramycin. In general, peak levels are used to determine whether the dosage is adequate; trough levels aid in ascertaining whether there is too much drug accumulation.

REFERENCE VALUES FOR AMINOGLYCOSIDES

Gentamicin (Garamycin) and tobramycin (Nebcin, Tobrex)	Therapeutic, 5–10 μg/mL Peak, <12 μg/mL Trough, <2 μg/mL
Amikacin (Amikin)	Therapeutic, 20–30 μg/mL Peak, <35 μg/ml Trough, <8 μg/mL
Netilmicin (Netromycin)	Peak, 6–10 μg/mL Trough, <2 μg/mL

▼ POSSIBLE NURSING DIAGNOSES FOR AMINOGLYCOSIDES

Risk for Injury Related to Dizziness or Hearing Loss

The nurse needs to be aware that the aminoglycosides may cause nerve damage (neurotoxicity). The eighth cranial nerve is often affected by this group of antibiotics. Ototoxicity manifests itself mainly as vestibular dysfunction, but loss of hearing can occur and can be irreversible (Katzung, 1995). Involvement of the vestibular branch causes a lack of equilibrium. The client should be examined for any dizziness or lack of balance. Clients should also be examined for any hearing impairment.

Risk for Altered Urinary Patterns

Aminoglycosides may cause kidney damage (nephrotoxicity). Nephrotoxicity is more likely if renal function is not normal. BUN and creatinine tests are often used to monitor renal function while the client is taking aminoglycosides. (See Chapter 4 on BUN and creatinine.) The client must remain well-hydrated, and the intake and output record must be carefully maintained.

▼ ANTIBIOTICS: VANCOMYCIN

Oral vancomycin is not well absorbed, so it is not used for systemic infections. However, it is very useful for some GI infections, such as those caused by *Clostridium difficile* (see Chapter 16). Intravenous vancomycin is used for serious gram-positive infections that do not respond to less toxic antibiotics such as penicillin or the cephalosporins. Although not an aminoglycoside, vancomycin can also cause damage to the eighth cranial nerve (ototoxicity) and renal damage (nephrotoxicity).

Preparation of Client and Collection of Sample

The laboratory needs 1 mL of serum. The peak should be drawn 60 min after the infusion is completed. Trough levels are drawn immediately before the next intravenous dose is started.

REFERENCE VALUES FOR VANCOMYCIN	
Therapeutic range	20–40 mg/L
Trough level	5–15 mg/L

▼ IMMUNOSUPPRESSIVE AGENT: CYCLOSPORINE ASSAY

As a potent immunosuppressive agent, cyclosporine has dramatically increased the success rate of organ transplants. In addition to having serum cyclosporine levels measured periodically, the client undergoes renal function tests (see Chapter 4 on BUN and serum creatinine) and liver function tests (see Chapter 12 on alanine aminotransferase [ALT]). Unwanted effects include nephrotoxicity, increased hair growth, and transient liver dysfunction (Katzung, 1995). Hyperlipidemia (Chapter 9) and hyperglycemia (Chapter 8) may also occur.

Preparation of Client and Collection of Sample

The laboratory needs 2 mL of serum in a green- or lavender-topped tube. Cyclosporine adheres tenaciously to plastic, so samples should not be drawn from any catheter that has been used for infusion of the drug.

REFERENCE VALUE FOR CYCLOSPORINE	
Therapeutic	100–200 ng/mL

Value varies widely based on laboratory method used (Kaplan et al., 1995).

▼ ANTICONVULSANTS

Phenytoin

Phenytoin, formerly called *diphenylhydantoin,* is the most common drug used to treat various types of epilepsy. It may be used alone or in combination with the other anticonvulsants in this section. Phenytoin is also used as an antiarrhythmic agent for certain types of cardiac irregularities. (See the section on antiarrhythmic drugs.)

Clients may have serum phenytoin levels measured to determine the proper dose for long-term therapy. Because it takes at least 1 week to achieve stable serum phenytoin levels, clients may have blood samples drawn several times.

Serum levels are related to certain side effects. In general, nystagmus (involuntary rapid movements of the eyeballs) appears when serum phenytoin levels are greater than 20 μg/mL. Gait ataxia occurs at about 30 μg/mL, and constant lethargy occurs when the level is about 40 μg/mL.

Preparation of Client and Collection of Sample

The laboratory needs 1 mL of serum. Record the time of the last dose, the route, and the amount of phenytoin. Intramuscular injection of phenytoin, rather than oral administration, reduces blood levels about 50%. Levels are usually drawn about 3 hr after the last dose. Caffeine, theophylline, probenecid (Benemid), warfarin, and quinidine interfere with the results.

REFERENCE VALUES FOR PHENYTOIN	
10–20 mg/L	As an anticonvulsant
10–18 mg/L	As an antiarrhythmic

Free Phenytoin

Some clinical abnormalities such as elevated BUN (Chapter 3) or bilirubinemia (Chapter 11) and drugs that displace phenytoin from albumin (e.g., salicylates) may cause the unbound fraction of phenytoin to rise. Thus, some laboratories may also report the unbound or free phenytoin as well as the total. An increase in free phenytoin increases the risk for toxicity.

REFERENCE VALUE FOR FREE PHENYTOIN
1–2 mg/L

Primidone (Mysoline, Primoline)

Primidone is not a barbiturate, but it is closely related and has similar actions. Primidone is used for the control of certain types of epilepsy. Doses higher than the therapeutic range can, however, cause ataxia and lethargy.

Preparation of Patient and Collection of Sample

The laboratory needs 1 mL of serum. A steady state occurs in 1–3 days. Because one of the metabolites of primidone is phenobarbital, phenobarbital levels may also be drawn at a later date when a steady state is reached.

REFERENCE VALUE FOR PRIMIDONE	
Therapeutic level	5–15 mg/L

Valproic Acid (Depakene)

Valproic acid is an oral anticonvulsant. Because valproic acid has a short biologic half-life, the time of the last dose and the time of the sampling must be considered carefully when judging the clinical effect from a certain concentration. Liver toxicity can occur. (See Chapter 12 on liver enzymes.)

Preparation of Client and Collection of Sample

The laboratory needs 0.5–1.0 mL of venous blood in a green-, gray-, lavender-, or blue-topped tube. A steady state is achieved in 2–3 days. There may be some fluctuation of serum values even with a steady state (Ravel, 1995).

REFERENCE VALUE FOR VALPROIC ACID	
Therapeutic range	50–100 mg/L

Free valproic acid is about 10–30% of the total (Kaplan et al., 1995).

Phenobarbital (Luminal)

Phenobarbital is a long-acting barbiturate (see later discussion of barbiturate panel) that is sometimes used in conjunction with other anticonvulsants.

Preparation of Client and Collection of Sample

The laboratory needs 1 mL of serum. The dose, the time of the last dose, and the time of the sampling should be recorded. Because phenobarbital is long-acting and cumulative, the client's daily dose also should be recorded. A tolerance to high levels of phenobarbital can develop if the increase is gradual. A steady state may take 8–15 days for children and 10–25 days for adults (Ravel, 1995). Phenobarbital has interactions with many other drugs.

REFERENCE VALUES FOR PHENOBARBITAL	
Therapeutic range	For anticonvulsant control 15–40 mg/L
Newborn	Levels greater than 40 mg/L may cause apnea

Carbamazepine (Tegretol)

Carbamazepine is used for seizure control but can itself cause seizures if the serum level is greater than the therapeutic range. The most widely feared side effect is bone marrow depression, which is rare but can occur. Clients need monitoring with a complete blood count (CBC) (Chapter 2) and platelet counts (Chapter 13).

Preparation of Client and Collection of Sample

The laboratory needs 0.5 mL of serum. It takes about 2 weeks for carbamazepine to reach a steady state. Many drugs can interfere with this test.

REFERENCE VALUE FOR CARBAMAZEPINE	
Therapeutic range	4–10 mg/L (some laboratories use 2–10 mg/L)

Free carbamazepine is about 25% of total (Kaplan et al., 1995).

Ethosuximide (Zarontin)

Ethosuximide is used to treat petit mal seizures. Toxic effects include GI disturbances, headaches, dizziness, and fatigue. A rarer side effect is a lupus-like syndrome.

Preparation of Client and Collection of Sample

Laboratory needs 0.5 mL of blood, which can be collected in a green-, lavender-, gray-, or blue-topped tube. The steady state occurs after several days, because the half-life may be as long as 40 hr.

REFERENCE VALUE FOR ETHOSUXIMIDE	
Therapeutic range	40–100 mg/L

▼ POSSIBLE NURSING DIAGNOSIS FOR ANTICONVULSANT THERAPY

Risk for Injury Related to Gait Disturbance and Seizure Activity

Most of the anticonvulsants in higher-than-therapeutic levels in the bloodstream can lead to ataxia, gait disturbances, dizziness, and drowsiness. Attention to safety is warranted. If the anticonvulsants are in the lower-than-therapeutic range, the client may be vulnerable to a return of seizures. However, if there are no side effects, long-term monitoring may not be needed. Over the years there is less of a tendency for fully controlled seizures to return, and it is likely lower serum levels will continue to be effective (Troupin, 1984).

▼ ANTIPSYCHOTIC AGENT: LITHIUM CARBONATE

Lithium (Lithane, Eskalith, Lithonate) is a psychotherapeutic agent used to treat the manic state of some types of bipolar disorder (manic depressive disorder). When the dosage is being adjusted, blood samples are drawn one to two times a week. Blood for the serum level may be drawn 8–12 hr after the drug is given. After a therapeutic dosage has been established, the client may have serum lithium levels measured monthly. Ravel (1995) noted that red-cell lithium levels may be more reliable indicators of noncompliance than serum levels. Electroencephalograms (EEGs) may be performed to evaluate the neurotoxicity from lithium.

Preparation of Client and Collection of Sample

The laboratory needs 1 mL of serum. Lithium samples are drawn 8–12 hr after dosage. Record the amount, the route, and the time of the last dosage on the laboratory request.

REFERENCE VALUES FOR LITHIUM	
Therapeutic range	0.5–1.5 mEq/L or 0.5–1.5 mmol/L (SI units)

▼ POSSIBLE NURSING DIAGNOSIS FOR LITHIUM LEVELS

Risk for Injury Related to Toxicity or Adverse Reactions

Lithium toxicity is a very serious problem. In some clients, particularly the elderly, neurotoxicity can develop even with normal serum levels. Hence clients must be assessed for such symptoms as diarrhea, vomiting, muscle weakness, and lack of coordination. An important nursing implication is to make sure that these clients have normal amounts of salt because lithium toxicity may be greater if serum sodium levels are low. (See Chapter 5 on diets with high-sodium content.) Hypothyroidism (Chapter 15) is one of the chronic adverse reactions.

▼ TRICYCLIC ANTIDEPRESSANTS

The tricyclic antidepressant drugs represent a frequent and serious problem in both unintentional and intentional overdosage. These drugs may take as long as 1 month to relieve depression, and dosage adjustments vary from person to person. The laboratory may measure both the drug and its active metabolite and report the sum of the active drugs. Some of the active metabolites are also available as primary drugs. For example, desipramine is an active metabolite of imipramine and nortriptyline of amitriptyline.

Preparation of Client and Collection of Sample

The laboratory needs 3 mL of serum in an orange-green-topped tube. For once-a-day dosages, the specimen should be drawn about 10–14 hr after dosage. For divided doses, the specimen can be drawn 4–6 hr after the last dosage. The steady state is obtained about 1 week after therapy is begun, but clinical improvement may not be noted for *several* weeks. Many drugs may interfere with the test.

REFERENCE VALUES FOR ANTIDEPRESSANTS	
Imipramine (Tofranil)	150–250 ng/mL
Desipramine (Norpramin)	125–300 ng/mL

Amitriptyline (Elavil)	80–250 ng/mL
Nortriptyline (Aventyl)	50–150 ng/mL
Doxepin (Sinequan)	150–250 ng/mL

See Depression Guideline Panel (1993) for a discussion of the limitations of these established ranges.

▼ POSSIBLE NURSING DIAGNOSIS FOR ANTIDEPRESSANTS

Risk for Injury Related to Possible Adverse Reactions of Antidepressant Drugs

A client taking antidepressant drugs needs careful assessment for adverse reactions, which can include cardiotoxicity and orthostatic hypotension. Clients who take these drugs are suffering from clinical depression, so usual client teaching may be difficult. Significant others must be educated about ways to decrease problems from long-term use. Deglin and Vallerand (1995) listed two pages of nursing implications for imipramine (Tofranil), the prototype for this classification of drugs. Boehnert and Lovejoy (1985) found that serum drug levels failed to identify clients with the toxic effects of ventricular arrhythmias or seizures. The prolongation of the QRS duration, noted by means of an electrocardiogram (ECG) was a better predictor. (See Chapter 24 on electrocardiography.) The Depression Guideline Panel (1993) discussed clients for whom blood level monitoring is most needed and summarizes unwanted effects.

▼ BRONCHODILATORS: THEOPHYLLINE PRODUCTS AND CAFFEINE LEVELS

Theophylline and its derivatives, such as aminophylline, dyphylline, and oxtriphylline, are all used as bronchodilators. Once used as a primary drug for asthma, theophylline is now used only if other drugs such as the corticosteriods and β-2-agonists are not effective (Katzung, 1995). There are many brand names for theophylline and the derivatives: Aminodur, Theo-Dur, Coledyl, Bronkodyl, Elixophyllin, and various others. Consult a pharmacology text for peak times and durations of the various products. For example, because aminophylline is 85% theophylline, aminophylline causes different theophylline levels from other theophylline products.

Because high serum levels of theophylline can result in life-threatening cardiac arrhythmias and seizures, the safest approach to individualize dosages of theophylline or theophylline products is to monitor serum levels. Clients who have abnormal liver function, who have congestive heart failure (CHF), or who are very young or very old may need very close monitoring of serum theophylline levels. Caffeine levels are sometimes ordered by neonatologists treating infants with theophylline because neonates quickly metabolize theophylline to caffeine.

Preparation of Client and Collection of Sample

The laboratory needs 3 mL of serum. The dose, the route, and the time of the last dose should be entered on the requisition. Note the specific times to draw peak and trough levels, which vary depending on the theophylline product being monitored. Because both theophylline and caffeine are xanthines, the client should not have coffee, colas, tea, chocolate, or any other source of caffeine for several hours before the serum specimen is drawn. Cimetidine, erythromycin, and propranolol may raise serum levels. In rare instances, ranitidine can raise serum theophylline to toxic levels (Gardner and Sikorski, 1985). A neonatal caffeine assay requires 0.5 mL of serum. After a steady state is achieved, serum peak levels should be drawn 30 min after intravenous dosage, 2 hr after a regular oral dosage, and 5 or more hr after the slow-release forms are given.

REFERENCE VALUES FOR THEOPHYLLINE	
Therapeutic range	10–20 µg/mL or mg/L
Risk of toxicity	>20 µg/mL or mg/L

REFERENCE VALUE FOR CAFFEINE ASSAY IN NEWBORN	
Therapeutic range	5–15 mg/L

▼ POSSIBLE NURSING DIAGNOSIS FOR THEOPHYLLINE LEVELS

Risk for Injury Related to Overdosage

Nurses should be aware of early clinical symptoms of theophylline overdose (Corbett and Yaros, 1994). Because theophylline is a xanthine, as is caffeine, some of the early symptoms of theophylline toxicity resemble a "coffee jag." Clients may have tachycardia with skipped beats. They may also be nervous and jittery, with tremors of the hands. Headache, dizziness, and vomiting may signal toxicity. The dosage of theophylline must be adjusted to prevent development of dangerous cardiac arrhythmias or seizures.

▼ CARDIAC DRUGS: DIGOXIN AND DIGITOXIN

Digoxin (Lanoxin) is a cardiotonic agent used to prevent or to treat CHF. Digoxin is also used to treat various types of atrial arrhythmias, such as atrial fibrillation. Digoxin and the other forms of digitalis, such as digitoxin, have a long half life, and thus serious toxicity can occur over time.

Preparation of Client and Collection of Sample

The laboratory needs 1 mL of serum. The dosage of digoxin or digitoxin, the route, and the time of the last dose should be included on the requisition. For digoxin, the sample may be drawn 4 hr after intravenous dosage and 6 hr after oral dosage. Some laboratories recommend at least 8 hr after either method of administration. For digitoxin, the sample should be drawn 6–12 hr after the last dose is given. Falsely elevated levels are caused by drugs such as spironolactone (Aldactone) and prednisone. Nifedipine, verapamil, and quinidine can increase serum digoxin levels, and barbiturates and cholestyramine can increase serum digitoxin levels (Howard, 1986).

REFERENCE VALUES FOR DIGOXIN AND DIGITOXIN

Therapeutic range	
Digoxin	0.5–2.0 μg/L
Digitoxin	10–30 μg/L

Slightly higher therapeutic ranges may be desirable for treating atrial fibrillation.

▼ POSSIBLE NURSING DIAGNOSIS FOR DIGOXIN

Risk for Injury Related to Digitalis Toxicity

To prevent digitalis toxicity, the key nursing implication is to monitor the client's pulse before digoxin is given. Digoxin, or other digitalis products, should be withheld and the physician notified if the adult's pulse is less than 60 beats per minute. Usually a pulse less than 70 beats per minute is the guideline for children, but this criterion varies depending on age. Clients should be taught to take their own pulses because, once digoxin is begun, it is usually continued on a long-term basis. Other symptoms of digitalis toxicity—such as nausea and vomiting, diarrhea, headaches, and visual disturbance—are also used to signal digitalis toxicity. An ECG also helps the clinician determine whether there is a toxic effect from digoxin. However, the symptoms of mild toxicity from digoxin may not be readily detected with clinical assessment or

ECG data. A measurement of serum levels of digoxin therefore aids in determining whether symptoms are due to a higher-than-necessary digoxin level.

Other laboratory tests important in assessing for digitalis toxicity are the serum potassium and the serum calcium levels. The nurse needs to be aware that a low serum potassium or a high serum calcium level tends to increase the risk of digitalis toxicity, even though the serum digoxin levels are not high. (See Chapter 5 on potassium and Chapter 7 on calcium levels.) Because digoxin is excreted by the kidneys, clients with poor renal function are prone to digitalis toxicity. (See Chapter 4 for tests of renal function; BUN and creatinine.)

▼ ANTIARRHYTHMIC DRUGS

Quinidine

Quinidine (Quinaglute, Cin-Quin, Quinidex, Cardioquin, and others) is an alkaloid obtained from the bark of the cinchona tree. Hence toxicity from quinidine products is sometimes referred to as *cinchonism.* Because quinidine depresses the excitability of the heart, it is used as an antiarrhythmic drug. Serum quinidine levels help the clinician adjust the dosage to the correct amount for the individual client. In fact, quinidine is the antiarrhythmic drug most often monitored with serum levels. Because the toxicity may not be readily apparent or may be attributed to other causes, serum levels can be used to ascertain whether a client's drug level is in a therapeutic range.

Preparation of Client and Collection of Sample

The dosage, the time of the last dosage, and the route should all be recorded on the lab requisition. The laboratory needs 1 mL of serum. Concurrent use of phenytoin or barbiturates may lower the serum quinidine level.

REFERENCE VALUES FOR QUINIDINE

Therapeutic range	1.2–4.0 mg/L
Toxic range	5–6 mg/L

▼ POSSIBLE NURSING DIAGNOSIS FOR QUINIDINE

Risk of Injury Related to Adverse Effects of Drug

Nurses should be aware that quinidine, a class I-A antiarrhythmic drug, can cause bradycardia and hypotension, so vital signs must be monitored. A few

(*continued*)

▼ POSSIBLE NURSING DIAGNOSIS FOR QUINIDINE (*continued*)

clients experience a syndrome called *quinidine syncope* because of a disorganized type of ventricular tachycardia (torsade de pointes). (See Chapter 24 on ECG assessments of arrhythmias.) Diarrhea and nausea are the most common noncardiac adverse reactions to quinidine. Headache, dizziness, and tinnitus, which may signify the development of cinchonism, should be reported immediately to the health care provider. As with all antiarrhythmic drugs, client teaching is crucial (Corbett, 1990).

Procainamide and NAPA

Procainamide (Pronestyl) is usually given orally for long-term prevention of arrhythmias. As with quinidine products, serum levels help prevent toxicity such as myocardial depression. Some laboratories also measure N-acetyl procainamide (NAPA), the active metabolite of procainamide.

Preparation of Client and Collection of Sample

The dosage, the route, and the time of administration of the last dose should be recorded on the laboratory request. The level is usually drawn just before the next dose is given.

REFERENCE VALUES FOR PROCAINAMIDE AND NAPA	
Procainamide therapeutic level	4–10 μg/mL
NAPA therapeutic level	2–8 μg/mL

▼ POSSIBLE NURSING DIAGNOSIS FOR PROCAINAMIDE

Risk for Injury Related to Adverse Effects of Drug

Monitoring of vital signs is essential to assess for adverse cardiovascular effects of this class I-A antiarrhythmic. Note that all antiarrhythmics may also be proarrhythmic. (See Chapter 24 on monitoring for arrhythmias.) Like quinidine, procainamide can also cause diarrhea and other GI symptoms. Because the drug may also cause a lupus-like syndrome, the client may have antinuclear antibody (ANA) titers (Chapter 14) drawn periodically.

Phenytoin

Although phenytoin (Dilantin) is more commonly used as an anticonvulsant, it is also sometimes used to control cardiac arrhythmias, such as those caused by digitalis toxicity. (See the reference values in the section on anticonvulsant drugs.)

Lidocaine and Tocainide

Lidocaine (Xylocaine) is given intravenously for the immediate control of premature ventricular contractions (PVCs). Because lidocaine is usually given only on an intermittent basis when the need arises, lidocaine levels are seldom measured. If clients have a continuous lidocaine drip, there may be a need to monitor serum levels if arrhythmias persist or if lidocaine toxicity is suspected. Tocainide (Tonocard), an oral analogue of lidocaine, may be used for long-term control of some arrhythmias.

Preparation of Client and Collection of Sample

Note the concentration of the drug and the rate of intravenous administration on the laboratory request. Lidocaine samples of 2 mL may be collected in a serum separator tube (SST), but green-, blue-, gray-, or lavender-topped tubes are also acceptable. Tocainide samples of 2 mL should not be in an SST. An orange-green-, green-, or lavender-topped tube is acceptable.

REFERENCE VALUES FOR LIDOCAINE AND TOCAINIDE

Therapeutic ranges	
Lidocaine	1.5–5.0 mg/L
Tocainide	4.0–10.0 mg/L

▼ POSSIBLE NURSING DIAGNOSIS FOR LIDOCAINE AND TOCAINIDE

Risk for Injury Related to Adverse Effects or Toxicity

Although unwanted cardiac effects are less likely than with the class I-A antiarrhythmic medications quinidine and procainamide, vital signs must be closely monitored as must the ECG when lidocaine is given intravenously. (See Chapter 24 on ECG monitoring.) Overdosages of lidocaine and tocainide, which are class I-B antiarrhythmics, tend to cause central nervous system depression, which can lead to slurred speech, confusion, and even convulsions. Tocainide can cause some blood dyscrasias, so the client may be followed with a CBC with differential (Chapter 2) and platelet counts (Chapter 13).

▼ SALICYLATES: ACETYLSALICYLIC ACID

Acetylsalicylic acid, or aspirin, is used as an analgesic, as an anti-inflammatory agent, and as a mild anticoagulant. ASA is a component of many over-the-counter (OTC) pain relievers, such as Anacin, Bufferin, and Excedrin. Aspirin poisoning is the most common type of poisoning in children. Adults may also take ASA or ASA-containing drugs in a suicidal gesture. In an overdose, the laboratory can screen a serum sample to see whether ASA is the culprit. (If an overdose has occurred, gastric contents and urine specimens should be sent to the laboratory, if available.)

Mild intoxication, or salicylism, causes a ringing in the ears (tinnitus) and gastric upsets. Because ASA acts as a respiratory stimulant, the hyperventilation that may result from aspirin overdose can cause respiratory alkalosis. (See Chapter 6 on acid–base balance.) Large doses of ASA also may cause GI bleeding, which is due to the irritant effect on the gastric mucosa and to interference with coagulation factors.

With its anticoagulant properties, ASA is sometimes used as a regular medication for clients who are at risk for thromboembolic episodes.

ASA is commonly used in high doses for clients who may benefit from the anti-inflammatory properties of ASA. For example, clients with rheumatoid arthritis may take large doses of ASA over a long period of time. It may take 12–20 325-mg aspirin tablets to keep the serum level at about 20 mg/dL. Serum ASA levels may be measured periodically to aid in maintaining a therapeutic but not a toxic range. Sometimes clients are afraid to take enough ASA to achieve therapeutic benefit. Serum levels may be used to evaluate whether a client is complying with the plan.

Preparation of Client and Collection of Sample

The laboratory needs 2 mL of plasma, collected in a heparin (green-topped) or EDTA (lavender-topped) tube. In the case of an overdose, urine, vomitus, or gastric lavage should be saved for laboratory analysis. For a routine assessment of salicylate level, the total daily dosage of ASA should be recorded, as should the time and amount of the last dose. Note exactly how many *tablets* the client says he or she takes a day. Do not rely on what the physician has ordered and assume that the client has followed this dosage at home.

REFERENCE VALUES FOR SALICYLATES

Therapeutic range (3 hr after dose)	
Children to 10 years of age	25–30 mg/100 mL
Adults	20–25 mg/100 mL
Toxic range	
Children and adults	>30 mg/100 mL
Older than 60 years	>20 mg/100 mL
Lethal range may be about 60 mg/100 mL	

▼ URINE TESTING: PHENISTIX

Phenistix (Ravel, 1995) are reagent strips used primarily to test for phenylketones in the urine. (See Chapter 18 for a discussion of phenylketonuria [PKU].) However, metabolites of aspirin, other salicylates, and phenothiazines also cause color changes in Phenistix. The color chart used to detect salicylates or phenothiazines shows tan for small amounts and brown for large amounts. (The color change for PKU uses a different color chart.) Phenistix can be used as a screening device of urine to check for overdose with aspirin or phenothiazines. (Phenothiazine testing is covered later in this chapter.)

▼ ACETAMINOPHEN

Serum levels are not necessary when acetaminophen is routinely used as an antipyretic and analgesic. Serum levels are measured if an overdose has occurred because toxic levels may cause liver damage. The level of the drug in the serum, 4 or more hr after ingestion, determines the need for acetylcysteine therapy to protect the liver (Kaplan et al., 1995). Follow-up care includes monitoring the liver enzyme ALT (Chapter 12) for several days.

Preparation of Client and Collection of Sample

Collect 1 mL of serum in a SST. Record time of ingestion and amount of drug ingested, if known. Samples drawn 4 hr and 12 hr after ingestion are used for treatment decisions. Acetaminophen is also part of a coma panel.

REFERENCE VALUES FOR ACETAMINOPHEN	
Therapeutic	10–20 mg/L
Toxic (4 hr after ingestion)	>120 mg/L
Toxic (12 hr after ingestion)	>50 mg/L

▼ BLOOD ALCOHOL

Ethanol, or grain alcohol, is the type of alcohol in alcoholic beverages. Ethanol, undoubtedly the most commonly abused drug, may often be one of the drugs involved in an overdose. As part of a toxicology screen, the laboratory may perform an alcohol panel that, in addition to ethanol, includes methanol (wood alcohol), isopropyl (rubbing alcohol), and acetone (an alcohol-related compound). A serum osmolality test (Chapter 4) may also be used to screen for ethanol or methanol. Alcohol and related toxic compounds may be ingested by drinking undrinkable solutions, such as cleaning fluids, shaving lotions, or disinfectants. Methanol is particularly dangerous because it can result in convulsions, blindness, and possibly death.

In addition to determining the cause of a coma, blood alcohol tests are also used to determine whether a driver was intoxicated at the time of a collision. The drawing of the blood specimen must be performed in a medically suitable environment according to the legal requirements of the state. (Breath analyzers are used at the scene of the collision, so nurses are not involved in obtaining samples.) Nurses who are trained in venipuncture may draw the blood for alcohol blood samples when the client is brought to the emergency department for medical treatment. The reluctance to involve hospital staff in drawing blood for legal evidence is based on the fact that the people drawing the blood may not know the exact legal ramifications of the procedure and that they will probably be subpoenaed to testify in a court case. Although it is permissible for qualified nurses to draw blood for the alcohol test, it is important that they understand the legal ramifications of the procedure and the policy for nurses in a particular institution. Blood may be drawn without consent in some states if the blood is drawn in a legally and medically accepted manner (Buley, 1986). A refusal to allow blood to be drawn may have legal consequences. Readers should consult current state laws.

Legal Definitions of Intoxication

Each state determines the exact blood alcohol level that is considered legally permissible for driving. Levels greater than 0.08% are considered proof of intoxication in most states. A few states have higher levels and a few have lower levels. For example, in California, it is a crime for adults to drive with a blood alcohol content of 0.08% or more, minors to drive with 0.05% or more, and commercial drivers with 0.04% or more. Some organizations, including the American Medical Association, have suggested adopting 0.05% as per se evidence of alcohol-impaired driving (Ravel, 1995).

Relation of Alcohol to Other Laboratory Tests

In addition to the usual symptoms of alcohol intoxication, a client who abuses alcohol may have severe hypoglycemia, because alcohol tends to inhibit the formation of glucose. (See Chapter 8 for symptoms and treatment of hypoglycemia.) Alcohol-induced hypoglycemia carries a high mortality if not identified and corrected. The mortality is particularly high for children. High blood alcohol levels are also an important cause of secondary hyperlipidemia. (See Chapter 9 on serum triglyceride levels.) High alcohol levels in a pregnant woman are of grave concern because of the fetal alcohol syndrome (Ouellette, 1984).

Preparation of Client and Collection of Sample

The client should give consent for collection of a blood specimen, but blood may be drawn without consent in some states if the blood is drawn in a legally and medically accepted manner. Be aware of the legal ramifications, state requirements, and the individual hospital's policy. No alcohol, such as alcohol wipes, should be used to obtain the blood specimen. Iodine or an aqueous germicidal solution such as benzalkonium can be used. Tinctures should not be used, because they have an alcohol base. The specimen should be refrigerated if it cannot be sent to the laboratory immediately.

REFERENCE VALUES FOR BLOOD ALCOHOL LEVELS

Ethanol or ethyl (grain) alcohol	
0.00%–0.05%	Sobriety is presumed
0.05%–0.10%	Gray zone
0.10%–0.15%	Legal limit, depending on state law (some states have lower levels)
0.30%–0.40%	Marked intoxication
0.40%–0.50%	Severe toxic effects with alcoholic stupor
0.50% and higher	Coma and death possible
Methanol or methyl (wood) alcohol	
25 mg/dL	Toxic level
80–115 mg/dL	Lethal

Although the legal definitions of intoxication are based on whole-blood figures, laboratories may use serum for the test, which gives 18–20% higher values. Ravel (1995) discussed the controversy about converting these figures.

▼ BARBITURATES

The barbiturates are used as anticonvulsants and infrequently as sedatives or hypnotics. The most severe effect of overdose with barbiturates is respiratory failure followed by circulatory collapse. Because the various barbiturates are often used in overdoses, the laboratory runs a barbiturate panel when clients are comatose from an unknown cause. The barbiturates usually measured include

1. Short-acting ones—pentobarbital (Nembutal) and secobarbital (Seconal)
2. Intermediate-acting ones—amobarbital (Amytal) and butabarbital (Butisol, Butacaps)
3. Long-acting ones—phenobarbital (Luminal)

A smaller amount of the short-acting barbiturates, as opposed to a larger amount for the long-acting barbiturates, causes coma. A toxicology screen for barbiturate overdose also includes an analysis of urine samples and, if requested, gastric contents. Any vomitus or gastric lavage products should be saved for laboratory analysis.

Preparation of Client and Collection of Sample

The laboratory needs 5 mL or less of serum, depending on the method used. Note any drugs that the client may have taken. Theophylline, for example, can cause a false elevation of the barbiturate level, as can valproic acid.

REFERENCE VALUES FOR BARBITURATES

Short-acting barbiturates	Coma level at about 5 mg/L
Long-acting barbiturates	Coma level at about 40 mg/L

See the section on anticonvulsants for the measurement of therapeutic levels of phenobarbital.

▼ TOXICOLOGY SCREENS IN BLOOD AND URINE

In addition to barbiturates, the following drugs may be tested for serum or urine screening:

1. Opioids (codeine, morphine, etc.)
2. Phenothiazines (prochlorperazine, chlorpromazine, etc.)
3. Tricyclic antidepressants (imipramine, amitriptyline, etc.)
4. Stimulants (amphetamines, methylphenidate, etc.)
5. Benzodiazepines (diazepam, etc.)
6. Phencyclidine (PCP)
7. Cocaine (as benzoylecgonine metabolite)
8. Other drugs, such as acetaminophen, marijuana

Preparation of Client and Collection of Sample

A urine sample of 50–100 mL is needed for a complete toxicology screen. Check with the individual laboratory. A large amount of blood, 20–30 mL, collected in several types of tubes is needed for a comprehensive drug screen or coma panel. These serum panels are expensive and may require specific approval from the laboratory. Individual screens of drugs may be performed if the type of drug is known.

▼ POSSIBLE NURSING DIAGNOSIS RELATED TO ELEVATED DRUG LEVELS, INCLUDING ALCOHOL

Altered Sensory Perception

The focus for nursing intervention is to promote a sense of reality by explaining environmental stimuli and also reducing those stimuli. Because the altered

(*continued*)

perceptions may be frightening, the client needs reassurance of safety and protection by health care workers (Carpenito, 1985). Long-term management of drug abuse necessitates other nursing diagnoses based on the individual client's needs and coping methods.

▼ BROMIDE

Bromide is an ingredient in several OTC drugs that are used as sleeping aids and "nerve tonics." Too often, clients and the health professionals consider all OTC drugs harmless. Bromide, a central nervous system depressant, in large doses can cause toxicity, which is called *bromism*. Some prescription drugs, such as pyridostigmine bromide used to treat myasthenia gravis, have been known to cause a bromide psychosis (Rothenberg et al., 1990). Clients with inadequate renal function are particularly susceptible to bromide overdosage.

The symptoms of bromism are nonspecific, but they usually include signs and symptoms of central nervous system toxicity, such as muscle incoordination and impaired intellectual functioning. The client may have vomiting and a rash. A public health nurse or clinic nurse may detect symptoms of bromism. A health history should contain a list of all drugs (including OTC drugs) that these clients take.

Preparation of Client and Collection of Sample

The laboratory needs 3 mL of serum. All medications that contain bromide should be noted.

REFERENCE VALUE FOR BROMIDE	
Toxic level in serum	>17 mEq/L

▼ LEAD

Among children, lead toxicity is second only to malnutrition as a public health problem in the United States. Exposure to lead is also an occupational hazard for some adults. The client usually has a variety of chronic symptoms, such as abdominal pain, weakness, and eventually neurologic dysfunction, with the potential for permanent brain damage. Because lead interferes with the normal synthesis of red blood cells, clients have anemia and characteristic changes in the peripheral blood smear (Chapter 2). However, many children do not look or feel sick even though they have lead levels that are associated with developmental defects. Public health departments and consumer groups have been active in promoting blood screening for all children at risk. Free testing is available in most communities. Levels should be measured at 12 months and 24 months of age with follow-up measurements as needed.

Preparation of Client and Collection of Sample

The laboratory needs 2 mL of blood. It is important that all the blood-drawing equipment be free from lead or lead particles. Special collection tubes are used that are lead-free. A complete history is needed concerning the client's exposure to toxic chemicals. Most public health surveys have a definite assessment guide that is to be followed when interviewing clients. The possible exposure of other people in the client's environment must be considered. Industrial pollution also is a public health problem.

REFERENCE VALUES FOR BLOOD LEAD LEVELS

In 1991 the Centers for Disease Control and Prevention (CDC, 1991) lowered the cutoff level for defining lead poisoning in children from 25 µg/mL to 10 µg/dL. The previous levels were from a 1985 recommendation.

▼ POSSIBLE NURSING DIAGNOSIS FOR LEAD POISONING

Impaired Health Maintenance Related to Unhealthful Environment

For many years, nurses have been involved in lead screening (Croft and Frenkel, 1975; Sharts-Hopko, 1993). The client most likely to experience lead poisoning is a child who lives in a poorly maintained home with peeling paint. Lead was banned as an ingredient in interior paints in 1978, but older houses may still contain particles that children ingest. In addition to the ban on lead in paints, environmental lead contamination in the United States has been lessened by the use of unleaded gasoline and a reduction in the amount of lead used in food and drink containers. Even though there has been a rather large decrease in lead exposure, approximately 1.7 million children younger than 5 years, still have unacceptable blood levels of lead (CDC, 1994). Thus, nurses still need to help educate parents about the need for screening in children who are at risk. Screening should be performed at 12 months and 24 months of age. Information about the process of reducing lead hazards can be obtained from the local public health department or by calling 1(800) LEAD-FYI. Nurses may also want to advocate for laws to eliminate lead hazards.

The treatment of lead poisoning is a process called *chelation*. For chelation, the client is given the calcium salt of *EDTA*. Lead replaces the calcium, and the lead–EDTA is excreted in the urine. (Note that other heavy metal poisoning may also be treated with various types of chelating products.)

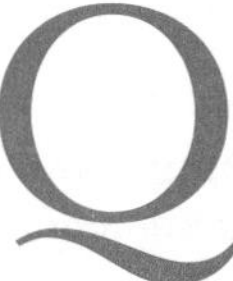

1. Serum levels of drugs may be needed when the risk of toxicity from a drug is increased. A factor that increases the toxicity of most drugs is

    a. Change in drug from a brand name to a generic
    b. Use of intramuscular or oral route rather than intravenous
    c. Hepatic dysfunction
    d. Increased urine output caused by increased intake of fluids

2. Mr. Telerechio is having blood drawn for peak and trough serum antibiotic levels. The nurse should be aware that the type of antibiotics that are commonly monitored by serum levels are the

    a. Penicillins b. Cephalosporins
    c. Aminoglycosides d. Tetracyclines

3. Bobby, 13 years of age, has epilepsy and the seizures are controlled by phenytoin (Dilantin). A serum phenytoin level drawn today was 23 µg/mL. Because this is slightly above the therapeutic range of 10–20 µg/mL, Bobby may begin to show a symptom of early phenytoin toxicity, which is

    a. Severe lethargy
    b. Cardiac arrhythmias
    c. Gait ataxia
    d. Nystagmus (involuntary rapid movements of the eyeballs)

4. Molley Faber is a psychiatric client being observed in a mental health clinic. Which of the following antipsychotic drugs requires monitoring with serum levels?

    a. Chlorpromazine (Thorazine) b. Lithium carbonate (Lithane)
    c. Fluphenazine (Prolixin) d. Thioridazine (Mellaril)

5. Johnny, 8 years of age, is receiving aminophylline 20 mg/hr by the intravenous route for treatment of an acute asthmatic attack that did not respond to β-2-agonists. Because aminophylline is a theophylline derivative, serum theophylline levels have been measured. The latest level of 30 µg/ml is considerably higher than the desired therapeutic range of 10–20 µg/mL. The nurse needs to make assessments of the client and be prepared for

    a. Cardiac arrhythmias and seizures b. Bronchospasms and dyspnea
    c. Renal and hepatic failure d. Hypertension crisis and stroke

6. Johnny has recovered from his acute asthmatic attack. The asthma is still not well controlled on other medications, so Johnny is being discharged with instructions to take a theophylline suspension (Elixophyllin 50 mg) every 6 hr. Johnny and his parents need to be taught that early symptoms of overdose of this drug may be similar to which of the following?

a. Deep sleep
b. Overuse of coffee
c. Another asthmatic attack
d. Cold or flu

7. Mr. Gardener, 78 years of age, is taking digoxin 0.25 mg/day because of congestive heart failure (CHF). He is being visited by a community health nurse. Which of the following information in Mr. Gardener's health history should alert the nurse to the fact that this client should be closely watched for digoxin toxicity?

a. Large intake of sodium in the diet, refusal of visit from dietician
b. Slightly low serum calcium level caused by a possible endocrine problem, evaluation in progress
c. Poor renal function as evidenced by increased serum creatinine level
d. History of noncompliance with physician's orders

8. Mrs. Ramos has a serum quinidine level of 6 mg/L, which is higher than the therapeutic range of 1.0–4.0 mg/L. Because there may be possible toxic effects of the quinidine, the nurse should assess and record which of the following?

a. Level of consciousness every 2 hr
b. Blood pressure and pulse every 2 hr
c. Lack of appetite or other gastrointestinal symptoms
d. Hourly urine output

9. Serum aspirin (ASA) levels may be a useful clinical assessment for

a. Mr. Fink, who uses ASA p.r.n. for a headache
b. Sally, 2½ years of age who was found in the bathroom playing with an empty bottle of acetaminophen
c. Mrs. Catalina, who takes ASA 650 mg q.i.d. for treatment of rheumatoid arthritis
d. Mr. Weber, who takes ASA 80 mg b.i.d. for an anticoagulant effect

10. In relation to blood alcohol levels, the emergency department nurse should know that

a. Alcohol should be used to wipe the skin before the blood specimen is drawn
b. A blood alcohol of 0.01% is usually considered legal evidence of intoxication, but this criterion may vary from state to state
c. The client's permission should be obtained for a blood specimen according to legal requirements
d. The person who draws the blood cannot be subpoenaed to testify in a court case

11. Mrs. Gearhart, 78 years of age, uses various over-the-counter (OTC) sleeping medications and nerve tonics. Mrs. Gearhart's niece reports to the home care nurse that her aunt has become very forgetful and irritable since she increased her nerve tonic. The niece thinks her aunt is taking "too much nonprescribed medicine." After looking at the ingredients in the OTC medicine, the nurse may need to refer Mrs. Gearhart for a medical evaluation of possible

    a. Salicylism (aspirin toxicity) b. Cinchonism (quinidine toxicity)
    c. Plumbism (lead poisoning) d. Bromism (bromide toxicity)

12. A public health nurse is preparing to speak to a community group about the problem of lead poisoning. Which of the following should be included in the talk?

    a. Screening of all children should be done at birth and repeated in 6 months
    b. Prevention is crucial because there is no treatment of lead poisoning
    c. Children with lead poisoning may not feel or act sick
    d. Elderly people are at the greatest risk for lead toxicity

▼ REFERENCES

Boehnert, M., and Lovejoy, F. (1985). Value of the QRS duration versus the serum drug level in predicting seizures and ventricular arrhythmia after an acute dose of tricyclic anti-depressants. *New England Journal of Medicine, 313* (8), 474–477.

Buley, D. (1986). When the burden of proof falls on you. *Nursing 86, 16* (2), 41.

Carpenito, L. (1985). Altered thoughts or altered perceptions? *American Journal of Nursing, 85* (11), 1283.

Centers for Disease Control. (1991). Preventing lead poisoning in young children: A statement of the Centers for Disease Control. Atlanta: Department of Health and Human Services, Public Health Services.

Centers for Disease Control. (1994). Blood lead levels—United States 1988–1991. *Morbidity and Mortality Weekly Report, 43* (30), 545–548.

Corbett, J.V. (1990). Classification system for antiarrhythmic drugs. *California Nursing, 12* (6), 42–43.

Corbett, J.V., and Yaros, P.S. (1994). Beta 2 agonists and maintenance drugs in the treatment of asthma. *MCN: American Journal of Maternal Child Nursing, 19* (6), 352.

Croft, H., and Frenkel, S. (1975). Children and lead poisoning. *American Journal of Nursing, 75* (1), 102–104.

Deglin, J.H., and Vallerand, A.H. (1995). *Davis's drug guide for nurses.* (4th ed.). Philadelphia: F.A. Davis.

Depression Guideline Panel. (1993). Depression in primary care: Volume 2. Treatment of major depression. Clinical practice guideline. Number 5. AHCPR Publ No. 93-0551. Rockville, MD: U.S. Department of Health and Human Services, Public Health Service, Agency for Health Care Policy and Research.

Food and Drug Administration. (1980). Dosage guidelines for theophylline products. *FDA Drug Bulletin, 10,* 4–6.

Gardner, M., and Sikorski, G. (1985). Ranitidine and theophylline. *Annals of Internal Medicine, 102* (4), 559.

Howard, P. (1986). A crash course in serum drug monitoring. *RN, 49* (4), 20–25.

Kaplan, A., Jack, R., Opheim, K.E., et al. (1995). *Clinical chemistry interpretation and techniques* (4th ed.). Baltimore: Williams & Wilkins.

Katzung, B. (1995). *Basic and clinical pharmacology.* (6th ed.). Norwalk, CT: Appleton & Lange.

Longe, R. (1989). Laboratory tests recommended by pharmacists in a skilled nursing facility. *American Journal of Pharmacy, 46* (5), 970–972.

McCormick, W., et al. (1978). Errors in measuring drug concentrations. *New England Journal of Medicine, 299* (20), 1118–1121.

Ouellette, D. (1984). The fetal alcohol syndrome. *Contemporary Nutrition, 9* (3), 1–2.

Ravel, R. (1995). *Clinical laboratory medicine: Clinical application of laboratory data.* (6th ed.). St. Louis: Mosby–Year Book.

Richens, A., and Warrington, S. (1979). When should plasma drug levels be monitored? *Drugs, 17,* 488–500.

Rothenberg, D., et al. (1990). Bromide intoxication secondary to pyridostigmine bromide therapy. *JAMA, 263,* 1121–1122.

Scala, R. (1978). The duty to report hazards: A toxicologist's view. *Bulletin of New York Academy of Medicine, 54,* 774–781.

Sharts-Hopko, N.C. (1993). Lead poisoning. *MCN: American Journal of Maternal Child Nursing, 18* (5), 288.

Squire, A., et al. (1984). Long-term antiarrhythmic therapy: Problem of low drug levels and patient noncompliance. *American Journal of Medicine, 77,* 1035–1038.

Troupin, A. (1984). The measurement of anticonvulsant agent levels. *Annals of Internal Medicine, 100* (2), 854–858.

TESTS PERFORMED IN PREGNANCY AND THE NEWBORN PERIOD

- Urine Pregnancy Tests: Biologic Tests for Pregnancy and Immunologic Tests for Pregnancy
- Serum HCG Levels: HCG Qualitative Pregnancy Test and HCG Quantitative Test
- α-Fetoprotein
- Prenatal Screening for Down Syndrome: Serum Markers
- Sickle Cell Anemia
- Thalassemia (Cooley's Anemia)
- Tay-Sachs Disease
- Estriol Levels
- Phenylketonuria
- Hypothyroidism
- Galactosemia
- Tests for Cystic Fibrosis

OBJECTIVES

1. Identify how a normal pregnancy changes the values of common laboratory tests in relation to prepregnancy values.
2. Explain the basic immunologic principle of tests for pregnancy.
3. Explain which of the autosomal recessive genetic diseases are commonly tested with screening programs for certain ethnic groups.
4. Explain why phenylketonuria (PKU), galactosemia, hypothyroidism and sickle cell are screened with routine tests for newborns even though the infants appear healthy.

5. Explain the use of the combination of human chorionic gonadotropin (HCG), α-fetoprotein (AFP), and serum estriol for prenatal screening.
6. Compare the types of tests for cystic fibrosis, including DNA probes.
7. Discuss the impact of the Human Genome Project on the field of genetic counseling and the role of the nurse.
8. Describe the appropriate nursing functions for a community health nurse who is working with a family that has a child with a genetic defect.

Previous chapters have described some tests important in pregnancy (Table 18–1). Appendix D summarizes the expected changes in laboratory values in a normal pregnancy and a list of references for values in pregnancy. Appendix B lists expected changes in newborns. Although integration of content from all clinical settings is emphasized in this book, some tests pertain *only* to the pregnant or to the newborn state. This chapter, therefore, focuses on common laboratory tests that are unique in maternal–child health settings.

Interwoven with all these advanced methods of testing is the nurse's involvement with the client as a person. The premise of this chapter is that pregnancy and childbirth should be joyous and healthy events. If tests must be used for a pregnancy, the health professionals must make sure that such tests are as nonthreatening as possible. The focus is what is normal about the pregnancy, not what may be abnormal.

PREGNANCY TESTS

Although pregnancy has early presumptive signs and symptoms, such as amenorrhea, nausea and vomiting, and skin changes, the positive signs are rarely present until a few months into the pregnancy. Any one of the following signs is both legal

TABLE 18–1. ROUTINE TESTS DONE DURING PREGNANCY

Name of Test	Assessment	Location in Book
Hb-hct	Anemia	Chap. 2 on CBC
Urinalysis	Possible urinary tract infection (UTI) and other conditions	Chap. 3 on routine urinalysis, nitrites, and LE
Urine for protein	Possible toxemia	Chap. 3 on proteinuria
Blood glucose at 24–28 weeks gestation	Possible diabetes	Chap. 8 on diabetes and pregnancy
Rh typing and unexpected antibody screen	Possible hemolytic disease of newborn (HDN)	Chap. 14 for Rh factor in pregnancy
STS	Possible congenital syphilis	Chap. 16 on syphilis and pregnancy
Rubella titer (*before* pregnancy)	Immunity to 3-day measles	Chap. 14 on why rubella titers are measured *before* pregnancy
Sickle cell	Also need to test father for trait	Chap. 28 on follow-up
Hepatitis B surface antigen	HBV carrier	Chap. 14 on HBV and pregnancy

Note: See this chapter for prenatal testing for Down syndrome, which has become more routinely offered. See Baldwin et al. (1994) on how most providers, including certified nurse midwives, follow practice guidelines for routine testing in pregnancy. Other tests, which are not routine, such as those for cytomegalovirus (CMV), AIDS, herpes (Chap. 14) and gonorrhea (Chap. 16) may be conducted if the pregnant woman is at high risk for these diseases.

and medical proof of pregnancy: (1) fetal heartbeat, (2) palpation of fetal outline, (3) recognition of fetal movements by someone other than the mother, and (4) ultrasonographic demonstration of the fetus.

In the modern world, few, if any, women are willing to wait a few months to know for sure if they are pregnant. The desire to know as soon as possible is strong, both for the woman who desires a child and for the woman who may choose to terminate a pregnancy. A pregnancy test and ultrasonography (Chapter 23) are also important if the client is believed to have an ectopic pregnancy, because immediate surgical intervention is needed (DeCherney and Pernoll, 1994). The rate of ectopic pregnancies increases as the rate of pelvic inflammatory disease increases (Devore and Baldwin, 1986).

All pregnancy tests are based on detecting the presence of HCG in the urine or serum of a pregnant woman. HCG, produced by the trophoblast cell component of the fetal placental tissue, can be measured as subunits of α and β. The α subunit is identical with that of luteinizing hormone (LH), follicle-stimulating hormone (FSH), and thyroid-stimulating hormone (TSH). The β subunit is unique for HCG and thus is a more sensitive test for pregnancy (Bock, 1990). HCG is present in the serum within 6–10 days after implantation, peaks in 12–14 weeks, and remains elevated all during pregnancy. HCG is also produced by some types of tumors of the testes or placenta. (See the quantitative test for HCG.) Although HCG can be measured directly in the serum to detect pregnancy (see the qualitative test for HCG), most pregnancy tests rely on indirect measurements of the amount of HCG in the urine.

▼ URINE PREGNANCY TESTS

Biologic Tests for Pregnancy

The older pregnancy tests used animals to test for pregnancy: Some of the woman's urine was injected into mice, rabbits, or frogs, and various changes in the animals were evidence that HCG was present. For example, HCG in the injected urine causes ovarian changes in rabbits (Friedman test) and in mice (Achheim–Zondek [AZ] test). In frogs (Galli Mainini test), sperm are found in the frog's urine if the injected urine contains HCG. With the advent of immunologic techniques, these older, biologic tests for pregnancy are only of historical interest.

Immunologic Tests for Pregnancy

Pregnancy tests now use monoclonal antibodies specific for HCG. A solution containing these antibodies is mixed with a small amount of urine. The presence of HCG causes a change of color in the urine. Urine pregnancy tests that used an older agglutination–inhibition technique were about 80% sensitive, whereas the immunoenzymetric assay with monoclonal antibodies is almost 100% sensitive.

Home Pregnancy Tests

Kits that can be used at home to detect pregnancy were introduced in 1976. Various manufacturers make the tests, which are widely advertised to the public. Some of these tests can detect pregnancy as early as the first day of the expected period.

All the tests recommend a second test if the first test is negative and if menses does not begin within a week. A second test may be needed because the urine did not have enough HCG yet, or because the woman may have miscalculated her period. If the test is positive, the woman can visit her physician or clinic to receive definite confirmation of the pregnancy.

All the kits emphasize that the kit does not replace the advice or care of a physician or midwife. If repeated tests are negative, the woman has saved the expense and time of consulting the health care system. Advertisements for the kits also make the point that a pregnancy test at home provides a way for a couple to learn the good news together. A test at home means no waiting for appointments and no suspense in waiting for an answer. A home pregnancy test may be a way for a woman to establish from the beginning that the baby belongs to her—not to a health professional. However, health professionals express concern that a woman may not perform the test correctly and thus function under the false assumption that she is not pregnant, continuing to take medicines that could be dangerous to the fetus. (Valanis and Perlman [1982] found that about one-fourth of their clients had a false-negative report because they did not follow instructions.) Various drugs such as aspirin may invalidate the test.

Preparation of Client and Collection of Sample

A first voided morning sample is ideal because the urine is concentrated. Some tests require a few drops of urine, and some are one-step, performed with a stick placed in the urine stream. The absorbent tip is recapped, and results are read in 3 min. Multiple-step tests take longer. All these pregnancy tests have an accuracy of about 98% if the test is performed exactly as outlined by the manufacturer.

▼ SERUM HCG LEVELS

HCG Qualitative Pregnancy Test

The laboratory can detect small amounts of HCG in the serum. There is some cross-sensitivity with LH and other pituitary hormones if the total HCG is measured. To reduce cross-sensitivity the laboratory measures the β subunit of HCG.

Preparation of Client and Collection of Sample

The test requires 0.5 mL of serum.

REFERENCE VALUE FOR HCG PREGNANCY TEST
The laboratory reports either positive or negative for pregnancy.

HCG Quantitative Test

The HCG level can be increased by some tumors, such as a hydatidiform mole (a benign adenoma) of the placenta, a choriocarcinoma (malignant) of placenta-like tissue, or some types of testicular carcinoma. If any of these conditions is suspected, the β subunit of HCG helps to confirm a diagnosis. Serial HCG levels are also used to monitor the response to surgical therapy or chemotherapy. In some cancers of the testes, the β subunit of HCG can be used as a tumor marker, as can AFP. For some types of testicular cancer (seminomas), there will be only a small elevation of HCG but never of AFP (Ostchega and Culnane, 1985).

HCG, in combination with AFP and serum unconjugated estriol, is used for prenatal screening for Down syndrome, as discussed later in this chapter. High levels of HCG are associated with Down syndrome. Because HCG is the most discriminating of these three maternal serum markers, researchers are investigating the possibility of urine screening for HCG as a routine procedure in pregnancy (Cuckle et al., 1994).

Preparation of Client and Collection of Sample

The test requires 0.5 mL of serum.

REFERENCE VALUES FOR HCG QUANTITATIVE (β-CHAIN-SPECIFIC)[a]

Tumor marker	
Any detectable levels are significant	
Abnormal pregnancy	
<5.0 mIU/mL	Not significant
5.0–25 mIU/mL	Borderline significance
>25 mIU/mL	Evaluate with serial determinations

[a]These values are β-chain-specific as discussed in the text. Bock (1990) noted that the use of both intact and β-HCG has raised issues about standardization of HCG tests.

▼ α-FETOPROTEIN

AFP is made by the liver of the embryo. If the fetus has a neural tube defect, the protein leaks out to the amniotic fluid. Between 15 and 20 weeks of pregnancy, AFP may be measured in the mother's blood. AFP was the first screening test of the pregnant woman's blood as a check for genetic defects in the child (Table 18–2). In some states, laws require that pregnant women be offered the test.

High levels of AFP in pregnant women do not always indicate a problem with neural tube defects because the fetal age may be incorrectly estimated, the woman may be bearing twins, or the rise could be caused by other reasons that are not yet

TABLE 18–2. COMMON GENETIC DISEASES THAT MAY BE DETECTED WITH SCREENING

	Types of Screen				
Defect	Detected in Carrier States in Blood Samples of Both Parents	Screening of Maternal Blood After Woman Is Pregnant[a]	Amniocentesis[b]	Fetal Blood Sampling (Research Studies)	**Comments**
Sickle cell anemia	X		X	X	Most common in black families. May be difficult to diagnose accurately in fetus or newborn, but new tests on cord blood are being tried.
Tay-Sachs disease	X		X		Most common in Jewish families of Eastern European origin. Wide-scale testing is conducted in Jewish populations.
Neural tube defects		X	X	X	Genetic defect that can be screened in maternal blood by use of AFP. Can occur in any pregnancy.
Cystic fibrosis	?		? or X	X	Gene can now be identified; also see sweat test. More common in Caucasians.
Galactosemia			X		Tests of newborns required by law in some states.
Hemophilia			? or X	X	Sex-linked gene. Amniocentesis cannot determine if disease present but can do so indirectly by showing sex of fetus.
Down syndrome		X	X		Incidence increases with maternal age. See text for use of HCG, AFP, and serum estriol as a screen for Down syndrome. Most common reason for amniocentesis is to check for Down syndrome.
Thalassemia (β)	X		X	X	Most common in families of Mediterranean descent. Screening of carriers not commonly performed on large-scale basis.
PKU	X		X	X	More common in Caucasians. All states require newborn testing.

[a]Nucleated cells of fetal origin have been reported to be present in most pregnancies so researchers are developing techniques to use DNA diagnosis on fetal cells in maternal blood samples (Takabayashi et al., 1995).
[b]See Chapter 28 for a discussion on amniocentesis and chorionic villus biopsy.

well understood. If the AFP blood screening test is abnormal, a repeat is done. If the test is positive on the second blood sample, the woman undergoes ultrasonography. If there is still doubt about the possibility of a defect, amniocentesis is performed. (See Chapter 28 for a detailed discussion on screening for neural tube defects. See Chapter 10 for discussion of AFP as a tumor marker.)

Low values of AFP may also be clinically significant because less AFP is present when the fetus has Down syndrome. (See the discussion on screening for Down syndrome.)

Preparation of Client and Collection of Sample

The laboratory needs 4 mL of serum in a serum separator tube (SST). The sample must be drawn between 15 and 20 weeks gestation. Check state laws regarding notification of client about the results.

GENERAL REFERENCE VALUES FOR MATERNAL SERUM[a]	
Week 19–21	2.1–9.6 µg/dL
31–33	8.4–34.4 µg/dL
37–40	6.3–16.5 µg/dL

[a]Check with AFP screening centers for specific values for the critical levels for 15–20 weeks gestation.

▼ PRENATAL SCREENING FOR DOWN SYNDROME—SERUM MARKERS

Maternal serum AFP levels tend to be lower than normal if the fetus has Down syndrome. Therefore, in 1984, maternal serum AFP, already in use as a screening test for neural tube defects, begin to be used as a screening test for Down syndrome (Cuckle et al., 1984). In the late 1980s, two additional maternal serum markers, an elevated HCG and a decreased unconjugated estriol level, were discovered to be associated with Down syndrome. The combined use of all three tests has made prenatal screening for Down syndrome more specific. The results of these three tests are considered useful for decision making by both younger and older pregnant women (Haddow et al., 1994). For example, since January, 1995, all pregnant women in California have this screening option through a program called California's Expanded Alpha-Fetoprotein Program. The screening is considered positive if there is more or less than the anticipated amount of each marker. Clients with positive results are offered genetic counseling and follow-up tests such as ultrasound (Chapter 23) and amniocentesis (Chapter 28). Research continues on the use of these tests in the first trimester, rather than the second, and the cost effectiveness of performing all three tests (Ravel, 1995).

▼ SICKLE CELL ANEMIA

Sickle cell anemia results from an autosomal recessive gene that produces an abnormal type of hemoglobin (hgb) called *hemoglobin S* (hgbS). (See Chapter 2 for tests on hgb.) HgbS does not function as normal hgb. The red blood cells have a sickle form, particularly when they are exposed to low oxygen concentrations or if the person is dehydrated. The abnormal cells are hemolyzed at an increased rate. The capillaries can become occluded by these sickled cells.

A person can either be a carrier of or have sickle cell disease. If the person has only one recessive gene for the sickle cell trait, the person is a carrier who has the trait. A person with the sickle cell trait usually has no symptoms, although exposure to very low oxygen concentrations may cause minimal symptoms. However, the effect of the trait, if any, is being studied because in the past some people with the trait were denied jobs, such as piloting planes. If only one parent is a carrier, there is no difficulty. If both parents are carriers, they face the one-in-four risk, for each pregnancy, that their child will have the disease. As shown in Table 18–3, the risk is also one-in-four that the child will not receive the trait from either parent, and the chance is one-in-two that the child will be a carrier. The carrier state is estimated to be present in about 8–10% of American blacks.

The Sickle Cell Disease Guideline Panel (1993) noted that screening programs that target a specific racial or ethnic group do not identify all infants with the disease, because health care professionals cannot always identify a client's racial or ethnic background on the basis of physical appearance, surname, or self report. Hence, the recommendation is for universal screening of newborns for sickle cell disease so that no infant is subjected to early death because screening was not performed. The collection method for blood for sickle cell screening is a heel stick. Like other routine newborn screening procedures for PKU, galactosemia, and hypothyroidism, the blood sample is put on filter paper for transportation to the laboratory.

TABLE 18–3. PROBABILITY OF AUTOSOMAL RECESSIVE GENETIC DISEASES WHEN BOTH PARENTS ARE CARRIERS

	Mother ↓ ND		Father ↓ ND	
NN		DD	ND	DN
1:4 have two normal genes, so no disease or carrier state.		1:4 have two defective genes, so have disease.	2:4 (or 1:2), have one normal and one defective gene, so will be carriers of the trait.	
25%		25%	50%	
of all children born to couples who are carriers.		of all children born to couples who are carriers.	of all children born to couples who are carriers.	

N, Normal gene; D, defective gene.

Note: Autosomal recessive diseases discussed in this chapter include (1) PKU; (2) cystic fibrosis; (3) sickle cell anemia; (4) Tay-Sachs disease; (5) thalassemia (Cooley's anemia).

Sex-linked recessive traits occur in different patterns. See the text for a discussion of hemophilia, which is transmitted by X chromosome.

Blood samples obtained from the umbilical cord or directly from a venipuncture are also acceptable, but collection is more expensive and the specimen is difficult to transport. The blood sample must be collected before any transfusions are given.

Although sickle cell disease is not curable, identifying newborns with the disease makes it possible for them to receive preventive vaccines for pneumonia, which can be lethal in children with sickle cell disease. Also, prophylactic penicillin is started and continued until at least 5 years of age (Hay et al., 1995).

▼ THALASSEMIA (COOLEY'S ANEMIA)

Thalassemia, like sickle cell anemia, is transmitted by autosomal recessive genes. Several variations of the defect can occur. Both the carrier state (thalassemia minor) and the presence of two recessive genes (thalassemia major) can be detected with hgb electrophoresis (see Chapter 2). In the United States, the thalassemia genes are most predominant in people of Mediterranean, Asian-Indian, Southeast Asian, and Chinese ancestry. Thalassemia minor, characterized by mild hypochromic, microcytic anemia does not require therapy, but does have implications for genetic counseling (Hay et al., 1995). Thalassemia major (Cooley's anemia) is a potentially fatal disease because the bone marrow cannot produce enough hgb to sustain life. The mainstays of treatment have been regular blood transfusions and the removal of iron with deferoxamine, an iron chelating agent. With proper treatment some clients with this disease live to 30–40 years of age. Bone marrow transplantation, gene therapy, and an agent to augment the production of fetal hgb all offer hope as ways to improve the prognosis for thalassemia major (Weatherall, 1993).

In recent years there has been great progress in determining the pathologic molecular structure of the different forms of thalassemia. Detection of carriers and the prenatal diagnosis with amniocentesis (Chapter 28) of the more severe forms has been accompanied by a reduction in the number of new cases. Many children, however, continue to be born with the disease, particularly in the developing world.

▼ POSSIBLE NURSING DIAGNOSES

Ineffective Coping Related to Chronic Illness

Both sickle cell anemia and thalassemia major are chronic conditions for which there is no cure. The child and the family need help coping with the disease. Families who have one child with the disease may greatly fear another pregnancy. (See the discussion at the end of this chapter.)

The cornerstone of treatment of children with serious chronic conditions is enrollment in a program that provides family education with comprehensive outpatient care and early treatment of acute complications. Nurses may

(*continued*)

▼ POSSIBLE NURSING DIAGNOSES (*continued*)

function as case managers for a group of clients in addition to giving direct care. Information about management of these diseases can be obtained from the national organizations. For further information, The Sickle Cell Disease Association can be reached at 1(800)-742-5530 and the Cooley's Anemia Foundation at 1(800)-522-7222.

Activity Intolerance Related to Anemia

Children with hemolytic anemias have a lowered hgb and hematocrit (hct), elevated reticulocyte counts, and, in some cases, abnormal red blood cells on a peripheral smear. (See Chapter 2 for a discussion on activity intolerance and other nursing diagnoses for a client with anemia.)

▼ TAY–SACHS DISEASE

Tay–Sachs disease, another inherited autosomal recessive condition, is most commonly found in Ashkenazi Jews of Eastern European origin. As with all other recessive diseases, both parents must have the gene to produce a child with the disease. The classic form of Tay–Sachs disease demonstrates a deficiency in an enzyme known as hexosaminidase A. The lack of this enzyme causes mental retardation, flaccid muscles, and death by 3–4 years of age. At present, there is no treatment. Some variants of this disease may proceed more slowly. Several similar disorders involving hexaminidase deficiency are not more common among Jews (Ravel, 1995).

There is a simple blood test to screen for carriers of Tay–Sachs disease, and it requires only a venous blood sample. The carriers of the recessive gene have lowered levels of the enzyme hexosaminidase A. The Tay–Sachs test is performed on couples to see whether both are carriers. If needed, the Tay–Sachs test can then be carried out on amniotic fluid (Chapter 28 on amniocentesis). Unless both parents have the gene, however, there is no need to test the amniotic fluid because the infant will not have the disease. Although the rate of Tay–Sachs is much lower in the non-Jewish population, the Tay–Sachs test can be performed on non-Jewish couples who are concerned about all possible risks. Mass screening programs are planned for Jewish people who may need to know if the trait is in their family. For example, in San Francisco, various synagogues, in conjunction with the genetic counseling center at the University of California at San Francisco, have offered mass screenings for a nominal fee.

▼ ESTRIOL LEVELS

During pregnancy, the fetus and the placenta function as a unit to produce estrogens, of which estriol (E_3) is the principal estrogenic compound. (See Chapter 15 for a discussion on other tests of estrogen compounds.) Estriol levels begin to increase about the eighth week of pregnancy and continue at high levels to term. Consistently high levels of estriol indicate a normally functioning fetal—placental unit.

Toxemia, suspected intrauterine growth retardation (IUGR), chronic hypertension, diabetes, and postmaturity are the common reasons for monitoring a pregnancy with estriol levels. To recognize a trend, however, there must be more than one serum or urine estriol measurement. A decrease over two or three samples, either as a slow downward trend or as an abrupt drop, is evidence of potential fetal distress because the placenta is not functioning normally. Ravel (1995) noted that estriol measurements are less commonly used as a primary method of assessing fetal well-being in high-risk pregnancies because nonstress testing (NST) is simpler, less expensive, and more accurate. (See Chapter 28 on NST.)

A new use of serum estriol levels is as one of the three tests used to screen for Down syndrome, as discussed earlier in this chapter. A lower than normal serum level of unconjugated estriol and AFP and a higher than normal HCG level are associated with this chromosomal abnormality (Haddow et al., 1994).

Preparation of Client and Collection of Sample

If the urine levels are to be monitored, the client must collect all urine for 24 hr. (See Chapter 3 for the key points to tell a client about a 24-hr urine specimen.)

If the estriol level is to be monitored with serum levels, there is no special preparation of the client. The test requires 2 mL of serum.

REFERENCE VALUES FOR ESTRIOL

Check with laboratory because values for estriol depend on week of gestation.

Urine (24-hr specimen)	At 16 weeks of pregnancy, the average excretion is 2 mg/day. At term, excretion is 35–40 mg/day (DeCherney and Pernoll, 1994). Interpretation of the values for an individual client must be performed on a series of tests to see whether there is a downward trend.

NEWBORN SCREENING

For many newborns, the symptoms of serious inborn errors of metabolism are evident at birth. Nurses who work with newborns need to be on the alert for any symptoms or signs that require medical assessment. Some of these characteristics may be noted by the parents. McCormack (1979) identified nine clinical hints for the diagnosis of inborn errors of metabolism:

1. Unexplained metabolic alterations in electrolytes with acidosis or dehydration
2. Progressive downhill course with central nervous system deterioration
3. Unexplained renal or cardiac failure

4. Unexplained large viscera
5. Abnormal urine odor
6. Marked change in features, large tongue, coarse features
7. Thrombocytopenia, neutropenia, or anemia
8. Renal colic or calculus
9. Idiosyncratic or unusual reaction to drugs

Different inborn errors of metabolism, of course, cause different symptoms. For example, the only symptom of PKU is a musty odor of the urine, which may not be noticed. Several other inborn defects give urine an odor that has been described as smelling like rotten cabbage, sweaty feet, stale fish, or burned sugar.

Although some genetic diseases produce symptoms at birth, others do not. Some of these "hidden" defects can cause serious damage if treatment is not begun early. Many tests can be performed to detect genetic abnormalities in the newborn, but conducting a large number of screening tests on all apparently healthy newborns is simply not feasible. A few genetic diseases are common enough, however, to warrant mass screening for all newborns. For a test to be used as a screening device in healthy newborns, the test must be accurate and highly reliable, it must be easy to perform in mass volume, and it must measure a genetic disease that is common enough to warrant the cost of mass screening and for which treatment is available.

Newborn Screening Tests Required by Law

The first newborn screening test, PKU, has been available since 1962. All states now require newborn testing for hypothyroidism and PKU (Hay et al., 1995), and many states require some other tests. For example, California requires tests for galactosemia and sickle cell anemia. All four of the tests use capillary blood placed on filter paper. The hospital is also authorized by state law to charge a fee for the tests. An information sheet is given to all new parents that explains in simple terms the reason for the tests. If the parents do not wish their child to have the tests, they must sign a statement relieving the physician and hospital of any liability for damages that may result from the lack of early detection of the four disorders. Parents are told that if they refuse the tests now, they can request the tests from a physician or a public health nurse later. The nurse can often be useful in further explaining how these tests are beneficial in helping the newborn get off to the best start possible.

The Human Genome Project, begun in 1988, and expected to take about 15 years, aims to identify and locate all human genes and their sequence. One of the early benefits of the project is the identification of defective genes responsible for about 4,000 known inherited disorders (Lessick and Williams, 1994). Advances in DNA-based diagnostic procedures (Chapter 1) will make it possible to screen for these newly found genes. As more testing becomes possible, society must decide whether the benefits are worth the costs. As noted earlier, any *mandatory* tests for newborns not only must be accurate and suitable for mass screening but also must detect diseases that can be controlled if early treatment is begun. Informed consent, legal liability, and quality assurance have been issues for some time (Chedd, 1981; Andrews, 1985;

Nyhan, 1985; Elias and Annas, 1994) and no doubt will continue to be. The reader is encouraged to learn the new screening tests that may be added to a newborn screen in the next few years.

▼ PHENYLKETONURIA

Phenylalanine is an amino acid found in all protein foods. An infant with PKU has a build-up of phenylalanine in the serum caused by the lack of an enzyme needed for the normal metabolism of this amino acid. Because the phenylalanine spills into the urine, the condition is called *phenylketonuria.* PKU is dangerous because the high levels of phenylalanine in the serum can cause brain damage and mental retardation. Originally, screening tests for PKU were performed on the urine, but the blood test (Guthrie test) is more valuable. PKU is much more common in Caucasians than in other groups.

Serum PKU Levels

Preparation of Client and Collection of Sample

The serum level may be abnormally elevated within 24 hr after the infant begins a milk diet. If the infant is not taking milk well, the test should be delayed. (See the discussion on the urine test that can be performed later at home.) The laboratory needs to know the date and time of birth as well as the date and time of the first milk feeding.

The usual procedure is to perform the PKU on the third day of life. If the baby is breast feeding, a second PKU may be performed after the milk supply is abundant. A screening test for PKU is performed on capillary blood drawn from a heel stick. (Chapter 1 describes the procedure for heel sticks for infants.) Serum levels are monitored if there is a positive first test. Some babies may have increased phenylalanine levels caused by immaturity of the liver. Not all infants with elevated serum phenylalanine levels have PKU, so a follow-up test measures tyrosine, an amino acid present after phenylalanine is metabolized. People with high tyrosine levels probably do not have PKU (Ravel, 1995). Prenatal diagnosis of PKU is often possible with DNA probes. Molecular approaches are also replacing serum measurements of phenylalanine and tyrosine to determine carrier status (Hay et al., 1995).

For serum phenylalanine, 1 mL of serum should be put in a plastic vial containing sodium fluoride (NaF) as a preservative. For serum tyrosine levels, 1 mL of blood is collected in a green-topped tube.

REFERENCE VALUES FOR PHENYLALANINE AND TYROSINE	
Serum phenylalanine	<4.0 mg/dL
Serum tyrosine	3.2–8.7 µmol/L

Urine PKU Levels (Phenistix)

Although PKU is better detected with the Guthrie blood test, urine can be used when blood testing is not feasible. The child's urine can be tested with a dip-and-read stick (Phenistix; Ames). Because the recommended times for urine checks for PKU are during the second, fourth, and sixth weeks of life, the urine screening may detect cases missed with early blood screening in the hospital. Any positive discoveries, indicated by a green color, should be verified with serum testing. (Urine should not be collected from disposable diapers because there may be chemical interference.) Urine tests may also be used to monitor the effectiveness of dietary management of PKU when it is not feasible to measure serum levels.

Because the Phenistix also detect the presence of *p*-aminosalicylates, they have been used to monitor clients who are taking *p*-aminosalicylates as treatment of tuberculosis. (A special color chart is used if the Phenistix are used to see if the client is taking *p*-aminosalicylates.) Phenistix react with aspirin metabolites and with phenothiazines and therefore may be of value in revealing or checking for the presence of aspirin or phenothiazines in cases of possible drug overdosage. (See Chapter 17 for more information on toxicologic testing.)

Preparation of Client and Collection of Sample

Phenistix may be used on any urine specimen either by dipping the stick into the urine or pressing it against a wet cloth diaper. Because salicylates and phenothiazines also cause positive reactions to the test, these drugs invalidate Phenistix as a test for PKU.

▼ POSSIBLE NURSING DIAGNOSES

Altered Nutrition

The treatment of PKU consists of limiting the intake of phenylalanine to a level appropriate for each child. (There are several varieties of PKU.) Products such as Lofenalac contain the essential amino acids with only a small amount of phenylalanine.

A restricted diet, tailored to the serum levels of phenylalanine, makes it possible for the child to develop normally without mental retardation. The nurse may have a role in helping the family meet the dietary needs of a child with PKU. The National Foundation of the March of Dimes gives a copy of *Low Protein Cookery for Phenylketonuria* to any family with a child with PKU. Some researchers believe children with PKU can stop the diet when they reach school age; others believe it is wise to continue the diet. Holtzman et al. (1986) had findings that suggest children should continue on the diet even after 8 years of age and that women should not terminate the diet until their reproductive goals have been met.

Anxiety Related to Planning for Future Pregnancies

PKU is an autosomal recessive genetic disease. So if a couple has one child with the disease, they have a one-in-four chance of having another child with the disease (Table 18–3). PKU can be detected with amniocentesis. Parents may choose to have a second child, however, even with the known risk, if they see that a first child is progressing well with dietary control. (See the discussion of genetic counseling at the end of this chapter.)

Knowledge Deficit Related to Danger of PKU for Newborn

When a woman who has PKU becomes pregnant, there is some risk that her infant will be retarded unless the woman follows the PKU diet before and during pregnancy. If a woman becomes pregnant without planning to, the damage may be done before the diet takes effect. Some women may have forgotten they ever followed a special childhood diet or were never told the reason why. Therefore, all women who have PKU need to be educated about the problems of maternal PKU and referred to a PKU clinic.

▼ HYPOTHYROIDISM

The pilot program for screening for hypothyroidism in newborns began in North America in 1972. The screening of more than 1 million infants resulted in the recommendation to use the thyroxine (T_4) filter paper test for screening and a follow-up of TSH for the 3–5% of low T_4 results (Fisher et al., 1979). The T_4 filter paper test requires only a drop of capillary blood. (See Chapter 1 for the discussion about heel sticks of infants.)

The tests used for hypothyroidism are discussed in Chapter 15. See the sections on hypothyroidism of the newborn for the symptoms of the disorder, on the medical treatment, and on the nursing implications.

▼ GALACTOSEMIA

The urine test used to screen the inborn metabolism of galactose is discussed in detail at the end of Chapter 8, where the treatment of the disease and the nursing diagnoses are also covered. Like other screening tests of the newborn, galactosemia screening tests can be performed by means of a heel stick to obtain capillary blood for filter paper. (Chapter 1 discusses heel sticks of infants.) Deficiency of the enzyme red blood cell galactose-1-phosphate uridyl transferase establishes the diagnosis.

▼ TESTS FOR CYSTIC FIBROSIS

Cystic fibrosis is a hereditary disease, caused by an autosomal recessive gene that affects the exocrine glands of the body. Because in this disease the mucous glands produce very thick mucus, the older name was mucoviscidosis. The thick mucus is the most troublesome in the lungs. The other problem in cystic fibrosis is the partial destruction and malfunction of the exocrine glands in the pancreas. Because cystic fibrosis also affects exocrine glands, such as the sweat glands, tests for its detection are based on determining the amount of sodium (Na) and chloride (Cl) in the sweat. The volume of sweat is not increased, even though the Na and Cl content is increased. A screening test involves the use of a paper patch test with a small battery-powered stimulator. The test is easily performed in the clinic or office (Coury et al., 1983). If the paper patch test is positive, a quantitative pilocarpine iontophoresis test (QPIT) is conducted (Yeung et al., 1984). In 1989, the gene responsible for cystic fibrosis was identified, and research continues to develop fast and accurate screening tests for cystic fibrosis. Not all the mutations of the gene have been identified, so the tests are not yet specific enough for mass screening. They are used, however, for screening in families who have an affected member (Hay et al., 1995).

Preparation of Client and Collection of Sample

A screening test is performed with gel pads containing pilocarpine. The small portable generator, easily held in place with a hook-and-loop (e.g., Velcro) strap, performs the sweat stimulation. (The pilocarpine in the gel pads causes some tingling.) The sweat is collected in a fill tab. High chloride levels cause a color change on the sweat tab.

REFERENCE VALUES FOR SWEAT TEST (QUANTITATIVE, NOT SCREENING)

In cystic fibrosis, the sodium and chloride levels may vary from 65 to >100 mEq/L, but the levels do not necessarily correspond to the severity of the disease (Wells and Meghdadpour, 1988).

Some clients who have chronic lung disease similar to cystic fibrosis have normal sweat levels and no common mutation in the gene at conventional genetic analysis. Diagnosis of cystic fibrosis with another type of mutation is possible with a DNA probe of nasal epithelial cells (Highsmith et al., 1994).

▼ POSSIBLE NURSING DIAGNOSIS FOR CF

Ineffective Airway Clearance

For a child with cystic fibrosis, the malabsorption problems may be partially overcome by the use of oral preparations of pancreatic enzymes. The problem with mucus in the lungs requires diligent and daily respiratory care. Refer to a pediatric text for details on nursing care.

HELPING THE FAMILY OF A CHILD WITH A GENETIC DEFECT

▼ GENERAL NURSING DIAGNOSES

Grieving Related to Loss of "Ideal" Infant

A family who has a child with a genetic defect needs help and encouragement to adjust to the changes that the disease requires. Because hypothyroidism can be controlled with the administration of thyroid hormone, and galactosemia and PKU can be made less severe by dietary restrictions, the family can be assured of a relatively healthy child. Still, the family needs time to mourn the "loss" of the perfect child.

Risk for Ineffective Family Coping Related to Chronic Illness

In the case of defects such as sickle cell anemia and cystic fibrosis, parents have no assurance that the child will be healthy. When a child is born with any disorder, treatable or not so treatable, nurses are in a position to focus their attention on the total needs of the family. They can, for example, be part of a team that conducts follow-up studies with the family. Kruger et al. (1980) studied the reaction of families to cystic fibrosis, and summarized five methods of assistance used by nurses and other health professionals to help families cope. These five measures are

1. Offering support, including the role of a listener
2. Guiding the parents, which involves use of available resources
3. Teaching so that all family members understand the disease
4. Providing physical care during bouts of illness
5. Providing an environment that promotes personal development to meet the demands of the situation

Surely the development of nursing needs to progress to match the technical advances that make it possible for children with defects to receive sophisticated medical intervention. Medical technology has certainly made it possible to increase the quantity of life. Nurses have a role of helping to improve the quality of life.

Knowledge Deficit Related to Risk of Future Pregnancies

One final important point in helping a family to adjust to the birth of a child with a genetic defect is the availability of genetic counseling to help the couple make a decision about future children. Tishler (1981) stated that during the presentation of genetic information, families often first experience denial of the problem, followed by anger and blame. The desirable final phase is inte-

(*continued*)

▼ GENERAL NURSING DIAGNOSES (*continued*)

gration and insight into the problem. The couple can then make their own decision about future pregnancies. (See Chapter 28 on amniocentesis and chorionic villus biopsy.)

As noted earlier in the section on newborn screening, the Human Genome Project will identify many defective genes and the use of DNA probes will make it possible to screen for most of them. Lessick and Williams (1994) noted that nurses must help assure that the technologies and knowledge brought about by this project are made available to clients and their families in a meaningful, understandable, and timely manner.

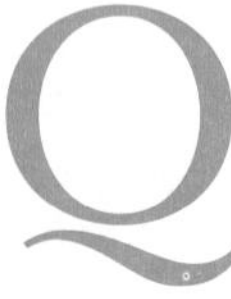

1. Elsie Fannin, who is 2 months pregnant, has come to the clinic for her first prenatal visit. Which of the following tests would be routine for this first visit?

   a. Blood glucose and serum electrolytes
   b. Urinalysis and hematocrit
   c. CMV titers and HIV status
   d. Alpha fetoprotein levels

2. The month after Mary underwent a hysterosalpingogram, she missed her period. When menses still had not occurred after 2 weeks, Mary bought a home pregnancy test kit. If Mary is pregnant, then

   a. The human chorionic gonadotropin (HCG) in her urine will react with sensitized cells in the test sample
   b. The test will be negative because it is only 14 days after an expected period
   c. The HCG antibodies in her urine will agglutinate the HCG in the test sample
   d. The gonadotropins LH and FSH may cause a false-*negative* result because the test is the direct agglutination type

3. A quantitative HCG measurement may be used to follow the course of

   a. Preterm labor b. Testicular cancer
   c. Breast cancer d. Preeclampsia

4. All the following are autosomal recessive genetic diseases. For which one is a screening test performed on Jewish people of Eastern European origin?

   a. Sickle cell anemia b. Thalassemia
   c. Tay–Sachs disease d. PKU

5. Mr. and Mrs. Green are both carriers of the autosomal recessive genes for sickle cell anemia. They have one child who has sickle cell anemia. What is the probability that a second pregnancy will produce a child who does not receive the defective gene from either parent (i.e., no sickle cell anemia or even sickle cell trait)?

   a. One-in-four chance
   b. One-in-two chance
   c. All children will have the trait
   d. Risk cannot be stated because one child has the disease

6. An expanded α-fetoprotein screening that also includes tests for HCG and serum unconjugated estriol is offered to pregnant women to screen for

   a. Down syndrome b. Neural tube defects
   c. Fetal maturity d. Endocrine disorders

7. Which of the following is *not* a rationale for conducting PKU, galactosemia, and hypothyroid screening on all newborns?

   a. Mass screening tests for all three disorders are accurate, technically easy to do, and considered cost-effective
   b. All three genetic defects cause mental retardation if treatment is not begun within weeks or months after birth
   c. All these diseases may cause symptoms within a day or 2 after birth
   d. All three diseases can be effectively controlled by dietary restrictions or hormone replacement

8. The 1993 guidelines from the Agency for Health Care Policy and Research (AHCPR) recommended testing for which of these diseases by means of universal newborn screening?

   a. Cystic fibrosis b. Thalassemia
   c. PKU d. Sickle cell anemia

9. Which of the following is an inappropriate role for the home care nurse who is working with a family who has a child with a genetic defect?

   a. Helping the family find and use available community resources
   b. Teaching the family about the effects of the disease
   c. Encouraging the family not to risk having another child
   d. Assisting with physical care if the child is ill

▼ REFERENCES

Andrews, L. (ed.) (1985). *Legal liability and quality assurance in newborn screening.* Chicago: American Bar Association.

Baldwin, L., Raine, T., Jenkins, L.D., et al. (1994). Do providers adhere to ACOG standards? The case of prenatal care. *Obstetrics and Gynecology, 84* (4), 549–556.

Bock, J. (1990). HCG Assays: A plea for uniformity. *American Journal of Clinical Pathology, 93* (3), 432–433.

Chedd, G. (1981). The new age of genetic screening. *Science, 81* (1), 32–40.

Coury, A., et al. (1983). Development of a screening system for cystic fibrosis. *Clinical Chemistry, 29* (9), 1593–1597.

Cuckle, H.S., Iles, R.K., and Chard, T. (1994). Urinary β-core human chorionic gonadotrophin: A new approach to Down's syndrome screening. *Prenatal Diagnosis, 14,* 953–958.

Cuckle, H.S., Wald, N.J., Lindenbaum, R.H., et al. (1984). Maternal serum alpha-fetoprotein measurement: A screening test for Down's syndrome. *Lancet, 1,* 926–929.

DeCherney, A.H., and Pernoll, M.L. (1994). *Current obstetric & gynecologic diagnosis & treatment.* (8th ed.). Norwalk, CT: Appleton & Lange.

Devore, N., and Baldwin, K. (1986). Ectopic pregnancy on the rise. *American Journal of Nursing, 86* (6), 674–678.

Elias, S., and Annas, G.J. (1994). Sounding board: Generic consent for genetic screening. *New England Journal of Medicine, 330* (22), 1611–1613.

Fisher, D., et al. (1979). Screening for congenital hypothyroidism: Results of screening one million North American infants. *Journal of Pediatrics, 94* (5), 700–705.

Haddow, J.E., Palomaki, G.E., Knight, G.J., et al. (1994). Reducing the need for amniocentesis in women 35 years of age or older with serum markers for screening. *New England Journal of Medicine, 330* (16), 1114–1118.

Hay, W.W., Groothuis, J.R., Hayward, A.R., and Levin, M.J. (1995). *Current pediatric diagnosis & treatment.* (12th ed.). Norwalk, CT: Appleton & Lange.

Highsmith, W.E., Burch, L.H., Zhaoqing, Z., et al. (1994). A novel mutation in the cystic fibrosis gene in patients with pulmonary disease but normal sweat chloride concentrations. *New England Journal of Medicine, 331,* 974–980.

Holtzman, N., et al. (1986). Effect of age at loss of dietary control on intellectual performance and behavior of children with phenylketonuria. *New England Journal of Medicine, 314* (10), 593–597.

Kruger, S., et al. (1980). Reactions of families to the child with cystic fibrosis. *Image, 12* (10), 67–72.

Lessick, M., and Williams, J. (1994). The Human Genome Project: Implications for nursing. *MEDSURG Nursing, 3* (1), 49–58.

McCormack, M. (1979). Medical genetics and family practice. *American Family Physician, 20* (9), 143–154.

Nyhan, W. (1985). Neonatal screening for inherited disease. *New England Journal of Medicine, 313* (1), 43–44.

Ostchega, Y., and Culnane, M. (1985). Tumor markers. *Nursing 85, 15* (9), 49–51.

Ravel, R. (1995). *Clinical laboratory medicine: Clinical application of laboratory data* (6th ed.). St. Louis: Mosby–Year Book.

Sickle Cell Disease Guideline Panel. (1993). Sickle cell disease: Comprehensive screening and management in newborns and infants: Quick reference guide for clinicians. No. 6. AHCPR Pub. No 93-0563. Rockville, MD: Agency for Health Care Policy and Research, Department of Health and Human Services.

Takabayashi, H., Kuwabara, S., Ukita, T., et al. (1995). Development of non-invasive fetal DNA diagnosis from maternal blood. *Prenatal Diagnosis, 15,* 74–77.

Tishler, C. (1981). The psychological aspects of genetic counseling. *American Journal of Nursing, 81* (4), 733–734.

Valanis, B., and Perlman, C. (1982). Home pregnancy testing kits: Prevalence of use, false-negative rates, and compliance with instructions. *American Journal of Public Health, 72* (9), 1034–1036.

Weatherall, D.J. (1993). The treatment of thalassemia: Slow progress and new dilemmas (Editorial). *New England Journal of Medicine, 329* (12), 877–878.

Wells, P., and Meghdadpour, S. (1988). Research yields new clues to cystic fibrosis. *MCN: American Journal of Maternal Child Nursing, 13* (3), 187–190.

Yeung, W., Palmer, J., Schidlow, D., et al. (1984). Evaluation of a paper-patch test for sweat chloride determination. *Clinical Pediatrics, 23* (11), 603–607.

CASE STUDIES

PRACTICE INTERPRETATION OF LABORATORY DATA

The following four case studies are presented:

- Mrs. Rita Rios, 38 years of age
- Sally Jamison, 14 years of age
- Mr. Jack Lee, 77 years of age
- Max Goldstein, 2½ years of age

These case studies give the reader an opportunity to practice interpreting laboratory data and using the data to formulate possible nursing diagnoses. The reader may select from the nursing diagnoses presented with each case study, although this is not meant to be an exclusive list of possibilities. (Reference values for the laboratory tests are found in Appendix A.) A discussion of the laboratory data follows each case presentation. Interpretation of each test is completed, and some suggested nursing diagnoses are given. Page numbers are listed in the discussion so the reader can refer quickly to the text for further elaboration on each test and possible nursing diagnoses.

RITA RIOS

Rita Rios, 38 years of age, was admitted last evening with possible pneumonia. She had completed a course of chemotherapy last week for cancer of the pancreas. She appears malnourished and states that she has no appetite. She is being maintained on intravenous fluids of D_5 0.45 NaCl with 20 mEq KCl/150 mL per hr. Her urine is orange, and her skin is slightly jaundiced. Current vital signs are: BP 130/80, P 130, R 28, T 102°F (39.2°C). The night nurse reports that Mrs. Rios keeps removing the O_2 cannula. The current laboratory results are:

1. Hgb 8 g; hct 25%; RBC 3 million/mm^3; MCV and MCH both low
2. WBC 4,000/mm^3 with 25% neutrophils and 5% bands (absolute count of neutrophils is thus 1,200)

3. Platelets 30,000/mm^3; PT 50%, 20 sec (control 12 sec)
4. Urinalysis: Positive for nitrites, leukocyte esterase, glucose, and bilirubin
5. BUN and serum creatinine WNL (within normal limits)
6. Lytes: K 3.0 mEq/L; Chlorides slightly elevated, 115 mEq/L
7. ABGs: pH 7.52; Pco_2 30 mm Hg; Po_2 60 mm Hg; and bicarbonate 20 mEq/L
8. FBS 190 mg/dL
9. Bilirubin: Total 5 mg/dL; indirect 0.5 mg/dL; direct 4.5 mg/dL
10. Alkaline phosphatase 150 U/L; GGTP 135 U/L

What Are the Priority Nursing Diagnoses for This Client?

- Ineffective airway clearance?
- Ineffective breathing pattern?
- Anxiety?
- Activity intolerance?
- Sensory perceptual alterations?
- Risk for injury? Infection? Bleeding?
- Altered nutrition?
- Fluid volume deficit? Actual or risk?
- Altered cardiac output?
- Altered comfort?

Discussion of Laboratory Data for Rita Rios

1. The values for hgb, hct, and RBC indicate anemia, most likely related to the malignant disease and the client's malnourished state. The anemia is not from acute blood loss alone because the low MCV and MCH are indicative of a microcytic, hypochromic anemia (see Chapter 2, p. 39). Chronic blood loss and iron deficiency are common reasons for changes in these two erythrocyte indices. Possible nursing diagnoses related to this chronic anemia would be *altered nutrition requirements* for *iron* and *protein,* risk for *activity intolerance,* risk for *infection,* and possible *altered comfort* related to feeling chilly. If iron supplements are prescribed later, Mrs. Rios may have a *knowledge deficit* regarding side effects (see Chapter 2, p. 32).
2. Mrs. Rios has neutropenia, not an unexpected side effect of chemotherapeutic drugs. The priority nursing diagnosis related to a lack of neutrophils is the *risk for infection* (Chapter 2, p. 52, discusses neutropenia).
3. Mrs. Rios has thrombocytopenia, also as a possible side effect of the chemotherapy. The PT is increased and the percentage is decreased; both show a lack of some of the coagulation factors manufactured by the liver. The changes in PT may be due to the obstructive jaundice (see the bilirubin levels) or less likely liver dysfunction from metastatic disease. Whatever the reason, these abnormal coagulation tests indicate that Mrs. Rios has a *risk for bleeding* (see Chapter 13, p. 324, on PT).

4. Positive tests for nitrites and leukocyte esterase are usually indications of a urinary tract infection (see Chapter 3, p. 77). The *risk for infection* is a high priority because the glucose in the urine increases the risk for urinary tract infection and perineal abscess. The spilling of sugar in the urine also alerts the nurse to a possible *fluid volume deficit,* although other data do not suggest that this is a problem at present, probably because Mrs. Rios is receiving intravenous fluids (see Chapter 3, p.76, on glycosuria).
5. A normal BUN and creatinine indicate no renal dysfunction from the chemotherapeutic drugs. Also, a normal BUN is evidence that there is no clinically significant fluid volume deficit at present (see Chapter 4, page 93, on BUN measurements).
6. The low potassium level may be due to a loss due to vomiting or a lack of intake. Hypokalemia is also found in alkalotic states. The chlorides are slightly elevated because another negative ion is slightly low (see Chapter 5, p. 135, on the electrolyte changes in acid–base imbalances). Because of the hypokalemia, Mrs. Rios has *altered nutrition.* The physician should be notified so additional potassium can be given, probably intravenously for now, and oral supplements or by means of dietary intake later.
7. By looking at the ABGs, one can see that Mrs. Rios is in respiratory alkalosis. The most likely cause for the respiratory alkalosis is hypoxia. The reason for the hypoxia is not immediately evident. The *impaired gas exchange* may be due to the pneumonia or even to metastatic disease. The hypoxia might also be due to *ineffective airway clearance* related to mucous plugs or fluid in the lungs. *Anxiety* and an elevated temperature may be contributing to the hyperventilation and thus an *ineffective breathing pattern.* Certainly, the present method of oxygen delivery is not satisfactory. A thorough respiratory and neurologic assessment must be completed to determine the best way to raise the Po_2 (see Chapter 6, p. 164, for possible nursing diagnoses related to hypoxia). In addition to the restlessness and anxiety from hypoxia, Mrs. Rios may also have *altered comfort* related to the neuromuscular irritability found in alkalotic states (see the symptoms of alkalosis on p. 150). In this case study, sedation would be appropriate given these blood gas values, but not with case study 3.
8. The elevated blood glucose levels, in the absence of hyperalimentation, is an indication of a lack of enough insulin to transfer glucose into the cells. The β cells in the pancreas may have been damaged by the pancreatic tumor. The physician may have to order insulin if hyperglycemia persists. Mrs. Rios may be a candidate for hyperalimentation if nutrition continues to be a problem. Continued hyperglycemia leads to a *fluid volume deficit* and increases the *risk for infection* (see Table 8–2, p. 208, on the effects of hyperglycemia).
9. The elevation of the direct bilirubin is an indication of obstructive jaundice. Direct bilirubin is the conjugated bilirubin (BC) that is increased in the bloodstream when the normal biliary pathway is blocked (see Table 11–2, p. 272, on the types of prehepatic and posthepatic jaundice). For Mrs. Rios, the obstruction is most likely due to the pressure of the pancreatic tumor

on the biliary tree. The dark orange urine with a positive test for bilirubin is further evidence that BC, which is water-soluble, is being eliminated by the urine rather than through the intestinal tract. (The urine would foam if shaken.) If the obstruction is complete, Mrs. Rios' feces will become clay-colored. Obstruction in the biliary tract also decreases the absorption of fat-soluble vitamin K, needed for the manufacture of prothrombin and other coagulation factors. Thus Mrs. Rios has the *risk for bleeding* (see Chapter 11, p. 281, on the relation of obstructive jaundice to the PT). Because of the biliary obstruction, Mrs. Rios will have *altered nutrition* caused by the inability to tolerate fats in the diet. As mentioned earlier, hyperalimentation may be needed during this acute phase until the obstruction is relieved with surgical intervention. The need to increase nutritional status will be a long-term goal. Two other nursing diagnoses related to the elevated direct bilirubin may be *altered comfort* caused by the pruritus from bilirubin deposits in the skin and *altered body image* related to the appearance of the jaundice (see Chapter 11, p. 278, for further discussion of the care of a client with obstructive jaundice).

10. The markedly elevated alkaline phosphatase and GGTP give further evidence that Mrs. Rios has biliary obstruction (see Chapter 12, p. 290, on enzymes used to assess for biliary obstruction). Needless to say, Mrs. Rios has many serious problems. She needs a caring, knowledgeable nurse to devise an individualized care plan. Mrs. Rios and her family are at *risk for ineffective coping* as they decide what further treatments, such as surgical intervention or chemotherapy, are wanted as palliative or, less likely, curative measures.

SALLY JAMISON

Sally Jamison, 14 years of age, has just been admitted to the hospital because of uncontrolled diabetes mellitus. She responds to questions but is drowsy if not stimulated. Her skin is flushed and dry. Her eyeballs are soft, and she reports blurred vision.

Vital signs are: BP 106/88, P 128, R 32, T 100°F (38.1°C). The physician is writing orders now. Sally's sister states that the client has been under a great deal of strain caused by a family conflict. The admission laboratory results show:

1. Hct 59%; RBC 5 million/mm^3; hgb 14 g; erythrocyte indices WNL
2. WBC 15,000/mm^3. No shift to the left
3. Platelets normal
4. Urinalysis: SG 1.040; sugar 2%; acetone moderate
5. Serum osmolality 316 mOsm
   Urine osmolality 1,400 mOsm
6. BUN 40 mg/dL; serum creatinine normal at 1.0 mg/dL
7. Lytes: K 5.8 mEq/L
8. ABGs: pH 7.30; Pco_2 30 mm Hg; Po_2 98 mm Hg; bicarbonate 15 mEq/L

9. Random blood sugar 450 mg/dL
   Plasma ketone 4+ in 1:1 diluted sample

What Are the Priority Nursing Diagnoses for This Client?

- Anxiety?
- Altered nutrition?
- Risk for injury? Infection? Bleeding?
- Altered urinary patterns?
- Fluid volume deficit? Actual or risk?
- Knowledge deficit?
- Ineffective coping? Individual or family?
- Ineffective breathing pattern?
- Activity intolerance?
- Altered cardiac output?
- Noncompliance?

Discussion of Laboratory Data for Sally Jamison

1. The elevated hct is an indication of a *fluid volume deficit.* The increase could be due to polycythemia (see Chapter 2, p. 27) but all the other laboratory data indicate fluid volume deficit. Normal erythrocyte indices indicate no apparent abnormalities with the size or amount of hgb content of the erythrocytes.
2. The elevated WBC count indicates that the body is responding to stress or infection. There is no shift to the left. Therefore there may not be a bacterial infection yet (see Chapter 2, p. 49, on the meaning of the shift to the left). Sally is vulnerable because of her diabetes; therefore *risk for infection* is a priority.
3. A normal platelet count indicates no potential problem with bleeding related to thrombocytopenia.
4. The elevated specific gravity is due to the presence of glucose in the urine and also reflects an *actual fluid volume deficit* as supported by other laboratory data. The urine osmolality is a better indicator of fluid imbalance because it is not affected by glucose. The moderate acetone level in the urine indicates that Sally's condition has progressed from hyperglycemia to ketoacidosis.
5. The elevated serum osmolality reflects the *fluid volume deficit* and the hyperglycemia that have made the serum very hypertonic. The elevated urine osmolality reflects an *actual fluid volume deficit* (see Table 4–4, p. 103, on serum and urine osmolality).
6. The elevated BUN with a normal creatinine is indicative of a *fluid volume deficit.* The ratio is 40:1 rather than the normal ratio (see Chapter 4, p. 93). The other factor that could elevate the BUN, but not the creatinine level, would be a marked increase in protein intake or gastrointestinal bleeding, but the hct shows no evidence of blood loss.

7. The hyperkalemia is expected because of the acidotic state (see Chapter 5, p. 127). Sally is at risk for altered *cardiac output* related to the development of arrhythmias. When the acidotic state is corrected, she will become hypokalemic unless her fluid and electrolyte balance is carefully monitored (see Table 6–6, p. 148, on usual electrolyte changes with acid–base imbalances). As Sally becomes able to resume oral intake, she may have *altered nutrition* related to the need for electrolyte replacement as well as other dietary modifications for her diabetes.
8. The ABGs indicate that Sally is in metabolic acidosis. The test for the plasma ketones indicates that the acidosis is ketoacidosis. She does not have an ineffective breathing pattern even though her respiratory rate is 32. These rapid and deep respirations (Kussmaul's respirations) have lowered the P_{CO_2} so that there is less carbonic acid to match less bicarbonate (see Table 6–3, p. 146 on the carbonic acid–bicarbonate ratio). The acidotic state can put Sally *at risk for injury* related to a change in her perceptual awareness and level of consciousness. Her weakness and fatigue cause *activity intolerance.*
9. The hyperglycemia is due to the uncontrolled diabetes mellitus. These levels of glucose and ketones are consistent with moderate ketoacidosis (see Table 8–4, p. 211). In addition to the other nursing diagnoses identified, others will become appropriate as Sally's diabetes is controlled. Does she have a *knowledge deficit* regarding the balance of food, insulin, and exercise? Or is the problem one of *noncompliance* that could be due to many factors? Sally's sister noted that there is a family conflict. Is there *ineffective individual or family coping?* What kind of referrals may be needed?

JACK LEE

Jack Lee, 77 years of age, was admitted to the hospital 4 days ago because of increased difficulty in breathing. He has had several previous admissions related to his chronic obstructive lung disease. He takes 0.25 mg digoxin a day and a mild diuretic.

Vital signs are stable. Mr. Lee states that he is ready to go home today. He lives alone and has no close relatives. The most recent laboratory findings are as follows:

1. Hct 60%; hgb 19.8 g; RBC 7.1 million/mm^3; erythrocyte indices WNL
2. WBC normal
3. Platelets 450,000/mm^3; PTT 28 sec (control 34 sec)
4. Urinalysis negative except for 2+ proteinuria and consistently low urine osmolality
5. BUN 45 mg/dL; creatinine 2.9 mg/dL
6. Lytes: K 4.0 mEq/L; Cl 90 mEq/L; bicarbonate 35 mEq/L
7. ABGs: pH 7.35; P_{CO_2} 58 mm Hg; P_{O_2} 60 mm Hg; bicarbonate 35 mEq/L
8. FBS 128 mg/dL
9. Serum digoxin 1.2 ng/mL

What Are the Priority Nursing Diagnoses for This Client?

- Activity intolerance?
- Impaired gas exchange?
- Ineffective airway clearance?
- Risk for injury? Thrombophlebitis? Infection? Bleeding?
- Altered urinary patterns?
- Anxiety?
- Impaired home management maintenance?
- Risk for fluid volume deficit or fluid volume overload?
- Knowledge deficit?

Discussion of Laboratory Data for Jack Lee

1. The elevated hct, hgb, and RBC are expected in response to chronic hypoxia. There are no laboratory data to support a fluid volume deficit, which would be another reason for an elevated hct, as noted in the second case study. Although Mr. Lee's erythrocytosis or polycythemia is most likely secondary to his hypoxia, he could have polycythemia vera because his platelet count is also elevated. The actual medical diagnosis is the puzzle for the physicians. From a nursing point of view, the presence of polycythemia or erythrocytosis should alert the nurse to the fact that this client is at *risk for injury* because the increased viscosity of his blood can lead to venous thrombi. Mr. Lee may have a *knowledge deficit* regarding ways to decrease the risk for deep venous thrombosis (see Chapter 2, p. 28, for appropriate nursing instructions about fluids and exercises).
2. A normal WBC count indicates that Mr. Lee is unlikely to have any current problems related to infection. However, elderly clients may not always have an increased WBC count as a response to infection; therefore careful assessment for any other signs of infection is warranted (see Chapter 16, p. 448, on infections in the elderly).
3. Mr. Lee's elevated platelet count could be due to many factors, including polycythemia, as discussed earlier. Compared with the normal (the control), the PTT is decreased. A decreased PTT can also be caused by many factors (see Chapter 13, p. 332). The decreased PTT gives additional data to suggest that Mr. Lee is at *risk for injury* related to the formation of venous clots. There is no evidence that his platelet count showed an abnormal type of platelets; if it had, bleeding could be a problem (see Chapter 13, p. 337).
4. The proteinuria indicates some renal dysfunction as verified by the other laboratory reports. The consistently low urine osmolality is evidence that the kidneys have lost the ability to concentrate urine. A urine osmolality is much more precise than a specific gravity in evaluating renal function (see Chapter 4, p. 102).
5. Elevations of both the BUN and the serum creatinine indicate that Mr. Lee does have renal insufficiency (see Table 4–1, p. 96). Because of this limited

renal reserve, there is a *risk for injury* or a worsening of renal function caused by infection, stress, fluid volume deficits, and some drugs. The use of contrast media for x-ray procedures also can be dangerous. (See Chapter 20, p. 549.)

6. Mr. Lee has no problem with hyperkalemia because his renal disease is not severe. The diuretic has not caused hypokalemia, which could be dangerous with the digoxin. The other electrolytes are consistent with compensated acid–base imbalance. The bicarbonate is elevated to balance the increased P_{CO_2}, as noted in the ABGs. Because bicarbonate, a negative ion, is elevated, another negative ion, chloride, is decreased in the serum to maintain an electrical neutrality (see Chapter 5, p. 110, on electrical neutrality).
7. Mr. Lee's ABGs show that he is in *compensated* respiratory acidosis. His pH remains within the normal range even though his P_{CO_2} is quite elevated. The P_{CO_2} level increased very gradually; therefore the kidneys have had time to retain enough bicarbonate to keep the bicarbonate–carbonic ratio at 20:1 (see Tables 6–3 and 6–4, pp. 146–147). Although Mr. Lee's condition is stable with regard to the chronic obstructive lung disease, the laboratory data suggest that Mr. Lee could have severe *impaired gas exchange* if he contracts a respiratory infection or is given high doses of oxygen or narcotics (see Chapter 6, p. 154, on the danger of oxygen therapy and drugs). Mr. Lee may have some *activity intolerance* and thus must learn how to conserve energy.
8. Mr. Lee does not have diabetes. This is important to know in an elderly client who already has several other problems common in the aged population. Elderly clients do have an FBS slightly higher than that of young adults (see Chapter 8, p. 202).
9. This serum digoxin level is within the usual therapeutic range for a dose of 0.25 mg/day. Because of Mr. Lee's renal insufficiency, however, he is *at risk for injury* related to his inability to excrete drugs at a normal rate (see Chapter 17, p. 488, on digoxin toxicity). Mr. Lee may have a *knowledge deficit* regarding the way to check his own pulse and watch for other symptoms related to adverse reactions to his medications. Mr. Lee's condition is stable now, and he is eager to go home; an astute nurse would recognize that Mr. Lee may have *impaired home maintenance management* unless he is aware of his health concerns. Perhaps a nurse should conduct a follow-up home visit.

MAX GOLDSTEIN

Max Goldstein, 2½ years of age, was brought to the emergency department an hour after he took an unknown number of his grandmother's pills. She had hydrochlorothiazide (50 mg), furosemide (Lasix) (40 mg), and aspirin on a shelf in the bathroom. On the advice of a neighbor, Max's father gave Max 3 teaspoons of *ipecac* syrup, but no pills were noted in the emesis. Admitting vital signs included P 160 and R 54. Max was drowsy and resisted further examination. He kept putting his hands over his ears. Initial laboratory results showed:

1. Hct 60%; RBC 6.5 million/mm^3
2. Urinalysis positive for salicylates, SG 1.030, negative for glucose and acetone
3. BUN 35 mg/dL; creatinine 1.0 mg/dL
4. Electrolytes: Na 130 mEq/L; K 2.6 mEq/L; Cl 90 mEq/L
5. ABGs: pH 7.30; Pco_2 25 mm Hg; Po_2 100 mm Hg; bicarbonate 18 mEq/L
6. Serum salicylates 45 mg/dL (toxic level in children is >30 mg/dL)

What Are the Priority Nursing Diagnoses for This Client?

- Risk for bleeding?
- Fluid volume deficit?
- Ineffective breathing patterns?
- Impaired family coping?
- Altered nutrition?
- Knowledge deficit related to safety needs of toddlers?
- Altered cardiac output?
- Anxiety?

Discussion of Laboratory Data for Max Goldstein

1. As in the case of Sally Jamison (case study 2), the elevated hct and RBC count are reflective of a severe *fluid volume deficit* (see Chapter 2, p. 30).
2. The urine specific gravity also supports a *fluid volume deficit*. Young children cannot concentrate urine as well as adults (see Chapter 3, p. 71, on specific gravity). The positive salicylate is expected, given the finding in the serum.
3. The elevated BUN and the normal serum creatinine level are further evidence of a *fluid volume deficit* (see Chapter 4, p. 93, on BUN–creatinine ratio).
4. The low values for electrolytes are evidence of a massive diuresis. Note that even with a fluid volume deficit, the sodium and chloride levels are low, and even with acidosis the potassium is low (see Chapter 6, p. 148). Hypokalemia is probably the greatest concern because of the risk for *altered cardiac output* related to the development of arrhythmias. The fluid volume deficit may also lead to shock and *altered tissue perfusion* as well as decreased *cardiac output.* Medical interventions are needed to restore fluid and electrolyte balance. Later on, Max may have *altered nutrition* because he may still need oral electrolyte replacements.
5. The ABGs for Max indicate metabolic acidosis. The salicylates are acid products that have used up the bicarbonate in the serum. The low Pco_2 is most likely a compensatory mechanism for the acidotic state. Aspirin is a respiratory stimulant and can cause respiratory alkalosis in the first stage of poisoning, particularly in adults (see Chapter 6, p. 148, on types of acidosis). In very young children metabolic acidosis occurs very rapidly. The *risk for injury* related to sensory–perceptual alterations and loss of consciousness should be considered. The *anxiety* levels of Max and his parents also are a high priority.

6. The effect of aspirin on the acid–base balance has been discussed. Large doses of aspirin may also cause gastrointestinal irritation and a decrease in clotting factors. Hence, Max should be monitored for *risk for bleeding*. As various medical interventions are used to stabilize Max, the nurse needs to keep in mind the risk for *ineffective coping by the family* related to their fear and possible guilt over the accident. After Max's condition is stabilized, attention may have to be focused on any *knowledge deficit* of the parents regarding the safety needs of toddlers. Active toddlers can often outwit even the most conscientious parents.

DIAGNOSTIC PROCEDURES

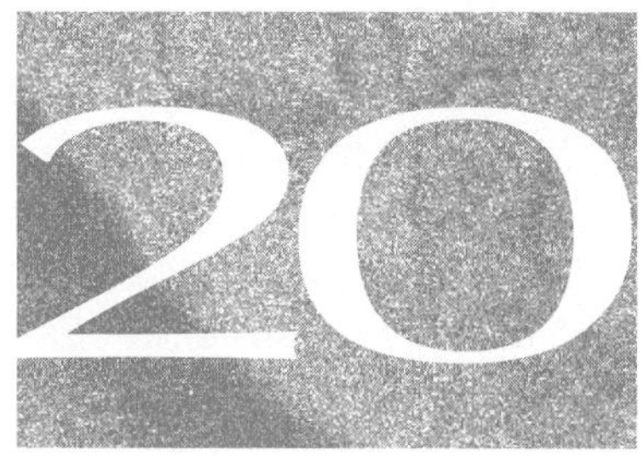

DIAGNOSTIC RADIOLOGIC TESTS

- Chest Radiographs or Chest X-rays
- Plain Radiographs of the Abdomen: Flat Plates, Three-way Films, and KUB
- Bone or Skeletal Radiographs
- Upper GI Series and Small-bowel Series
- Barium Enema Radiographs
- Oral Cholecystogram or Gallbladder Series
- Cholangiograms: Intravenous, Operative, Transhepatic, and Endoscopic
- Intravenous Pyelograms
- Arteriograms and Digital Subtraction Angiograms
- Venograms
- Lymphograms
- Hysterosalpingograms
- Mammograms
- Myelograms
- Arthrograms

OBJECTIVES

1. Describe the difference between fluoroscopy and routine radiography.
2. Explain how the four densities of air, fat, water, and bone are represented on x-ray film.

3. Identify three methods to reduce the hazards of exposure to x-rays.
4. List several important points to teach clients on how to protect themselves from unnecessary x-ray exposure.
5. Identify possible nursing diagnoses for clients undergoing radiologic studies.
6. Identify possible nursing diagnoses when clients return from undergoing radiologic studies.
7. Identify radiologic tests that require dye or a contrast medium, and explain how the dye adds additional nursing implications.
8. Name specific nursing actions appropriate in assisting a radiographic technician using portable equipment obtain a high-quality radiograph of a client in bed.
9. Compare the diagnostic tests described in this chapter, and identify the tests that cause pain, which often necessitates the use of analgesics.

The first part of this chapter briefly describes the three ways in which x-rays are used in diagnostic testing and how the hazards of radiation can be reduced when diagnostic radiographs are needed. The second part discusses the general nursing diagnoses to prepare a client for x-ray studies and to take care of the client after the radiographs are obtained. The last part of this chapter describes each of the common x-ray studies and the key nursing implications in caring for the client before and after each test. Although the preparation for each test is outlined in this book, the reader is advised to consult with the radiology department regarding the exact protocol to be followed at the particular institution, especially the guidelines given for pre- and posttest care. Most radiology departments have printed guidelines on the preparations needed for each test. The nurse should never hesitate to consult with members of the radiology department if a question arises about what is or is not necessary before a test. In addition, the nurse may need to consult the radiology department when several different tests are ordered for a client. For example, a radioactive iodine (RAI) test must be completed before radiographs are obtained with iodine contrast medium. Also, barium studies may make it impossible to perform other abdominal tests for 1–2 days.

Although rare, some radiology departments have a nurse as part of the staff. If a nurse is employed by the radiology department, she or he may have several roles, including (1) extended temporary floor nurse and guardian, (2) teacher, (3) consultant on how to deal with intravenous bottles, chest tubes, and other materials, (4) liaison with the clinic staff, and (5) team helper for a critical care nurse who may accompany the client to the radiology department.

HOW X-RAYS ARE USED IN DIAGNOSTIC TESTS

X-rays (or roentgen rays) were discovered in 1895 by the German physicist Roentgen, who received the first Nobel Prize in Physics (1901) for his discovery. By 1896, the first x-ray machines were in use. Since that time, much has been learned about both the benefits and risks of x-rays and radiographs. X-rays are electromagnetic radiation of very short wavelengths, which are commonly generated by passing a current of high voltage (from 10,000 volts up) through a Coolidge tube. X-rays can penetrate most substances, including human tissues, by strongly ionizing the tissue through which they pass. They cause some substances to fluoresce and affect photographic plates, qualities extremely useful for diagnostic tests. X-rays are, however, harmful to living tissue. X-rays can alter cells so they cannot reproduce. Consequently, radiation therapy is used to treat various types of cancer. (See Chapter 22 for further examples of diagnostic and therapeutic use of radiation in the form of radioisotopes.)

At present, there are three principal ways in which x-rays are used as diagnostic tests: (1) radiography, (2) fluoroscopy, and (3) tomography. Tests using the first two methods are discussed in this chapter, and tomography is discussed in Chapter 21.

Radiographs

Radiographs or x-ray pictures of body structures, are like negatives of photographs. X-rays that go through the body and the x-rays that reach the film positioned on the other side of the body turn the film black. X-rays penetrate air easily; therefore, areas filled with air or gas appear very dark on the film. For example, lungs, which contain a large amount of air, appear very dark on a plain x-ray film. In contrast, bones or the dyes used as contrast media appear almost white on the film because the x-rays cannot penetrate these substances to reach the sensitive x-ray film. Organs and tissues appear as shades of gray because they have more mass than air but not as much as bone. For example, heart tissues contain a large amount of water, and the heart appears lighter on film than fatty tissues, for example. From the blackest to the whitest, the four densities of substances on radiographs are

1. Air—blackish
2. Fat—dark gray
3. Water—lighter gray
4. Bone—whitish

Fluoroscopy

In fluoroscopy, the client is placed in front of an x-ray tube, and a fluoroscopic screen is held over the body part to be examined. Recall that x-rays have the ability to make certain substances, such as those used to coat the screen, fluoresce, or give off light. As with radiographs, different structures of the body allow different amounts of x-ray beam to project on the fluoroscopic screen. The image remains on the monitor for continuous observation; therefore, any movements in the body can be monitored. For example, as a client swallows barium, the flow of barium can be monitored on a fluoroscopic screen. Fluoroscopy is valuable in cardiac catheterizations to help the physician see the exact position of the catheter in the heart. (See Chapter 26 on cardiac catheterization.) Fluoroscopy is performed in the dark, so that images of the various densities are seen in sharper outline. Before fluoroscopy is performed, the physician puts on goggles with red lenses, which help the eyes adjust to the dark. Fluoroscopy prolongs the time of exposure to radiation; therefore it is used only when it is deemed very important to observe the change in position or movement in the body. Videotapes of the fluoroscopic procedure (cineradiography) enable the movements to be studied at later times. Cineradiography is also valuable as a teaching tool.

Tomograms and Computed Tomography

A tomogram, also called *laminagram* or *planogram,* is a special type of radiograph that is taken with both the x-ray tube and film in motion during exposure. The camera takes pictures of several different planes of tissues. With each change in the position of the camera, a slightly different level of tissue is in focus. Computed tomography (CT) uses computers, scanners, and tomography to obtain a three-dimensional, cross sectional view of any body structure. (CT scans are discussed in Chapter 21.)

REDUCING THE HAZARDS OF RADIATION EXPOSURE

Probably the most important point for the nurse to remember about radiation is that exposure to any type of radiation is cumulative. The nurse must be aware of the serious risks to clients or personnel who are repeatedly exposed to radiation. Some of the risks associated with cumulative doses of radiation are (1) increased risk for cancer or genetic damage, (2) sterility, (3) alterations in the composition of individual cells, and (4) depression of the production of bone marrow. Leukemia and skin cancer are more common in people who use radioactive substances in their occupations. The amount of radiation in one radiograph is not enough to cause these problems, but radiation exposure must always be as limited as possible.

The effect on humans of any kind of radiation, natural or synthetic, is measured in a unit of quantity called *rem* (*roentgen equivalent for man*). A millirem is 1/1,000 of a rem. Most references estimate that the average American receives 100–200 mrem of radiation a year from the sun, cosmic rays, television sets, and diagnostic radiographs. Medical irradiation is probably between 50 and 70 mrem per person per year. For radiographs 1 rem is equivalent to 1 rad (radiation absorbed dose); the SI unit is the gray (1 Gy-100 rad). X-ray exposure is designated in millirad. Berger and Hübner (1983) listed the high, moderate, and low doses of x-rays in relation to the gonad dose and the bone marrow dose. For example, a radiograph of the lower gastrointestinal (GI) tract has a high gonad dose (>100 mrad) and a high bone marrow dose (400–2,000 mrad).

The exact amount of radiation allowed for the general public cannot be expressed in millirem. The general guide of the National Council on Radiation Protection and Measurements is that all radiation exposure be held to the lowest practical level. The permissible level of radiation incurred under occupational circumstances is 5 rem or 5,000 mrem/year. The allowable amount for workers in nuclear plants or in radiology or nuclear medicine departments, however, is not a simple numerical rule. The formulas used to calculate the allowable radiation exposure for these workers takes into account the lifetime exposure of workers. People who work with radiation must wear badges to monitor the exact amount of exposure to ensure that these limits are not exceeded. For example, the increased use of x-rays and fluoroscopes in the operating room has increased the number of nurses who are exposed to radiation on a daily basis and thus need to wear badges (Driscoll, 1989).

Time, distance, and shielding are three ways to offer radiation protection. For example, the time of exposure to x-rays should always be as short as possible. Fluoroscopy is not performed if a simple radiograph will suffice—exposure is shorter with a conventional radiograph. Keeping a distance from the x-ray machine is a second way to avoid radiation exposure. Thus, all personnel should leave the room when x-ray studies are being conducted. California law states that only personnel required for the radiographic procedure shall be in the radiographic room during exposure, and except for the client, all such people shall be equipped with appropriate protective devices (Henry, 1982). Occasionally a nurse may be asked to help with a radiographic procedure being performed at a client's bedside. (See the discussion on portable chest radiography.) If the nurse must be involved in the procedure, shielding is important. Shielding (the third method of protection from radiation) involves the use of lead as a barrier to the x-rays (e.g., lead aprons and sometimes lead gloves). The walls of the radiography room are also shielded with lead, as are containers for radioactive materials.

It is sometimes difficult for health personnel to remember that x-rays are present, because the rays cannot be seen, heard, or felt. One type of monitor gives an audible beep when the wearer is exposed to a specified level of radiation. The use of an audible beeper has helped new radiology residents and other health workers gain an immediate awareness of radiation safety in clinical areas (Gray, 1979). Ingegno et al. (1994) measured the amount of radiation to which resident physicians were exposed when they applied bilateral arm traction or maintained the airway in clients undergoing radiography of the neck. None of the resident physicians, who all wore lead aprons but no thyroid shields or lead gloves, had any measurable radiation exposure.

Teaching Clients About X-rays

In 1984, the House of Delegates of the American Nurses Association passed a resolution that the Association educate its constituents about the new criteria for chest radiographs and the role of the consumer in reducing the number of unneeded radiographs. Clients should be encouraged to keep their own record of all x-ray exposures. This x-ray record can be carried to the physician, clinic, or hospital. The card should be filled in each time the client undergoes a radiologic examination. It should include the date, type of examination, address where the films are kept, and the name of the referring physician. Other tips for the public from the Department of Health and Human Services (1984) are

1. Do not decide on your own that you need a radiograph.
2. Do not insist on a radiograph as part of a routine physical.
3. If your physician orders a radiograph, ask how it will help with the diagnosis.
4. Tell your physician about any similar radiographs you have undergone.
5. Ask if gonad shielding can be used for you and your children. (A lead apron should be routinely provided.)
6. Tell your physician if you believe you are pregnant.

As an additional precaution, Gofman (1987) emphasized that consumers should ask the dosage of the proposed radiograph and how this compares with the typical dose.

Pregnant and Potentially Pregnant Women: The 14-Day Rule

Ideally, a woman in her childbearing years should undergo radiography only during her menses or 10–14 days after onset to avoid any exposure to a fetus. The routine use of lead aprons offers some protection to the fetus of the woman who is aware that she is pregnant. It may be wise to postpone *elective* x-ray examinations of a pregnant or potentially pregnant woman.

Benefit Versus Risk, Including Costs

Over time the public has become aware of the health risks of unnecessary radiographs. The controversy about nuclear plants caused an increased awareness by the public of the potential dangers of radiation. In addition to the health hazards from overuse of x-rays, the cost of unnecessary radiographs should be considered. As more stringent criteria are used to control insurance payments, consumers are now becoming aware of costs. If consumers can take more responsibility for avoiding unnecessary radiography, there may be a financial gain as well as a decreased risk of illness or mutations from radiation exposure.

The point does need to be emphasized that if a client needs a radiograph for diagnostic purposes, the benefit far outweighs the risk, and cost should not be a deciding factor. It is beyond the scope of nursing practice to evaluate the usefulness and safety of specific tests ordered for a client. If the nurse encounters a client who is refusing a radiograph because of a fear of radiation, it would probably be better to have the radiologist or physician explain the benefits of the test in relation to the small risk of radiation. An informed public can cooperate with health professionals to reduce the risks and increased costs of x-ray tests. When radiography is performed, the client should feel confident that the benefit of a specific test far outweighs the risk. The nurse can be instrumental in educating the public to have a healthy respect for x-rays as diagnostic tools. The work by Jankowski (1986) is an excellent reference for putting the risks of radiation in perspective for pregnant clients.

▼ PRETEST NURSING DIAGNOSES RELATED TO RADIOGRAPHIC PROCEDURES

Knowledge Deficit Related to Test Procedures

When radiologic tests are necessary for a client, the physician or nurse practitioner is responsible for informing the client why the tests are needed and describing the benefits and risks associated with the specific tests. If radiograph is part of an invasive test, a special permit must be signed (see Chapter 25). Most radiology departments have printed material that gives information about how the test is carried out and what is necessary for client preparation. The role of the nurse is primarily to clarify the information the client has received and to follow up on anything that seems unclear. If there are no printed instructions or if the client is unable to read, the nurse explains the information. If the client does not speak English, an interpreter is needed. The nurse must understand enough about the test to be able to give simple, accurate information to the client. (Key points about specific tests are discussed later in this chapter.)

Anxiety Related to Unknown Sensations of the Procedure

Often the client may be more concerned about what the test feels like than a technical explanation of the test itself. Hartfield and Cason (1981) studied the effects of procedural information, sensation information, and no information on the anxiety levels of clients undergoing barium enema radiography. Clients who received sensation information reported less anxiety than the other groups. Nursing research for many years has suggested clients cope better with discomfort and pain if they are told what sensations to expect (Johnson and Rice, 1974).

On the basis of nursing research about preparing clients for painful procedures, McHugh et al. (1982) suggested several guidelines:

- Physical sensations should be described, but not evaluated.
- Clients should be told what causes the sensations (i.e., dye causes flushing), so they will not conclude something has gone wrong.
- Clients should be prepared for aspects of the experience that are noticed by most clients.

Anxiety Related to Possible Findings of Test

The nurse can often relieve much of the client's anxiety by making sure that the client has received all the information he or she needs about the test, including any preparations that are needed. However, even with adequate information many clients are anxious about x-rays. In addition to the fear of pain and discomfort from some radiographic procedures, there is often a

(*continued*)

▼ PRETEST NURSING DIAGNOSES RELATED TO RADIOGRAPHIC PROCEDURES (*continued*)

certain amount of worry about what might be found. The nurse must not overlook the psychological needs of the client when focusing on the physical preparation. Clients may be relieved to find a nurse who not only listens but also actively encourages them to express any feelings they have about the upcoming test. Specific questions about the interpretation of the test should be referred to the physician who is diagnosing the problem. The nurse may help the client think of specific questions that should be answered.

Altered Comfort Related to Lack of Preparation for the Procedure

A study carried out in a hospital in England identified four factors that clients labeled as being stressful during barium x-ray studies (Barnett-Wilson, 1978): (1) waiting time in the radiology department, (2) moving about on the hard x-ray table, (3) darkness and noise during the screening, and (4) enemas or suppositories that made the clients sleepless and exhausted before the test. An awareness of the physical factors likely to cause stress during x-ray studies should help the nurse plan care that is nurturing and supportive both before and after what many clients may experience as an ordeal.

The waiting time in the radiology department may be exhausting to some clients. The nurse can alert the department personnel that the client is confused or incontinent or in a great deal of pain so that the client with a serious problem is not left waiting for a long time. If a very weak client must wait, a gurney should be used for transportation rather than a wheelchair. If permissible, pain medications may be given before the trip. Because a number of x-ray tests require lying or moving about on a hard table, the client should be well-rested. Enemas or suppositories should be introduced early enough so that the client can rest before going to the radiology department. If possible, the nurse can promise to let the client rest once the examination is finished. For some clients, the waiting time in the radiology department causes boredom. The nurse can encourage the client to take some reading material or other activity, such as knitting, to help pass the time.

The nurse should see if the client is ready for the examination. Glasses, dentures, and hearing aids should not be removed before the examination if they are needed. X-ray personnel should be informed that a client is hard of hearing or has other communication problems. The client needs to empty his or her bladder. A robe should be worn for privacy and warmth, as should slippers if the client is to stand during the test.

These suggestions for ensuring client comfort are basic and thus often not mentioned. However, unless the nurse attends to these details, the radiography experience may be more uncomfortable than necessary. If the x-ray examination is being performed on an outpatient basis, the nurse can give the client tips on how to come prepared for the procedure. It is also important the client know the approximate duration of the test so business or home affairs do not present problems.

Risk for Fluid Volume Deficit Related to n.p.o. Status

The nurse must make sure that the client understands when he or she is not allowed to eat or drink before a test (n.p.o.). If feasible, having the client drink eight glasses of water for 1–2 days before the test decreases the risk for a fluid volume deficit. With some tests, a light breakfast or clear liquid may be allowed. Clients may need clarification that clear liquids means just that. Orange juice, milk, and so on are not clear liquids—one cannot see through them. Because of dehydration, especially in the very young or the elderly, the nurse must find out if the test requires strict n.p.o. status or if clear liquids are permissible. Most hospitals put an n.p.o. sign in the card file and on the client's door, but a well-informed client is the best guarantee that the client will observe n.p.o. status, if necessary. For children the restrictions of n.p.o. status may be for only 3 hours rather than the usual 6–8 hours for adults.

Altered Elimination Pattern Related to Need for Intestinal Preparations

X-ray studies that involve structures in the lower abdomen may require intestinal preparation before the procedure. Table 20–1 summarizes the criteria needed to maximize intestinal preparation. Note that clients with ileostomies are not given enemas or laxatives as intestinal preparation. The preparation may be accomplished by cleansing enemas, cathartics, or suppositories. For example, a client may be given a bisacodyl tablet (Dulcolax) or castor oil the night before the radiograph and a suppository the next morning. It is important for the nurse to assess the effectiveness of the intestinal preparation. If the method used did not cause evacuation of the intestine, other methods may be needed before the client goes to the radiology department. A poorly prepared client may mean that the radiographs have to be repeated.

An extensive intestinal preparation involves a total intestinal irrigation with a mixture of electrolytes and polyethylene glycol. The glycol prevents transfer of electrolytes into or out of the solution and also prevents production of gas in the intestine. This type of preparation is more often used for colonoscopy (Chapter 27) or surgical procedures, but it may be used for some radiographic preparations. The solution is prepared by adding tap water to a powder to make 1L of solution. The solution tastes better if refrigerated. The client drinks one glass of solution every 10–15 minutes or about 1.5 L an hour until the bowel return is clear or until the maximum of 4–6 L is ingested. The first bowel movement usually occurs about 1 hr after the last of the solution is ingested, and

(*continued*)

TABLE 20–1. SUMMARY OF CRITERIA NEEDED FOR INTESTINAL PREPARATION[a]

1. Restriction of diet to clear liquids (check for times)
2. Hydration of the client with adequate clear liquids (check for amounts)
3. Use of an evacuant that stimulates the small intestine (check for laxative ordered)
4. Use of an evacuant that stimulates the colon (check for laxative or suppositories ordered)
5. Use of an enema as an additional cleansing method (check for orders for tap water enemas or small medicated enemas)

[a]See text for more details on specific preparations for various procedures and the use of total intestinal irrigation.

▼ PRETEST NURSING DIAGNOSES RELATED TO RADIOGRAPHIC PROCEDURES (*continued*)

the intestine is clear in 4–6 hours. The intestinal preparation is quicker if the client follows a clear-liquid diet for 24 hours, but the client may require potassium replacement (Murray et al., 1992). Serum potassium levels may be checked 2 hours after the lavage and again before the procedure.

Children and Elderly. A series of cleansing enemas or strong cathartics or repeated suppositories may be very taxing to elderly, frail clients. Also, the irrigation method with an electrolyte solution results in many trips to the bathroom. The nurse should question "standard" orders for intestinal preparation when the client is very small or frail. Smaller doses may be sufficient. Cathartics or enemas may be contraindicated if the client has had severe diarrhea or bleeding. Children younger than 1 year are usually not given any suppositories as intestinal preparation. Children 1 to 9 years of age may be given half a suppository. Any dose of laxative must be calculated on the basis of the weight of the child.

Teaching at Home. When intestinal preparation is to be conducted in the home, the client must be taught exactly what to do if the procedure does not clean out the intestine. The client also needs to be shown exactly how to insert the suppository or how much fluid may be needed for the irrigation method. Often what is obvious to the health professional may not be to the client. Written instructions are standard, but a time for verbal interaction is often needed and much appreciated.

Risk for Injury Related to Adverse Reactions to Contrast Medium

Many contrast media contain iodinated compounds, which can provoke allergic reactions (Table 20–2). Some newer agents contain less iodine, but they are more expensive. The radiology department should be notified if the client

TABLE 20–2. NURSING IMPLICATIONS WHEN CONTRAST MEDIUM OR DYE IS USED FOR X-RAY TESTS

Examples of Common Radiologic Tests Using Iodine Contrast Medium or Dye

1. Intravenous cholangiograms (IVC)
2. Intravenous pyelograms (IVP)
3. Arteriograms

Prettest	Posttest
Assess for allergy to iodine	Assess for any allergic reactions
Instruct on sensations of dye	Encourage fluids
	Do not use urine tests, such as specific gravity, for 24 hr
	Assess for phlebitis at injection site

Note: In addition to allergic reactions, a vasovagal reaction may occur during instillation of dye. See text for details.

has any allergies to iodine substances. Nurses should ask clients if they have any other allergies. For example, an allergy to seafood may be due to an allergy to iodine.

Clients with any preexisting renal problems are at risk for nephrotoxicity from the dye. Blood urea nitrogen (BUN) or creatinine may be measured to assess renal function (see Chapter 4). Acute renal failure after the use of contrast medium is limited to clients with complicating factors and is usually reversible (Cruz et al., 1986). Even in elderly clients, contrast medium–induced renal failure is often transient. Careful attention to the hydration status of the elderly may lessen the occurrence (Berkowitz and Cassell, 1992).

Before the radiologist injects the dye intravenously, the client again is questioned about possible allergies. Many of the dyes have an antihistamine in the preparation, but the radiologist still watches carefully for any signs of allergy, such as nausea, vomiting, palpitations, dyspnea, and dizziness. Sometimes antihistamines, such as hydroxyzine, and the H_2 blocker cimetidine are ordered at bedtime and in the morning before the procedure. Radiology departments are always equipped with drugs (epinephrine, antihistamines, and corticosteroids) and equipment to treat anaphylactic shock, which can result from the dye. The intravenous radiographic contrast material can also cause a vagal reaction marked by profound bradycardia and hypotension. Treatment of a vagal response includes intravenous atropine (Bush et al., 1985). Serious thromboembolic events have also been reported with contrast media (Food and Drug Administration [FDA], 1989.)

Clients need to understand that normally the dye causes a flushing, warm sensation when it is injected intravenously. The dye may also cause a salty taste in the mouth. Some references suggest to use the term *contrast medium* rather than dye when explaining tests to the client. The word *dye* may give the impression that the material permanently changes body color, which it does not.

▼ POSTTEST NURSING DIAGNOSES RELATED TO RADIOGRAPHIC PROCEDURES

The nurse or the client performing self care needs to know exactly what type of procedure was carried out, because specific implications are related to specific tests. (Care after a test is detailed in the descriptions of the tests later in this chapter.) Some hospitals may have a small recovery room for clients who need special observation, such as neurologic checks. More commonly, clients are returned to their rooms as soon as the procedures are finished. Many clients undergo radiography on an outpatient basis; therefore the client or a significant other needs careful instruction on possible complications.

Risk for Injury Related to Use of Contrast Medium

Usually if the client is allergic to the contrast medium, an immediate allergic reaction occurs in the radiology department, but delayed reactions are possible. Consequently, any symptoms such as urticaria, nausea, vomiting, or dyspnea should be reported immediately. Oral antihistamines or corticosteroids may be ordered for allergic reactions not acute enough to require epinephrine. Occasionally, the vein used for the dye injection may become inflamed. Any local tissue reactions should be reported. Warm compresses may be used for phlebitis.

Altered Fluid and Food Requirements

Dyes given intravenously for radiographic diagnostic tests are excreted in the urine. The dye acts as an osmotic diuretic. Thus, if other conditions allow, a client who has a dye injection should be given extra fluid to replace the fluid lost with excretion of the dye. Some clients may report bladder irritation or burning on urination caused by the dye. As noted earlier, the dye poses a risk of nephrotoxicity in clients with preexisting renal problems. The dye is not visible in the urine, but it does elevate the specific gravity of the urine. (Dye does not change the osmolality of the urine, so a urine osmolality test would be a valid test of fluid balance [Chapter 4].) Some of the newer dyes have less osmotic effect.

The contrast medium barium sulfate, used for studies of the GI tract, may cause constipation; therefore consumption of fluids should be encouraged after these radiographic examinations. The barium is visible in the stool as white streaks.

The client may be very hungry or thirsty from being on n.p.o. status for a long time. If allowed and tolerated, a cup of tea or some milk is appreciated until more solid food can be obtained. The liquids can help eliminate the dehydration, which may develop from the extended n.p.o. status.

For many people, food is more than just physically satisfying. Food can be a symbol of love and care. Concern about the client's lack of food may be interpreted by the client as a sign of warmth and caring. (One of the cornerstones of professional nursing is nurturing.) It becomes routine for the nurse to withhold food and fluids because of diagnostic procedures. It is not routine for the client to go without food or fluids, and mere acknowledgment of this deprivation may be satisfying to the client.

Altered Comfort Related to Pain After Procedure

Waiting in the radiology department and the test procedures themselves may be exhausting. Clients should therefore be allowed to rest and be disturbed only for necessary procedures, such as checking vital signs and inspecting dressings for bleeding. Lying on a hard table causes a backache for some people. A backrub often is appreciated. A heating pad may also be helpful if muscles or joints hurt from the positioning during the test. (A physician's order is needed for heat applications.) Some procedures cause pain severe enough to require the use of analgesics. The nurse must assess whether the pain is the expected type for the procedure. For example, pain at the site of arterial puncture is expected, whereas pain in the foot may be a symptom of an embolus from the puncture site.

After diagnostic tests, an outpatient may need to rest before going home. (Monitoring may also be needed for a few hours.) If advisable, clients should be told in advance to have someone available to drive them home. The client should be informed about the level of pain to be expected. For example, hysterosalpingography may cause severe abdominal pain a few hours after the procedure. The client should be alerted that if the pain is not relieved with analgesics, she should notify the clinic or physician because pain can be a sign of a complication, such as a perforation. Arthrography also can cause considerable pain after the test. The manipulation of the joint entailed in the procedure can cause severe pain when the local anesthetic wears off. Instruction on the use of warm compresses or sitz baths to relax the tense, tired muscles from the painful radiographic session may be helpful. Mild analgesics may be needed.

Anxiety Related to Waiting for the Results of the Test

Interpretation of the test results is usually not available for 1–2 days. The client may be concerned about the results of the test. The nurse can act as a sounding board and help the client formulate questions to ask the physician. The nurse can also let the client express feelings about any pain or discomfort experienced during the test.

Nursing Implications for Future Care

By listening to the client's personal account of the test, the nurse not only helps the client put the experience in perspective but learns something that might help in preparing the next client for a radiologic test. As noted earlier, clients should be prepared for sensations experienced by most clients who undergo a diagnostic procedure. McHugh et al. (1982) suggested that nurses make lists of all aspects of a client's experience. Then using the list, the nurse can interview clients to learn what aspects of the experience are noticed by at least 50% of clients. The nurse also learns the words clients use most often to describe the sensations. Clients' descriptions are usually less technical and complex than nurses'.

▼ CHEST RADIOGRAPHS OR CHEST X-RAYS

Description. Chest radiographs are obtained not only in the radiology department but also at the client's bedside if the client cannot be transported to the radiology department. However, bedside, portable chest x-ray machines are not of as good a quality as those in the radiology department. In the radiology department, the client stands 6–9 feet from the x-ray machine, whereas, the small, portable chest x-ray machines must be at most 3 feet from the client. In the radiology department, a conventional chest radiograph is a posteroanterior (PA) view because the client stands with the anterior part of the body next to the film. A portable chest x-ray machine provides only an anteroposterior (AP) view because the film is behind the client's back. In describing positions of the client, the first part of the term refers to the site of entry and the second to the exit of the x-ray beam, which is captured on the film. Note the basic working principle: The part that needs to be studied should be next to the film. Chest radiographs may be lateral views or oblique views as well. If there is question about the presence of free pleural fluid, the radiograph is taken with the client supine or in a lateral decubitus position, so the fluid pools. (*Decubitus* means lying down; hence, a decubitus ulcer results from a sustained lying-down position.) If the presence of air is suspected, the client is kept sitting up. For most chest radiographs, the client is asked to take a deep breath and hold it so that the lungs are fully expanded and the diaphragm is descended.

Purposes. Radiographs of the chest are used to identify abnormalities of the lungs and structures in the thorax. In addition, the size of the heart and abnormalities in the ribs or diaphragm can be determined. The three most common abnormalities diagnosed with chest radiographs are pneumonia, atelectasis, and pneumothorax. A chest radiograph is sufficient to help diagnose pneumonia, which is the most common cause of infectious death in the elderly (Berkowitz and Cassel, 1992). Unfortunately, in early stages of tuberculosis or asthma, the client may have a normal chest radiograph. Also in chronic obstructive pulmonary disease (COPD), the chest radiographic findings may not correlate with the clinical status. Expiration radiographs are used to detect a small pneumothorax or to demonstrate alterations in ventilation caused by emphysema or partial bronchial obstructions. Tumors of the lung can be identified with chest radiographs but CT scans (Chapter 21) give much more detail. Chest radiographs are also used to validate correct placement of central venous catheters and pacemaker leads.

Client Preparation

A chest radiograph obtained in the radiology department requires no special preparation. The client should not wear jewelry or any metal around the neck or on the hospital gown. Most clients are very familiar with chest x-rays and realize that there is no pain or discomfort.

Nurse's Role with Portable Chest Radiography

If portable chest radiography is used at the client's bedside, the nurse may have a more active role in preparing the client than when the client goes to the radiology department. For example, chest electrodes need to be temporarily removed so the metal does not interfere with the picture. Intravenous tubing and arterial lines may cause shadows; thus, nothing should be lying on top of the client's chest. The client's back must be in even contact with the film holder. If the client is slumped in bed, the picture may be of poor quality. Sometimes the nurse may be asked to hold the client while the radiograph is being obtained. California law states that no individual occupationally exposed to radiation shall be permitted to hold clients during exposures except in emergencies, nor shall any individual be regularly required to perform this service (Henry, 1982). If it is absolutely necessary for someone to help hold the client in a position, the helper should wear a lead apron. (Lead gloves may also be used for protection.) As discussed earlier, although the radiation from one chest radiograph is minimal, the nurse must remember that radiation exposure is cumulative over a lifetime. Pregnant nurses should definitely not be exposed to any x-rays during a client's examination. Nurses who could be pregnant should follow the 14-day rule discussed earlier (i.e., radiation only up to 14 days after onset of menses).

▼ POSTTEST NURSING IMPLICATIONS RELATED TO CHEST RADIOGRAPHY

There are no special implications for nursing care after chest radiography. If the x-ray film shows atelectasis, the client needs vigorous pulmonary toilet for ineffective airway clearance.

▼ PLAIN RADIOGRAPHS OF THE ABDOMEN: FLAT PLATES, THREE-WAY FILMS, AND KUB

Description. Plain, or scout-view, radiographs, also known as "flat plates," of the abdomen may be obtained as the first step in assessing a variety of abdominal problems. They may be obtained with the client lying flat, turned to the left, and upright. These three positions are called a *three-way abdominal radiograph.* If the main focus is on the kidneys, ureters, and bladder, the radiograph is called a *KUB.*

Purposes. Abdominal radiographs can help detect loops of dilated intestine, patterns of gas, and possible obstructions. Stones and calcified areas in the pancreas, biliary system, or urinary system may be detected, but radiographs with contrast medium are needed for diagnosis. Perforations in the GI tract result in the escape of air into the peritoneal cavity, which causes an elevation of the diaphragm on the affected side. The elevated diaphragm is seen on the plain radiograph.

Client Preparation

In abdominal trauma, a flat-plate radiograph is ordered as a stat procedure. If there are questionable abdominal injuries, there will not be any attempt to clear the intestine of feces and gas. In nontraumatic conditions, however, the client may need an intestinal preparation before the radiograph is obtained. (See the introductory remarks on types of intestinal preparation that may be performed.)

▼ NURSING IMPLICATIONS RELATED TO PLAIN RADIOGRAPHY OF THE ABDOMEN

There are no special nursing implications related to a flat-plate radiograph of the abdomen. However, the nurse should be aware that the client may be scheduled for other radiographs that involve the use of a contrast medium to identify particular structures. The nurse should also assess and record the exact nature of any abdominal pain and absence or presence of bowel sounds, which could be useful in the differential diagnosis of acute abdominal problems.

▼ BONE OR SKELETAL RADIOGRAPHS

Description and Purpose. Skeletal radiographs are routinely used to detect fractures. They may also be used to detect tumors of the bone, but scans are more useful. (See Chapter 22 for the use of bone scans with radionuclides to detect tumors.) Simple radiographs are useful in assessing skull fractures; however, the presence or absence of a skull fracture does not correlate with the possible severity of any underlying brain damage. (CT scans, discussed in the next chapter, are extremely valuable in detecting soft-tissue injuries.) Skeletal radiographs are also used to assess arthritic conditions and to detect osteomyelitis.

Client Preparation

Skeletal radiographs require no special preparation. If the radiographs are being obtained to assess a possible fracture, the client should be treated as having a fracture until it is ruled out. The client needs careful handling and immobilization of the affected part. Pain relief may be needed before transportation. If skull radiographs are required, the client should undergo a neurologic assessment before transportation to the radiology department. If any drainage is present, a check for the presence of glucose reveals if the fluid is cerebral fluid. Glucose in cerebral fluid makes the test positive. Mucus contains no glucose. The nurse should notify the members of the radiology department of any instability in the client's vital signs, so that the radiographs can be obtained immediately and the client watched carefully.

▼ NURSING IMPLICATIONS RELATED TO SKELETAL RADIOGRAPHS

Exercise the precautions regarding care of potential fractures. If the client is undergoing skeletal radiography because of arthritis, the client may need an analgesic after the manipulation.

▼ UPPER GI SERIES AND SMALL-BOWEL SERIES

Description and Purposes. Barium swallows are used for radiographs of the upper GI tract. The client drinks barium sulfate, which is a chalky radiopaque substance. Its nonwater-soluble quality prevents it from being absorbed by the GI tract. If there is a possibility of a leak or an obstruction, the radiologist uses a contrast agent, meglumine diatrizoate (Gastrografin), which is water-soluble. Fluoroscopy during the barium swallow outlines the esophagus and any structural defects. Esophageal varices may also show on the radiograph.

The swallowed barium coats the stomach wall so that defects, such as tumors or ulcers, are seen as dark areas with a white background. An endoscopic examination (Chapter 27) is the definitive test for gastric and duodenal ulcers. The time it takes for the barium to empty out of the stomach is important in some cases because duodenal ulcers may cause pyloric obstruction or gastric outlet obstruction. As the barium goes through the small intestine, another series of radiographs may be taken, called a *small-bowel series.*

An upper GI series takes about 45 min. If a small-bowel series is performed, it may take as long as 5 hr to complete the examination. Also, a follow-up series may be performed in 24 hr.

Drugs may be given during an upper GI series. For example, glucagon may be given to relax the intestinal tract. Drugs may also be used to accelerate the passage of barium through the stomach and small intestine to promote better visualization of the jejunum and ileum. Metoclopramide (Reglan) is such a promotility agent. These drugs are given intravenously after the client reaches the radiology department.

Client Preparation

The client usually eats a light meal the evening before the radiograph is obtained and ingests nothing by mouth from midnight until the test. Food or medicine in the GI tract interferes with the barium coating the walls. Sometimes oral medications may be continued until 2 hr before the scheduled examination if gastric emptying is normal. However, any administration of medication should be authorized by the physician. Some parenteral medications, such as antibiotics, are continued; others may not be (e.g., regular insulin would be withheld, whereas a longer-acting insulin may be given). Because narcotics and anticholinergic drugs, such as atropine, slow the mobility of the intestinal tract, the radiologist should be notified if these drugs have been given to the client. Sometimes atropine might be ordered before an upper GI series if the client has a hyperactive intestine. The client should be told that fluoroscopy is performed in the dark and that the table is tilted to help the flow of barium. If a small-bowel series is to be performed, the client needs to know that it is a long procedure that requires two trips to the radiology department. The client should also be told that the barium has a chalky taste. Many radiology departments use flavored barium sulfate (e.g., peppermint or chocolate), but most clients still find it unpleasant to drink.

▼ POSTTEST NURSING IMPLICATIONS RELATED TO UPPER GI RADIOGRAPHY

The client may need to wait for a second series of radiographs to be taken. Food and water should not be allowed until the radiologist completes the test. If the client has an ulcer, the lack of food in the stomach may aggravate abdominal pain, so food or antacids should be resumed as soon as possible. The client should be informed that his or her stool will be light-colored because of the barium being excreted. For some clients, the barium may be constipating, so laxatives or enemas may be needed. Barium in the intestine interferes with other abdominal tests, so the others should be scheduled first; otherwise, the client may need an enema so that other structures can be visualized with these other tests.

▼ BARIUM ENEMA RADIOGRAPHS

Description. For examination of the lower colon, an enema of barium sulfate is given. This enema is performed in the radiology department. The client must retain the barium while a series of radiographs are obtained. After the barium is excreted, a final radiograph of the intestine is obtained. Sometimes air is put into the empty colon afterward for a double-contrast examination. The introduction of air may cause slight discomfort. A barium enema examination takes about 1–1½ hr to complete.

Purpose. A barium enema examination is commonly used when any kind of lower intestinal problem is suspected. Tumors, strictures, polyps, and diverticula can all be well-visualized with this method. Sometimes a barium enema is also therapeutic; it may reduce an obstruction caused by intussusception or telescoping of the intestine.

Client Preparation

The lower colon must be prepared with the bowel preparation used in a particular setting. As noted in Table 20–1, bowel preparations may include enemas, laxatives, electrolyte irrigations, or suppositories. It is essential that there be no fecal matter in the lower colon. The client may be given a cleansing enema early the morning of the radiograph. Some institutions do not schedule enemas the day of the radiograph. If the client has a severely inflamed intestine or active bleeding, strong cathartics or other bowel preparation is contraindicated.

A liquid diet may be ordered for the day before the examination. Clients are given a light breakfast the day of the examination because the food does not reach the large intestine by the time of the examination. However, if there is any question about complications, food may be withheld. Perforation of the colon is an unlikely complication, but it can occur if the intestine is diseased and friable. When there may be complications, it is always better that the client not have a full stomach. Adequate ingestion of liquids is important so that the client is well-hydrated. An example of client instructions for use with outpatients is shown in Table 20–3.

If a client is unable to retain the fluid of the enema, the nurse needs to inform the radiology department so a special tube can be used to instill the contrast medium. A client who can retain the enema fluid can be spared this extra discomfort. Most people can retain the amount of fluid used for a barium enema, but it is often a concern for the client.

A barium enema can be administered through a colostomy. Usual bowel preparations are completed, and the colostomy is irrigated before the procedure. Alterescu (1985) noted that mechanical bowel cleaning differs for clients with ileostomies because enemas and laxatives are not used.

TABLE 20–3. INSTRUCTIONS FOR BARIUM ENEMA

THE SUPPOSITORY AND LAXATIVES MAY BE PURCHASED AT THE PHARMACY. (*Senokot* and *X-prep* are brand names for senna preparations; bisacodyl [*Dulcolax*] may also be used.)

ON THE DAY BEFORE YOUR APPOINTMENT—EAT AND DRINK ONLY THE FOLLOWING:

LUNCH	This meal may include clear broth, white chicken meat sandwich (no butter, lettuce, or other additive), or two hard-boiled eggs, strained fruit juices, Jello or other gelatin (without fruits or nuts), coffee or tea (without cream or milk), or carbonated beverages.
3 PM	Take 2 ½ oz of the prescribed laxative and drink one full glass of water.
SUPPER	Limit your evening meal to liquids without milk products. This meal may include clear broth, strained fruit juices, Jello or other gelatin (without fruits or nuts), coffee or tea (without cream or milk), or carbonated beverages.
10 PM	Insert one suppository into your rectum.

ON THE DAY OF YOUR APPOINTMENT:

BREAKFAST	Limit to coffee or tea (without cream or milk), strained fruit juices, and continue to drink water until 1 hr before the test.

Two (2) hours before your scheduled examination, insert one suppository into your rectum.

PLEASE REPORT TO THE X-RAY DEPARTMENT ON ______________________ AT ______________

WHAT IS A BARIUM ENEMA?

This is an x-ray examination of the large intestine. For this study it is most important to clean the bowel of all retained fecal matter. A tube is placed into your rectum, and the barium liquid flows easily into your bowel. The radiologist studies the bowel with a fluoroscope. Several x-rays are taken.

NOTE: If you have severe diarrhea or considerable rectal bleeding, consult your physician before taking the laxative or suppository. If you have any questions, or require a change of appointment, please call the x-ray department.

X-ray departments may modify these instructions as to whether 12-, 24-, or a 48-hr prep is needed.

▼ POSTTEST NURSING IMPLICATIONS RELATED TO BARIUM ENEMA EXAMINATION

A barium enema can be exhausting physically and psychologically. It is embarrassing to many people to be given an enema in the radiology department and then to be asked to assume awkward positions in front of other people. If the client did not retain the barium well, a bath may be in order. Although most clients do expel the barium in the radiology department, some, particularly the elderly, may become constipated from barium still in the intestine. Fluids should be encouraged, 2,000 mL a day for adults, unless contraindicated. Cleansing enemas or a laxative may be given if there is a problem with defecation. If the barium was instilled via a colostomy, irrigations can rid the intestine of the residual barium. As mentioned earlier, the client's first stool will be a light color or will have white streaks.

▼ ORAL CHOLECYSTOGRAM OR GALLBLADDER SERIES

Description. For an oral cholecystogram (OCG), six dye tablets are taken orally 1 or 2 nights before the radiograph is obtained. The tablets contain iodinated compounds, such as iopanoic acid (Telepaque) or ipodate sodium (Oragrafin). The radiopaque dye or contrast medium is excreted by the liver into the biliary system and concentrates in the gallbladder. Dye is not given if the client has any liver dysfunction. For example, a bilirubin greater than 3 or 4 mg/dL would be a contraindication to a gallbladder series. (See Chapter 11 on bilirubin levels.)

Purposes. A gallbladder series is used to determine if a gallbladder can fill, concentrate, and empty bile properly. The presence of stones is seen as light shadows in the gallbladder. If the gallbladder is not visualized on the x-ray film, the test may be repeated with a double dose (12 tablets) of dye. If the gallbladder is still not visualized, this may indicate an obstruction in the biliary tree or a diseased gallbladder. The client may be given a fatty meal after the OCG, and more radiographs may be later taken to see how well the gallbladder empties. (Ultrasonography also is used to detect gallstones [Chapter 23], and is fast replacing OCG.)

Client Preparation

Most radiology departments start client preparation for an OCG 2 days before the examination. On the first evening, the client eats a high-fat meal (milk, eggs, and bread with butter) and then takes the dye tablets. The next evening, a normal meal without fats is eaten, followed by a second dose of six dye tablets. This double dose of tablets may eliminate some cases of nonvisualization of the gallbladder, which are due to lack of dye and not to gallbladder disease.

Because the oral tablets contain iodine, the client must be examined for any sensitivity to iodine compounds. The six tablets are taken after the evening meal, one every 5 min with water. After the six tablets are taken, the client ingests nothing by mouth. The tablets may cause nausea, vomiting, and diarrhea in some clients. If the client vomits the tablets, the test must be rescheduled. Diarrhea does not cause loss of the dye. Preparation with enemas or suppositories may be ordered to clean out the intestine. If the client has received morphine sulfate, the radiologist should be notified, because morphine may cause spasm of the sphincter of Oddi.

▼ POSTTEST NURSING IMPLICATIONS RELATED TO ORAL CHOLECYSTOGRAPHY

As mentioned earlier, the client may be given a fatty meal if more radiographs are planned to see how well the gallbladder empties. Otherwise, the client can resume whatever diet is tolerated. Actually a fat-restricted diet is often needed because of the client's fat intolerance caused by an obstruction of the biliary system. (See Chapter 11 for the nursing diagnoses when a client has an obstruction of the biliary system.)

▼ CHOLANGIOGRAMS: INTRAVENOUS, OPERATIVE, TRANSHEPATIC, AND ENDOSCOPIC

Description and Purposes. A cholangiogram is a radiograph of the biliary tree obtained with contrast medium so the cystic, hepatic, and common bile ducts can be visualized. In contrast, an OCG is used to assess the ability of the gallbladder to concentrate and excrete the dye.

Intravenous Cholangiogram. When the dye is given intravenously, the liver excretes the dye into the biliary tree. X-ray pictures are taken at intervals after the dye is injected. The dye begins to appear in the biliary tree about 10 min after the intravenous administration of the contrast agent. It takes about 4 hr but sometimes 8 hr for the dye to be totally excreted, so the client may be in the radiology department for several hours.

T-tubes Cholangiography. Cholangiograms are also obtained during surgical procedures to check for stones in the common bile duct, which might not be seen or felt. With the operative method, the dye is injected directly into a drainage catheter (T tube) placed in the common bile duct during a surgical procedure. X-ray films are taken immediately after the dye is instilled. A T-tube cholangiogram may also be obtained several days postoperatively to evaluate the patency of the biliary tree. Clients who undergo exploration of the common bile duct have T tubes for bile drainage until the edema in the common bile duct is relieved.

Transhepatic Cholangiography. Transhepatic cholangiograms are obtained by means of percutaneous insertion of a needle into the common bile duct. The insertion is carried out with the aid of fluoroscopy. After the needle is in the common bile duct, dye is injected.

Endoscopic Cholangiopancreatography. A fourth way to inject dye into the biliary system is with the use of an endoscope passed into the GI tract through the sphincter of Oddi into the biliary tract. (See Chapter 27 for a discussion of endoscopic procedures.)

Client Preparation

Of the four procedures described, intravenous cholangiography is most commonly used. The client takes nothing by mouth for 6–8 hr before the test. A preparation is ordered to clear the intestinal tract. Intravenous cholangiography is performed in the radiology department and is not particularly uncomfortable except for the sensation of dye being injected intravenously.

If cholangiograms are part of an operative procedure, the client receives the routine preoperative preparation. A percutaneous transhepatic cholangiogram is conducted in the radiology department. Because this is an invasive procedure, the physician must explain the specific risks to the client. The endoscopic procedure is also invasive and entails risks; consequently, institutions have special protocols to follow regarding permission. (See Chapter 25 for nursing implications for invasive tests.) Because obstructions in the biliary system tend to increase bleeding, the client usually has a prothrombin time (PT) performed before any type of invasive procedure on the biliary tree. If the PT is increased, vitamin K must be given parenterally before traumatic tests are done. GI absorption of vitamin K, a fat-soluble vitamin, is hampered when there is a biliary obstruction and thus a lack of the bile salts for fat absorption. Chapter 11 discusses laboratory tests used to assess for biliary obstruction and the nursing diagnoses for clients with elevation of direct bilirubin (obstructive jaundice).

▼ POSTTEST NURSING IMPLICATIONS RELATED TO CHOLANGIOGRAPHY

The aftercare for a client who has had dye instilled for an intravenous cholangiogram would be the routine nursing diagnoses discussed at the beginning of this chapter.

See Chapter 25 for the nursing implications when a client has undergone an invasive procedure that may cause bleeding. Frequent checking of vital signs and bed rest for a specified amount of time are important. Just as in a liver biopsy, complications such as leakage of bile into the peritoneal cavity can occur when a needle is inserted into the common bile duct. Any abdominal pain, which could mean bile peritonitis, should be called to the attention of the physician. Chills and fever may be due to inflammation of the bile duct.

▼ INTRAVENOUS PYELOGRAMS

Description. Diatrizoate sodium (Hypaque) and diatrizoate meglumine (Renografin) are dyes used for pyelograms because they are excreted by the urinary system. Another name for intravenous pyelography (IVP) is excretory urography because it demonstrates the ability of the entire urinary tract to excrete dye. After the dye or contrast medium has been injected intravenously, radiographs are obtained every minute for 5 min, allowing visualization of the cortex of the kidney. Approximately 15 min later, radiographs are obtained as the dye collects in the pelvis of the kidney and is excreted via the ureters into the bladder. The dye outlines the bladder in about 45 min. The client is asked to void, and a postvoiding radiograph is obtained to see how well the bladder empties. The entire set of radiographs takes about an hour. If the dye is not well-excreted, a 24-hr follow-up radiograph must be obtained.

Purposes. Structural defects or tumors can be observed when the urinary system is outlined with dye. A retrograde introduction of dye, through ureteral catheters, to outline the urinary system is carried out with a cystoscope. (See Chapter 27 for endoscopic procedures.) Renograms, conducted with radionuclides (Chapter 22), can be performed if clients are allergic to the contrast medium used for IVP.

Client Preparation

The client is given a light meal the evening before the test. Different radiology departments may have different instructions regarding nothing-by-mouth status. Some radiologists prefer that the client not take in any fluids so the dye will not be diluted. Other radiologists want the client to be given clear liquids so that the client is not dehydrated before the examination. A lack of normal renal function may make it hazardous for a client to receive dye that is excreted via the kidney; therefore, serum creatine and BUN levels are assessed before the test is begun (Chapter 4). The intestinal preparation for an IVP must be thorough. A cathartic agent as well as suppositories the evening before and the morning of the examination may be necessary. Enemas may be necessary if the client has undergone a barium study in the preceding 48 hr.

The client should be instructed about the sensation of the dye being injected. (See the general implications about contrast medium discussed earlier in this chapter.) There may be more than one venipuncture. The only other discomfort results from lying in one position during the series of radiographs. Voiding in the radiology department may be embarrassing for clients who must use a urinal or bedpan if they cannot go to the bathroom.

▼ POSTTEST NURSING IMPLICATIONS RELATED TO IVP

See the general implications for dye use, including a fluid intake of 2,000–3,000 mL of fluids. The client should be observed for any signs of urinary problems, such as difficulty voiding or bladder irritation. Note that the serum creatinine levels and creatinine clearance tests may be used to assess any loss of renal function.

▼ ARTERIOGRAMS AND DIGITAL SUBTRACTION ANGIOGRAMS

Description. *Angiography* is a broad term meaning visualization of blood vessels that are either arteries or veins. *Arteriography* is a more precise term designating visualization of arteries. Digital subtraction angiography (DSA) uses a computer to select only certain parts of images to be displayed at one time. This computerized application of angiography results in a very sophisticated way of viewing the vascular system. The most common site of dye injection for an arteriogram is the femoral artery. Arterial catheters are positioned with a guidewire that is used to advance the catheter to a specified location in the arterial tree. Because the arterial catheter is radiopaque, movement of the catheter is noted with fluoroscopy. After correct placement is obtained, dye is injected into the catheter to outline a portion of the artery. In this way the circulation in the lower extremity can be visualized. Also, the catheter can be threaded via the femoral artery into the abdominal aorta to the level of the renal arteries for renal arteriograms. The arteries of the GI tract can be visualized if the dye is instilled in the celiac axis. The brachial artery can be used for upper extremity visualization. Carotid arteriography may also be performed but can disrupt atherosclerotic plaques, which can become cerebral emboli. Therefore, the carotid arteries are usually visualized with dye administered through a catheter threaded through other arteries.

Purposes. Arteriograms are extremely valuable for observing the blood flow to a part of the body and to detect lesions that may be amenable to surgical treatment. The catheter used to administer the contrast agent used to confirm the diagnosis of a suspected kidney or liver lesion may also become a vehicle for the selective delivery of chemotherapeutic drugs or drugs to stop bleeding. Catheters in arteries are also used to remove atherosclerotic plaques in a procedure called *percutaneous transluminal angioplasty* (PCTA).

Client Preparation

The client must sign a special permission form. At some hospitals it is routine to discuss the possibility of angioplasty and obtain informed consent at the time a client signs a consent form for arteriography because the therapeutic maneuver may immediately follow the diagnostic procedure. After premedication is administered the client cannot legally consent to a procedure not cited on the original consent form. (See Chapter 25 for the nurse's role in preparing clients for invasive procedures.) Because arteriography involves intravenous administration of an iodinated dye, the implications for dye use should be considered. The client's weight is used to determine the dose of the dye. (See the discussion on dyes at the beginning of this chapter.) The client ingests nothing by mouth for 6–8 hr before the procedure; some institutions do allow liquids before an arteriogram. There may be an order to shave an area, but usually any preparation of the puncture site is performed in the radiology department.

▼ POSTTEST NURSING IMPLICATIONS RELATED TO ARTERIOGRAPHY

The client stays supine for a minimum of 4–6 hr to decrease the possibility of bleeding from the puncture site; some institutions may instruct the client to stay supine longer. The nurse should make an observation of the puncture site as soon as the client returns from the radiology department. This serves as

(*continued*)

▼ POSTTEST NURSING IMPLICATIONS RELATED TO ARTERIOGRAPHY (*continued*)

a baseline comparison if later there is blood on the dressing or swelling around the site. There may be more than one site if one puncture was not successful. The pressure dressing on the site should not be removed. An ice bag may also be placed on the site to decrease the possibility of bleeding or hematoma formation. Vital signs should be taken every 15 min for the first hour and then every 2–4 hr as ordered or deemed necessary. Frequent temperature checks are not necessary but temperature should be recorded every 4 hr to detect beginning septicemia or a reaction to the dye. Pulses distal to the arterial puncture must also be checked with the vital signs. Thrombus formation, emboli release, nerve damage, or spasms of the artery are all possible complications. Pain at the puncture site is not uncommon and may require analgesics, but pain distal to the puncture site may indicate an embolism. A false aneurysm, a cystic-like mass that communicates with the damaged arterial wall, may develop immediately after the trauma or develop weeks later (Fahey and Finkelmeier, 1984).

Femoral Arteriogram. For a *femoral* arteriogram, the pedal pulses are checked. (See Chapter 23 for the use of a Doppler probe to assess arterial pulses.) The client may not have had detectable pulses before the arteriogram; this must be taken into account. The color, sensation, and warmth of the foot on the side examined should be compared with the other foot. Any pain in the foot or leg should be carefully assessed and compared with the pain before the arteriogram.

Brachial Arteriogram. If a *brachial* arteriogram is obtained, there is concern not only for spasm, embolism, or thrombus formation but also for nerve compression. Pain or numbness in the fingers or hand should always be reported immediately. Blood pressure readings should not be taken on the examined arm because they temporarily compromise arterial circulation in the lower arm.

Carotid Arteriogram. For a *carotid* arteriogram, both temporal pulses should be checked. In addition, the client should be assessed for any signs of transient ischemic attacks (TIA), such as facial weakness, visual disturbances, or slurred speech. The client's head should be kept elevated about 30 degrees. A light ice collar may be used to reduce swelling. Pressure on the carotid arterial site should be avoided; this can cause a vagal response that can slow the heart. Tracheal obstruction can result from swelling, so the client should be observed for any difficulty breathing or swallowing. A tracheostomy set should be nearby.

Renal Arteriogram. If a *renal* arteriogram is performed, hypotension may result from a decrease in the formation of renin for a short time. Renal function must be closely monitored. BUN and serum creatinines may be ordered (Chapter 4).

Fortunately, all these complications of arteriograms are rare, but the nurse who makes skilled assessments may detect a problem before it becomes serious.

▼ VENOGRAMS

Description. A dye or contrast medium can be injected into a vein by means of venipuncture or cutdown to view the venous system of particular organs or to evaluate flow to a particular area (e.g., radiographs taken as the dye goes through the venous system of the leg). Dye may be injected into a catheter in the femoral vein or inferior vena cava, and the catheter can be threaded to various organs to inspect details in the venous supply of the organ.

Purposes. Venograms may be useful in detecting deep venous thrombosis (DVT) or to assess other venous abnormalities, such as congenital abnormalities or incompetent valves. Venograms show only structure and flow. Radioisotopes (Chapter 22) are sometimes injected into veins to assess for the presence of DVT.

Client Preparation

Food and fluids may be withheld for 4 hr before the test. A consent form is needed. (See earlier discussion of contrast medium.)

▼ POSTTEST NURSING IMPLICATIONS RELATED TO VENOGRAPHY

There are no restrictions on eating. The client is usually not instructed to maintain bed rest, as with an arteriogram. If the client has DVT, bed rest may be maintained and anticoagulants used. (See Chapter 13 for tests for heparin regulation.) There are fewer complications of venous puncture than of arterial puncture. However, the nurse should carefully assess vital signs and check for any signs of hematoma formation. Phlebitis may result, and warm compresses can be used to ease the pain of an irritated vein. The implications for the use of a dye must be noted as discussed earlier in this chapter. If a cutdown was necessary, the area must be assessed for infection.

▼ LYMPHOGRAMS

Description. Visualization of the lymphatic system can be achieved by means of injection of dye or contrast medium into the lymphatic system of an arm or leg. A dye (Evans blue) is first injected into the web of skin between the first and second toes or between the fingers. The blue dye is picked up by the lymphatic system. After approximately 30 min the lymphatic system is outlined, and a lymphatic vessel is then dissected and a small catheter inserted for the injection of an iodine dye (Ethiodol). Radiographs are taken after the iodine dye is injected and again 24 hr later. Other x-ray pictures may be taken later because the lymph nodes retain the contrast medium for several weeks, even months.

Purposes. Enlarged and diseased lymph nodes can be identified on the radiographs. The lymphogram can show not only the extent of the disease, such as a lymphoma or Hodgkin's disease, but also the effectiveness of therapy.

Client Preparation

The client may be instructed to ingest nothing by mouth or may be allowed to eat. A consent form is signed, and precautions for use of contrast medium are noted. The client should be prepared for some discomfort when the hand or foot is given a local anesthetic. The most difficult part of the procedure may be lying still for the extent of the procedure, which may be as long as 3 hr. Because of the long waits during the test, the client may need reading material or other quiet diversions.

▼ POSTTEST NURSING IMPLICATIONS RELATED TO LYMPHOGRAPHY

To prevent edema, the client should keep the affected limb elevated for 24 hr. Vital signs should be checked to detect any signs of bleeding, infection, or adverse reactions to the dye.

The site of the dissection may become painful as the local anesthetic wears off, and mild analgesics may be needed for the incisional pain. Any numbness in the extremity distal to the incision should be reported immediately because of possible nerve damage. The site has a few stitches, which are removed in 7–10 days. The site should not get wet for 1–2 days. The site should be examined for any sign of infection, and warm compresses should be applied to ease any discomfort from inflammation. If dye travels to the lung, via the thoracic duct, pneumonia may develop. Thus, respiratory problems should be evaluated by the physician. Skin discoloration from the blue dye fades in a few days. Stool and urine also show some discoloration. The client may even note a bluish tint in vision.

▼ HYSTEROSALPINGOGRAMS

Description. The client is placed in the lithotomy position, and a vaginal speculum is inserted. Dye is injected through the cervix into the uterus and fallopian tubes. The client is awake during the procedure. There is likely to be some abdominal discomfort from the pressure of the dye, even though only about 5–10 mL is used. Water-based dye tends to cause less cramping than oil-based dye (DeCherney and Pernoll, 1994). Fluoroscopy is used to monitor the progression of the dye through the fallopian tubes. Ultrasonography (Chapter 23) with dye may be used to establish tubal patency so that there is no exposure to radiation. The examination is scheduled within a week to 10 days after the client's menstrual period, to ensure that the client is not pregnant. The test takes about half an hour.

Purposes. The test is used to detect blocked fallopian tubes. Other abnormalities in the uterus, such as fibroid tumors, also are demonstrated on the radiograph. This is one of the tests performed as part of an infertility evaluation. (See Chapter 28 for a discussion of the five basic tests for infertility.) Occasionally, the injection of the dye may also be included to evaluate the success of a tubal ligation.

Client Preparation

A hysterosalpingogram is often carried out on an outpatient basis. There are no restrictions of food or fluid. The client should have finished a menstrual period within the preceding 7–10 days. The client must void immediately before the procedure. Although some institutions have the client take an enema or suppository before the examination, no special intestinal preparation is usually necessary. The client must remove her clothes from the waist down. Some clients are given a mild analgesic. (See Chapter 25 on ways nurses can help prepare clients to cope with painful procedures.)

▼ POSTTEST NURSING IMPLICATIONS RELATED TO HYSTEROSALPINGOGRAPHY

A few hours after the procedure, the client may have severe uterine cramps that require analgesia. Warm sitz baths may be soothing. Although rare, perforation of the uterus can occur, so any severe cramping or profuse bleeding should be called to the attention of the physician or clinic. The client may have some vaginal spotting for a day or two, so she should be informed about the possible need for sanitary napkins. There is a slight chance of infection. Very rarely a pulmonary embolism could result from the entrance of the oil-based dye into the bloodstream.

▼ MAMMOGRAMS

Description. A mammogram is a radiograph of the breast to detect the presence of tumors too small to be discovered at palpation. Mammograms may include injection of a dye into the mammary ducts, but routine screening procedures do not include the use of a contrast medium. Dye is useful in identifying intraductal papillomas. During the examination, the client stands or sits with breasts pushed against the film holder. An inflated rubber cushion is used to decrease the discomfort of the flattened breasts against the film holder. The procedure takes about 30 min.

Purposes. Because breast cancer is the leading type of cancer in women, mass screening for this disease is needed. Mammograms became popular in the early 1960s as a tool to detect early breast cancer. In the late 1970s, however, concern about radiation risks caused a reevaluation of whether mammograms should be performed routinely. The American Cancer Society issued a statement in 1980 and revised it in 1983 to state that in addition to breast self-examinations and regular medical examinations, a baseline mammogram should be performed between the ages of 35 and 40 years. From 40 to 49 years of age, mammograms should be done every year or two. After 50 years of age, a yearly mammogram is recommended. (Clients at high risk may need more frequent checks at younger ages.) The consensus continues to be that screening mammography does decrease mortality from breast cancer among women 50 years and older (Bassett et al., 1994). However, there is a range of opinion about the value of screening mammography among women 40–49 years of age who do not have symptoms. Some studies have suggested that mammography does not reduce mortality in this population (Kerlikowske et al., 1995). Young women and elderly women need to confer with their health care providers to see what assessments are most appropriate for them. In addition to screening, mammography is also used to guide the placement of a needle or wire in a lump as a guide to a biopsy. (See Chapter 25 on invasive procedures.)

Barriers to Mammograms

Unfortunately many women do not undergo mammography because of fear or denial, cost, accessibility, or the lack of a physician's recommendation (Lauver, 1992). Since 1990, Medicare has paid for the examination, and many insurance companies have added the test as the focus on preventive care has increased. Mobile mammographic clinics have increased access. More publicity also is being given to the high incidence of breast cancer in the United States. Nurses can be effective in educating women about the value of mammograms and the need for continued research in this area. Consumer groups, such as Breast Cancer Action, have been involved in calling attention to the need for more attention to this disease.

Nurses can also help educate consumers about quality control for mammography. Beginning in October, 1994, all mammographic facilities in the United States were required to be certified by an FDA–approved accreditation body. This certificate must be prominently displayed (FDA, 1995).

Client Preparation

The client should not use deodorant, perfume, or powder on the day of the test; these chemicals may interfere with the x-ray picture. The client should wear clothing easy to remove from the waist up. The client should be prepared for some physical discomfort related to the manipulation of the tender tissue, particularly if the breasts are pendulous and much compression must be performed. Otherwise, the test is not physically painful, but it may be traumatic to be exposed. Suggestions to reduce the pain of a mammogram include scheduling the examination during the first 2 weeks after menses, reducing caffeine intake for 3 months before the mammogram, and working with the technician to have more control with the compression of the breasts (Nielsen et al., 1993). Women who have considerable breast pain may be advised to take a mild analgesic an hour before the mammogram (Bassett et al., 1994). The potential diagnosis of cancer may cause much anxiety; thus attention to psychological needs also helps the woman have a more pleasant experience with mammography. A mammogram performed to place a needle or wire marker in the lump as a guide to subsequent biopsy is anxiety producing.

▼ POSTTEST NURSING IMPLICATIONS RELATED TO MAMMOGRAPHY

There are no specific nursing implications; however, the nurse should assess if the client knows how to perform a self-examination of the breast. (See Chapter 25 on breast biopsies for follow-up of lumps in the breast.) Breast self-examination should be viewed as an adjunct to mammography, yet many women do not examine their breasts on a regular basis, even though the incidence of breast cancer is steadily rising (Sternberger, 1994).

▼ MYELOGRAMS

Description. A myelogram is a radiograph of the subarachnoid space of the spinal column in which air or dye may be used as a contrast medium. The dye may either be an oily contrast agent or a water-soluble medium. Water-soluble dye is most often used and is suitable for both inpatient and outpatient procedures. If an oil-based dye is used, it is removed at the end of the procedure. The water-soluble dye is not. The dye or air is injected by means of lumbar puncture. The client lies on a tilted table to allow the dye to flow into different parts of the spinal column.

Purposes. Radiography and fluoroscopy performed after the contrast medium is instilled can show distortions of the spinal cord caused by tumors or changes in bone structure. Herniations or protrusions of intervertebral disks can also be visualized. CT or magnetic resonance imaging (MRI) may give more detail (Chapter 21).

Client Preparation

The client's allergy history is important if iodine is being used. The client should ingest nothing by mouth for 4–6 hr, and an intestinal preparation may be ordered. Intravenous fluids may be used to hydrate the client. The client should be prepared for the positioning necessary for a lumbar puncture. (See Chapter 25 on lumbar punctures.) Sedatives may be ordered. Phenothiazines are not used because they lower the seizure threshold. Consent forms are needed. Flam et al. (1989) found that a 5-min tape about the procedure for a myelogram reduced the anxiety level of those undergoing the test.

▼ POSTTEST NURSING IMPLICATIONS RELATED TO MYELOGRAPHY

If an oil-based dye is used, the client should be instructed to stay flat in bed 6–8 hr after the dye is removed. If water-soluble dye was used, the head of the bed should be kept elevated for at least 8 hr to keep the dye from irritating the cerebral meninges. The client may need analgesics if headache, pain, and stiffness in the neck occur. About 20% of clients experience headaches, nausea, and vomiting after the test. Fewer than 1 in 1,000 have a seizure. If conditions permit, fluids should be encouraged to at least 2,000 mL for adults to help with the production of adequate cerebrospinal fluid (CSF). The motor sensations of the lower extremities should be assessed to make sure there was no nerve damage. The voiding pattern of the client should be assessed because urinary retention may be a problem in the first 24 hr.

Outpatient clients are monitored for at least 2 hr and accompanied home by a friend or family member.

▼ ARTHROGRAMS

Description. For an arthrogram, dye is injected into a joint, usually the knee and sometimes a shoulder or other joint. The procedure is performed under local anesthesia in the radiology department. After the needle is inserted into the joint space, fluid is usually aspirated for analysis. Then the dye, and sometimes air, is injected. The client may be asked to run in place to spread the dye around the knee joint. Also, the joint is manipulated to spread the dye. (Some clients find the movement of the joint uncomfortable.) Radiographs are taken with the joint in various positions.

Purposes. Arthrograms help evaluate suspected joint damage such as tears in the cartilage of the knee. If surgical intervention is anticipated, arthroscopy may be performed in place of the arthrogram. Arthroscopy allows the physician to examine the joint directly and even perform simple repairs (Chapter 27).

▼ PRETEST NURSING IMPLICATIONS RELATED TO ARTHROGRAPHY

Precautions related to the use of contrast dye should be noted. If the procedure is being performed on an outpatient basis, and many are, a friend or family member may have to drive the client home.

▼ POSTTEST NURSING DIAGNOSIS RELATED TO ARTHROGRAPHY

Altered Comfort Related to Knee Manipulation

Mild-to-moderate discomfort may be present after the procedure. The joint should rest for about 12 hr. The knee may be wrapped in an elastic bandage for 12–24 hr. Ice bags can be used to reduce swelling, and mild analgesics may be needed. Some slight grating may be present for a day or two after the procedure. Strenuous activity, such as jogging, should not be resumed until advised by the physician. Exercises to strengthen the knee may be prescribed, depending on the results of the examination. Two possible complications after arthroscopic surgical procedures are hemorrhage and thrombophlebitis, but the incidence of either is quite low.

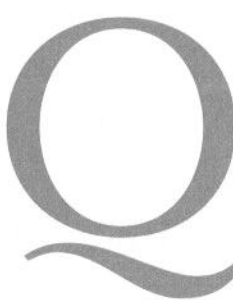

1. Which one of the following is *not* useful in providing radiation protection?

   a. Scheduling radiographs a few days apart so there is a time interval between exposures
   b. Shielding the client with lead aprons to protect uninvolved areas
   c. Having all personnel maintain distance when the x-ray machine is in use
   d. Making the exposure of the client as short as possible

2. The American Cancer Society's recommendation for the use of mammograms as screening devices for breast cancer is that all women have *annual* mammograms after age

   a. 35 b. 40
   c. 50 d. 60

3. Which of the following is an inappropriate action by a client?

   a. Asking for a lead apron to be used if dental x-rays are needed
   b. Carrying a card that lists all x-rays that have been performed
   c. Asking the physician to explain how x-rays will help with the diagnosis
   d. Refusing care until x-rays are obtained to validate any unexplained symptoms

4. Which of the following factors probably creates the least stress for a client undergoing a barium enema?

   a. Moving about on a hard x-ray table
   b. Being rushed through the x-ray procedure
   c. Darkness and noise during fluoroscopy
   d. Enemas or suppositories given before the test

5. General nursing implications for clients undergoing any type of radiologic test would *not* include

   a. Helping the client prepare for waiting by giving a magazine or other diversion
   b. Making sure that the client has slippers if he or she must stand during the test
   c. Instructing the client about any restrictions on food and fluids
   d. Listing the complications that may occur

6. General nursing implications when a client returns from a radiologic test would *not* include

   a. Offering a back rub to relieve the discomfort from lying on a hard table
   b. Encouraging extra fluids (if the pathophysiologic condition allows) if dye was used as a contrast medium
   c. Finding out if the client can eat, and if so, offering food as soon as possible
   d. Instructing the client to maintain bed rest for 4–6 hr

7. The specific gravity of urine will be unchanged after a client has undergone which one of the following x-ray tests

   a. KUB b. Cholangiography
   c. Arteriography d. IVP

8. Which of the following nursing actions should *not* be considered part of a routine procedure for a client who is undergoing portable chest radiography?

   a. Helping the client sit up as straight as possible before the radiograph is obtained
   b. Removing electrodes from the chest before the radiograph is obtained
   c. Helping the technician place the film holder behind the client's chest
   d. Holding the client in a fixed position while the radiograph is obtained

9. Sally is an adolescent who has a history of severe epigastric pain relieved by food or milk. Which of these nursing actions is routine when Sally undergoes an upper GI series (barium meal)?

a. Telling Sally to take nothing by mouth before the examination
b. Telling Sally that when fluoroscopy is performed (as the barium is swallowed) the room will be very bright
c. Giving an enema to Sally after radiography is completed
d. Informing Sally that the barium sulfate often causes diarrhea

10. Mr. Somorini is undergoing a barium enema because of slight rectal bleeding. Which of these nursing actions is *not* routine for a client undergoing a barium enema?

a. Administration of cathartics or suppositories the evening before the examination
b. Informing Mr. Somorini that he will need to hold the barium in the colon while a series of radiographs are taken
c. Giving a light diet the evening before the examination
d. Withholding food when Mr. Somorini comes back from the radiology department because a second set of radiographs is obtained in 3–4 hr

11. The nurse in the emergency department should be aware that a routine radiograph will most likely be the primary diagnostic tool for

a. Ricardo Lopez, 72 years of age, who has a fever and a productive cough
b. Ruth Tyler, 44 years of age, who has abdominal pain that occurs after eating a large amount of fats
c. Bobby, 8 years of age, who has acute pain in the right upper outer quadrant
d. Jason Bonehart, 21 years of age, who has a severe head injury from a motorcycle accident

12. Mr. Leonard has just returned to his hospital room after a femoral arteriogram. Which nursing action would be inappropriate?

a. Allowing him to stand if he cannot void in bed
b. Checking vital signs every 15 min for the first hour, then every 2 hr if vital signs are stable
c. Keeping an ice bag on the puncture site
d. Checking pedal pulses and the color and warmth of the feet when vital signs are taken

13. The possible need for a mild oral analgesic for procedure-related pain is least likely for a client undergoing

a. Mammography **b.** Arthrography
c. Small-bowel series **d.** Hystosalpingography

▼ REFERENCES

Alterescu, K. (1985). What about special procedures? *American Journal of Nursing, 85* (12), 1363–1367.

Barnett-Wilson, J. (1978). Patients' response to barium X-ray studies. *British Medical Journal, 1,* 6122.

Bassett, L.W., Henrick, R.E., Bassford, T.L., et al. (1994). High-quality mammography: Information for referring providers. Quick reference guide for clinicians No. 113. AHCPR Publication No. 95-0633. Rockville, MD: Agency for Health Care Policy and Research, Public Health Service, U.S. Department of Health and Human Services.

Berger, M., and Hübner, K. (1983). Hospital hazards: Diagnostic radiation. *American Journal of Nursing, 83* (9), 1155–1159.

Berkowitz, J.F., and Cassell, I. (1992). Diagnostic imaging: Special needs of older patients. *Geriatrics, 47* (3), 55–68.

Bush, W., et al. (1985). Adverse reactions to radiographic contrast material. *Western Journal of Medicine, 132,* 95.

Cruz, C., Hricak, H., Samhouri, F., et al. (1986). Contrast media for angiography: Effect on renal function. *Radiology, 158* (1), 109–112.

DeCherney, A.H., and Pernoll, M.L. (1994). *Current obstetric & gynecologic diagnosis & treatment.* (8th ed.). Norwalk, CT: Appleton & Lange.

Department of Health and Human Services. (1984). *Are routine chest x-rays really necessary?* HHS Publication No. 84-8205. Washington, DC: U.S. Government Printing Office.

Driscoll, J. (1989). Reducing exposure to radioactivity in the O.R. *Ethicon: Point of View, 26* (3), 4–6.

Fahey, V., and Finkelmeier, B. (1984). Iatrogenic arterial injuries. *American Journal of Nursing, 84* (4), 448–451.

Flam, B., Spice-Cheery, P., and Amsel, R. (1989). Effects of preparatory information for a myelogram on patients' expectations and anxiety levels. *Patient Education and Counseling, 14* (2), 115–126.

Food and Drug Administration. (1989). Warning added to labeling of iodinated contrast agents. *FDA Bulletin, 19* (2), 19.

Food and Drug Administration. (1995). Mammography quality deadline. *FDA Medical Bulletin, 25* (1), 3.

Gofman, J. (1987). What nurses need to know about ionizing radiation. *California Nurse, 83* (2), 6–7.

Gray, J. (1979). Radiation awareness and exposure reduction with audible monitors. *American Journal of Roentgenology, 133,* 1200–1201.

Hartfield, M., and Cason, C. (1981). Effects of information on emotional responses during barium enema. *Nursing Research, 30,* 151–155.

Henry, T. (1982). Radiation exposure and margins of safety. *California Nurse, 78* (11), 5–7.

Ingegno, M., Nahabedian, M., Tominaga, G.T., et al. (1994). Radiation exposure from cervical spine radiographs. *American Journal of Emergency Medicine, 12* (1), 15–16.

Jankowski, C. (1986). Radiation and pregnancy: Putting the risks in proportion. *American Journal of Nursing, 86* (3), 261–265.

Johnson, J., and Rice, V. (1974). Sensory and distress components of pain. *Nursing Research, 23,* 203–209.

Kerlikowske, K., Grady, D., Rubin, S.M., et al. (1995). Efficacy of screening mammography: A meta-analysis. *JAMA, 273* (2), 149–154.

Lauver, D. (1992). Addressing infrequent cancer screening among women. *Nursing Outlook, 40* (5), 207–212.

McHugh, N., et al. (1982). Preparatory information: What helps and why. *American Journal of Nursing, 82* (5), 780–782.

Murray, S., Preuss, M., and Schultz, T. (1992). How do you prep the bowel without enemas? *American Journal of Nursing, 92* (8), 66–67.

Nielsen, B., Miaskowski, C., and Dibble, S.L. (1993). Pain with mammography: Fact or fiction. *Oncology Nursing Forum, 20* (4), 639–642.

Sternberger, C. (1994). Breast self-examination: How nurses can influence performance. *MEDSURG Nursing, 3* (5), 367–371.

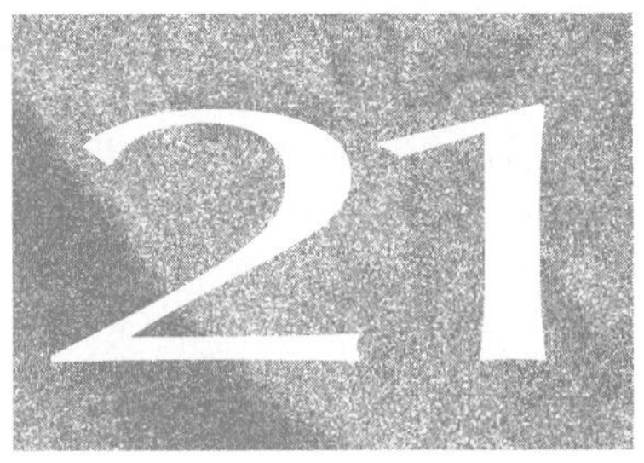

TOMOGRAPHY AND BODY SCANS

- Computed Tomography
- Magnetic Resonance Imaging
- Positron Emission Tomography
- Single Photon Emission Computed Tomography

OBJECTIVES

1. Discuss the basic advantages and disadvantages of computed tomography (CT), magnetic resonance imaging (MRI), positron emission tomography (PET) and single photon emission computed tomography (SPECT) as body scans.
2. Compare and contrast the preparations needed for infants, children, and adults who undergo various body scans.
3. Describe the usual preparations for CT scans with and without contrast medium.
4. Describe the special precautions needed for clients undergoing MRI.
5. Describe how PET and SPECT allow clinicians to examine metabolic functions rather than structure.
6. Identify priority nursing diagnoses for clients undergoing various types of scans.

Tomography is a method of body-section radiography. A specially designed x-ray machine and film holder move around the client in an arc, focusing at various angles, each with a slightly different depth. With each change in the angle of tomography, a selected body plane becomes sharply defined while the areas above and below the focal point become slightly blurred.

Computed tomography uses the principle of tomography with the addition of detectors, computers, and a scanner, which make possible a three-dimensional cross-sectional view of the body. The basic principles of computerized image reconstruction of an object are common to all four types of scans (CT, PET, SPECT, and MRI). On the horizon but still remote from clinical practice are other types of imaging, including microwave tomography, infrared imaging, and electron spin resonance imaging (Steiner, 1990).

Cormack, an American physicist, and Hounsfield, an English research engineer, working independently conducted the research that culminated in the development of CT. They shared the 1979 Nobel Prize for Physiology or Medicine. The Nobel committee acknowledged that no other method of x-ray diagnostics had led to such remarkable success in such a short time. Another type of body imaging, which uses a magnetic field and no radiation, MRI, became the success story of the 1980s. Boch and Purcell received a Nobel Prize in 1952 for the work that led to the development of MRI.

ADVANTAGES AND DISADVANTAGES

These sophisticated imaging modalities are noninvasive examinations that require a skilled technician to operate the machine. Much research is being conducted to compare the advantages and disadvantages of scans with those of invasive procedures (Chapter 25), sonography (Chapter 23), and radionuclide scans (Chapter 22) for assessing various pathophysiologic conditions. The advantage of the scans and MRI is the exquisite detail of the images. Now computers may be used to tie together the results of MRI and CT to give incredibly detailed pictures of all parts of the body.

CT does have two disadvantages. One is the cost of the test, which must be considered if other less expensive tests can provide satisfactory results. Although CT scans are expensive, the cost may be less than the combined charges for the tests they replace. The controversy about the cost of scans led to laws that made it necessary for institutions to certify the need for the machines. The second disadvantage of CT is the time of exposure to radiation. Although the amount of radiation is very small, all radiation exposure is cumulative through life. (See Chapter 20 for a detailed discussion on the role of the nurse in relation to the radiation hazards of repeated diagnostic tests.) Fear of radiation is easily evoked, so it is important that clinicians realize that the radiation dose from high-resolution chest CT is actually less than that for conventional CT and only slightly more than that for chest radiograph (van der Bruggen-Bogaarts et al., 1995).

MRI does not create any radiation exposure, but it costs more than CT and is not available in all health care settings. As noted later, some clients must not enter the MRI area because of problems that can arise from the presence of ferromagnetic materials in the imager. Compared with CT, MRI excels in demonstration of some pathologic conditions, such as those of the central nervous system. Artifacts of bone do not interfere with MRI as they may with CT.

PET and SPECT have the advantage of detailing metabolic function rather than structure. Both require minute amounts of radioisotopes, so radiation exposure is minimal. At present, PET is available only in large medical centers and is very expensive. SPECT is more widely available; a brain scan costs about the same as a CT brain scan (Souder and Alavi, 1995).

If angiography with contrast medium is part of a CT scan, the risks associated with the dyes must be acknowledged. (See Chapter 20 on nursing precautions with contrast medium.) The type of contrast medium used with MRI does not have as great a disadvantage as that used with CT. The radioisotopes used with PET and SPECT do not cause untoward reactions.

▼ COMPUTED TOMOGRAPHY

Description. *CT*, *CAT scan*, and *EMI scan* all refer to the use of what used to be called *computerized axial tomography*. The EMI scanner was developed by Electrical and Musical Industries, a British-based group of international companies (Seeram, 1976). The preferred term is *computed tomography* (CT), which produces a *CT scan*.

A CT scan is obtained with an x-ray machine that rotates 180 degrees around the client's head or body. Detectors read the amount of radiation each body tissue or organ absorbs. A computer processes these readings and converts them to an image shown on a screen and stored on disks. The resulting pictures show a three-dimensional cross section of all body parts. A CT scan divides each area of tissue being viewed into an area 3 mm square and 13 mm thick for most imaging examinations. The results are available in a few minutes. A CT scan can depict almost all types of tissue except nerves. In older scans of the head, the client's head was fitted in a rubber bag so there was no cushion of air between the hair and scalp. This is not necessary with the newer scans.

A CT scan, a noninvasive procedure, causes no pain. The client simply lies still while the machine goes around the body. As emphasized before, no risks are entailed, other than being exposed to a small amount of radiation. The procedure takes 15–30 min. If contrast medium is used, the procedure takes 30–60 min, and there are the usual risks associated with an iodine contrast medium.

Purposes. Around 1972, the first CT scans were used for identifying brain abnormalities and head injuries (Pohutsky and Pohutsky, 1975). CT was found to be much more valuable in diagnosing problems in the brain than the older x-ray tests such as pneumoencephalograms or cerebral arteriograms. The details available with a CT scan are remarkable. For example, a CT scan can clearly show if a brain abscess is becoming smaller after treatment with antibiotics. CT scans are also used to locate foreign objects in soft tissue, such as the eyes. For example, a piece of metal lodged in an eyeball can be precisely mapped out so the surgeon has to do much less probing. Intracranial lesions, such as neoplasms or hematomas, can be located without a craniotomy. The surgeon thus has a much better understanding of the location and extent of brain disease before performing an operation.

Body scanners, which came into use later than head scanners, in 1976, had a less dramatic impact. Controversy arose about how many CT scanners were needed in one community, and if each hospital needs a machine. There was also a debate about whether a body scan offered more diagnostic help than other less expensive diagnostic tests (van Dyk et al., 1980). Since that time, CT body scans have become an integral part of health care and may be the first line test for evaluating malignant neoplasms of solid organs as well as unexplained masses, abscess collections, and trauma (Berkowitz and Cassell, 1992).

Cine CT can provide moving images of the heart. This ultrafast scan can also be used to measure blood flow to the brain and to look at airways in newborns.

Coronary Artery Screening. Ultrafast CT is highly sensitive in detecting calcium in coronary arteries, a possibly useful marker for the presence of coronary atherosclerosis. Healthy arteries do not show calcium deposits, but small amounts of calcification may occur with aging. A normal screening virtually rules out clinically significant atherosclerosis, particularly in young people. An abnormal scan does not have a specific correlation with critical coronary artery stenosis, although more calcium usually means more widespread atherosclerosis (Wong et al., 1994). The use of coronary artery screening is being investigated at several research centers, and the procedure is available for clinical use.

▼ PRETEST NURSING DIAGNOSES RELATED TO CT

Knowledge Deficit Related to Preparation for a Head Scan

Unless contrast medium is to be used, the client can eat and drink before the examination. Some clinicians may even allow clear liquids if a dye is to be used. Wigs and any objects in the hair, such as bobby pins, are removed. The client can be assured that the procedure is not painful and is much like putting one's head in a hair dryer. Although CT is not painful, the thought of having one's head immobilized can be frightening. The person must lie still during the procedure. A two-way intercom allows communication with the radiology personnel. (See the discussion on claustrophobia in the section on MRI.)

Radiopaque dye may be given intravenously to outline the cerebral vessels. If dye is given, the client may need preparation. (See Chapter 20 on how to prepare for reactions to dye, which include flushing and possible allergic reaction.)

Risk for Ineffective Coping of Children and Confused Adults

One suggestion is to encourage a child to play at home by lying still with head flexed toward chest. The parent can dim the lights in the room and move an arm around the child's motionless head. By humming softly, parents give children an idea of the sounds they will hear during the test. Children should be taught that they can open and close their eyes but not move their head. This preparation may work for children older than 3 years. Infants sleep during the procedure if kept awake and then fed just before the test. The greatest problems is with toddlers and confused adults: Sedation may be required. (See Chapter 27 for a discussion of adverse reactions to sedatives.)

Knowledge Deficit Related to Preparation for CT Body Scans

Scans of the thorax or pelvic region may or may not require special preparation. The nurse must ask the radiologist what specific preparations are required. A tampon may be used as a vaginal marker. The client may be required to have a full or empty bladder. A contrast medium may be given to outline various organs. Low-density barium solutions and dilute water-soluble iodinated contrast materials are used (Ball et al., 1986). The client must be assessed for allergies and prepared for a flushing sensation and possible nausea (Chapter 20). However, some of the newer contrast media made for CT scans contain less than 10% of the iodine found in older products. The client may eat a low-residue diet for a few days before the examination. Intestinal preparations vary in importance with the various parts of the body being scanned. Contrast medium can be given by means of enema. Drugs may be used to decrease peristalsis during the test, including propantheline and glucagon. Synthetic cholecystokin (Sincalide) may also be given to increase peristalsis to cause filling of the gastrointestinal (GI) tract with swallowed contrast medium. These medications are given during the procedure and require an intravenous injection. If a biopsy is planned, guided by the scan, the general nursing implications (Chapter 25) for invasive procedures should be heeded.

▼ POSTTEST NURSING IMPLICATIONS RELATED TO CT

There are no specific nursing implications related to the scanning procedure. If a radiopaque dye has been given, the nursing implications about dye should be followed. (See the general nursing diagnoses discussed in Chapter 20.) The nurse must be aware of any sedatives or other drugs given as part of the procedure because untoward effects from drugs are always possible. (See the discussion of the side effects of medications used for endoscopic procedures in Chapter 27.) If invasive procedures were performed, vital signs and the other assessments described in Chapter 25 are appropriate.

▼ MAGNETIC RESONANCE IMAGING

Description. MRI uses a huge magnet and radio waves to produce an energy field that can be transferred to a visual image. Use of the older term, *nuclear magnetic resonance* (NMR), was discontinued in 1984. The word *nuclear* may be frightening to clients because it may conjure up a vision of the nuclear fission of the atomic bomb. Nuclear in the sense of NMR simply refers to the dense core of the atom. Not only is the test not related to atomic bombs, it does not involve any kind of radiation hazard. Clark (1983) noted that perhaps NMR should stand for *no more radiation*. The richness of detail of the images without the use of contrast medium and the lack of radiation hazard are advantages of MRI over CT. MRI costs about one-third more than CT.

The huge magnet in the imager produces a magnetic field. The magnetic field causes atoms in the tissues and more particularly the nuclei of the hydrogen ions to line up in a parallel configuration. When the technician pushes a switch, radio waves are sent into the magnetic field and the lined-up ions pick up some of this energy. When the radio wave is switched off, the atoms revert back to their lined-up configuration influenced by the magnet. The change in the energy field is sensed and converted to a visual display on a computer screen.

The entire MRI machine must be enclosed in a room to protect the image from interference with outside radio signals. The magnetic field around the imager is always present and stops watches, erases credit cards, and even pulls stethoscopes out of pockets. In an emergency, the magnet can be turned off, but it is expensive to restart it. MRI disrupts some intravenous drip regulators, but others may not be affected (Engler and Engler, 1986). Special routine and emergency equipment compatible with MRI have been developed, but may not be generally available. Thus, a client may have to be moved out of the MRI room for resuscitation. If a ventilator-dependent client needs an MRI, an alternative to the MRI-compatible ventilator is the use of extended ventilator tubing and the presence of a critical care nurse and a respiratory therapist (Rotello et al., 1994). Many articles have been written about the potential projectile effects of numerous ferromagnetic items, including one that warns that guns could be accidentally discharged by the force of the magnet in the MRI suite (Kanal and Shaibani, 1994).

The client is put on a moving pallet that is pushed into the large cylinder that contains the magnet. As the radio signals are switched off and on the client hears a variety of noises. The sound has been described as initially like the slow beat of an Indian drum and then with abrupt stops and starts like a muffled jackhammer (Osaki et al., 1985). Ear plugs are available if the client wishes them. MacPhie (1983) noted the sounds as dull and lulling and then sometimes as thunderous bombardments, but at no time unbearable.

Purposes. Although the MRI is relatively expensive, the detailed scan may be well worth it. In March 1985, Blue Shield of California approved payments for MRI and thus paved the way for Medicare also to consider the test no longer only an experimental or research tool. MRI can do some things CT cannot. For example, MRI not only clearly defines internal organ structure but also helps detect changes in tissue such as edema or infarcts. Blood flow patterns and detailed information on blood vessel integrity can give an earlier warning than ever before of developing atherosclerotic disease (Marchette and Holloman, 1985). Because of the lack of bone artifacts, MRI can help identify tumors in the pituitary gland (Glaser et al., 1986).

Another use of MRI is to differentiate normal kidney tissue from acute tubular necrosis (ATN) and acute rejection in a transplanted kidney. Ultrafast MRI, called *cine MRI,* can produce a complete image of the heart at the rate of 30–40 images *per* one heart beat. Conventional MRI produces an image about every 1 or 2 sec. Cine MRI, like cine CT, is really a movie of the heart.

Advances in MRI hardware and software have resulted in better resolution and faster screening techniques. For example, MRI may be a sensitive imaging technique for high-resolution images of great-vessel anatomy and for mapping of blood vessel flow. The results may be very close to actual cardiac catheterization measurements (Hardy et al., 1994). Perfusion imaging is faster than that done with PET, which is discussed later. Abdominal screening has been improved by techniques for fat suppression. As MRI use continues to grow, methods for storage and transmittal of data are being developed to establish diagnostic networks. Images from different clinics can be sent to one point where experts can view the images and send back a report (Angelidis, 1994).

▼ PRETEST NURSING DIAGNOSES RELATED TO MRI

Knowledge Deficit Related to Needed Preparation

Watches, tapes, and credit cards are damaged by the magnetic field; therefore, clients must shed these items. Clients must also remove jewelry, clothing with metal fasteners, and hair clips. Objects containing ferrous metal produce artifacts. Also, the movement of the object can be detrimental to the client. For example, clients who have metal implants such as surgical clips, heart valves, or orthopedic clips cannot undergo MRI because the magnet may move the object within the body. Implantable ports made from stainless steel may produce artifacts during MRI. Titanium ports reportedly produce minimal artifacts, but this should be checked with the imaging department. Artificial joints that are not ferrous present no problems. Clients should also be asked about any injuries that could have left some metal embedded in a sensitive place such as an eye. Any movement of even a small fragment could cause permanent damage. Clients may feel odd sensations from dental work in their teeth if a filling or a bridge contains ferrous material. The machine can deactivate pacemakers, so clients with pacemakers cannot undergo MRI.

The nurse should check with the MRI department to determine if contrast medium is to be used because the material may affect whether the client needs

(*continued*)

▼ PRETEST NURSING DIAGNOSES RELATED TO MRI (*continued*)

to have any food or beverage restrictions. Various oral contrast agents, including barium sulfate, antacids, or supplements such as Geritol, which contains iron, may be used to improve the contrast between the GI tract and the surrounding organs. Glucagon may be given to decrease peristalsis. Blueberry juice, rich in manganese, is an inexpensive and effective oral contrast agent (Hiraishi et al., 1995). Drugs such as gadoteridol (Prohance) and gadopentetate dimeglumine (Magnevist) are given intravenously to increase the detectability of some lesions. Unlike the iodinated contrast media used for CT, these agents are not commonly associated with adverse reactions, but nausea and taste disturbances may occur.

Many scans take as long as 45 min to an hour so the client should void before entering the cylinder.

Anxiety Related to Feelings of Claustrophobia

Hricak and Amparo (1984) found a 1–5% incidence of claustrophobia in adults undergoing MRI and that using the prone position so the client could see out reduced the claustrophobia. Other measures to decrease claustrophobia are visualization of peaceful scenes or other relaxation techniques. One nurse recalled prepared childbirth exercises and thus was able to overcome her initial claustrophobia and anxiety (Marchette and Holloman, 1985). Special prism glasses are available so a client can have a view outside the cylinder. Also some cylinders are now made of see-through plastic material.

Osaki et al. (1985) conducted a descriptive study to assess the perceptions of 45 children and their parents of the MRI experience. Some parents were concerned about claustrophobia. Both children and their parents emphasized the benefit of sensation information and liked that there were no shots or intravenous catheters (some injectable sedation may be used for the young). Having the parent present was another advantage during the procedure. Parents may read or talk to the child, because there is no risk of radiation from the procedure. (Parents must be debriefed about watches, credit cards, and such, which may be damaged by the magnet).

Because clients must lie still for a long time, young children and very anxious adults may need sedation. Drugs do not interfere with the examination.

▼ POSTTEST NURSING IMPLICATIONS RELATED TO MRI

There is no special aftercare of the client. (See the discussion in Chapter 20 on the anxiety related to waiting for results that may take 1–2 days.) Although there are no known hazards from the test, clients with tumors may be concerned about any possible effect on the tumor (MacPhie, 1983).

▼ POSITRON EMISSION TOMOGRAPHY

Description. The PET scanner is the latest in diagnostic imaging equipment. Until recently, CT and MRI were used to diagnose internal problems, but they primarily looked at the structure of the body. PET and SPECT give additional information because they measure the functions of the body. More than 50 PET cameras have been operating in the United States since 1980, most in research centers, but many are now being considered for clinical use. Reimbursement by insurance companies is on a case-by-case basis because PET costs about one-third more than MRI.

For PET studies, the client receives an injection of a biochemical substance tagged with a radionuclide, which emits positrons. PET used to be limited to institutions with access to a cyclotron for the production of the special isotopes. However, one isotope, rubidium-82, has the advantage of being produced by a generator rather than by a cyclotron (Zaret and Wackers, 1993). When the radioactive particles combine with the negatively charged electrons normally found in the cells of tissue, they emit gamma rays that can be detected with a scanning device. The PET scanner translates the emissions into color-coded images. For example, radioactive glucose can be used to map biochemical activity in the brain. The half-life of the isotopes used is short, so there is minimal radiation dosage. The radiation is usually less than one-fourth that of a CT scan. However, the gamma rays that are the byproduct of all positron-emitting isotopes are more penetrating than the type of gamma rays emitted by other isotopes (Chapter 22), so thicker shields are used for the holders and containers (Daghighian et al., 1990).

Purposes. PET, as a measure of brain activity, is used to study the effects of stroke, epilepsy, migraine headache, Parkinson's disease, dementia, and other disorders, such as schizophrenia. PET studies of the heart have three general uses. First, and perhaps most important, is assessment of myocardial viability. Other uses are to measure regional myocardial perfusion and to assess cardiac metabolism (Zaret and Wackers, 1993). PET may also be used to evaluate malignant tumors. Theoretically, any physiologic substance can be tagged and traced as it is metabolized in the body. Much research is being undertaken to make these theoretic possibilities real.

▼ PRETEST NURSING IMPLICATIONS RELATED TO PET

Some scans require avoidance of food and fluids, others do not. Alcohol, caffeine, and nicotine should be withheld for most types of scans. Check with the radiology department about any medications to be used or temporarily discontinued. Two intravenous lines may be needed, one for serial arterial blood samples and one for intravenous injection of the isotope. The client should void because the scan may require more than 1 hour.

(*continued*)

▼ PRETEST NURSING IMPLICATIONS RELATED TO PET (*continued*)

For some types of cardiac scans, the client uses a treadmill or exercise bicycle (Schultz et al., 1991). (See Chapter 26 for more information about stress tests.) For brain scans, blindfolds and earplugs are used to reduce external stimuli to the brain. For some PET brain scans the client may be asked to recite passages or perform other intellectual tests to see how the brain activity changes with remembering or reasoning. Lights or other stimuli may be used to stimulate the brain.

▼ POSTTEST NURSING IMPLICATIONS RELATED TO PET

See Chapter 22 for the discussion of general nursing implications for intravenous radioisotopes, such as (1) observing the site for phlebitis, (2) relieving anxiety, and (3) encouraging ingestion of fluids to hasten urinary excretion of the isotope.

▼ SINGLE PHOTON EMISSION COMPUTED TOMOGRAPHY

Unlike PET, which uses a radiopharmaceutical labeled with a positron-emitting isotope, SPECT uses several of the common radionuclides discussed in Chapter 22 that are commercially prepared. SPECT is becoming readily available in hospitals of all sizes. A brain SPECT costs about as much as a CT brain scan.

SPECT has become the scan of choice for a diagnostic evaluation for dementia and some other types of central nervous system disorders (Souder and Alavi, 1995). SPECT is used to measure blood perfusion in the brain, in contrast to the neuronal uptake of glucose in PET. The reader is encouraged to consult current literature for advances in the use of SPECT and other types of imaging.

▼ PRETEST AND POSTTEST NURSING IMPLICATIONS RELATED TO SPECT

There are no restrictions on food or fluids. (See Chapter 22 on general nursing implications for clients receiving radionuclides.)

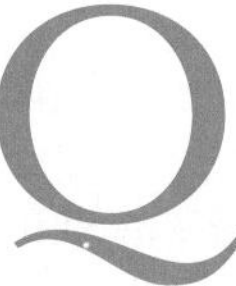

1. Which of the following is the main disadvantage of CT scans as compared with MRI or ultrasound procedures?

   a. The number of personnel needed to run the machine
   b. The amount of preparation required for the client
   c. The amount of radiation exposure to the client
   d. The lack of detailed images

2. The priority nursing intervention after a client is finished with a body scan is to assess

   a. Vital signs because of possible adverse effects, such as bleeding
   b. Level of anxiety related to outcome of procedure
   c. Pain level caused by the procedure
   d. Effects of radiation, such as nausea

3. Which one of the following would be *inappropriate* for a 3-year-old child who is undergoing CT head scanning that does not involve the use of any contrast medium?

   a. Nothing-by-mouth status for 3–4 hr before the examination
   b. Use of sedation 30 min before the test
   c. Removal of bobby pins or other items in the hair
   d. Have the child practice keeping his or her head still while a humming noise is made

4. Some types of CT scans require specific client preparations. Which of the following types of CT scan requires the most physical preparation of the client?

   a. Brain scans **b.** Pelvic scans **c.** Thoracic scans **d.** Abdominal scans

5. Nursing implications related to the use of intravenous radioisotopes are appropriate for a client undergoing

   a. MRI **b.** PET
   c. CT **d.** Tomography

6. Mr. Lagerquist is scheduled for MRI today. Which of the following is an essential part of pretest teaching?

   a. Mr. Lagerquist will have an intravenous infusion started before the examination
   b. Any objects containing ferrous metal interfere with the test

c. Food and fluids are withheld for 4–6 hr before the test
d. Mr. Lagerquist may turn side-to-side during the scan, but he must not sit

7. In educating a client about the sensations of MRI the nurse would *not* need to prepare the client for the possibility of

a. A strange feeling around tooth fillings
b. Slight redness of the skin
c. A variety of noises, some rather loud
d. Claustrophobia or a closed-in feeling

▼ REFERENCES

Angelidis, P.A. (1994). MR image compression using a wavelet transform coding algorithm. *Magnetic Resonance Imaging, 12* (7), 1111–1112.

Ball, D.S., Radecki, P.D., Freidman, A.C., et al. (1986). Contrast medium preparation during abdominal CT. *Radiology, 158* (1), 258–260.

Berkowitz, J.F., and Cassell, I. (1992). Diagnostic imaging: Special needs of older patients. *Geriatrics, 47* (3), 55–68.

Clark, M. (1983). NMR = No more radiation? *American Journal of Nursing, 83* (9), 1371–1372.

Daghighian, F., Sumida, R., and Phelps, M. (1990). PET imaging: An overview and instrumentation. *Journal of Nuclear Medical Technology, 13* (1), 5–13.

Engler, M., and Engler, M. (1986). Hazards of magnetic resonance imaging. *American Journal of Nursing, 86* (6), 650.

Glaser, B., et al. (1986). Magnetic resonance imaging of the pituitary gland. *Clinical Radiology, 37* (1), 9–14.

Hardy, C.E., Helton, G.J., Kondo, C., et al. (1994). Usefulness of magnetic resonance imaging for evaluating great-vessel anatomy after arterial switch operation for D-transposition of the great arteries. *American Heart Journal, 128,* 326–332.

Hiraishi, K., Narabayashi, I., Fujita, O., et al. (1995). Blueberry juice: Preliminary evaluation as an oral contrast agent in gastrointestinal MR imaging. *Radiology, 194,* 119–123.

Hricak, H., and Amparo, E. (1984). Body MRI: Alleviation of claustrophobia by prone positioning. *Radiology, 152* (3), 819.

Kanal, E., and Shaibani, A. (1994). Firearm safety in the MR imaging environment. *Radiology, 193,* 875–876.

MacPhie, C. (1983). Apudoma, NMR imager and me. *California Nurse, 79* (6), 8.

Marchette, L., and Holloman, F. (1985). A first-hand report on the new body scanners. *RN, 48* (11), 28–31.

Osaki, L., Tessler, M., and Higgins, S. (1985). The ABC's of your child having a MRI. San Francisco: University of California Department of Radiology.

Pohutsky, L., and Pohutsky, K. (1975). Computerized axial tomography of the brain: A new diagnostic tool. *American Journal of Nursing,* 75 (8), 1341–1342.

Rotello, L.C., Radin, E.J., Jastremski, M.S., et al. (1994). MRI protocol for critically ill patients. *American Journal of Critical Care, 3* (3), 187–190.

Schultz, S.J., Foley, C.R., and Gordon, D.G. (1991). Preparing your patient for a cardiac PET scan. *Nursing 91, 21,* 63–64.

Seeram, E. (1976). The EMI scanner. *Canadian Nurse, 72* (11), 40–42.

Souder, E., and Alavi, A. (1995). A comparison of neuroimaging modalities for diagnosing dementia. *Nurse Practitioner, 20* (1), 66–74.

Steiner, R. (1990). Radiology at the crossroads. *Clinical Radiology, 42,* 161–163.

van der Bruggen-Bogaarts, B.A., Broerse, J.J., Lammers, J.J., et al. (1995). Radiation exposure in standard and high-resolution chest CT scans. *Chest, 107* (1), 113–115.

van Dyk, J., et al. (1980). On the impact of CT scanning on radiotherapy planning. *Computerized Tomography, 4,* 55–65.

Wong, N.D., Vo, W., Abrahamson, D., et al. (1994). Detection of coronary artery calcium by ultrafast computed tomography and its relation to clinical evidence of coronary artery disease. *American Journal of Cardiology, 73,* 223–227.

Zaret, B.L., and Wackers, F.J. (1993). Nuclear cardiology. *New England Journal of Medicine, 329* (12), 855–863.

DIAGNOSTIC TESTS WITH RADIONUCLIDES OR RADIOISOTOPES

- Bone Scans
- Brain Scans
- Gallium Scans
- Indium Scans or Leukocyte Imaging
- Gallbladder Scans
- Gastrointestinal Scans
- Liver and Spleen Scans
- Lung Scans—Perfusion Images and Ventilation Studies
- Cardiac Scans
- Renal Scans
- Thyroid Scans
- RAI Uptake Study
- Compatibility and Red Blood Cell Survival
- Blood Volume Studies
- Schilling Test

OBJECTIVES

1. Differentiate between the use of common radionuclides for diagnostic testing and for therapy.
2. Compare and contrast the procedures used for in vitro and in vivo testing.
3. Explain why pregnant women and children are advised not to undergo radionuclide studies if other nonradioactive tests can suffice.

4. State the general nursing implications for preparing a client for any organ scan with technetium (Tc-99m).
5. State the principal use of a bone scan performed with radionuclides.
6. Explain the purpose of a gallium scan in a client with a fever of undetermined origin.
7. Plan a teaching program for a client who is to undergo a radioactive iodine uptake study in 2 weeks.
8. Explain the purpose of administration of potassium iodine before an iodine-125 (I-125) scan for sites other than the thyroid.
9. Describe the nursing functions when a client undergoes a Schilling test.

The terms *radionuclide* and *radioisotope* are both used to describe the radiopharmaceuticals used for diagnostic tests in the nuclear medicine department. Often in general practice, the older term *radioisotope* is still used. However, recent literature uses the more precise term *radionuclides*, and this term is used in this chapter. The term *radionuclide* conveys that the element has a nucleus that has been made radioactive.

In diagnostic nuclear medicine, the radionuclide is given to the client and the radiation emitted from a particular organ is measured. The basic rationale for the use of radionuclides is to observe the function—not the structure—of an organ. However, PET and its cousin, SPECT, do assess both structure and function because radionuclides and a sophisticated computer are used to record and plot the effect of the radioactive substance in the body. PET and SPECT are discussed in Chapter 21.

RADIONUCLIDES AS RADIOACTIVE ELEMENTS

Radiation occurs where there is a lack of stability in the nuclei of atoms. As the atom spontaneously disintegrates, radiation is emitted in the form of α-, β-, and γ-rays. Some of the synthetic radionuclides are purified so that only γ-rays are emitted. About 50 of the roughly 350 isotopes of all elements in nature are naturally radioactive. Isotopes of an element are slightly different molecular forms of the same chemical element. The discovery that certain natural elements were radioactive was made in 1896 by Becquerel, who was working with uranium compounds. In 1903, Becquerel shared a Nobel prize with Marie Curie and Pierre Curie, who discovered another naturally occurring radioactive substance, radium. The unit used to measure the activity of radionuclides is the curie (Ci) named in honor of the Curies. The SI unit is the becquerel (Bq; 1 Ci = 37 gigabecquerels [GBq]).

In the early part of the 20th century, scientists discovered that it was possible to make naturally nonradioactive elements radioactive by bombarding the nucleus with subatomic fragments to make it unstable. The invention of the cyclotron (atom smasher) in 1931 made it possible to make many elements radioactive. Some of these synthetic radionuclides, such as iodine-131 (I-131), have been used extensively for therapy and diagnostic testing. Therapy with I-131 for cancer of the thyroid was begun in 1943—a time when both peaceful and war uses of nuclear products were being explored. The use of I-131 for cancer of the thyroid was dubbed the "atomic cocktail" (Myers and Wagner, 1974). Because of the length of its half-life, I-131 is infrequently used for diagnostic tests. Newer shorter-lived substances have replaced I-131, as discussed later.

USE OF RADIONUCLIDES AS THERAPEUTIC AGENTS

This chapter focuses on the use of radionuclides for diagnostic tests, but it should be pointed out that radionuclides are also used frequently in therapy. Two commonly used radionuclides are I-131, used to treat some cases of thyroid cancer and hyperthyroidism, and phosphorous-32 (P-32), used to treat malignant neoplasms that produce pleural and peritoneal effusions. P-32 is also used to treat polycythemia vera and other myeloproliferative disorders in adults.

METHODS OF DIAGNOSTIC TESTING WITH RADIONUCLIDES

In Vitro Testing

With in vitro testing (sample testing), the radionuclide is given intravenously or orally, and at a later date, samples are taken from the blood or urine. Blood volume studies, red blood cell (RBC) studies, and the Schilling test are examples of tests that use samples, not scans, to measure radionuclides. Sample tests are discussed at the end of this chapter, with specific points about nursing implications. Although radioactive iodine uptake testing (RAI) may also involve the collection of urine samples, it is primarily an in vivo test because the radioactivity of the thyroid gland is measured with a counter. Table 22–1 lists in vitro sampling tests. Many other laboratory tests such as those for antibodies (Chapter 14) and hormones (Chapter 15) are in vitro tests that use radionuclides for tagging the substance to be measured.

TABLE 22–1. IN VITRO SAMPLING TESTS

Test	Example of Radionuclide Used	Timing of Test After Dosage	Special Preparation
Red blood cells (RBCs)			
Compatibility	Cr-51	1 hr	Blood drawn from client, then re-injected after tagged
Survival and sequestration	Cr-51	3–4 wk	Blood samples drawn 2–3 times a week
Blood volume studies			Blood drawn from client, then re-injected after tagged
RBC plasma volume	Cr-51 Radioiodinated human serum albumin (RIHSA)		Record height and weight Must have normal hydration
Schilling test (test for absorption of vitamin B_{12})	Vitamin B_{12} tagged with Co-57 (oral)		Nothing-by-mouth status before test; urine saved for 24 hr; see text for details, such as intramuscular administration of vitamin B_{12} by nurse

Co, cobalt; Cr, chromium.

In Vivo Testing

The in vivo method (organ scan or scintigram) of measuring the amount of radionuclide in the body is performed by means of organ scanning. Table 22–2 lists in vivo tests. The scan of an organ is referred to as a scintigram because a scintillation camera is used to make a scan or picture. The scintillation camera, which came into use in 1964, has made testing with radionuclides a very useful method of

TABLE 22–2. IN VIVO TESTING (ORGAN SCANS OR SCINTISCANS)

Scan	Examples of Radionuclides Type and Route	Timing of Scan After Dosage	Special Preparation
Bone	Tc-99m tagged phosphate compounds (IV)	Immediately and 2–4 hr (takes 1 hr to scan entire body)	Push fluids 2–4 hr before Void before ?Intestinal preparation
Brain			
Perfusion	Tc-99m pertechnetate (IV)	Immediately	None
Static views	Tc-99m glucoheptenate (IV)	Immediately 15 min 1–4 hr	None
	Radioiodinated human serum albumin (RIHSA) (IV)	18–48 hr	None
Functional	IMP or HMPAO	Varies	None
Cardiac			
For infarction	Tc-99m pyrophosphate (IV)	90 min–3 hr	See text
Perfusion scan	(Th-201) (IV)	3–5 min; also in 3–6 hr	See discussion of dipyridamole and stress tests
Ejection–fraction studies	Albumin or red blood cells tagged with Tc-99m	Immediate with first pass analysis	
Gated cardiac pool imaging	Same as above	Continuous over 1–2 hr	See text
Gastrofunctional studies	Tc-99m sulfur colloid	Varies with part of GI tract studied	Maintain nothing-by-mouth status. See text about medications
Hepatobiliary			
Liver and spleen (reticuloendothelial cells)	Tc-99m sulfur colloid	10–15 min	None
Gallbladder	Tc-99m with HIDA or PIPIDA (IV) Tc-99m DISIDA (IV) (Hepatolite)	Immediate and intervals to 24 hr	Maintain nothing-by-mouth status for 2 hr before Fat restriction during time of test
Lung	Tc-99m with albumin (IV)	15 min	None
Perfusion	Xe-133 (inhalation)	Immediate	None
Ventilation	Kr-85 (inhalation)	Immediate	None
Renal[a]			
Perfusion	Tc-99m DTPA, DSMA Glucoheptanate (IV)	Immediate (20 min)	Hydrate as ordered
Static views	As above	Up to 4 hr	

TABLE 22–2. (*Continued*)

Scan	Examples of Radionuclides Type and Route	Timing of Scan After Dosage	Special Preparation
Function	I-131 or I-123 tagged to orthoiodohippurate (IV)	Immediate and up to 1 hr as continual scan	Hydrate as ordered Potassium iodide solution as ordered
Thyroid screening	Tc-99m pertechnetate (IV) I-123 (oral)	30 min 24 hr	No prep Maintain nothing-by-mouth status 8 hr before No iodine for 4 wk pretest and 2 hr posttest
RAI (radioactive iodine uptake)	I-123 or I-131 (oral)	2 hr, 6 hr, 24 hr	As above; see text
Total body scans			
Inflammatory lesions and neoplasms	Gallium citrate, Ga-67 (IV)	4–6 hr and 24–72 hr or longer (up to 5 days)	Usually needs intestinal preparation
Inflammatory only	Tagged leukocytes with In-111 (IV)	4–24 hr	None
Thyroid malignancy	I-131	3–7 days	See text

HMPAO, Tc-99m exametazine; IMP, I-123 iodoamphetamine; In, indium; IV, intravenous; Kr, krypton; Th, thallium; Xe, xenon.

[a]A triple renal study uses two IV injections to obtain perfusion, static views, and excretory function of the kidney.

diagnostic testing. The client is given a radionuclide compound (radiopharmaceutical) intravenously, orally, or by inhalation, depending on the organ to be scanned. Minutes or hours later, or sometimes the following day, the scintillation camera takes a radioactivity reading from the target organ and feeds these readings into a computer. The computer translates these readings into a two-dimensional image or scan. The scintigram is printed in a gray scale so there is more variation than in a black-and-white picture. Scintigrams may also be produced in color. These varying shades of gray or color show the relative distribution of the radionuclide in the different parts of the organ. Very dark spots on the scintigram are called *hot spots* because more of the radionuclide was deposited in that spot. Parts of the tissue that do not pick up the radionuclide are seen as light-colored areas. Spots without radionuclide uptake are *cold spots* or *cold nodules*. The scintigram is interpreted by a physician trained in nuclear medicine, and a written report of the scan is put in the client's chart. Some common findings on scintigrams are discussed for each scan in this chapter. In general, imaging with radionuclides is most useful where there is disturbance of function rather than a structural defect.

Types of Radionuclides Used in Diagnostic Testing

In the past, I-131 was used not only for diagnosis of and therapy for thyroid disorders but also as a radioactive tag carried to other organs. For example, rose bengal can be tagged with I-131. When the rose bengal is excreted by the liver into the biliary tract, the radioactive substance outlines the hepatobiliary system. Other forms of iodine are also used as radionuclides, including I-123, which has a half-life of 13 hr compared with a half-life of 8 days for I-131. (The importance of half-life is discussed in the section on hazards.) Other radionuclides, such as gallium and thallium, are used for certain types of scanning. Sodium chromate (Cr-51) is used to tag RBCs, and cobalt (Co-57) is used to tag vitamin B_{12} for the Schilling test. Although various radionuclides are useful for certain tests, Tc-99m is the most commonly used for nuclear medicine diagnostic testing.

Technetium

There are several isotopes of technetium, and all are naturally radioactive. A very unstable form of technetium, Tc-99m, has a half-life of only 6 hr (Bettelheim and March, 1991). Tc-99m is combined with various compounds that carry the radionuclide to various target organs. For example, bone uses most of the phosphorus in the body, so Tc-99m combined with pyrophosphate is used for a bone scan. Technetium-99m combined with albumin is used as a lung scan because the radio-tagged albumin disperses in the pulmonary precapillary arterioles. Other compounds can carry Tc-99m to other specific organs, such as the hepatobiliary system, thyroid, or brain. If Tc-99m is given without another compound (straight), it is excreted in the urine and in the saliva. Thus, straight Tc-99m can be used to study the parotid glands or immediate flow through the cerebral vessels. Tc-99m is always administered intravenously. The timing of the scans after the administration of the radionuclide depends on the target organ to be viewed. Some organs may take up the substance in a few hours so scans are performed relatively soon, whereas others may not be completed for 24 hr or longer. RBCs can be tagged with Tc-99m to help diagnose gastrointestinal (GI) bleeding.

RADIATION HAZARDS FROM RADIONUCLIDES

The radiation hazard from radionuclide diagnostic testing is very slight because the doses used are usually very small. Also, duration is brief because of the short half-life of the radionuclides used. It was mentioned earlier that the curie (Ci) is the unit used to measure the activity of radionuclides. The curie is based on the radioactivity of a standard gram of radium. The dosages used in therapy are in millicurie (mCi) levels (0.001 Ci). In contrast, dosage levels for the radiopharmaceuticals used for diagnostic testing are in microcurie (μCi) levels (0.001 mCi). Thus, the radiation from diagnostic testing is roughly a thousand times less than with therapy (Rummerfield and Rummerfield, 1970). When millicurie levels are being used for therapy, other clients and personnel should be protected from the radiation in the client. The National Council on Radiation Protection and Measurements has guidelines that the hospital *must* follow when therapy is being performed with radionuclides. The guidelines for diagnostic procedures are less complicated than those for therapeutic procedures; however, nuclear medicine personnel must take precautions in handling samples. If urine or fecal matter must be saved for sample testing, the worker should wear waterproof gloves when putting the samples in containers or in cleaning bedpans. If urine can be disposed of by means of dilution in the sewage system, no special precautions are needed. Thus, from a nursing point of view, the usual precaution with urine is not to touch the urine, and if samples must be obtained, waterproof gloves should be worn to handle the sample. (See the discussion of Posttest Nursing Diagnoses Related to Radionuclide Studies.) Velchik's research (1990) found the amount of radiation exposure to medical personnel to be minimal when working with clients who had just undergone eight common scans. Still he concluded that the ALARA rule (*a*s *l*ow *a*s *r*easonably *a*chievable) is appropriate for any diagnostic test that uses radioactive material.

Waste Disposal for Diagnostic Testing Materials

The minimal radiation hazard from radionuclide diagnostic testing is brief because the half-life of most diagnostic radiopharmaceuticals is short. Half-life is the time in which it takes a radioactive element to lose half of its radioactivity. An unstable radioactive element continuously disintegrates, but some take much longer than others to "physically decay." I-123 has a half-life of only 13 hr compared with 8 days for I-131. Tc-99m has a half-life of only 6 hr, and disposal is not a problem. In dramatic contrast, radium has a half-life of 1,590 years. In addition to less exposure for the client, the shorter the half-life, the less is the problem of waste disposal. For nuclear medicine diagnostic testing, the waste disposal problem is not acute because wastes can be held until physical decay occurs.

Radionuclides as Low-Level Radioactive Wastes

Because radiation from any source is cumulative, it should always be kept at a minimum for clients, personnel, and the general public. The Nuclear Regulatory Commission grants a license to a physician or an institution to conduct research, therapy, or diagnostic testing with radioactive material. Specific standards must be maintained, and they are the responsibility of a person designated as the Radiation Protection Officer.

Problems with a Long Half-Life

Large research centers may conduct research that involves the use of carbon-14, which has a half-life of 5,750 years. Radioactive waste that has a very long half-life is picked up by private carriers and taken to specified sites for dumping in several states. (Nuclear plants have their own waste disposal systems.) These dumping sites may not be enough as more radionuclides are used in testing. The nurse as a health professional and as a concerned citizen should keep abreast of the regulations the government provides for all nuclear wastes because the health of entire communities may be threatened when rigid controls are not followed.

Radionuclide Diagnostic Testing During Pregnancy

Radiation destroys or alters cells as they go through the dividing stages of growth. In the fetus, and to a lesser degree in the child, cell growth is rapid; thus, many cells are vulnerable to alteration by radiation. (This, of course, is why radiation is used as a therapeutic agent for cancer cells, which divide and grow at an increased rate.)

As a rule, radionuclides are not used for diagnostic testing during pregnancy if other tests suffice. Although the amount of radioactivity in diagnostic testing is small, it is prudent to protect the fetus from any radiation whenever possible. As with radiography, elective diagnostic tests with radionuclides should be performed during menses or within 10–14 days after onset of menses for women who could become pregnant. When a test cannot be postponed, pregnant women may need to sign a special consent form for radionuclide testing (McDonagh, 1991). Jankowski (1986) compared the risk of radiation to other risks of pregnancy and noted that low levels of radiation used for screening are of negligible risk. If testing is conducted, the pregnant woman should empty her bladder frequently after the test is begun.

Radionuclide Tests for Infants and Children

Women who are nursing should not breast feed the infant until the radionuclide has been eliminated. If children need scans, the dosages of the radiopharmaceuticals are calculated to provide maximum results with the minimum dose possible (Shore and Hendee, 1986).

Radionuclide Tests for Elderly Clients

Radionuclide testing is noninvasive and well tolerated by elderly clients. For some clinical situations such as acute GI bleeding or pulmonary embolus, these tests may be the first used in older clients (Berkowitz and Cassell, 1992).

▼ PRETEST NURSING DIAGNOSES RELATED TO RADIONUCLIDE STUDIES

Knowledge Deficit Related to Procedure

The nurse should be familiar with the particular procedure being used for the test so that the client's questions can be answered. If the client is not sure why the test is needed, the nurse can help the client obtain the correct information from his or her physician. The nurse can assure the client that the scans do not hurt. The nurse should also inform the client that he or she will have to lie still during the scan, but the positioning is usually not uncomfortable. The scans may take 30–60 min. The machine makes clicking noises at times. Some scanners can be brought to the client's bedside, but usually it is preferable to obtain the scan in the nuclear medicine department. A parent can accompany a child. Some clients may need a sedative or pain medication before the scan, but this is not a common practice. Sedatives do not interfere with the test. Most of the radionuclides are given intravenously, so the client should be told that a venipuncture will be performed in the nuclear medicine department. All the Tc-99m compounds used for organ scans are given intravenously. Iodine compounds may be given orally or intravenously, depending on the test. If radioactive iodine is being used for studies other than of the thyroid, potassium iodide is given before and after the scan to block uptake by the thyroid gland. For some lung studies, the radio-tagged substance is inhaled.

Anxiety Related to Timing of Scans

The length of time between the administration of the radioisotope and the scan varies depending on the type of scan (see Table 22-2). A member of the nuclear medicine department notifies the nurse of the specific time the client should return for the scan or if the client is to remain in the nuclear medicine department for the entire time of the test. Clients should know if they are to stay in the nuclear medicine department for an extended length of time so they can bring reading material or handwork. For ambulatory care, the client may be given the radiopharmaceutical and told when to return for the scan. Specific written instructions should be given.

Anxiety Related to Possible Effects of Radiation

The nurse needs to understand fully the standard procedures for diagnostic radionuclide testing in a specific setting so the client is not confused about inconsistencies. The nurse can reassure the client that the dose of radiation used for diagnostic testing is small and that all necessary precautions for safety are being taken. It may also be helpful to point out that only the radioisotope is radioactive. The scintillator acts as a detector of the radiation emitted *from* the client as opposed to a conventional x-ray machine, from which radiation is emitted to penetrate through the body. Thus, the long time, sometimes as much as an hour, spent in front of a scintillator does not cause any radiation effects as would long exposure to x-rays. The clicking of the scintillator reflects only measurements of radioactivity already present. (Even health workers may need education about the relative safety of procedures performed in the nuclear medicine department.)

▼ POSTTEST NURSING DIAGNOSES RELATED TO RADIONUCLIDE STUDIES

Risk for Injury Related to the Procedure

Involved assessments are not needed after most scanning procedures because there is no risk for most of the procedures. If a stress test is performed as part of a thallium scan for coronary perfusion, there are specific posttest considerations. (See Chapter 26 on stress tests.) If the radionuclide is given intravenously, and almost all are, the site of the needle puncture should be assessed for inflammation. Warm packs can be used for any phlebitis that develops. The medications used for testing are unlikely to cause any side effects.

Anxiety Related to Test Results

As discussed in Chapter 20, the nurse is often able to act as a sounding board for a client who has anxiety about his or her condition. The results of the scan are not usually available for a day or two, so the nurse can help the client formulate specific questions to ask the physician. For example, if a liver scan is obtained to assess for possible metastasis, the client may be anxious while awaiting the results. The nurse can help the client express feelings and identify the main areas of concern regarding choices about treatments.

Altered Fluid Requirements Related to Need to Excrete Isotopes

As noted in the pretest preparations, most of the scans do not require any restrictions in diet, either before or after the scan. If there are no contraindications, the client should be encouraged to drink extra fluids to help expedite excretion of the radionuclide. This is particularly advised for pregnant clients.

Disposing of Urine

Although the amount of diagnostic radionuclide excreted in the urine is low, urine should not be used for any laboratory tests. Clients should be told to flush the toilet three times after voiding. Rubber gloves are recommended if the urine must be handled. The nuclear medicine department must supply the information about the timing of the precautions with urine, based on the half-life of the radionuclide used.

Some hospitals have developed specific guidelines and appointed safety advisors for personnel who care for clients who must stay in bed and who are undergoing nuclear medicine diagnostic procedures. Infants also pose a problem for disposal of wastes because the nurse must handle the urine. Common guidelines may be

1. Wear disposable gloves (not sterile ones) when handling wastes
2. Flush the toilet three times after excreta is discarded
3. Rinse reusable containers twice before general cleaning

4. Rinse disposable containers twice before discarding in the general waste
5. Wash hands with gloves on. Remove gloves and wash hands again. Dispose of gloves in general waste
6. For infants and incontinent clients, use disposable diapers, wear disposable gloves when changing diapers, and discard gloves and waste as described above

Readers are encouraged to talk to nuclear medicine personnel in their own setting to obtain accurate up-to-date information about guidelines used for clients undergoing tests with radionuclides. The nurse should not unduly alarm clients. If urine is accidentally spilled or touched, this is not an emergency. Immediate disposal of the waste is not of the same urgency as when clients undergo therapy with radioactive substances. The nurse should act in a prudent manner so that any and all exposure to radiation is minimized. (See Chapter 20 for more discussion on radiation hazards for health workers.)

▼ BONE SCANS

For a bone scan, Tc-99m pyrophosphate is given intravenously. In 2–4 hr, the radionuclide concentrates in the bone tissue. It takes about an hour for the scintillation camera to scan the entire body, front and back. If there is increased bone activity, the bone tissue takes up more of the radionuclide. The scan outlines areas of osteoblastic and osteolytic processes in the bones, such as malignant tumors or osteoporosis.

Purposes. A bone scan is most often performed to check for silent metastasis to the bone. A metastatic lesion in the bone shows up on a scan about 6 months earlier than on a conventional radiograph. Bone scans may be obtained on a routine basis after detection of malignant tumors of the breast or prostate, because bone metastasis is a strong possibility with these tumors. A bone scan may reveal the reason for an elevated level of alkaline phosphatase (ALP), an enzyme associated with bone activity (Chapter 12).

▼ NURSING IMPLICATIONS RELATED TO BONE SCAN

Consumption of large amounts of fluids should be encouraged for 2–4 hr before the test to ensure that the client is well-hydrated and thus will quickly eliminate the radionuclide not absorbed by the bones. The client must void before a bone scan so the pelvic bones can be seen. If the client cannot void, a Foley catheter must be inserted before the client goes to the nuclear medicine department (Lull, 1991). Pain medications or a sedative may be required so the client can lie still for the prolonged scanning time.

▼ BRAIN SCANS

Brain scans are conducted as perfusion scans and static views of the brain tissues. A cerebral perfusion scan is performed 30 sec after intravenous injection of Tc-99m. If straight Tc-99m is used, some of it is excreted in the saliva; the client must not touch the saliva and then put his or her hands near his or her head. Tc-99m pertechnetate static scans of the brain are obtained at intervals, such as 15 min, 1 hr, and 24 hr. Potassium perchlorate in solution or capsule may be given 30–60 min before the procedure to prevent uptake by saliva and other tissues. If a lesion has damaged the blood-brain barrier, the radionuclide localizes in that area. The blood-brain barrier is a complex system of membranes and fluid spaces that keeps substances in the blood from diffusing into the brain tissue. Tumors and other lesions destroy this protective barrier; consequently, more of the radionuclide diffuses into the brain tissue. Radio-iodinated human serum albumin (RIHSA) may be used to evaluate changes in the blood-brain barrier. The advent of lipid-soluble radiopharmaceuticals that can cross the intact blood-brain barrier has made it possible to study the perfusion of the brain and to document the distribution of the tracer over several hours. These agents are a breakthrough in brain imaging because the older tagging agents only localized in the disrupted area of the brain barrier. In addition, the use of SPECT (Chapter 21) has improved the quality of brain scans.

▼ GALLIUM SCANS

Gallium citrate (Ga-67) is useful in diagnostic scanning because gallium localizes in inflammatory lesions and in some tumors. A gallium scan may be used to detect a hidden abscess or metastatic nodules. Ultrasonography (Chapter 23) may show the presence of a mass, but is not useful in determining if a mass is benign or malignant. A gallium scan can be a complementary procedure in studying the nature of a mass found with other diagnostic modalities. Chronic osteomyelitis may be detected with a gallium scan. (See indium scans for acute infections.) Gallium scans have become very useful for identifying the diffuse pulmonary inflammation that occurs with *Pneumocystis carinii* pneumonia.

If the purpose is to identify an abscess, the client may be screened in 6 hr and then again in 24, 48, or 72 hr. For malignant neoplasms such as melanoma or lymphoma, the scans may be performed at 24, 48, and 72 hr. Gallium has a half-life of 78 hr (Plankey and Plankey, 1990).

A dual isotope scanning can be performed with Ga-67 and Tc-99m to enhance the specificity of the scan. Otherwise the interpretation of the scan is limited by the complex distribution of Ga-67 (Karl et al., 1985).

▼ NURSING IMPLICATIONS RELATED TO GALLIUM SCAN

Enemas or laxatives are sometimes given before a gallium scan to empty the GI tract. The intestinal tract collects gallium, and confusing results may occur if there are shadows in the GI tract. Not all institutions require intestinal preparation, and the dual isotope scanning reduces the amount of confusing results.

▼ INDIUM SCANS OR LEUKOCYTE IMAGING

Indium (In-111) is used to label leukocytes, which then go to infected areas of the body. In contrast to gallium, In-111-labeled leukocytes are not taken up by neoplastic lesions. Any infected area in the body can be visualized in 4–24 hr. Indium is also used to label platelets and RBCs for other types of studies. For white blood cell (WBC) imaging, 40 mL of the client's blood is withdrawn 2 hr before the scan so the WBCs can be labeled with indium. Thus this test may also be called *indium-labeled autologous leukocytes*. If the client's granulocyte count is less than 2,000/mm^3 (Chapter 2), WBCs from a compatible donor may be tagged and used for the test. These tagged WBCs tend to localize in acute infections that are less than 8 days old. Gallium scans are more useful for chronic infections, but sometimes both scans may be performed for a client who has a persistent fever of undetermined origin (FUO). There is no special preparation of a client for an indium scan except for the blood drawing before the test. Indium may be labeled to other substances. For example, In-111 pentetreotide (OctreoScan) is a radiolabeled analog of somatostatin. This agent is used to help locate neuroendocrine tumors that bear somatostatin receptors (Sandler and Delbeke, 1993).

▼ GALLBLADDER SCANS

The older technique to screen the biliary tract used rose bengal or bromosulfophthalein (BSP) dye tagged with I-131. These substances are excreted by the liver into the biliary tree and concentrate in the gallbladder. The newer method of evaluating biliary function is with Tc-99m combined with chemicals, such as HIDA and PIPDA. These scans are obtained immediately, every 5 min for 30 min, and at intervals over a 24-hr period. If clients have consumed nothing by mouth for more than 24 hr, the nuclear medicine department gives a drug, sincalide (the synthetic active octapeptide of cholecystokinin), to empty the gallbladder 30 min before the radionuclide is given (Lull, 1991). During the test, morphine may be given to differentiate between delayed visualization and nonvisualization. The morphine causes contraction of the sphincter of Oddi.

When information about organs adjacent to the gallbladder is not desirable, the radionuclide scan of the hepatobiliary tree may become the first procedure performed to evaluate acute cholecystitis. Hepatobiliary scans are obtained in conjunction with ultrasonography (Chapter 23) and x-ray studies of the gallbladder (Chapter 20) for chronic cholecystitis or for assessment of obstructive jaundice (see Chapter 11 on bilirubin).

▼ NURSING IMPLICATIONS FOR GALLBLADDER SCAN

The client stops consuming anything by mouth a few hours before the test. Sometimes clear liquids are allowed. The client may eat after the initial scan, but fats are restricted during the 24-hr test period to decrease rapid emptying

(*continued*)

▼ NURSING IMPLICATIONS FOR GALLBLADDER SCAN (*continued*)

of the gallbladder. The client should be assessed for any allergies to morphine, because the drug may be given as part of the gallbladder scan. The use of morphine can cause posttest sedation.

▼ GASTROINTESTINAL SCANS

Several different tests can be performed to evaluate the functional ability of the GI tract. A test also can be performed to assess for active GI bleeding.

Gastrointestinal Function Studies

Esophageal Motility Studies (Transit Time). The measurement of the transit time through the esophagus can be measured by having the client drink a liquid tagged with Tc-99m sulfur colloid. The study takes approximately 30 min.

Gastroesophageal Reflux Studies. The client is given Tc-99m sulfur colloid in acidic orange juice, and images are taken with the client in a supine position. An abdominal binder is used to obtain increasing predetermined external pressure gradients (Lull, 1991).

Gastric Emptying Studies. The client is given Tc-99m sulfur colloid mixed with scrambled eggs and eaten with bread. Images are taken to evaluate the time for gastric emptying, which should be 70–125 min. A longer time indicates impaired gastric emptying, and a shortened time indicates hypermotility (Lull, 1991). If there is no gastric outlet obstruction, metoclopramide (Reglan) may be given to assess if the drug will help improve gastric motility.

Gastrointestinal Bleeding Studies. Radionuclide studies are more commonly used to assess active lower GI bleeding, but they also may be useful for upper GI bleeding. Two types of scans, both with Tc-99m, are used. For acute bleeding, labeled sulfur colloid is injected intravenously, and if the bleeding is rapid, the scan may be positive at the spot of blood loss. The colloid disappears within minutes after injection so it does not detect slow bleeding. To detect slow bleeding, labeled RBCs are used as markers in the circulation for 1–2 days, so they may help pinpoint the bleeding site (Bongard and Sue, 1994). A positive scan indicates the need for repeat endoscopy. (See Chapter 27 on endoscopy for bleeding.) Because a client with active GI bleeding may need careful monitoring, a nurse or physician may be required to go to the nuclear medicine department with the client.

▼ NURSING IMPLICATIONS RELATED TO GASTROINTESTINAL FUNCTION TESTS

Consult with the nuclear medicine department to see how long the client should abstain from food and drink before a specific test. Also note that anticholinergic drugs and narcotics should not be given before the test because they decrease GI motility.

▼ LIVER AND SPLEEN SCANS

Hepatobiliary scans are used primarily to note biliary function; however, liver function is assessed, too, because the agents used to outline the biliary tree are excreted by the liver. Many different radiopharmaceuticals can be used for specific liver scans to assess the reticuloendothelial system or the structural changes in cirrhosis. A liver scan is a common procedure for clients in whom liver metastasis is suspected. Tc-99m is combined with sulfur colloid to assess for neoplasms in the liver. Liver scans may also be useful in assessing trauma to the liver or the presence of an abscess. The spleen is visualized simultaneously, if desired. The scan is obtained 10–15 min after the radionuclide is injected intravenously. No special preparation is needed.

▼ LUNG SCANS—PERFUSION IMAGES AND VENTILATION STUDIES

Lung scans may be performed either as perfusion studies or as ventilation scans. Perfusion studies use macroaggregated albumin (MAA) tagged with Tc-99m, which disperses in the pulmonary precapillary arterioles. Perfusion lung scans are used to evaluate the possibility of pulmonary embolisms. Ventilation lung scans are performed with radioactive gas. The client inhales a bolus of xenon-123. The lungs are then scanned for about 5 min to determine how much gas enters each lobe of the lung and how long it takes the gas to be expelled. Krypton is another radioactive gas used for ventilation studies. Radionuclide perfusion studies and ventilation studies are usually correlated with other pulmonary function tests (Chapter 24) and blood gas studies (Chapter 6). Ventilation–perfusion studies may be performed in clients who have possible smoke inhalation injury even though a bronchoscopy appears normal (Bongard and Sue, 1994).

▼ NURSING IMPLICATIONS RELATED TO LUNG SCANS

A current chest radiograph should be sent to the nuclear medicine department with the client. Clients need to be prepared for the sensation of the mask used for the ventilation study.

▼ CARDIAC SCANS

Infarction Scans

A test for detecting myocardial infarction uses Tc-99m pyrophosphate (the same compound used in bone scans). If there is an infarction in the myocardium, the uptake of radionuclide is increased in this "hot" spot. The scan of the myocardium is obtained 1½–3 hr after intravenous injection of the radionuclide. The test can be performed at the client's bedside to prevent exertion on the part of the client. The hot-spot myocardial imaging test is most helpful 1–3 days after the infarction. This test may be useful when the more traditional ways of diagnosing myocardial infarction, cardiac enzymes (Chapter 12), and electrocardiographic (ECG) readings (Chapter 24) have not given enough information.

▼ NURSING IMPLICATIONS RELATED TO INFARCTION SCANS

There is no special preparation of the client. A physician or critical care nurse may be required to go with the client to the nuclear medicine department. SPECT is desirable if available (Chapter 21).

Perfusion Scans

A thallium scan is useful for evaluating coronary perfusion. Thallium is a physiologic analogue of potassium in regard to distribution in the myocardium. A thallium scan may show the site of an old infarction or demonstrate partial obstructions to coronary blood flow. Poorly perfused regions of the myocardium are depicted as low levels of thallium uptake. These "cold" spots may be seen in both acute and old infarctions. A stress test is commonly performed as part of a thallium scan because coronary perfusion may only decrease with a certain amount of exertion. Research has suggested that combining a thallium scintigram with a stress test improves the prognostic ability of the tests (Kaul et al., 1988). (See Chapter 26 for a description of the protocol for stress tests.) The client may actually exercise, or the heart may be paced to obtain the tachycardia associated with exercise. Scans are performed a few minutes after the thallium is injected and within 3–4 hr after the exercise or pacing to see the redistribution of the thallium. If there are still areas of poor distribution, scans are performed again in 18–24 hr to differentiate ischemia from infarction. Many institutions also use SPECT (Chapter 21) in conjunction with thallium treadmill testing to obtain three-dimensional images of the heart.

Pharmacologic Stress Testing

For clients who have orthopedic, neurologic, or other limitations that preclude an exercise stress test, the dipyridamole–thallium test is a safe and reliable substitute (Lam et al., 1988). The test is conducted in a specialized cardiac laboratory where the client can be carefully monitored for both cardiac and noncardiac effects of the drug used to elicit stress on the heart. Dipyridamole (Persantine) is given intravenously followed by an intravenous injection of thallium. Dipyridamole is a coronary vasodilator for healthy arteries. If the client has coronary artery disease, the diseased arteries do not respond to the drug, so certain areas take up less thallium. Aminophylline may be given to reverse the effect of dipyridamole. Other alternatives to a stress test are the use of dobutamine or adenosine with either thallium or Tc-99m sestamibi (Cardiolite).

Tc-99m–labeled agents with better imaging characteristics, combined with advances in equipment, provide better image quality. The problem of breast artifacts with myocardial imaging is considerably lessened with these newer agents as compared with thallium-201 imaging (Wackers, 1992). Another advantage of Tc-99m sestamibi (Cardiolite) is that it allows direct measurement of both myocardial perfusion and ventricular function (Keeys, 1994).

▼ PRE- AND POSTTEST NURSING IMPLICATIONS RELATED TO MYOCARDIAL IMAGING

Imaging scans require the client to abstain from food and drink for 6–8 hr. Check with the cardiologist to see what medications should be withheld. For a dipyridamole–thallium scan, the client should not have had any theophylline preparations for 48 hr or dipyridamole (Persantine) for at least 24 hr. Clients with a history of bronchospasms should not undergo the dipyridamole test. Posttest care is usually uneventful; adverse reactions, such as nausea, headaches, and angina, tend to occur during the test. If needed, cardiac monitoring may be maintained after the test (Chapter 25). The precautions for handling urine are appropriate for a few hours after the test. If the thallium or another radionuclide is given as part of an exercise stress test, there are more specific nursing implications, which are discussed in Chapter 26. The client should be prepared for having about 10 electrodes connected to the body.

Multiple Gated Acquisition Scan—Wall Motion Studies and Ejection Fractions

A multiple gated acquisition scan (MUGA scan) is a sophisticated study of heart function that includes wall motion studies and ejection fraction studies. The scan is performed in conjunction with ECG monitoring of cardiac function. Signals from the ECG trigger the scintillation camera to record the flow of blood at precise times in the cardiac cycle. A computer is used to break down the time from one R wave to the next into fractions of a second called *gates*. These scans from multiple gates within the cardiac cycle can be used to assess if the motion of the ventricular walls is normal. For example, a ventricular aneurysm causes abnormal wall motion. Computer analysis of the data also determines the percentage of ejection of blood from both ventricles. A normal ejection fraction is more than 55% for the left ventricle and more than 45% for the right ventricle (Barkett, 1988). Clients with severe cardiomyopathy have very low ejection fractions. Measurement of ejection fraction is now standard in clients who have had a myocardial infarction. The ejection fraction at peak exercise, rather than its change with exercise, may provide valuable prognostic information (Zaret and Wackers, 1993).

A MUGA scan is done in a specialized cardiology laboratory. The client is first given an intravenous injection of a nonradioactive material that binds with RBCs in the plasma. In about 30 min, a second intravenous injection of Tc-99m is given, and this radioactive substance binds to the material coating the RBCs. The monitoring of the first pass of the radionuclide through the heart is completed, and then scanning may continue over an hour or two.

▼ NURSING IMPLICATIONS RELATED TO WALL MOTION STUDIES OR MUGA SCANS

There are no special preparations other than the general ones for all clients undergoing radionuclide scans. Usually the test is not performed less than 3 hours after a meal. The client should be told why there are two injections and that ECG monitors are used. Some parts of the study may require special approval. The scan is usually performed in the nuclear medicine department, but the equilibrium studies can be performed at the bedside if the client is too ill for transportation.

▼ RENAL SCANS

Scans of the kidneys evaluate both renal perfusion and function. Tc-99m is tagged to a compound such as dimercaptosuccinic acid (DMSA). The tagged compound is administered intravenously, and a series of scans is taken to assess the dynamic perfusion of the kidneys. Static scans are taken for 20 min–4 hr to assess the structure of the kidneys. Another type of compound orthoiodohippurate (Hippuran) tagged with radioactive iodine can be given as a second intravenous injection so continuous images can be obtained over approximately an hour to measure the time it takes to travel through the cortex and pelvis of each kidney. The times of uptake, transit, and excretion of the radionuclide by each kidney can be plotted on a graph called an *isotopic renogram curve*. Plotted curves are compared with normal reference curves to determine abnormalities in either kidney. The use of two intravenous injections to assess the perfusion, structure, and excretory ability of the kidneys is sometimes called a *triple renal study*. A loop diuretic, furosemide, may be used to stimulate a large urine output. Captopril, a drug that inhibits an angiotensin-converting enzyme, is used with a renal scan to assess for renal arterial stenosis. Captopril produces a transient decrease in perfusion to the kidney that has severe renal arterial stenosis. The client's blood pressure must be carefully monitored after the drug is given.

Intravenous pyelography (IVP) involves the use of a radiopaque dye to evaluate the excretory ability of the renal system (see Chapter 20 for IVP). For clients allergic to the contrast medium used for IVP, renograms can be used as a substitute to assess the excretory pattern. Renal imaging to assess renal dysfunction is used in conjunction with various other diagnostic studies. Renal biopsies (Chapter 25) are sometimes performed in conjunction with renal scans.

▼ NURSING IMPLICATIONS RELATED TO RENAL SCANS

See the general nursing diagnoses in the introduction. In addition, the client should be well-hydrated. If a captopril study is planned, the client should not have had any antihypertensive drugs for 24 hr and no angiotensin-converting enzyme inhibitors for at least 48 hr before the test. For aftercare, see the discussion on safety precautions for disposing of urine.

▼ THYROID SCANS

Several different isotopes of iodine are used for thyroid scans. Iodine, such as I-123, can be given either orally or intravenously. Scans of the thyroid are performed to assess nodules, which may be felt in the thyroid gland. Benign nodules appear as "warm" spots on the scan because they tend to take up the radionuclide. Conversely, malignant tumors appear as "cold" spots because they do not tend to take up the radionuclide. The actual presence of a malignant neoplasm must still be determined with a biopsy. (A special type of scanning of the thyroid called an *RAI uptake* is discussed in a separate section because the RAI uptake scan is different from organ scans in general.)

For someone with no symptoms of thyroid problems, thyroid scans can be obtained with Tc-99m because the screening can be completed faster with less radiation exposure because of the short half-life of Tc-99m. Thyroid scans are also performed on people who have no thyroid problems but do have a history of radiation to the face and neck. Until the late 1950s, x-ray therapy was used in the treatment of acne and thymus gland disorders, and this past radiation exposure may promote malignant growths in the thyroid gland. Thyroid scans with Tc-99m require no special preparation. Ultrasound is also used to screen the thyroid (Chapter 23).

I-131 Whole Body Imaging for Thyroid Tumor Metastasis

A whole-body scan with I-131 uses a dose 100 times greater than the dose normally used for thyroid imaging (Lull, 1991). The whole-body scan is used to detect metastasis from a proved malignant tumor of the thyroid. Scans are taken 3 and 7 days after the client is given the oral dose of I-131.

▼ NURSING IMPLICATIONS RELATED TO WHOLE BODY SCANS WITH I-131

Inform women of childbearing age that a pregnancy test is performed to rule out pregnancy and that the test should be performed during the first 10 days of the menstrual cycle. Consult with the physician concerning the schedule for withdrawing all thyroid medication before the test. See precautions for urine handling discussed at the beginning of this chapter.

▼ RAI UPTAKE STUDY

For an RAI uptake study, the client is given radioactive iodine either in an oral capsule or intravenously. The uptake by the thyroid gland is measured with a scanner at several time intervals, such as 2–4 hr and 24 hr. A person with hyperthyroidism has increased uptake of iodine, more than 35%. Conversely, a person with hypothyroidism has decreased uptake of iodine by the thyroid gland. The values of the RAI uptake are expressed in percentages: the amount of thyroid uptake divided by the amount of the dose given. The reference values vary depending on the locality because normal iodine consumption varies in different locales.

REFERENCE VALUES FOR RAI	
Scan (uptake)	1–13% after 2 hr 4–19% after 4 hr 11–30% after 24 hr

▼ NURSING IMPLICATIONS RELATED TO RAI UPTAKE

Because the amount of iodine consumption before the test affects the uptake of radioactive iodine, it is important that the client not have additional iodine uptake for several weeks before the test. A list of medications currently being taken by the client should be recorded on the laboratory request. Thyroid medications and amiodarone (Cordarone) interfere with the test.

As mentioned in Chapter 20, most contrast media used for x-ray studies have an iodine base. A client should undergo a RAI uptake study before studies that use iodine dye. Clients need to be instructed to avoid all sources of iodine. Some foods, such as kelp and enriched breakfast cereals, are high in iodine. Vitamin preparations may contain iodine, as do most cough syrups. Even suntan lotion and nail polish can be be sources of exogenous iodine. Such a small amount of iodine is used for the RAI uptake scan that it does not cause any allergic problems, even in people who are allergic to iodine. (In contrast, x-ray dyes that contain iodine can cause anaphylactic shock in people with allergies to iodine.

The client abstains from food and drink by mouth 6–8 hr before the test but can resume food 1 hr after the oral dose is taken. Scans are performed a few hours after administration of iodine and the next day. For outpatients, make sure the client knows what time to return for scans.

▼ COMPATIBILITY AND RED BLOOD CELL SURVIVAL

Sodium chromate (Cr-51) readily binds with the protein of hemoglobin (Hgb) so RBCs can be tagged to evaluate the rate of hemolysis or RBC survival in some hemolytic diseases. A sample of blood is withdrawn from the client, tagged with the radioactive Cr-51, and injected back into the client. A collection of blood samples are drawn at various time intervals. One sample may be drawn within 1 hr to measure compatibility and then two to three times a week to assess survival. No special preparation of the client is required. No blood transfusions should be given 48 hr before the study.

▼ BLOOD VOLUME STUDIES

Cr-51 is used to tag the RBCs, and RIHSA is used to tag plasma. A measured amount of blood is withdrawn from the client, tagged with radionuclides, and injected back into the client. After 30–60 min, samples of blood are drawn and the amount of dilution of the original sample is calculated. The total blood volume of a client can thus be estimated.

▼ NURSING IMPLICATIONS RELATED TO BLOOD VOLUME STUDIES

It is important that the hydration of the client be normal before the blood studies are performed. Intravenous solutions invalidate the test, as does abstinence from food and drink. The nurse must record the height and weight of the client before the test is conducted.

▼ SCHILLING TEST

The Schilling test is used to assess the ability of the small intestine to absorb vitamin B_{12}. (Clients with a deficiency in vitamin B_{12} will have macrocytic anemia; Chapter 2.) An oral preparation of vitamin B_{12} is tagged with Co-57. The test measures how much of the tagged vitamin B_{12} is eliminated in the urine. The client is given a loading dose of untagged vitamin B_{12} intramuscularly to saturate the cells with vitamin B_{12} so that much of the tagged vitamin B_{12} can be excreted. Nurses usually give the intramuscular dose. The oral cobalt-tagged vitamin B_{12} is given by the nuclear medicine personnel. A dual isotope technique may be used, so that tagged vitamin B_{12} and intrinsic factor are given with tagged vitamin B_{12} without intrinsic factor. Thus the Schilling test is conducted in one step.

▼ NURSING IMPLICATIONS RELATED TO SCHILLING TEST

All urine is collected for 24 hr and should be kept on ice. No preservative is needed. If renal function is questionable, the test may last longer. The precautions for urine handling should be observed, as discussed earlier in this chapter. The client must be fasting before the test begins and for 2 hr after the oral vitamin B_{12} is given.

REFERENCE VALUES FOR SCHILLING TEST (24-HR URINE EXCRETION)	
Vitamin B_{12} without intrinsic factor	10–40%
Vitamin B_{12} with intrinsic factor	10–40%

Clinical Significance. Intrinsic factor is found in the gastric mucosa and is essential for the proper absorption of vitamin B_{12}. If urine values increase when intrinsic factor is given with vitamin B_{12}, a diagnosis of pernicious anemia is likely. In pernicious anemia and some gastric lesions, the 24-hr excretion of tagged vitamin B_{12} without intrinsic factor is usually less than 7%, and the excretion of tagged vitamin B_{12} with intrinsic factor is considerably greater than 7–20% (Lull, 1991). If defective absorption is low both with and without intrinsic factor, other types of intestinal malabsorption must be considered, such as sprue. Some unusual and unexplained anemias may be assessed with bone marrow biopsies. If bone marrow studies are ordered, these are performed before any injections of vitamin B_{12} because vitamins change the appearance of the bone marrow. (See Chapter 25 on bone marrow studies; see Chapter 2 for nursing diagnoses related to macrocytic anemias.)

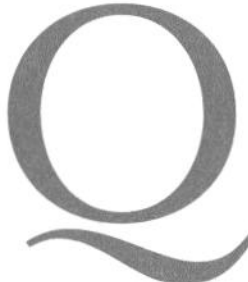

1. Technetium (Tc-99m) is useful as an agent for diagnostic testing because this radioactive element
   a. Has a half-life of only 2 days
   b. Can be tagged to go to the brain, bone, liver, or lung
   c. Is radioactive only when it reaches the target organ
   d. Is excreted only in the urine

2. Scintigraphy involves taking the reading of radioactivity from a body organ and transforming the reading into
   a. Audible sounds (Geiger counter)
   b. Quantitative measurements
   c. A two-dimensional image of the organ
   d. A vertical graph

3. The radiation hazard from the radionuclide diagnostic testing is much less than when radionuclides are used for therapy because the dose used for diagnostic testing is about
   a. Half as much as used in therapy
   b. 10 times less than in therapy
   c. 100 times less than in therapy
   d. 1,000 times less than in therapy

4. Which of the following would be a reason to postpone, if possible, radionuclide diagnostic studies in a female client? She is
   a. Seven days past onset of menstrual period
   b. Pregnant in first trimester
   c. Menstruating
   d. Allergic to iodine

5. Which of the following nursing actions is appropriate in preparing a client for any organ scan with technetium (Tc-99m)?
   a. Explain to the client that all urine must be monitored after the test
   b. Make sure the client ingests nothing by mouth
   c. Explain that the test involves intravenous administration of a very small dose of a radioactive substance
   d. Shave the area that will be viewed during the scan

6. The main use of a bone scan with radionuclides is to detect
   a. Silent metastasis from the breast or prostate gland
   b. Silent metastasis from the liver or kidney
   c. Utilization of phosphorus by the body
   d. Fractures

7. Mrs. Lourdes is going to undergo a gallium scan this morning because of a fever of undetermined origin (FUO). Gallium is useful as a radionuclide for scintigraphy because gallium localizes in

   a. Inflamed tissue and some types of tumors
   b. The lungs
   c. The brain and spinal column
   d. The hepatobiliary system

8. Mrs. Hunter is scheduled for a radioactive iodine uptake (RAI) scan in 4 weeks, so she is to have no iodine intake. Therefore, which one of the following would be allowed because it contains no iodine?

   a. Suntan lotions
   b. Vitamin preparations
   c. Contrast medium for x-ray test
   d. Soft drinks, such as colas

9. Mrs. Langerdorf is undergoing a Schilling test today. Which of the following is an appropriate nursing function in regard to this test?

   a. Saving all urine for 24 hr after the oral cobalt-tagged vitamin B_{12} is given
   b. Giving an ordered intramuscular injection of vitamin B_{12} as a loading dose after the oral cobalt-tagged vitamin B_{12} is given
   c. Keeping the client isolated from other clients because radioactive cobalt is used
   d. Drawing two blood samples for serum levels of vitamin B_{12} before and after the injection

▼ REFERENCES

Barkett, P. (1988). Cardiac M.U.G.A. scan. *Nursing 88, 18* (10), 76–78.

Berkowitz, J.F., and Cassell, I. (1992). Diagnostic imaging: Special needs of older patients. *Geriatrics, 47* (3), 55–68.

Bettelheim, F.A., and March, J. (1991). *Introduction to general, organic and biochemistry.* (3rd ed.). Philadelphia: Harcourt Brace Jovanovich.

Bongard, F.S., and Sue, D.Y. (1994). *Current critical care diagnosis & treatment.* Norwalk, CT: Appleton & Lange.

Jankowski, C. (1986). Radiation and pregnancy: Putting the risks in proportion. *American Journal of Nursing, 86* (3), 261–265.

Karl, R., Hartshorne, M.E., Cawthon, M. (1985). Dual isotope scanning with gallium-67 citrate and technetium-99m radiopharmaceuticals. *Clinical Nuclear Medicine, 10* (7), 507–512.

Kaul, S., Lilly, D., Gascho, J., et al. (1988). Prognostic utility of the exercise thallium-201 test in ambulatory patients with chest pain: Comparison with cardiac catheterization. *Circulation, 77,* 745–758.

Keeys, M.U. (1994). Nuclear cardiology stress testing. *Nursing 94, 24* (1), 63–64.

Lam, J., Chaitman, B., Glaenzen, M., et al. (1988). Safety and diagnostic accuracy of dipyridamole-thallium imaging in the elderly. *Journal of the American College of Cardiology, 11* (3), 585–589.

Lull, R.J. (1991). *Nuclear medicine manual.* San Francisco: San Francisco General Hospital.

McDonagh, A. (1991). Getting your patient ready for a nuclear medicine scan. *Nursing 91, 21* (2), 53–57.

Myers, W., and Wagner, H. (1974). Nuclear medicine: How it began. *Hospital Practice, 9* (2), 103–113.

Plankey, E., and Plankey, M. (1990). A nuclear approach to cancer detection. *American Journal of Nursing, 90* (6), 107–108.

Rummerfield, R., and Rummerfield, M. (1970). What you should know about radiation hazards. *American Journal of Nursing, 70* (4), 780–786.

Sanders, M.P., and Delbeke, D. (1993). Radionuclides in endocrine imaging. *Nuclear Medicine, 31* (4), 909–921.

Shore, R., and Hendee, W. (1986). Radiopharmaceutical dosage solution for pediatric nuclear medicine. *Journal of Nuclear Medicine, 27* (2), 287–297.

Velchik, M. (1990). Radiation exposure associated with the performance of radiologic studies in radioactive patients. *Journal of Nuclear Medicine Technology, 18* (3), 211–213.

Wackers, F.J. (1992). Diagnostic pitfalls of myocardial perfusion imaging in women. *Journal of Myocardial Ischemia, 4* (10), 23–37.

Zaret, B.L., and Wackers, F.J. (1993). Nuclear cardiology. *New England Journal of Medicine, 329* (12), 855–863.

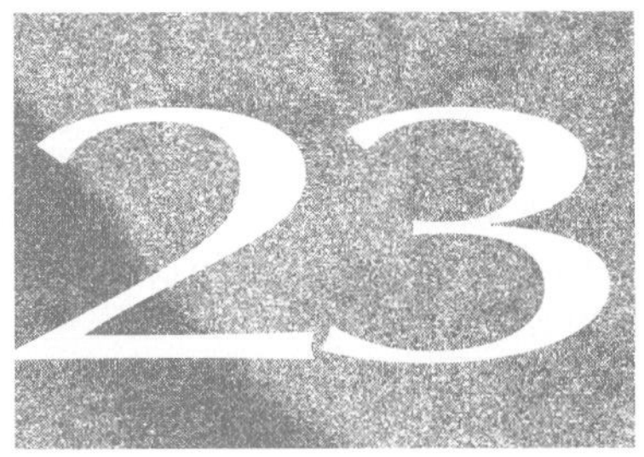

DIAGNOSTIC ULTRASONOGRAPHY

- Doppler Techniques
- Pelvic Sonograms: Ultrasound Scans in Pregnancy and Gynecologic Conditions
- Transvaginal Ultrasound Scanning
- Abdominal Sonograms
- Transrectal Ultrasound Scanning
- Echocardiograms: Transthoracic and Transesophageal
- Echoencephalograms
- Thoracic Sonograms

OBJECTIVES

1. Explain the differences between A-mode, B-mode, and real-time scans as methods of pulse–echo recordings.
2. Describe three clinical situations in which the nurse uses Doppler ultrasound for assessment.
3. Describe the preparation of the client for pelvic and abdominal sonograms.
4. Compare and contrast the pre- and posttest care of clients undergoing transthoracic and transesophageal echocardiograms.
5. Describe the responsibilities of the nurse when a child undergoes echoencephalography.
6. Explain why ultrasound examinations of the thorax are of limited usefulness.
7. Identify at least two nursing diagnoses for clients undergoing sonography.

Ultrasound, a noninvasive method of diagnostic testing, uses sound waves to detect physical changes in the client. Sound is a physical force, and thus sonograms are in no way related to radiographs (Chapter 20), CT scans (Chapter 21), or radionuclide scans (Chapter 22).

Ultrasound, first used in industry to detect flaws in metal, is used as a sonar system to locate objects in the water and for depth sounding of the ocean floor. For health care, ultrasound first gained importance as a diagnostic tool in pregnancy (Meire, 1977). Sonograms of the heart (echocardiograms) soon followed, and later ultrasound became commonly used to view many areas of the body. Fields and Calvert-Hill (1985) compared ultrasound to a sophisticated physical assessment. Common tests using both pulse–echo recordings and Doppler methods are described in this chapter (Table 23–1). The Doppler method of assessment is often used by the nurse in obstetric settings, in medical–surgical units, and in home care.

ULTRASOUND PRINCIPLES

Although this chapter focuses on the use of ultrasound as a diagnostic tool, ultrasound waves are also used in therapy. Ultrasound, in large and continuous doses, can generate heat in tissues; therefore, ultrasound treatments are used for various kinds of low back pain. Ultrasound has also been tried as a method to promote tissue regeneration and to generate heat to kill malignant growths. A procedure called *percutaneous ultrasonic lithotripsy* (PUL) has become well established as a therapeutic use of ultrasound to pulverize kidney stones (Ruge, 1986) and now may also be used for gallstones.

Description

Ultrasonics is part of the science of acoustics that deals with sound waves that are beyond the range of audible sound. The human ear can hear sounds that are of a frequency between 16,000 and 20,000 cycles/sec. The unit of frequency is a hertz (Hz), which is equal to one cycle per second. Thus, ultrasound waves are of a frequency higher than 20,000 Hz. Sonograms are performed with transducers, which produce sound waves of varying strength or intensity. Intensity is the measurement

TABLE 23–1. ULTRASOUND METHODS USED FOR ASSESSMENT

Method	Example of Use
Pulse-echo methods	
1. A-mode (amplitude modulation)	Echocardiogram
2. B-mode (brightness modulation)	Sonograms of fetus, pelvic and abdominal structures
Doppler method	
1. Doppler stethoscope	1. Monitoring of fetal heart rate
2. Doppler instrument	2. Monitoring of peripheral pulses
3. Pulse volume recorder	3. Assessing extent of vascular disease
4. Color flow imaging	4. Assessing direction of blood flow

See Hanson et al. (1990) and Rudolphi (1990) for examples.

of the strength of a sound wave and is measured as the amount of power per cross-sectional area. However, more useful to the nurse than figures of frequencies and intensities is the comparison of dosages used in tests. Intensities used for treatment are at least 20 times the intensities used in diagnostic testing (Ziskin, 1980).

For diagnostic purposes, ultrasound waves are sent into the body with a small transducer pressed against the skin. Technically, the transducer is the piezoelectric crystal, which changes electric energy to sound waves and vice versa. However, the unit that houses the crystal is also called the *transducer* in general terms. A transducer changes one form of energy into another. An electric signal from the machine is converted to ultrasound waves. Air almost completely impedes the transmission of the ultrasound waves into the body; thus the transducer must be in good contact with the skin as it is being moved. A lubricant, such as mineral oil, glycerin, or a water-based jelly, is used to ensure good contact with the skin. The lubricant is called the *coupling agent.* The transducer not only sends the sound waves into the body but also receives any returning sound waves, which are deflected back as they bounce off various structures. Some sound waves pass through the body. The transducer converts the returning sound waves into electric signals that can then be transformed with a computer into either scans or graphs (pulse–echo methods) or into audible sounds (Doppler method).

Pulse–Echo Method of Displaying Ultrasound

All the pulse–echo techniques measure the time it takes the sound waves to reach various structures and return to the transducer. There are various ways that the readout can be presented. In A mode (amplitude modulation), the echoes are displayed in a graphic form (e.g., the graph completed for an echocardiogram). In B mode (brightness modulation), the echoes appear as different intensities of brightness. B-mode scans use dots of brightness to show a two-dimensional cross-sectional view of the various structures. Thus, with a B-mode scan, one can actually see a "picture" of the fetus in the womb, for example. B-mode scans may be still (static scans), or motion may be added.

Real-time Imaging

The terms *real-time* and *real-time imaging* describe scanners that are capable of scanning so rapid that motion is displayed. In other words, real-time scanning is like a movie. A fetus can be seen moving around, sucking a thumb, or performing other motions. The use of a scanner with rapid sequencing is valuable in observing heart action. For real-time imaging, there is no need for the client to suspend respiration during the scan, as was true of older static scans.

Gray Scale, Color, and Magnification

The first sonograms were black and white. In 1979 gray-scale imaging became possible. Now computerized sonographic machines can magnify a selected area five to seven times and thus give a view as powerful as with low-power microscopic techniques (Birnholz, 1985). Color-coded sonography became available (Goldman, 1986) in the 1980s. In the 1990s the first contrast agent for ultrasound became available, as did three-dimensional viewing techniques.

POSSIBLE RISKS FROM ULTRASOUND

There are two known effects of ultrasound in tissue: the production of heat and cavitation. Cavitation is the appearance of gas-filled bubbles in a sound field. Ultrasound waves greater than 100,000 Hz cause formation of gas bubbles in bacterial cells, killing the bacteria. As far as is known, the low-intensity dose of ultrasound used for sonograms is harmless to humans; there is no heat formation or cavitation in the tissues. The sound waves are delivered intermittently for sonograms and not continuously as with therapy.

Sonograms have been used in pregnancy since the mid-1960s, and there have not been reports of damage to either the woman or the fetus. In the past some authorities questioned the risks of ultrasound to the developing fetus (Mendelsohn, 1983). The Doppler devices used in fetal monitoring are of low enough dosages to be free of adverse heating effects or cavitation in tissues. However, the Doppler instrument used in arterial studies does use intensities of sound that produce some heat in tissues; consequently, arterial Doppler monitors are not considered suitable for fetal investigation. As far as is known, routine Doppler monitoring and other uses of ultrasound in pregnancy have no adverse effects on the fetus (DeCherney and Pernoll, 1994).

Cost Versus Benefits of Routine Screening

Although routine ultrasound screening is often conducted during pregnancy to detect fetal abnormalities and to estimate gestational age, it is not certain if ultrasound screening is useful for pregnant women who are at low risk for perinatal morbidity or mortality. In one large study, 15,151 pregnant women were randomly assigned to either (1) undergo two routine ultrasound examinations during pregnancy—at 15–22 weeks gestation and again at 31–35 weeks, or (2) undergo ultrasound examinations only for medical indications identified by a physician. The routine use of screening sonograms did not improve perinatal outcome as compared with the selective use of ultrasonography based on clinical judgment (Ewigman et al., 1993).

▼ DOPPLER TECHNIQUES

With the Doppler method, returning sound waves are transformed into audible sounds, which can be heard with earphones. Not only are sound waves produced by moving objects, but sound waves that are bounced off different moving objects have slightly different frequencies. The sound produced by an artery is pulsatile and multiphasic, whereas the sound from a vein is intermittent and varies with respiration. Doppler ultrasound is used to assess the movement of the opening and closing of the heart valves and the flow of blood. This technique is used for bedside assessments and as a laboratory diagnostic aid. A Doppler stethoscope can detect the presence of fetal heartbeats, even when the heartbeat is inaudible with a conventional stethoscope.

Doppler ultrasound can be used for fetal monitoring during labor and delivery. It is also used to monitor the fetus during an oxytocin challenge test (OCT) or a nonstress test, which may be performed during the last trimester of pregnancy (Chapter 28).

In addition to the use of a Doppler stethoscope or monitor for evaluating fetal status, the nurse may also use a Doppler instrument to monitor blood flow in clients who have altered arterial circulation. A portable Doppler instrument is about the size of a tissue box. A small flat transducer is placed over the vessel to be assessed, and when the unit is turned on, transmitted sound waves bounce off the moving blood, producing a pulse heard with earphones. The portable Doppler unit, useful in the first few days after an arterial graft to assess the continued patency of the graft, may also be used in a clinic to assess chronic perfusion problems. Another type of Doppler unit is sometimes used to monitor blood pressure in shock when the blood pressure is barely audible. Pulses can be detected with a Doppler unit when they are too faint to be felt with the fingertips. A Doppler unit with blood pressure cuffs also can be used to measure the pulse volume of both arteries and veins and obtain a pressure index by means of comparison of leg and arm pressure readings.

Color Flow Imaging

Doppler flow imaging is sometimes called *color flow imaging* or *mapping* because the color is used primarily to detect the direction of blood flow and to assist in determining whether the flow is laminar or turbulent. For example, valvular regurgitation can be displayed in vivid colors that dramatically emphasize the areas of turbulence. Color flow imaging is also useful in documenting the shunts seen in some congenital heart defects. Color flow imaging technique also can help differentiate the true and false lumens in aortic dissection.

Duplex Scanning

Duplex scanning uses both real-time imaging and Doppler flow imaging to obtain information about many vascular problems, such as plaques in arteries or the presence of aneurysms. The real-time imaging shows how the veins and arteries function. The Doppler technique shows flow as well as the velocity within the vessels. Duplex scanning may also be used to scan renal transplants for rejection (Rudolphi, 1990). A duplex scan may be performed in a specialized vascular laboratory or in the radiology department. The procedure usually lasts less than an hour. If an abdominal scan is obtained, the client may need to fast for 12 hr.

▼ PELVIC SONOGRAMS: ULTRASOUND SCANS IN PREGNANCY AND GYNECOLOGIC CONDITIONS

Purposes. Sonograms were originally used for evaluating the position of the placenta and the status of the fetus. Before amniocentesis (Chapter 28) is performed, the position of the placenta is determined with ultrasound. The fetal growth rate can also be determined by measurements of the images obtained with ultrasound. Ectopic pregnancies, hydatidiform moles, or structural abnormalities in the fetus can be detected with ultrasound, as can death of the fetus. For ectopic pregnancies, ultrasound scans are easier to interpret after 6 weeks gestation (Schwab, 1988). The presence of twins can almost always be detected. It is possible, however, for one twin to "hide" behind the other, so the two-dimensional scan does not show the second fetus. For some situations, a Level II ultrasound scan may be ordered. This type of scan takes longer and is more expensive than a conventional scan, but the quality of resolution is better. For example, a Level II scan is performed if a pregnant woman has a positive α-fetoprotein (AFP) test (Chapter 18). One of the advantages of ultrasound is that repeated scans are not usually considered risky. If necessary, sonograms may be taken several times during a pregnancy. Ultrasound scans may also be obtained after delivery to check for any retained placenta. Pelvic sonograms are also used to evaluate pelvic inflammatory disease and abscess formation. Pelvic masses can also be detected with ultrasound.

▼ PRETEST NURSING DIAGNOSES RELATED TO PELVIC SONOGRAMS

Anxiety Related to Well-being of Fetus

The movement of the transducer over the abdomen is not at all painful. The client can see the scan on the monitor. Mot pregnant women are thrilled to be able to see an image of the fetus on the monitoring screen. The technician can point out the head, feet, and other features as the fetus moves about. The heartbeat is seen as a blip of light. At many centers, any woman who wishes a picture of her fetus is given a copy of the sonogram. It is also understood, however, that watching the monitor can be an unbelievable, chilling moment for a woman whose fetus is dead of if the scan is being performed to assess malformations.

Altered Comfort Related to Full Bladder and Positioning

Besides the anxiety of finding possible abnormalities with the sonogram, two other factors may make a sonogram uncomfortable. One factor is the need to have a full bladder during the procedure. A full bladder is an acoustical window so that other structures can be seen in relation to the bladder. Sound waves travel well through liquid. Some institutions do not require a full bladder if the fetus is more than 26 weeks gestation. The other factor is the need to lie flat for 20 or so min. Some pregnant women experience hypotension due to the pressure on the vena cava. It may be necessary for the woman to turn on her left side to relieve this pressure.

Knowledge Deficit Related to Physical Preparation

There is no need to restrict medications or alter the client's diet before the test. If it is essential that the client's bladder be full during the sonogram, the client

TABLE 23–2. PREPARATION OF CLIENT FOR SONOGRAPHY

Test	Nothing By Mouth?	Intestinal Preparation	Other
Pelvic sonogram	No	No	May need full bladder
Abdominal sonogram	Usually but not always	Varies	See text for medication and other preparation
Echocardiogram	No	No	None
Echoencephalogram	No	No	Sedation for children?
Thoracic sonogram	No	No	None
Transrectal sonogram	No	No	None
Vaginal sonogram	No	No	None

must drink about 750 mL of water before the test. A full bladder is an acoustical window. If the client has an intravenous infusion going, the nurse needs to check to see how much the rate of infusion should be increased. If the client has a Foley catheter, the catheter must be clamped so that the bladder is full for the pelvic sonogram (Table 23–2).

▼ TRANSVAGINAL ULTRASOUND SCANNING

Vaginal ultrasonography uses a probe placed inside the vagina to pinpoint ovulation, diagnose tubal pregnancies, or evaluate other gynecologic problems, such as endometriosis. Transvaginal ultrasonography may be particularly useful in differentiating acute appendicitis from pelvic inflammatory disease (Pelsang et al., 1994). Transvaginal ultrasonography combined with transfundal pressure has been used to detect an incompetent cervix in pregnant women at risk for this condition (Guzman et al., 1994).

▼ PRETEST NURSING IMPLICATIONS FOR TRANSVAGINAL SONOGRAMS

The woman needs to be told that the transvaginal approach is only minimally uncomfortable. A lubricant is used for the probe. For this approach the woman does not need to have a full bladder, an appreciated advantage for a client who may undergo ultrasonography for 10 days in a row to assess ovulation (see Chapter 28 on infertility tests.)

▼ POSTTEST NURSING IMPLICATIONS RELATED TO PELVIC SONOGRAMS

There are no special nursing implications after the client has undergone pelvic or transvaginal sonography. If the sonogram was obtained to assess for fetal abnormalities or fetal death, the nurse must be sensitive to helping the woman find support to cope with the distressing news. (See Chapter 28 for a discussion on the role of the nurse in helping couples deal with loss.)

▼ ABDOMINAL SONOGRAMS

Purposes. Sonography of the abdomen is being used more and more as the equipment becomes more sophisticated and clinicians become more adept at identifying abdominal problems with a sonogram. A sonogram of the abdomen may mean the client does not undergo exposure to radiation or invasive procedures to diagnose a problem.

For some abdominal conditions, ultrasonography may be the first examination performed. For example, ultrasonography is a first test for conditions such as appendicitis and cholelithiasis (Berkowitz and Cassell, 1992). In other clinical conditions, abdominal sonograms are complementary to other examinations, such as radionuclide studies (Chapter 22), x-ray studies (Chapter 20), or CT and MRI (Chapter 21). In addition to no radiation hazard, sonography has the advantage of being less expensive than CT or MRI, and is readily available in most health care settings.

▼ PRETEST NURSING DIAGNOSIS RELATED TO ABDOMINAL SONOGRAMS

Knowledge Deficit Related to Preparation

The actual procedure for an abdominal sonogram is similar to that for a pelvic sonogram. However, the client does not need to have a full bladder for an abdominal sonogram as for a pelvic sonogram. The client may be instructed to abstain from food and drink or may be allowed only liquids, depending on the exact nature of the abdominal sonogram. For example, if the gallbladder is the focus, the client must take nothing by mouth for 12 hr and may have a fat-free meal the evening before the examination. If the client eats before a sonogram of the gallbladder, the gallbladder is not full and thus is not easily visualized. For other scans, the purpose of allowing only liquids is to reduce gas formation in the colon, because gas does interfere with the scan. Another way to reduce gas in the gastrointestinal (GI) tract is by administering drugs that contain simethicone (e.g., Mylicon). Smoking and gum chewing are prohibited because they increase gas formation. Sometimes an enema is needed to clear the intestine. Barium used for other tests interferes with a sonogram. (See Chapter 20 for principles of intestinal preparation.) Abdominal scars and obesity make it difficult to obtain a good abdominal sonogram. Abdominal dressings must be removed before a sonogram. Contrast medium may be given.

Risk for Ineffective Coping of Child

Children should be accompanied by a parent if possible. Even young children can cooperate if they are not overly anxious. Also, the transducer can be first placed on a doll and the child allowed to see the shadows on the screen. (See Chapter 25 on preparing children for diagnostic procedures.)

▼ POSTTEST NURSING IMPLICATIONS RELATED TO ABDOMINAL SONOGRAMS

The client may be ill from the pathophysiologic condition that necessitated the sonogram, but there is no concern over the direct effects of a sonogram. Occasionally, a sonogram may only be a preliminary test to an invasive procedure, such as liver or renal biopsy. If so, the invasive procedure has some nursing implications (Chapter 25).

▼ TRANSRECTAL ULTRASOUND SCANNING

Transrectal ultrasound scanning produces a clear image of the prostate gland so tumors can be detected at an early stage. Ultrasound also helps localize the tumor and thus makes it possible for radiation to be used as an alternative to prostatectomy. Transrectal examination of the prostate may be combined with the prostate-specific antigen (PSA) test discussed in Chapter 14 for screening for prostatic cancer.

▼ PRETEST NURSING IMPLICATIONS RELATED TO TRANSRECTAL SCREENING

The man needs to be told that the rectal probe will be well lubricated and will cause only minimal discomfort.

▼ ECHOCARDIOGRAMS: TRANSTHORACIC AND TRANSESOPHAGEAL

Purposes. Ultrasound has become a well-established diagnostic tool for valvular defects. Ultrasound was first used to detect abnormalities in the mitral valve and has become the standard method for diagnosing mitral valve prolapse (Labovitz et al., 1988). An echocardiogram is also used to measure the diameters of the cardiac chambers and evaluate other structural abnormalities of the heart such as atrial septal defect and patent ductus arteriosus. Pleural effusion and cardiac tamponade are other abnormalities identified with ultrasound. An ECG is often run simultaneously, therefore echographic findings can be correlated with the cardiac cycle. Earlier echocardiograms used the M mode (motion) to conduct time–motion studies of the heart. Newer types can also produce cross-sectional scans, which can be used to detect some changes in coronary vessels. Echocardiograms also use the color flow imaging discussed earlier. The color is useful in detecting the direction of blood flow and whether the flow is laminar or turbulent. Echocardiograms, in combination with other tests, may eliminate the need for more invasive procedures, such as a cardiac catheterization (Chapter 26).

A transthoracic echocardiogram (TTE) may have to be followed up with a transesophageal echocardiogram (TEE), which gives more detail because there is no impedance by the lungs and chest-wall structures. Unlike a TTE, a TEE is invasive.

▼ PRETEST NURSING IMPLICATIONS RELATED TO TRANSTHORACIC ECHOCARDIOGRAMS

The client needs no special preparation. The echocardiography technician directs the transducer at specific points on the client's chest to obtain images of the mitral valve and other structures. During the test the client may be asked to perform the Valsalva maneuver. Also, the client may be given a vasodilator, such as amyl nitrite, which can have the side effect of tachycardia. If an ECG is performed, the client needs instruction about the procedure (Chapter 24).

▼ POSTTEST NURSING IMPLICATIONS RELATED TO TRANSTHORACIC ECHOCARDIOGRAPHY

There is no specific care of the client after a TTE because it is a noninvasive procedure.

▼ TRANSESOPHAGEAL ECHOCARDIOGRAMS

The introduction of the transesophageal approach to echocardiography has given clinicians a new "window on the heart," because this approach is unimpeded by chest-wall structures and lung interference. A TEE can be safely performed on critically ill clients at the bedside and demonstrates abnormalities that are missed with TTE (Pearson et al., 1990). For example, a TEE allows clear visualization of posterior structures of the heart, such as the left atrium and the aortic root, which are needed to evaluate prosthetic heart valves (Alton et al., 1992). Other clinical uses of TEE are for the diagnosis of infective endocarditis, the diagnosis of aortic abnormalities, such as aortic dissection, the assessment of a cardiac source of an embolus, monitoring of atrial fibrillation, and the evaluation of clients who have had a myocardial infarction.

A TEE is obtained with a transducer mounted on the end of a gastroscope. The physician inserts the scope and has the client swallow as the scope goes down the esophagus. Over the next 5–20 min the probe is manipulated and then gently withdrawn to provide various views of the heart. A video camera records the findings. Special contrast medium may be given intravenously.

Although a TEE is clearly superior to a TTE in detecting many potential cardiac abnormalities, it carries a small risk related to esophageal intubation and the use of drugs. Therefore, a harmless and painless TTE may be used as a screening test with a follow-up TEE if deemed necessary by the physician (Pearson, 1993).

▼ PRETEST NURSING IMPLICATIONS RELATED TO TRANSESOPHAGEAL ECHOCARDIOGRAMS

The client needs to fast for 4–6 hours before the examination. If the client has a prosthetic valve, antibiotics are given prophylactically before and after the procedure (Hibner et al., 1993). An informed consent should be obtained and eyeglasses and dentures removed before the procedure begins. If present, a nasogastric tube is usually removed to prevent entanglement with the endoscopic probe. If the client has an endotracheal tube, a special latex cover may be used to protect the probe (Sullivan-Witterschein et al., 1992). The client is usually sent to a specialized room, but bedside units are available for critically ill clients.

The client needs to know that before the scope is inserted, a local anesthetic is used to numb the throat and the gag reflex. The client is asked to lie on the left side during the procedure, which usually takes 5–20 min. Clients may also be given small intravenous doses of narcotics or antianxiety agents to reduce the discomfort of the procedure. Occasionally, glycopyrrolate may be used to reduce

(*continued*)

▼ PRETEST NURSING IMPLICATIONS RELATED TO TRANSESOPHAGEAL ECHOCARDIOGRAMS (*continued*)

respiratory secretions. A bite block in the client's mouth protects the patient's teeth if he or she does not have removable dentures. Oxygen saturation is monitored, and oxygen may be administered. (See Chapter 6 on pulse oximetry.) Cardiac rhythm is monitored. (See Chapter 24 on cardiac monitoring.)

▼ POSTTEST NURSING IMPLICATIONS RELATED TO TRANSESOPHAGEAL ECHOCARDIOGRAMS

After the probe is removed, the client may need to cough to clear secretions. Nothing is taken by mouth until the gag reflex returns. Throat lozenges or saline rinses may be used to soothe the sore throat. Observations of vital signs, cardiac rhythm, and oxygenation may continue for 45 min after the probe is removed. (See Chapter 27 for more on monitoring for unwanted effects of drugs.) Outpatients should have someone drive them home.

▼ ECHOENCEPHALOGRAMS

Purposes. Ultrasonic visualization of the head may be used to evaluate some head injuries, but the adult brain cannot be well-imaged because ultrasound cannot penetrate bone. CT and MRI are more valuable in identifying masses and tumors because these studies give a three-dimensional cross section of the entire brain (Chapter 21). Echoencephalograms are effective to monitor certain cerebral abnormalities that cause shifts of cerebral midline structures. For example, ultrasound has been useful in monitoring the state of hydrocephalus in young infants. The size of the ventricles and the functions of the shunts are monitored with echoencephalograms or echoventriculograms. Because the newborn's skull is not completely fused into a solid bony structure, ultrasound is a useful tool for detecting intracranial hemorrhage.

▼ PRETEST NURSING IMPLICATIONS RELATED TO ECHOENCEPHALOGRAMS

As with most other ultrasound procedures, there is no pain or risk for the client. The head is placed on a foam sponge. If the echoencephalogram is performed on a small child, the nurse may need to hold the child's head. Then, a water-soluble gel is applied to the skull. Thick hair may make it difficult to obtain a sonogram, but any cutting of the hair must be completed according to hospital procedure. During the sonogram the client must remain motionless. If the client cannot lie still during the examination, the physician may order a sedative. Drugs, food, and fluids can be taken normally. Portable ultrasound units may be wheeled to neurologic units or newborn nurseries to avoid transporting critically ill clients.

▼ POSTTEST NURSING IMPLICATIONS RELATED TO ECHOENCEPHALOGRAMS

There is no special aftercare, but the nurse should be aware of the underlying pathophysiologic problem, which may indicate a need for frequent neurologic assessment. The nurse should assess if the gel has been washed off the scalp or is matted in the hair.

▼ THORACIC SONOGRAMS

Purposes. Because ultrasound does not penetrate air, sonograms are not as useful for thoracic disease as for abdominal disease. For a lesion to be identified with ultrasound, there must be no air-filled lung between the chest wall and the lesion. Sonograms of the chest may be useful in identifying pleural fluid, abscess formation, or malposition of the diaphragm.

▼ NURSING IMPLICATIONS RELATED TO THORACIC SONOGRAMS

There is no special preparation of the client and no special care after the procedure.

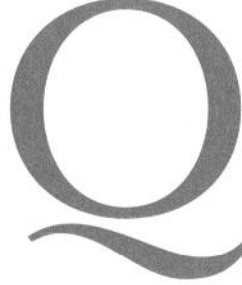

1. Sonograms or ultrasound scans are performed with ultrasound waves, which are
   - **a.** Waves of energy closely related to the γ-rays of radiographs
   - **b.** High-frequency sound waves, which are beyond the range of audible sound

c. Sound waves of very low frequency that are undetectable by the human ear
d. Part of a still undefined physical force

2. The type of ultrasound scan that demonstrates motion, such as the movement of a fetus is

a. A-mode scan b. B-mode scan c. Real-time scan d. Doppler scan

3. The nurse is *least* likely to use Doppler ultrasound to assess which of these clients?

a. Mrs. Jarvis, who is in the first stage of labor
b. Mr. Bixby, who has had an aortofemoral bypass
c. Mr. Tucker, who had a pacemaker inserted yesterday
d. Mrs. Horn, who is undergoing an oxytocin challenge test (OCT)

4. The nurse should be aware that abdominal sonography is particularly useful as first-line testing for

a. Cholelithiasis and appendicitis
b. Gastrointestinal bleeding
c. Metastasis to the liver or other abdominal organs
d. Renal arterial stenosis

5. Which of the following is necessary before a pelvic sonogram? The client must

a. Maintain nothing-by-mouth status b. Be given an enema or suppository
c. Not take any medication d. Have a full bladder

6. Which of the following preparations is necessary when a client is undergoing an abdominal sonogram?

a. Reinforcing abdominal dressings
b. No smoking or gum chewing for several hours before the examination
c. Use of drugs for sedation
d. Having the client drink two to three glasses of water before the examination

7. Mr. Love, 78 years of age, underwent a transthoracic echocardiogram (TTE) yesterday and is now scheduled for a transesophageal echocardiogram (TEE). The nurse preparing him for the TEE should emphasize that

a. A TEE is much the same as a TTE
b. The radiation exposure is minimal
c. Food and fluids do not need to be withheld
d. Dentures need to be removed before the procedure

8. Baby Dabney is undergoing an echoencephalogram to monitor a ventricular shunt that was inserted for hydrocephalus. The responsibilities of the nurse who accompanies the baby to the ultrasound department may include

   a. Explaining the results of the sonogram to the parents
   b. Reassuring the mother that anesthesia is used
   c. Giving an ordered contrast medium before the examination
   d. Holding the baby's head while the sonogram is being done

9. The use of ultrasound in the thorax is difficult because

   a. The transducer cannot be moved evenly on the chest wall
   b. Ultrasound does not penetrate air
   c. Thoracic tumors are solid masses
   d. The movement of the heart interferes with the sound waves

REFERENCES

Alton, M.E., Pasierski, T.J., Orsinelli, D.A., et al. (1992). Comparison of transthoracic and transesophageal echocardiography in evaluation of 47 Starr-Edwards prosthetic valves. *Journal of American College of Cardiology, 20,* 1503–1511.

Berkowitz, J.F., and Cassell, I. (1992). Diagnostic imaging: Special needs of older patients. *Geriatrics, 47* (3), 55–68.

Birnholz, J. (1985). Evolution of the ultrasonic exam. *Journal of Clinical Ultrasound, 13* (2), 83–84.

DeCherney, A.H., and Pernoll, M.L. (1994). *Current obstetric & gynecologic diagnosis & treatment.* (8th ed.). Norwalk, CT: Appleton & Lange.

Ewigman, B.G., Crane, J.P., Frigoletto, F.D., et al. (1993). Effect of prenatal ultrasound screening on perinatal outcome. *New England Journal of Medicine, 329* (12), 821–827.

Fields, S., and Calvert-Hill, M. (1985). Clinical efficacy of screening the entire abdomen during real-time ultrasound examination. *Journal of Clinical Ultrasound, 13* (6), 411–413.

Goldman, M. (1986). Real time two dimensional Doppler flow imaging: A word of caution. *Journal of American College of Cardiology, 71* (1), 89–90.

Guzman, E.R., Rosenberg, J.C., Houlihan, C., et al. (1994). A new method using vaginal ultrasound and transfundal pressure to evaluate the asymptomatic incompetent cervix. *Obstetrics & Gynecology, 83* (2), 248–252.

Hanson, F., Happ, R.L., Tennant, F.R., et al. (1990). Ultrasonography guided early amniocentesis in singular pregnancies. *American Journal of Obstetrics and Gynecology, 162* (6), 411–413.

Hibner, C.S., Moseley, M.J., and Shank, T.L. (1993). What is transesophageal echocardiography? *American Journal of Nursing, 93* (4), 74–80.

Labovitz, A.J., Pearson, A.C., McClusky, M.T., et al. (1988). Clinical significance of the echocardiographic degree of mitral valve prolapse. *American Heart Journal, 115,* 842–849.

Meire, H. (1977). Ultrasound: Current status and prospects. *British Journal of Radiology, 50,* 379–380.

Mendelsohn, R. (1983). The risks of ultrasound. *RN, 46* (5), 101.

Pearson, A.C. (1993). Transthoracic echocardiography versus transesophageal echocardiography in detecting cardiac sources of embolism. *Echocardiography: A Journal of CV Ultrasound & Allied Technology, 10* (4), 397–403.

Pearson, A.C., Castello, R., and Labovitz, A.J. (1990). Safety and utility of transesophageal echocardiography in the critically ill patient. *American Heart Journal, 119,* 1083–1089.

Pelsang, R.E., Warnock, N.G., and Abu-Yousef, M. (1994). Diagnosis of acute appendicitis on transvaginal ultrasonography. *Journal of Ultrasound Medicine, 13,* 723–725.

Rudolphi, D. (1990). Duplex scanning. *American Journal of Nursing, 90* (4), 123–124.

Ruge, C. (1986). Shock (wave) treatment for kidney stones. *American Journal of Nursing, 86* (4), 400–401.

Schwab, R. (1988). Ultrasound versus culdocentesis in the evaluation of early and late ectopic pregnancy. *Annals Emergency Medicine, 17,* 801–803.

Sullivan-Witterschein, K., Hussey, R., and Perry, M. (1992). Using transesophageal echocardiography to assess the heart. *Nursing 92, 22* (9), 63–64.

Ziskin, M. (1980). Basic principles of ultrasound. In R. Sanders (ed.). *Principles and practices of ultrasonography in obstetrics and gynecology.* Norwalk, CT: Appleton-Century-Crofts.

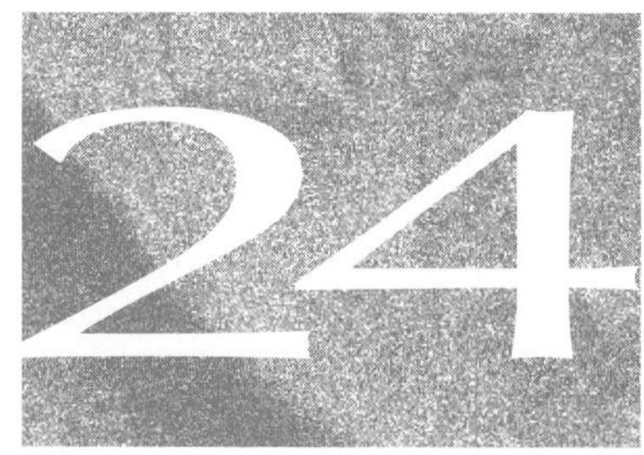

COMMON NONINVASIVE DIAGNOSTIC TESTS

- Electrocardiography
- Telemetry and Cardiac Monitoring
- Ambulatory Electrocardiography
- Electroencephalography
- Electromyelography
- Pulmonary Function Tests: Spirometry
- Peak Flow Testing
- Thermography

OBJECTIVES

1. Identify two general nursing diagnoses useful in preparing clients for noninvasive diagnostic testing.
2. Describe five basic characteristics of a normal sinus rhythm on a lead II ECG strip and how common arrhythmias change these characteristics.
3. Given an ECG of a normal sinus rhythm, calculate the heart rate of the client.
4. State what nursing assessments are useful in monitoring the mechanical events of the heart when the client has an abnormal ECG or is undergoing telemetry.
5. State four important nursing functions to help prepare a client for an electroencephalogram (EEG).
6. Describe what a nurse should teach a client about an electromyelogram (EMG).

7. Explain how the pulmonary function tests (forced vital capacity [FVC], forced expiratory volume [FEV], maximum voluntary ventilation [MVV], and forced expiratory flows [FEF]) are used in assessing lung ventilation defects that are obstructive or restrictive.
8. Describe the importance of peak flow meters in promoting self-care for clients with asthma.
9. Describe how the measurement of heat is accompanied with diagnostic thermography.

The preceding four chapters describe noninvasive procedures that use x-rays (Chapters 20 and 21), radionuclides (Chapter 22), and ultrasound (Chapter 23). This chapter discusses several types of noninvasive tests, including measuring such diverse things as electric events (ECG, EEG, and EMG), air flow (pulmonary function tests), and body surface heat (thermography) (Table 24–1). The unifying theme throughout all these tests is that because they are noninvasive, there is little or no risk to the client. These tests give an indirect assessment of an organ and its structure or function. Most are fairly easy to perform (usually completed by a skilled technician) and are relatively inexpensive.

Invasive diagnostic tests are those that use methods that invade the body, such as cardiac catheterization (Chapter 26) or an endoscopic procedure (Chapter 27). Other common invasive procedures are the subject of Chapter 25. The nurses must realize that this division of invasive and noninvasive tests is strictly from the professional's view. For the client, *any* test is an invasion of his or her personal space and privacy. Although health professionals consider an ECG noninvasive (because the body is not entered), the client may (because of the use of electrodes on the body) perceive it as being invasive.

TABLE 24–1. NONINVASIVE DIAGNOSTIC PROCEDURES USING VARIOUS TYPES OF MEASUREMENTS

Tissue	Electricity	Ultrasound	Magnetic Field	Air Flow	Heat	X-Rays
Heart	ECG Telemetry Holter monitors	Echocardiogram	Magnetic resonance imaging (MRI)			Chest radiographs Cine computed tomographic (CT) scan
Brain	EEG	Echoencephalogram	MRI			Skull radiographs CT scan
Muscles	EMG					
Lungs		Thoracic sonogram	MRI	Spirometry		Chest radiographs CT scan
Tumors or inflammation		Abdominal and pelvic sonograms	MRI		Thermography	Flat plates of abdomen CT scan

Note: See this chapter for nursing diagnoses for most noninvasive tests, Chapter 20 for radiographs, Chapter 21 for CT and MRI, and Chapter 23 for sonograms.

▼ GENERAL NURSING DIAGNOSES RELATED TO NONINVASIVE TESTS

Knowledge Deficit Related to Test Procedures and Preparation

It is the nurse's responsibility to see that the client is both physically and psychologically ready for the test. Preparation of the client should include reassurance that the test is neither painful nor harmful. Special consent forms are not needed because there is no anticipation of any complications from the test itself. There are specific physical preparations for several of the tests, such as a shampoo before an EEG. Some drugs affect the results of several of these tests; thus, the nurse must be aware of the information required on laboratory requests. Also, the nurse must make sure the client understands any restrictions on drugs, food, or liquids. Preparation for a child must take into account children's concepts of illness (Pidgeon, 1985). School-age children are very receptive to teaching. (See Chapter 25 for more on children's reactions to procedures.)

Anxiety Related to Outcome of Test

The focus of nursing care after a noninvasive test is to let the client rest once an assessment has been performed. It is important for the nurse to validate that the client is physically stable and not psychologically upset by the test performed. The results of the test may not be known immediately, and this may be a source of anxiety for the client. (See the discussion in Chapter 20 on posttest anxiety.) With few exceptions, there are no specific nursing implications after noninvasive testing. Although these tests are relatively simple to perform and there is practically no risk to the client, the client may be quite ill from the basic pathologic problem. The aftercare of the client is therefore geared to the underlying problems.

▼ ELECTROCARDIOGRAPHY

Description. An electrocardiogram (ECG) comprises the electrical impulses generated by the heart during its depolarization and repolarization. The impulses are picked up by electrodes and displayed on a strip of graph paper. The electrodes are fastened to all four of the client's extremities by means of rubber straps. A jelly or paste is used under each electrode to help conduction of the electrical impulse. The electrodes on both arms and the left leg are used to record impulses. The electrode on the right leg is a ground. A suction bulb is moved across the client's chest to obtain recordings for six different areas of the heart (precordial leads).

A common lead used for monitoring (and the one usually displayed in nursing textbooks) is lead II, which records the electrical activity of the heart with the negative electrode on the right arm and the positive electrode on the left leg. As the electrical current moves through the heart, the current moving toward the positive electrode shows as a positive deflection on the graph (above the baseline). If the electrical current moves away from the positive electrode, the graph shows a negative deflection (below the baseline). In lead II, as the electrical current goes through the atrium and the ventricles, there are two positive deflections: the P wave and QRS complex. In other leads, such as the augmented leads, the P wave and QRS complex are seen as negative deflections because of the placement of the electrodes. Lead I uses both arm electrodes and lead III uses the left arm and left leg electrodes. In addition to these three leads (I, II, and III) and the six precordial leads (V_1–V_6), there are also three augmented unipolar leads (VR, VL, and VF), which make up the standard 12-lead ECG. Six-inch recordings of each lead are taken. With all 12 leads of the ECG, a clinician can gain a great deal of knowledge about the total electrical activity of the heart. However, for basic monitoring or for an assessment of an arrhythmia, lead II may suffice.

Purposes. The ECG is a diagnostic tool used very frequently for clients with chest pain or other cardiac symptoms. Toxicity to certain drugs, such as tricyclic antidepressants, can be monitored with ECGs (Boehnert and Lovejoy, 1985). The ECG is the definitive way to diagnose the various arrhythmias. Rhythm strips are almost always first scanned by nurses (Boltz, 1994). It is also very helpful in differentiating myocardial infarction from myocardial ischemia. A cardiologist interprets the ECG and writes a formal summary of the findings. This summary is put in the client's chart with samples from the various leads of the ECG. Although a 12-lead ECG can tax the skill of even an experienced cardiologist, nurses in expanded roles may conduct an initial analysis. Purcell and Haynes (1984) described a five-step analysis used to detect ischemia or necrosis.

Characteristics of a Normal Sinus Rhythm

All nurses need to have a basic understanding of what a normal sinus rhythm looks like (Figure 24–1), so arrhythmias can be detected on a rhythm strip. Electrolyte imbalances of potassium, calcium, and magnesium cause characteristic changes in rhythm, so nurses need to be able to identify these changes (Raimer, 1994). The characteristics of a normal ECG are as follows:

1. The heart rate is 60–100 beats per minute in an adult (two ways to calculate rates are discussed later)
2. The rhythm is regular
3. A P wave precedes each QRS complex
4. The PR interval is 0.12–0.20 sec (shorter in children)
5. The QRS complex is normal and less than 0.12 sec
6. The T wave is normal.

Describing Arrhythmias

In describing arrhythmias, a normal sinus rhythm means that the heart rate is under the control of the sinoatrial node (SA node). A *sinus* tachycardia means that the rate is faster than 100 beats per minute in an adult, but the SA node is still controlling

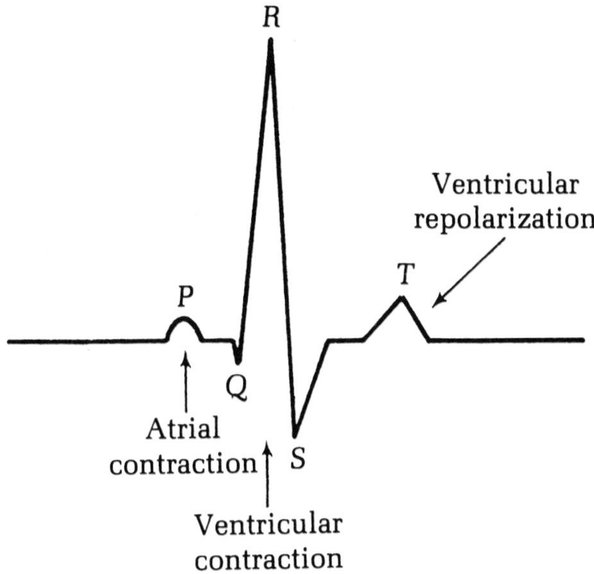

Figure 24–1. Basic components of an ECG tracing. (Note that atrial repolarization is hidden in the QRS complex.) See text for definition of P wave, PR interval, QRS complex, T wave, QT intervals, and ST segment.

the rate. *Atrial* tachycardia means the atrium is controlling the heart rate, whereas *ventricular* tachycardia means the ventricle is controlling the heart rate. In *nodal* or junctional arrhythmias, the atrioventricular (AV) node is controlling the rate. Thus, by simply reading the name of the arrhythmia from the ECG report, the nurse can assess something about the origin of the arrhythmia.

Ectopic or Premature Beats

A premature ventricular contraction (PVC) occurs when the ventricle originates a beat before the normal conduction of the impulse from the SA node. In rhythms with an occasional premature beat, the cardiac rate is still being controlled by the SA node. Another name for premature beat is *ectopic beats*, which means *displaced* or *malpositioned*. (An ectopic pregnancy occurs outside the uterus.) Ectopic or premature contractions can arise from the atrial tissue (premature atrial contraction [PAC]), ventricular tissue (PVC), or from AV junctional tissue.

P Wave

The P wave occurs at the beginning of each contraction of the atria (depolarization). The rounded P wave is the impulse that spreads through muscle, not through conductive tissue in a straight line. (In contrast, the QRS complex is a straight line with a peak because the impulse travels straight through conductive tissue.)

Abnormal P Wave

In a PAC, the P wave does not demonstrate the usual sequence seen with normal sinus rhythm. In arrhythmias, such as atrial fibrillation, the P waves cannot be distinguished on the ECG because the atria are quivering or fibrillating. In atrial enlargement, the P wave looks different from normal because the impulse travels through more tissue.

PR Interval

The PR interval is the time it takes the impulse to travel from the atrium to the ventricle through the AV node and the bundle of His. Normally the PR interval is 0.12–0.20 sec. (One large square on the ECG paper measures 0.20 sec.)

A PR interval longer than 0.20 sec indicates a slowing of the impulse through the AV node and bundle of His. Drugs, such as digitalis, can cause a widening PR interval or first-degree heart block. Other types of drugs may also prolong the PR interval. In one type of second-degree heart block, the PR interval becomes longer and longer until the ventricular beat is dropped. In complete heart block, the PR interval cannot be measured because the ventricles are originating beats that are totally independent of the SA impulses, which generate the atrial beats. Thus, in complete heart block, the P waves may be normal, but no QRS complex follows. The P waves and QRS complexes are totally independent of each other.

QRS Complex

The QRS complex reflects the contraction (depolarization) of the ventricles. Normally, the QRS complex is less than 0.12 sec.

A PVC causes a distorted and widened QRS complex. A PVC usually looks very different from the other QRS complexes in the strip. Often, the QRS complex is a negative deflection rather than the positive deflection seen in lead II. All these changes in the QRS complex are due to an impulse that originated in ventricular tissue and traveled through the ventricle differently from the normal impulse, which comes from the SA node.

In myocardial infarction, the appearance of the QRS complex is one part of the ECG that is changed. Abnormal Q waves are characteristic of some types of myocardial infarction.

In ventricular tachycardia, the ventricles have taken control of the heart rate, and the ECG shows only spikes of QRS complexes, which are wide and rather bizarre looking.

ECG Documentation of the Type of Cardiac Arrest

In ventricular fibrillation, there are only wavy lines on the ECG with nothing that resembles a P wave or QRS complex. Ventricular fibrillation causes cardiac arrest—when the ventricles are fibrillating (quivering), there is no cardiac output—and the

ECG shows chaotic electrical activity. For the other type of cardiac arrest, cardiac standstill or asystole, the ECG shows a straight line—even the quivering or fibrillation of the ventricle has stopped. Only the ECG can be used to differentiate whether a cardiac arrest is due to asystole or fibrillation.

T Wave

The T wave occurs as the ventricles recover from the contraction period. This period of electrical recovery is called *repolarization*. (The repolarization of the atrium is not seen on the ECG graph because it is hidden in the larger electrical event of the QRS complex.)

Myocardial damage may cause inversion of the T waves. High levels of serum potassium (hyperkalemia) cause tall, peaked T waves. An ECG on an oscilloscope is sometimes used to monitor potassium replacement in severe cases of hypokalemia. Low levels of potassium (hypokalemia) cause inverted T waves. A flattened T wave means the ventricle is not able to repolarize normally. (See Chapter 5 for a discussion on the effects of potassium on cardiac function.)

QT Interval

The QT interval covers the period of both ventricular depolarization and repolarization. Its normal duration is 0.36–0.44 sec.

The QT interval is useful in evaluating the effects on the heart of drugs such as quinidine. Ischemia or electrolyte changes may prolong or shorten the QT interval.

ST Segment

The ST segment is the time between completion of depolarization and the beginning of repolarization of the ventricles. One often interprets only a nonspecific ST abnormality on an ECG.

A decidedly depressed or downward slope of the ST segment is somewhat characteristic of myocardial ischemia. Digitalis depresses the ST segment. (See the Stress Test in Chapter 26 for more explanation about ST changes from exertion and other factors.) Conversely, an elevated ST segment is one of the characteristics of a myocardial infarction. As with all other changes in the ECG, the meaning of the changes may be open to several interpretations, depending on other clinical data.

DETERMINING HEART RATE WITH AN ECG

Because the ECG paper is horizontally marked for time, heart rate can be determined by looking at an ECG strip. (The vertical deflections reflect the amplitude of the voltage, but this is not of great use to a nurse who is just beginning to learn about ECGs.) As seen in Figure 24–2, each tiny square of ECG strip measures 0.04 sec, and each larger square (which consists of five tiny ones) is 0.20 sec. By

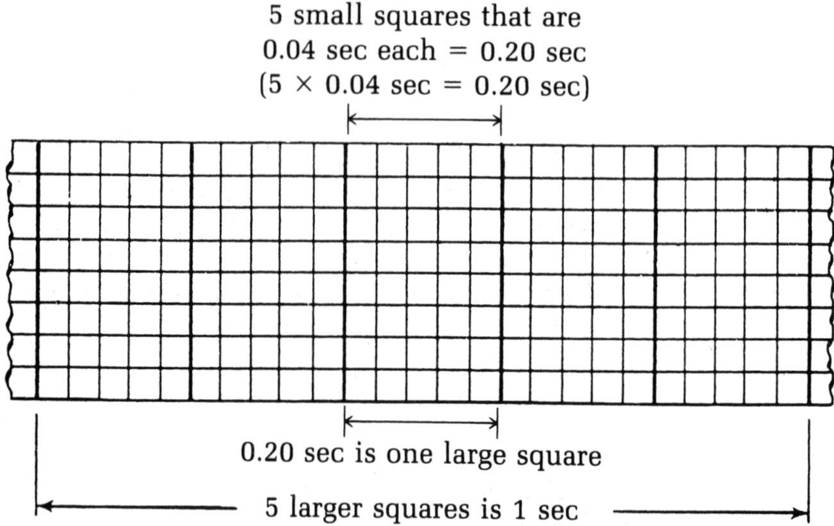

Method A: Count the number of large squares that occur between each QRS complex.

Formula: $\dfrac{\text{60 sec}}{\text{Number of squares between beats} \times 0.2\text{ sec}} = \text{Beats per min}$

Method B: Count the number of beats in 30 large squares.

Formula: Number of beats in 30 squares × 10 = Beats per min

Figure 24–2. Two methods to determine heart rate from an ECG tracing. See text for examples of use.

remembering that each large square signifies 0.20 sec, one can calculate the heart rate by means of several different formulas. Two simple methods that a nurse can use to time a heart rate by scanning an ECG strip are described in the following sections. Both methods assume a steady rate of impulses.

Method A: Counting the Squares Between the Beats

The squares between each QRS complex can be counted to determine the time between each beat. For example, if there are three large squares between each beat (QRS complex), this implies a time interval of 0.6 sec (3 squares × 0.2 sec) between each beat. Thus, in 60 sec, there would be 100 beats (60 sec ÷ 0.6). If there were five large squares between each beat, this would mean 1 sec (5 × 0.20 sec) between each beat. In 60 sec, there would be 60 beats (60 sec ÷ 1 sec per beat). Thus, when a client has a normal rhythm on an ECG strip, which has no fewer than three squares and no more than five squares between beats, the rate is within the normal adult range of 60–100 beats per minute. The formula for calculating heart rate by this method is

$$\frac{\text{60 sec per min}}{\text{Number of squares between beats} \times 0.20 \text{ sec}} = \text{Beats per minute}$$

Example:

$$\frac{60}{\text{3 (squares between beats)} \times 0.20} = \frac{60}{0.6} = 100$$

Method B: Counting the Beats in 30 Squares

Another way to calculate heart rate from an ECG strip is to count the number of QRS complexes in a certain number of squares. Recall that the large square measures 0.20 sec. By counting the beats in 30 large squares, one has counted the number of beats occurring in 6 sec because 30 squares times 0.20 sec equals 6 sec. The number obtained for 6 sec is multiplied by 10 to obtain the number of beats per minute. The time markings on the ECG strip designate 3-sec intervals and can also be used to determine 6-sec segments. For example, if the total number of beats in 30 squares is 5, the heart rate is 50 beats per minute (5 beats in 0.6 sec × 10). The formula for this method of calculating heart rate is

Number of beats in 30 squares (or 0.6 sec) × 10 = Number of beats per minute

Example:

5 beats (in 30 squares) × 10 = 50 beats per minute

▼ PRETEST NURSING DIAGNOSES RELATED TO ECG

Knowledge Deficit Related to Preparation for ECG

It is not necessary for a client to discontinue drugs or abstain from food and drink before an ECG. The client should not wear metal jewelry. Clothing must be loose so the electrodes can be fastened on the arms and legs and the suction bulb moved across the chest. Women need to remove hose because the electrode paste must be applied directly to the skin. The jelly or paste used with the electrodes is nonallergenic, but it may feel messy to the client. Clients may be skeptical about "being strapped to an electrical box," as a client once said. Therefore, the client may need reassurance that the machine only detects electrical signals *from* the client not to the client. Because many drugs, such as quinidine or digitalis, affect certain aspects of the ECG, it is important that the cardiologist who interprets the test be aware of any cardiac drugs the client has received. ECG requests have a place to note the cardiac drugs that the client has received.

(continued)

▼ PRETEST NURSING DIAGNOSES RELATED TO ECG (*continued*)

Risk for Injury Related to Malfunctioning Equipment

From a safety point of view, any electrical equipment does present an electrical hazard if the machine is defective and not properly grounded. As a rule, all electrically operated appliances should be plugged into the same wall outlet so there is no difference in grounding points. Improperly grounded or defective equipment can cause a current leakage through the client if the two pieces of equipment are plugged into outlets more than 12 feet (3.6 m) apart (Meth, 1980). The ECG technician has the responsibility of checking the machine to make sure that there are no frayed cords or other problems and that the machine is properly grounded. With a changing economic climate, nurses may find that running a 12-lead ECG becomes a nursing task. The nurse needs to keep in mind that for very ill clients, such as those with electrodes placed into the ventricle, all electrical equipment must be checked and grounded properly, including ECG machines. The nurse should consult with the hospital's electrical engineer about any problems that occur and how to perform safety checks of routine equipment.

▼ POSTTEST NURSING DIAGNOSIS RELATED TO ECG

Risk for Altered Cardiac Output Related to Underlying Pathophysiologic Condition

The ECG technician or nurse helps the client wipe off the electrode paste or jelly. Aside from this, there is no other special client care related directly to the test. However, if the ECG was done to evaluate a possible myocardial infarction, cardiac precautions should be continued until other diagnostic tests, such as cardiac enzymes (Chapter 12), are interpreted by the client's physician. If the ECG was performed to evaluate an arrhythmia, the nurse may need to inquire about any changes in medication orders. Usually the ECG technician scans the graph for blatant abnormalities and calls this to the attention of the physician. An experienced nurse can often differentiate between benign supraventricular abnormalities and potentially dangerous ectopic beats arising from the ventricle (Cudworth, 1986). Sometimes the ECG strip is kept with the client's chart; thus, the client's personal physician can immediately evaluate the strip. Otherwise the ECG is interpreted by a cardiologist, and a typed summary appears on the client's chart.

Heart rate, rhythm, and the presence or absence of a pulse deficit should be routinely monitored by the nurse if there is any question of arrhythmias.

The nurse must remember that the ECG measures only the electrical events in the heart and not cardiac output. The quality of peripheral pulses, capillary filling time, and color of the client are all signs of adequacy or inadequacy of cardiac output. Dyspnea, angina, abnormal heart or breath sounds, and a decrease in urine output are all detected by the nurse—not from an ECG reading. Therefore, even when a monitor is used to show ECG pattern, the nurse must still collect information to obtain a complete idea of the efficiency of the heart.

DIAGNOSTIC MONITORING IN INTENSIVE CARE UNITS

Clients at risk for serious cardiac arrhythmias are connected to cardiac monitors, which provide continuous surveillance of the electrical impulses of the heart. The ECG pattern is displayed on an oscilloscope, and when needed, on graph paper for a permanent record. When the client is connected to a monitor in an intensive care unit (ICU) or coronary care unit, the nurse must have special training on how to recognize arrhythmias that need immediate medical attention. Critical care units have standardized orders that permit a nurse who has had special training to administer antiarrhythmic drugs, such as lidocaine (Xylocaine) when a client has certain patterns of PVCs. Today's critical care nurse also focuses on early recognition of potentially lethal cardiac conduction defects by recognizing electrical axis deviations on the ECG. The reader is encouraged to consult one of the many excellent textbooks that focus on critical care nursing. (See Chapter 26 on electrophysiologic studies.)

▼ TELEMETRY AND CARDIAC MONITORING

Telemetry is taking measurements at a distance from the client by the use of radio signals. Telemetry has been extensively used in physiologic assessments during space travels. In the hospital setting, telemetry is used to monitor the ECG of a client without the client having to be hooked up to a monitor. The telemetry nurse monitors the monitor.

Small electrode disks are applied to the client's chest to obtain a good reading on the monitor. Disposable prelubricated disks can be kept on the client for several days unless skin irritation is noted. The wires from the electrodes are connected to a portable transmitter. The portable transmitter is about the size of a small tissue box and can be left lying in bed by the client or can be strapped to an ambulatory client's waist. Telemetry, like a conventional ECG, measures only the rate and electrical events of the heart. The nurse is still needed to assess the mechanical events (i.e., cardiac output) in the client.

Telemetry with Telephone and Facsimile

Telephone recordings of ECGs originated in 1971. A special instrument is used with the telephone. The graphic representation of heart rhythm is fed into a computer and a duplicate is made for analysis by a cardiologist. The response time for emergency requests is 10–15 min for a complete reading. Clients with pacemakers may have phone checks completed every 3 months or so to supplement office visits (Witherell, 1990). The telephone transmitter is supplied through the physician or pacemaker clinic.

Facsimile technology has made it possible to send complete ECGs to a cardiologist on call, making a well-organized 24-hour system for ECG interpretation available in even small community hospitals or clinics (Bertrand et al., 1994).

▼ AMBULATORY ELECTROCARDIOGRAPHY

In outpatient settings, clients may be given a portable recorder (sometimes referred to as Holter monitor) to wear, which records the ECG on magnetic tape. When the tapes are returned to the cardiology laboratory, a computer scans the tapes to identify points of interest. This method is expensive, but it can be helpful in pinpointing the type of arrhythmia causing the client's symptoms. Also, the ambulatory ECG can be used to evaluate the effects of some treatments. The usual duration of Holter monitoring is 24 hr. However, some arrhythmias, such as those associated with syncope, may not be detected in the first 24 hr, so a 48-hr strip may be needed (Bass et al., 1990). Holter monitoring may be as useful as the more expensive electrophysiologic studies (Chapter 26) to predict the efficacy of antiarrhythmic drugs for ventricular tachyarrhythmias (Mason, 1993).

New types of monitors for ambulatory ECGs, called arrhythmia event recorders, allow the client to record an electrocardiogram during a symptomatic episode with a small device that is capable of transtelephonic transmission. Some units look like a wristwatch; one electrode forms the back of the monitor worn around the wrist. When symptoms occur, the client activates the record button and rests a hand on top of the other electrode. A high quality ECG strip is recorded. This stored ECG can be sent by phone anywhere in the world. Readers should consult current literature on the various items available, since technologic advances continue at a fast pace.

▼ NURSING DIAGNOSIS RELATED TO AMBULATORY ECG

Knowledge Deficit Related to the Procedure for Monitoring

The client is not to swim or bathe when the monitor is in place. Also the client must not have any radiographs taken while the monitor is being used—radiographs erase the tape. Metal detectors, remote control TV, CB radios, microwave ovens, and even electric blankets may interfere with the readings.

The client should be instructed to keep a diary of any events that cause symptoms such as shortness of breath, dizziness, or angina. The client should also keep a record of such activities as sleeping time, exercise, eating, bowel movements, cigarette smoking, sexual activity, and emotional stress, which may be related to the cardiac symptoms.

It has been observed that clients are often unaware that symptoms, such as dizziness, are due to arrhythmia. In addition to the usual cardiac symptoms, symptoms such as headache, indigestion, or weakness may be linked to the specific time of an arrhythmia. Thus, a 24-hr strip may elucidate the cause of vague client symptoms so that the symptoms can be treated.

Often, nurses instruct clients in the use of Holter monitors or other cardiac event recorders when it is necessary to evaluate arrhythmias related to physical reconditioning at home after a cardiac operation or myocardial infarction.

▼ ELECTROENCEPHALOGRAPHY

Description. An electrocephalogram (EEG) is a recording of the electrical activity of the brain. The EEG primarily records activity of the superficial layers of the cerebral cortex. Approximately 20 surface electrodes are applied to the client's scalp. A jelly may be used to help conduction of the electrical signals. The electrode wires are attached to the EEG machine that records the electrical signals on a piece of graph paper.

If the client is comatose, the EEG can be performed at bedside. However, for routine diagnostic studies, the client is taken to the EEG laboratory, where the environment can be better controlled. The recording takes an hour or two and includes a nap. The first part of the recording is obtained with the client as relaxed as possible to obtain a baseline reading. The client is then asked to hyperventilate for several minutes, to see how this changes the patterns of the brain. The client may become light-headed from hyperventilating. Evoked potential studies evaluate changes in the brain in response to various stimuli such as flickering light and auditory signals. In addition, somatosensory signals may be generated by skin electrodes. Sleep may evoke abnormal patterns that are not present when the brain is more active, so sleeping patterns may also be obtained.

Purposes. Although the EEG is nonspecific, it can help identify a focus of disturbance in the brain. Most clients with cerebral seizures have abnormal EEGs, but a normal EEG does not rule out a seizure disorder. Normal EEGs are seen in about 20% of children and 10% of adults who have epilepsy. However, these percentages are reduced when serial tracings are obtained (Hay et al., 1995).

When the brain is dead, the electrical activity of the brain is absent, and the EEG is flat. The EEG is one way to detect brain death in a comatose client. Other tests for brain death and written statements by physicians are based on current local standards because there is not a national standard for brain death in adults (Bongard and Sue, 1994). Studies performed on comatose clients show that the findings of the EEG have a high correlation with the survival or death of a client in a coma.

EEGs may be performed to evaluate narcolepsy, sleeping patterns, and sleep apnea. These types of studies are conducted in a specially equipped sleep laboratory. Concurrent measurement of the client's oxygen level can be measured with a pulse oximeter (Chapter 6). EEGs to evaluate sleep disturbances are called *somnograms*. To evaluate abnormal EEG waves, clients may also be connected to an ambulatory EEG system. As with the Holter monitors used for ambulatory ECGs, clients keep a journal of their activities and any symptoms that occur during the 24-hour monitoring period.

▼ NURSING DIAGNOSIS RELATED TO EEG

Knowledge Deficit Related to Preparation

For routine EEG testing, the client should have no medicines for 24–48 hr before the test, except medicines particularly ordered by the physician. Tranquilizers, stimulants (including coffee, tea, colas, and cigarettes), and alcohol all cause changes in brain patterns. The client should have normal meals because hypoglycemia can cause changes in brain patterns. The client's hair should be shampooed the day before the test, and no oils, sprays, or lotions should be applied to the hair. It may be desirable that the client not have much sleep before the EEG recording, because sleep deprivation may evoke abnormal brain patterns. The last part of the EEG recording may be conducted with the client asleep, and the client may have trouble falling asleep if he or she has just slept. Therefore, the adult client may be instructed to go to bed late the night before the test and to awake early. Children and infants should not be allowed to nap before the scheduled test. For ambulatory EEG monitoring, the client needs instructions on how to keep the electrodes in place. A journal of activities is needed for this type of monitoring.

If an EEG is being performed to evaluate the possibility of brain death, it is important that artifacts be kept to a minimum. Artifacts can be caused by manipulation of the electrodes or by electrical interference. The nurse should follow the specific guidelines of the institution when EEGs are performed at the client's bedside. (The electrical hazards for ECG also apply to EEG, in which several electrical appliances may be in use at once.)

▼ POSTTEST NURSING DIAGNOSIS RELATED TO EEG

Risk for Injury

The only specific care after an EEG is a shampoo to remove electrode gel from the hair. If seizure activity is a possibility, seizure precautions should be noted.

▼ ELECTROMYELOGRAPHY

Description. An electromyelogram (EMG) measures the electrical activity of muscles. Needle electrodes are inserted into selected skeletal muscles. (Although in one sense the test is somewhat invasive, it is discussed here because of the similarities between ECGs and EMGs.) This procedure does cause some pain. The skin is cleaned with alcohol or iodine, but no local anesthetic is used. The muscle activity is recorded at rest, during voluntary activity, and with electrical stimuli. The findings from the EMG are recorded and usually summarized in narrative form for use on the client's chart. Informed consent is needed for this test.

Purposes. In nerve atrophy, there may be characteristic fibrillation, even in the resting muscle. Usually a resting muscle has no electrical activity. The test can be useful in determining the extent of peripheral nerve injuries and differentiating paralysis of psychological origin.

EMG cannot be used to diagnose specific neuromuscular diseases, but it can differentiate between neuropathy and myopathy. All neuromuscular abnormalities are classified in two categories:

1. *Myopathy* is a disease or disturbance of striated muscle fibers or cell membranes. Myasthenia gravis or primary muscular dystrophy are examples of myopathies that produce abnormal EMGs.
2. *Neuropathy* is a disease or disorder of the lower motor neuron. Toxic effects of drugs, hypothyroidism, polio, and diabetes can all cause neuropathy.

▼ NURSING DIAGNOSES RELATED TO EMG

Knowledge Deficit Related to Procedure for EMG

No special physical preparation of the client is required before or after the test. Premedications for sedation or pain relief are avoided to assess a normal neuromuscular pattern. Muscle aches after the procedure may be relieved with mild analgesics. The procedure may take 1–2 hr if extensive testing is performed. The nurse should prepare the client for the discomfort and sounds of an EMG. The client may feel pain on insertion of the needle electrodes and hears audio amplification that sounds like firecrackers. If nerve conduction studies are carried out, the feelings may be similar to static electricity.

Risk for Impaired Mobility

Before and after an EMG the nurse can be very useful in evaluating the functional capacity of the client with an unknown neuromuscular problem. Thus,

(*continued*)

▼ NURSING DIAGNOSES RELATED TO EMG (*continued*)

the gait of the client, ability to perform range-of-motion (ROM) exercises, and any motor–power–sensory deficits should be recorded. Clinical data are always used as part of the base for interpreting EMG reports.

▼ PULMONARY FUNCTION TESTS: SPIROMETRY

Description. Pulmonary function tests (PFTs) can be classified as (1) ventilation tests and (2) specialized PFTs of gaseous diffusion and distribution. PFTs, performed in a pulmonary function laboratory, cover the entire range of respiratory volume and capabilities. On the other hand, PFTs performed on the unit or in ambulatory care settings are modified to ventilation tests of FEV, vital capacity (VC), and MVV. This section focuses only on the more common ventilation studies. Chapter 22 includes information about lung perfusion scans. The clinical significance of blood gas analysis, an important aspect of most pulmonary studies, is discussed in Chapter 6.

For ventilation studies of lung volume and capacity, the client breathes into a machine called a *spirometer*. A spirometry system consisting of a plug in a spirometric module connected to a computer graphic, such as blowing out birthday candles, is used to test pulmonary function. The computer analyzes the results and prints a report. Reports are stored so that comparisons of tests can be made over time. (The nurse sometimes uses a portable spirometer, the Wright spirometer, for clinical assessment of the client's ventilation status.)

Purposes. PFTs for lung volume and capacity help identify whether the client has an obstructive defect, a restrictive defect, or a combination of both. When there is an increase in airway resistance, the defect in ventilation is called an *obstructive defect*. Asthma, bronchitis, and emphysema cause obstructive defects in ventilation. When the defect in ventilation is due to a limitation on chest expansion, the defect is called a *restrictive defect*. Pathologic conditions that limit chest expansion include fibrosis of the lungs, muscle dystrophy, obesity, and abnormal curvature of the spine. Conditions such as pulmonary congestion may cause both obstruction and restriction of ventilation. The ventilation tests help delineate the type of defect present and whether the defects are reversible with therapy such as bronchodilation. Ventilation tests are often ordered before a client undergoes an operation, so any respiratory problems can be anticipated and better treated or prevented. Nurses in ambulatory settings may be actively involved in conducting ventilation tests as part of a nursing assessment. Nurse-directed clinics for clients with chronic lung disease have routinely measured FEV, FEV_1 to VC ratios, and MVV for many years (Nield, 1974). Petty (1986) noted that measurement of volume and flow should be as common as measuring vital signs, because these pulmonary function tests are helpful in assessing clients who have to be protected from the development of acute problems. PFTs are an important tool in neonatal intensive care and may be performed by nurses skilled in this area (Cullen et al., 1994). Home testing can even be conducted by clients with inexpensive peak flow monitors that can be used by people with asthma to assess a worsening of their status. More expensive handheld spirometers can also be purchased by clients to measure FVC, FEV, and MVV.

▼ PRETEST NURSING DIAGNOSIS RELATED TO PULMONARY FUNCTION TESTS

Knowledge Deficit Related to Procedure

The clinician conducting a PFT gives the client specific instructions for each step of the test. The client must breathe only through his or her mouth. A noseclip is used on the nose. The client needs to rest before the test so that he or she can perform as well as possible. The client should not take any bronchodilators or narcotics before the test because they can change breathing capabilities. Because the various breathing maneuvers require the maximal cooperation of the client, the test is not reliable in young children or confused adults. Food and fluids may be consumed.

▼ POSTTEST NURSING DIAGNOSIS RELATED TO PULMONARY FUNCTION TESTS

Risk for Ineffective Breathing Patterns

The client may be discouraged if the tests showed less than optimal lung functioning. Poor test results may be an incentive for the client to stop smoking to prevent further damage. Also, the test results can help guide the clinician in determining what breathing exercises may be beneficial for the client and whether drugs such as bronchodilators are effective. Clients with restrictive defects may need help to maximize respiration. Clients with obstructive defects need to learn how to get more air out by using techniques such as pursed-lip breathing. Nurses skilled in teaching breathing techniques may foster positive changes in the client.

Summary of Findings from Ventilation Studies

VC and FVC. The vital capacity (VC) is the maximum amount of air that can be expired after a normal inspiration. The vital capacity when the breathing is forced is the forced vital capacity (FVC).

REFERENCE VALUES FOR VC AND FVC
Must be determined with charts, which are specific for sex, age, and height. A value less than 75–80% the predicted value is abnormal.

Clinical Significance. For most clients the results of VC and FVC are similar. VC increases with physical fitness. In fact, FVC may be a good indicator of overall good health. In restrictive diseases, the VC or FVC is always decreased—this test is the best assessment of restrictive defects. In obstructive defects, the VC may not be appreciably decreased. However, the more severe the obstruction, the more likely it is that the air trapping will reduce VC.

FEV. The FEV is the percentage of vital capacity that can be expressed in 1, 2, or 3 sec. The figures are expressed as FEV_1, FEV_2, and FEV_3. The test is useful to evaluate the severity of airway obstruction and to evaluate the effectiveness of bronchodilators.

REFERENCE VALUES FOR FEV

Normally 65–85% of the vital capacity can be expressed in the first second and up to 95–97% by 3 sec. For FEV_1, less than 75% of the predicted value is considered abnormally low.

Clinical Significance. In obstructive disease, FEV_1 is decreased. In restrictive disease, FEV_1 is normal or can be decreased. In some restrictive diseases in which there is an increase of elastic resistance, the FEV_1 may be normal or elevated.

REFERENCE VALUES FOR FEV_1 COMPARED WITH FVC

Younger people can expel 75–85% of the VC in 1 sec. Older people can normally expel about 65–75% in the first second. This is the only PFT in which age is an important determinant and in which increases as well as decreases may be abnormal.

Clinical Significance. The ratio of the total FVC to FEV_1 is decreased with obstructive disease, and increased, normal, or sometimes decreased with restrictive disease. The amount of disability from obstructive disease may be rated by the ratio of the FEV_1 to the VC. For example, one such rating considers 60–70% a mild disability, 40–60% a moderate disability, and less than 40% a severe disability (Carroll, 1986).

VE, MVV, or MBC. These tests measure the volume exhaled in 1 min. The volume exhaled per minute at rest is volume exhaled (VE). The volume exhaled in 1 min when the person breathes as deeply and rapidly as possible is called the maximal voluntary ventilation (MVV) or the maximal breathing capacity (MBC). Usually the minute volume is 15–20 times the one time volume of the FVC.

REFERENCE VALUES FOR VE, MVV, OR MBC

Values are matched on a chart for age and weight. Less than 80% of predicted value is considered abnormally low.

Clinical Significance. Clients with obstructive defects have volumes less than 80% of the predicted values. In restrictive disease, the values usually are normal. Severe ventilation defects may show less than 35% of predicted value.

FEF. FEF measures how fast a person can exhale a specified amount of air. This test is useful in screening clients for subclinical obstructive disease. The person breathes in as deeply as possible and then times how many seconds it takes to exhale through an open mouth. The test is performed three times, and the fastest time is recorded. Most people can expel all the air in 2–5 sec. If clients perform a simple version of this test at home they should contact a doctor if it takes longer than 5 sec to expel the air.

REFERENCE VALUES FOR FEF

Values are matched on a chart for age and weight. Less than 75% of the predicted value is abnormally low.

Clinical Significance. A long-time smoker may have no symptoms of respiratory problems, but the FEF is less than 75% of the predicted values.

In summary, the test used most often for restrictive defects is FVC. The tests used for obstructive defects are the FEV, FEV_1 to FVC ratio, MVV, and FEF for subclinical disease. For mixed types of defects, all these tests are helpful (Petty, 1986).

▼ PEAK FLOW TESTING

In the past several years, small easy-to-use devices called *peak flow meters* have become available for home monitoring of clients with asthma. To test peak flow, the client sets the flow tab at the predetermined normal rate and then blows into the tube-shaped monitor as hard and as fast as possible. A whistle blows if the flow rate achieves the predetermined set rate of flow. Some meters have more sophisticated gauges than others. Prices vary considerably depending on the design and whether the device is made from cardboard or plastic. The less expensive meters are reliable, but they may not last long. Most come with a carrying case and daily record charts.

If these meters are used on a regular basis, the client can detect the beginning reduction in air flow that warns of an impending asthma attack. Stelzer (1989) noted that the reductions in air flow may precede an asthma attack by hours or even a day or two, so the client has ample time to consult the health care provider and make needed adjustments in medication. Or the client may be instructed to go to the emergency department if the peak flow drops below a certain point. For example, a goal for a client with asthma may be to maintain peak expiratory flow rate (PFFR) greater than 80% of the personal best and with less than 20% variation during a 24-hour period (Borkgren and Gronkiewicz, 1995).

▼ NURSING IMPLICATIONS RELATED TO USE OF PEAK FLOW MONITORS

The sooner an asthma attack is treated, the easier it is to stop, so detailed instructions on how to use the monitor are warranted. Encouraging the use of a peak flow meter helps clients and parents of young children with asthma become partners with the health care team in managing a frightening and unpredictable disease. This approach makes the client much more in control of the problem with more self-assurance in leading a normal life. One brochure for a peak flow meter notes that children enjoy making the whistling sound and give it their all, including following physician orders, so they can keep a normal peak flow rate.

▼ THERMOGRAPHY

Description. Thermography is a technique that uses an infrared camera to photograph the surface temperature of the body. The pictures of the temperature of the skin's surface can show variations from blue cold to red hot. The body part to be photographed is exposed to air. The client is disrobed in a 68–70°F (20–21°C) environment for 15 min. Some methods involve spraying the area with 95% alcohol. Inflammation and malignant processes, in which there is an accelerated local metabolism, generate additional heat, which may be detected on the body surface.

Purposes. Some research has suggested that thermography might be useful for breast cancer prognosis (Isard et al., 1988). At present, thermography is not recommended as a screening device for breast cancer because the results are not conclusive and mammography is much more effective (Chapter 20).

Some research has been completed to see if thermography can help detect bone tumors, vascular disease, or conditions in which inflammation is present. For example, thermography has been suggested as a possible way to measure reactions to skin tests and the change in skin temperature when there is nerve impairment. Thermography has been used to assess areas of pain in the body. The locus of pain is often cooler than the rest of the body. Because thermography is noninvasive, with no risk to the client, it may be a diagnostic tool that will become more useful in clinical practice in the future. The reader is encouraged to consult current research literature.

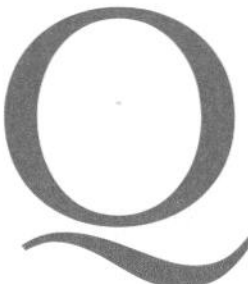

1. Special consent forms for noninvasive diagnostic tests are
   a. Usually required and are obtained by the physician in charge
   b. Always required if the client has not undergone the test before
   c. Not usually required because there is no risk to the client
   d. Completed if the client is fearful of the procedure

2. The repolarization of the ventricle is shown on the ECG as the
   a. QRS complex b. QT interval
   c. ST segment d. T wave

3. A characteristic of a normal ECG for an adult is
   a. A PR interval less than 0.10 sec
   b. A heart rate between 70 and 80 beats per minute
   c. A positive deflection of the QRS complex on lead II
   d. A P wave after each QRS complex

4. Premature heartbeats change the appearance of the ECG. Which of the following is a characteristic of a premature ventricular contraction?
   a. A P wave precedes the QRS complex
   b. A T wave is absent after the QRS complex
   c. The QRS complex is wider than normal
   d. The QRS complex is absent

5. Mr. Smiley has just undergone an ECG. The nurse has noted that the rhythm is regular and that there are eight QRS complexes in 30 large squares of the ECG graph. Therefore, Mr. Smiley's heart rate is
   a. 50 b. 60
   c. 70 d. 80

6. Another way to figure Mr. Smiley's pulse rate on the ECG graph would be to count the large squares between each QRS complex. If there were four large squares between each QRS complex, Mr. Smiley's rate would be
   a. 55 b. 65
   c. 75 d. 85

7. Mr. Faber has a history of angina. He had some nonspecific changes on an ECG performed today. He is now undergoing telemetry. Which of the following measures of cardiac activity could be eliminated by the nurse because telemetry is being used? (Assume the telemetry equipment has been checked and is functioning properly.)

   a. Counting the apical rate and noting the rhythm
   b. Noting any dyspnea, angina, or abnormal breath sounds
   c. Checking the quality of peripheral pulses
   d. Noting the amount of urinary output

8. Which of the following nursing actions is *inappropriate* when a client is to undergo an EEG?

   a. Allowing a child to nap before the procedure
   b. Seeing that the client has a shampoo
   c. Allowing regular meals but no coffee, tea, or colas
   d. Checking to see if tranquilizers and sedatives should be withheld

9. Mrs. Tooler is to have an EMG to assess a weakness in her left leg. Which of the following statements is correct to tell Mrs. Tooler when she asks about the test?

   a. There is no pain or discomfort during an EMG
   b. The test can specifically determine the type of muscular disorder present
   c. The client must remain on bed rest for a while after the test
   d. The test can help the physician determine whether the muscular problem is due to nerve or muscle dysfunction

10. Which one of the following pulmonary function tests is most useful for detecting subclinical cases of obstructive defects in ventilation?

    a. FVC (forced vital capacity)
    b. FEV_1 (forced expiratory volume in 1 sec)
    c. MVV (maximum voluntary ventilation)
    d. FEF (forced expiratory flow)

11. Education about the use of a peak flow meter would be of the greatest benefit for

    a. Mr. Harris, who is to undergo an exploratory thoracotomy
    b. Mr. Warzyniak, who is a heavy smoker
    c. Mr. Leonard, who took an overdose of a narcotic and had respiratory depression for a few hours
    d. Sandy Blake, aged 15, who has a history of severe asthma attacks

12. Thermography is based on the principle that inflammation and some malignant processes cause accelerated heat production. This increase in heat is measured by

a. Rectal and oral thermometers
b. Pictures with an infrared camera
c. Heat-sensitive electrodes attached to the body
d. Immersion in a water bath of a certain temperature

▼ REFERENCES

Bass, E., Curtiss, E.L., Arena, V.C., et al. (1990). The duration of Holter monitoring in patients with syncope: Is 24 hours enough? *Archives of Internal Medicine, 150* (5), 1073–1078.

Bertrand, C.A., Benda, R.L., Mercando, A.D., et al. (1994). Effectiveness of the fax electrocardiogram. *American Journal of Cardiology, 74*, 294–295.

Boehnert, M., and Lovejoy, F. (1985). Value of the QRS duration versus the serum drug level in predicting seizures and ventricular arrhythmias after an acute overdosage of tricyclic antidepressants. *New England Journal of Medicine, 313* (8), 474–477.

Boltz, M.A. (1994). Nurse's guide to identifying cardiac rhythms. *Nursing 94, 24* (4), 54–58.

Bongard, F.S., and Sue, D.Y. (1994). *Current critical care diagnosis & treatment.* Norwalk, CT: Appleton & Lange.

Borkgren, M.W., and Gronkiewicz, C.A. (1995). Update your asthma care from hospital to home. *American Journal of Nursing, 95* (1), 26–34.

Carroll, P. (1986). What you can learn from pulmonary function tests. *RN, 49*, 24–26.

Cudworth, K. (1986). Is that funny looking beat dangerous? *RN, 49* (5), 32–35.

Cullen, J.A., Greenspan, J.S., Antunes, M.J., et al. (1994). Pulmonary function testing in the critically ill neonate. Part II: Methodology. *Neonatal Network, 13* (2), 7–13.

Hay, W.W., Groothuis, J.R., Hayward, A.R., and Levin, M.J. (1995). *Current pediatric diagnosis & treatment* (12th ed.). Norwalk, CT: Appleton & Lange.

Isard, H., Sweitzer, C., and Edelstein, G. (1988). Breast thermography: A prognostic indicator of breast cancer survival. *Cancer, 62*, 484–488.

Mason, J. (1993). A comparison of electrophysiologic testing with Holter monitoring to predict antiarrhythmic-drug efficacy for ventricular tachyarrhythmias. *New England Journal of Medicine, 329* (7), 445–451.

Meth, I. (1980). Electrical safety in the hospital. *American Journal of Nursing, 80* (7), 1344–1348.

Nield, M. (1974). A nurse directed chest clinic. *Nursing Clinics of North America, 9*, 147–155.

Petty, T. (1986). ABC's of simple pulmonary function assessment. *Nurse Practitioner, 11* (6), 50–60.

Pidgeon, V. (1985). Children's concepts of illness: Implications for health teaching. *Maternal-Child Nursing Journal, 14* (1), 23–33.

Purcell, J., and Haynes, L. (1984). Using the ECG to detect MI. *American Journal of Nursing, 84* (5), 628–642.

Raimer, F. (1994). How to identify electrolyte imbalances on your patient's ECG. *Nursing 94, 24* (6), 54–58.

Stelzer, D. (1989). Peak flow meters. *Lung Line Letter, 3* (4), 2.

Witherell, C. (1990). Permanent pacemakers: Questions nurses ask. *American Journal of Nursing, 90* (12), 20–28.

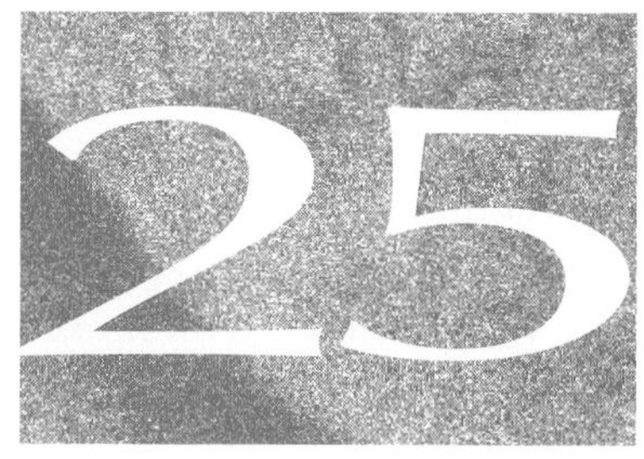

COMMON INVASIVE TESTS

- Lumbar Puncture
- Bone Marrow Aspiration or Biopsy
- Thoracentesis (Pleural Tap)
- Paracentesis (Abdominal Tap)
- Gastric Analysis
- Papanicolaou Smears or Exfoliative Cytologic Studies: Papanicolaou Smears of the Uterus
- Cervigram
- Colposcopy, Cervical Biopsy, and Endometrial Biopsy
- Breast Biopsy and Needle Aspiration
- Liver Biopsy
- Renal Biopsy

OBJECTIVES

1. Identify nursing diagnoses related to preparing adults and children for invasive diagnostic procedures performed at their bedsides, in a treatment room, or in the outpatient department.
2. Identify the key nursing implications for clients undergoing bone marrow aspirations.
3. Describe the usual procedure for the collection of spinal fluid and the normal characteristics of cerebrospinal fluid (CSF) as demonstrated at routine laboratory analysis.

4. Compare and contrast the pre- and postcare of clients undergoing thoracentesis or paracentesis.
5. Describe the procedures needed for a gastric analysis, including the use of medications, which may be administered by the nurse.
6. Identify the key nursing diagnoses for clients undergoing breast and cervical biopsies for suspected malignant tumors.
7. Compare and contrast the pre- and postcare of clients undergoing renal and liver biopsies.
8. Identify what is important in informing consumers about the Papanicolaou smear as a cancer detection tool.

As discussed in Chapter 24, the division of diagnostic tests into invasive and noninvasive is somewhat artificial because all testing may be considered as an invasion to the person to some degree. The term *invasive* is usually used to describe diagnostic tests that entail the use of needles or instruments inserted inside the body to directly record or assess the structure and function of an organ. Some invasive diagnostic procedures are performed at the client's bedside, such as a thoracentesis or pleural tap. Others are performed in specially equipped treatment rooms, radiology suites, or even in a specialized laboratory, such as a cardiac catheterization laboratory. Invasive tests require specialized equipment and highly skilled clinicians. When invasive procedures are performed by experienced, skilled clinicians, the incidence of serious side effects is low. But there is always the possibility of complications when the body is invaded with needles and other types of probes. The possibility of complications ranges from simple problems to severe injury and even death. After the physician explains the possible risks to the client and the expected benefits of the test, the client or guardian must sign a consent form specific to the test. Hogue (1986) noted that a tape recording of the discussion with the client or a guardian can substitute for a written document. However, institutions almost always use written forms. *The policy of informed consent is essential for all invasive tests.* A general form used at admission is not acceptable.

The invasive tests covered in this chapter are those that are usually performed in the hospital unit or in an outpatient clinic. A nurse is often present during these procedures and actively assists the physician and supports the client. These tests include needle aspirations or taps and various kinds of biopsies performed with the aid of local anesthesia. Nurse practitioners may actually perform some procedures on clients whose condition is stable.

The second broad type of invasive procedures are those performed in a special laboratory or specially equipped procedure room, such as endoscopic procedures or cardiac catheterizations. The role of the staff nurse for these procedures is to prepare the client for the test and to care for the client afterward. If a nurse wants to assist with endoscopic procedures or cardiac catheterization, special clinical training is required. Cardiac catheterizations and electrophysiologic studies are discussed in Chapter 26 and endoscopic procedures in Chapter 27.

▼ GENERAL PRETEST NURSING DIAGNOSES

Risk for Injury

As mentioned earlier, the physician must have the client or guardian sign a specific consent form for any invasive procedure. The usual risks are mentioned on the form. The nurse must be aware of the policy of the institution. Most institutions require one or more routine laboratory tests before invasive procedures. The nurse coordinates the collection of any samples needed for laboratory analysis such as hematocrit (hct) and urinalysis. The nurse also assesses the physical and mental status of the client before the test; these are baseline assessments, which are referred to after the test. One of the most critical baseline assessments is the client's normal blood pressure and heart rate. For some of these tests, the blood pressure cuff is left on the client's arm during the procedure so the nurse can take readings throughout the procedure.

Altered Comfort Related to Pain of Procedure

All invasive procedures are to some degree uncomfortable for the client, and most cause some pain. At the very least, the pain is confined to the prick accompanying the injection of the local anesthetic. Some procedures also cause momentary pain or unpleasantness during the test. If the nurse is with the client during the procedure, he or she can be valuable in assisting the client in dealing with any expected momentary pain. For example, various breathing techniques or pain distractors can be taught to the client. Sometimes simply squeezing the nurse's hand helps the client cope. Depending on the interest of the client and the skill of the nurse, the client may be taught techniques, such as imaging or other methods to divert his or her attention from the present situation. For example, if the client has learned the Lamaze breathing technique to reduce discomfort during labor, this technique could be used to lessen the discomfort during a painful procedure. The nurse should find out what the client believes will help ease discomfort. For some clients sedatives may be needed, but accurate information about the test may alleviate anxiety and make sedatives unnecessary. The key points to emphasize are that (1) the duration of pain is brief and (2) local anesthesia is used. Pretest information should include what the client will see, smell, taste, or feel to lessen the dread of the unknown. Some clients may want a lot of technical information. Others may want to know only how much it will hurt. Research studies have suggested that adult clients who receive information about the sensations of a procedure appear to have less anxiety than clients who receive no information or only procedural information (Johnson and Rice, 1974).

Sometimes systemic drugs are needed to control the anxiety and pain of invasive procedures. For example, meperidine (Demerol) and a phenothiazine

(*continued*)

▼ GENERAL PRETEST NURSING DIAGNOSES *(continued)*

may be given before the procedure is started. These drugs may have an effect for several hours. Sometimes, midazolam (Versed) may be given just before the procedure. Sedation occurs within 3–5 min after an intravenous slow push and usually lasts only for about 30 min. Suderman (1990) noted that children remain awake after receiving midazolam but are relaxed and often have nearly total amnesia of the procedure. If many tests are performed and some need to be repeated, such as bone marrow aspirations and lumbar punctures for leukemia, some amnesia may be desirable.

Anxiety and Fear in Children

Preparing children for invasive tests means preparing the parents, too. The use of a booklet designed for children is helpful (Waidley, 1985). It is sometimes better to let the parents explain the procedure to the child. It has been suggested that it is better to speak to adolescents when they are alone. The nurse's assessment of the child's growth and developmental stage is essential for appropriate health teaching. For example, school-age children are usually receptive to teaching (Pidgeon, 1985). Encouraging a child to play with some of the equipment may help alleviate anxiety. Research studies have suggested that, as with adults, telling children about the sensations they will feel may lower distress (Suderman, 1990). Adolescents may be particularly interested in seeing what equipment will be used during the test. Children, as well as adults, need to know how they can help during the test. Young children may have to be restrained; thus, they deserve explanations. By the age of 3 years, children may be able to undergo procedures without the use of restraint if (1) the parent holds the child, (2) the child is allowed to participate, and (3) acceptable behavior is rewarded (Beckemeyer and Bahr, 1980). Keeping a security blanket or favorite toy nearby may also help relieve the child's anxiety. Distraction, such as with the use of a kaleidoscope, has ameliorated children's perceptions of pain during needle sticks (Vessey et al., 1994).

Knowledge Deficit Related to Test Procedure

Some of the tests require the client to maintain nothing-by-mouth status, whereas others do not. Medications may or may not be withheld; specific medications may be part of the test. The client should be physically comfortable; thus, he or she should be given a chance to void before the procedure begins. (For some of the procedures, such as a paracentesis, an empty bladder is essential.) Physical preparation is described in the discussions of each test. (Table 25–1 lists key points about the tests.) The nurse also needs to explain what aftercare will be needed. Thus, children and parents will not be concerned because the child is being carefully watched after the test. By the same

TABLE 25–1. COMMON INVASIVE TESTS: SUMMARY OF KEY POINTS FOR NURSING CARE[a]

Test	Nothing by Mouth Before Test	Local Anesthetic Used	Restricted Activity After Test	Assess for Complications
Lumbar puncture	No	Yes	Varies, usually several hours	Spinal headache; nerve damage to legs or bladder
Bone marrow biopsy	No	Yes	No	None likely; infection possible
Thoracentesis	No	Yes	1 hr on unaffected side	Pneumothorax; subcutaneous emphysema
Paracentesis	No	Yes	No	Hypovolemia; peritonitis
Gastric analysis	Yes	No	No	Rare allergic reaction to drugs
Papanicolaou smears of uterus	No	No	No	None likely
Cervical biopsy—endometrial biopsy	No	Sometimes	No	Bleeding from biopsy site
Breast biopsy	No	Yes	No	None likely; infection at site or bleeding possible[b]
Liver biopsy	Yes	Yes	Up to 24 hr	Internal bleeding; bile peritonitis
Renal biopsy	Yes	Yes	Up to 24 hr	Hematuria and internal bleeding; urinary tract infection

[a]See text for detailed discussions about all preparations before and after each test and for possible nursing diagnoses.
[b]If breast biopsy performed under general anesthesia, client needs routine postanesthesia assessments.

token, the adolescent or adult needs to be told before the test that his or her blood pressure will be taken, say, every 15 min so there is no misconception that something is amiss.

Preparation of Equipment

For all these procedures, special trays are used. For example, the basic equipment for a lumbar puncture is sterilized on one tray. A check must be completed to see if the necessary slides, chemistry tubes, culture tubes, and other equipment are included on a special procedure tray. Someone may need to check with the laboratory to determine what tubes are necessary.

In some institutions, the nurse may be responsible for setting up equipment for a procedure. In other settings, the person who performs the procedure is responsible for acquiring all needed equipment. Many procedure trays are now packaged commercially with all disposable items. The nurse must check with the particular institutions to see exactly what procedures are followed in that setting. Most prepared trays contain packets of skin antiseptics, such as povidone–iodine (Betadine), which has broad-spectrum microbicidal action.

Injectable Local Anesthetics

The two most common injectable local anesthetics used for invasive diagnostic testing are procaine (Novocain) and lidocaine (Xylocaine). Procaine, which is shorter acting, lasts about $\frac{3}{4}$–$1\frac{1}{2}$ hr; lidocaine lasts for $1\frac{1}{2}$–2 hr. Sometimes a very small amount of epinephrine is combined with lidocaine to promote local vasoconstriction. Two reasons why some local vasoconstriction may be desirable are (1) the vasoconstriction slows the absorption of the drug to lengthen its duration, and (2) the vasoconstriction may cause decreased bleeding at the injection site. Epinephrine is not used in areas of the body supplied by end-arteries, such as fingers, toes, penis, or nose. Epinephrine is never used with a local anesthetic if tissue circulation is compromised. Also, epinephrine is not used if a client is taking β-blockers.

The syringes and needles used for the local anesthetic are included on the various trays. These routine types of needles on a procedure tray are (1) 25-gauge $\frac{5}{8}$-inch needles for local skin infiltration, (2) 22-gauge $1\frac{1}{2}$-inch needles for deeper structures, and (3) spinal needles, which are various gauges and extra long (3 inches) for very deep injections. (Trays such as a bone marrow or paracentesis tray include cutting needles or trocars for different test procedures.) Sterile towels are also on prepared procedure trays. Usually the vial of anesthetic is not included on the equipment tray and must be added.

Adverse Reactions to Local Anesthetics

Systemic effects can arise from local injections that contain epinephrine. Nurses should assess for any skin flush or increased pulse when epinephrine is used. Anaphylaxis can occur from lidocaine or procaine if the client is allergic to local anesthetics, but this is very rare (Katzung, 1995).

Local Anesthetic Cream

EMLA, a *e*utectic *m*ixture of *l*ocal *a*nesthetics, has decreased the use of needles for local anesthesia. *Eutectic* means to melt well at a low temperature. Although lidocaine and prilocaine are crystalline solids as individual components, a mixture of these two local anesthetics in equal amounts fuses as a liquid at room temperature (Gajraj et al., 1994). The cream, actually very small droplets, penetrates the skin and blocks neuronal transmission of pain.

This relatively new anesthetic cream, introduced in 1993, is effective for both adults and children who must undergo painful procedures such as lumbar punctures or bone marrow taps. Modifying the pain experience has been especially helpful for clients who must undergo repeated painful procedures.

The cream is not rubbed in, but an occlusive dressing such as Tegaderm or Saranwrap is placed over the area to promote penetration. After the designated application time, which is usually 1 hour, the cream is wiped off and the area is prepared for the procedure. Duration of the analgesic effect after removal of the cream is 1–2 hours.

A newer form of EMLA contains the emulsion in a patch surrounded by an adhesive ring. The patch may not adhere as well as the occlusive dressing, but it is equally effective with no substantial differences in side effects. Parents and nurses should be aware that young children may remove dressings or patches, so use of a secure extra covering may be prudent.

Common side effects of EMLA are erythema, blanching, or slight edema in the area. Allergic reactions are very rare with this type of local anesthetic, but clients must be assessed for any possible allergic reactions, including contact dermatitis. Metabolites of prilocaine can cause methemaglobinemia in newborns and in older infants receiving other methemaglobin-inducing agents, such as sulfonamides and acetaminophen. Nurses have a role in helping patients cope with painful procedures. EMLA combined with the caring attitude of a skilled nurse seems to be a winning combination (Corbett, 1995).

Arranging Environment for the Test

The nurse or clinician performing the procedure must check the lighting in the area. Most hospitals or clinics have a treatment room, which ensures adequate lighting and privacy. If the procedure is performed at the client's bedside, a treatment light should be brought to the room. A good light is needed so doors do not have to open—closed doors ensure privacy for the client. In a multiple-bed unit, it is better to take the client to a treatment room, otherwise, the bed should be screened and perhaps the other client can go to a waiting room, if possible. Clients should not be exposed to another client's invasive procedure. Emergency equipment and drugs should be readily available. For example, atropine may be needed for the bradycardia that can occur from a vasovagal reaction.

Nurse's Role During Procedure

The nurse may remain with the client to offer support. It has already been emphasized that the nurse can help prepare the client for the procedure by exploring, with the client, the best way to cope with any pain or discomfort. The nurse can explain that the antiseptic feels cold to the skin and the injection of the local anesthetic causes a stinging sensation. The nurse can offer to hold the client's hand or let the client squeeze his or her hand. Hand holding also helps remind the client not to put his or her hands on the sterile field. For a child, special restraining procedures may be required to ensure the safety of the child and the sterility of the procedure. The parent may help hold the child. If the parent is not present, the nurse can hold the child. The nurse may be essential in helping the client maintain a certain position, such as with a lumbar puncture. The nurse also assists the physician or the clinician who performs the procedure. This may require pouring an antiseptic into a basin, opening extra gauze packages, or holding collection tubes. The nurse must make sure all collected samples are clearly marked in the order collected. Also, the nurse is needed to observe any untoward effects of the procedure (e.g., check the blood pressure several times during a procedure).

Nurse practitioners perform bone marrow aspirations and other invasive procedures. However, the focus of this chapter is for nurses in general practice, who usually assist during invasive diagnostic procedures. Guarriello (1984), a nurse and a lawyer, cautioned nurses to (1) never perform any act that is beyond the established scope of nursing and (2) never attempt procedures they have not been trained to perform. No one else, including the physician, can assume responsibility for an error because the nurse was told to perform a procedure.

▼ GENERAL POSTTEST NURSING DIAGNOSES

Risk for Injury Related to Adverse Reactions

One of the nursing implications for any invasive test is to carefully check vital signs before, during, and after the procedure. Routines may vary for different procedures, depending on the policy of the institution and the procedure performed. Regardless of the stability of the vital signs, they should be taken at regular intervals as long as there is any possibility of the client bleeding or having other complications. Vital signs after an invasive test include blood pressure, pulse, and respiration. (The client's temperature is *not* taken every 15 min. The client's temperature may become more important later if there is any possibility that the procedure has caused an infection.) If there is any indication of a possible febrile reaction, temperature should be checked routinely every 4 hr. All vital signs must be documented on the client's record and should be graphed so trends (e.g., decreasing blood pressure and increasing pulse rate) are readily apparent. Blood for a hct may be drawn a few hours after the procedure. (See Chapter 2 for an explanation of why hct is only accurate several hours after any bleeding has occurred.)

The time at which the procedure was performed and the name of the clinician who performed it should be recorded. The amount of any fluid withdrawn and its color and characteristics (e.g., cloudy or bloody) should be documented. The number of specimens sent to the laboratory also should be documented.

In addition to the specific items, such as the vital signs and other items discussed later, the nurse should record the general condition of the client after the test. For example, if there were no untoward reactions, this should be recorded as "client tolerated procedure well with no complications noted at present." *Specific* assessments of the client's condition depend on the test. These are emphasized in the discussion about each test.

Risk for Activity Intolerance Related to Need for Bed Rest

The positioning of the client after the procedure may be important. If the client is to remain in a certain position or maintain bed rest for a specified amount of time, the client needs to know this information. Also a sign can be placed at the foot of the bed. For example, the sign may say "Flat in bed until 7 PM." Information about positioning should also be recorded in the card file. Clients may be dizzy when first allowed to walk. Ambulatory care clients often need someone to drive them home.

Altered Comfort Related to Pain and Complications

The nurse must know what type of pain is usual after a procedure so ordered analgesics can be used for relief without masking what could be a symptom of a complication. The nurse must also know any specific complications associated with a procedure so the posttest assessment is appropriate. For example, listening for breath sounds after a pleural tap or thoracentesis is necessary to detect a pneumothorax. There may be a need for medical follow-up if pain persists after the use of mild analgesics.

Risk for Infection

The dressing over the site of an invasive procedure should remain sterile. The nurse must use sterile technique if the dressing becomes wet and must be changed. Some procedures may require a pressure dressing, whereas others only require a small adhesive dressing.

Altered Fluid or Nutritional Requirements

Any limitations on eating after the procedure are discussed for the specific tests. For some tests, encouraging fluids is beneficial.

▼ LUMBAR PUNCTURE

Description. Positioning of the client for a lumbar puncture (LP) is very important. Clients are turned on their sides and told to curl up into a ball with head and feet as close to each other as possible (fetal position). This position allows for the maximum separation of the vertebrae. A LP can be performed with the client sitting, but pressure readings cannot be obtained. The usual preparation of the skin with antiseptic and local anesthetic is completed. The clinician inserts a spinal needle into a lumbar space, which is below the end of the spinal cord. The spinal cord usually terminates at the second lumbar vertebra. Thus, the spinal cord is not touched with the needle. Sometimes the needle does graze a spinal root, causing a sharp pain, which radiates down the client's leg. If the client has pain in one of the legs, the clinician needs to know which leg, so the needle position can be slightly readjusted. Once the needle is positioned in the subarachnoid space, a pressure reading is taken with a three-way stopcock and a manometer (standard equipment on a LP tray). The client must relax and straighten out his or her legs before the opening pressure is performed because intra-abdominal pressure increases CSF pressure. After a baseline pressure has been obtained, the physician may want the client to strain slightly (Valsalva maneuver) to see if the increased abdominal pressure causes an increase in CSF pressure. If there is a blockage in the spinal canal, the CSF pressure may not change. The Queckenstedt test is also used to see if there is a block in the flow of CSF. The physician may ask an assistant to apply finger pressure to both internal jugular veins of the client. Obstruction of these veins causes a rise in CSF pressure, unless there is a block somewhere in the spinal column. The Queckenstedt test can be dangerous if too much pressure is put on the carotid receptors. The assistant must know exactly how and where to apply the pressure. After the pressure readings are completed, a few milliliters of CSF are obtained in tubes for (1) chemistry, (2) cell counts, and (3) microbiologic examination. A closing pressure may be obtained. The CSF pressure drops 5–10 mm of water pressure for each milliliter of fluid removed. Usually only about 10 mL is removed, but this can reduce pressure by 50–100 mm. The needle is withdrawn, and a dry sterile dressing is placed over the site.

Purposes. A LP or spinal tap measures CSF pressure and is used to obtain CSF for laboratory examination. A LP also is performed to inject dye into the spinal column (see myelograms, Chapter 20). A LP performed for a spinal tap is similar to that performed for spinal anesthesia.

Spinal fluid is formed in the lateral ventricles of the brain. The fluid bathes the brain and spinal cord and protects the central nervous system (CNS) from injury. Measurements of the various CSF components helps in the diagnosis of various conditions of the CNS. A special summary about the clinical significance of CSF changes is discussed at the end of this section. Nurses should be aware of the normal characteristics of CSF because the laboratory results are usually sent to the unit.

Contraindications to LP

Measurement of CSF pressure helps detect any obstruction in the normal flow of CSF. However, if increased intracranial pressure is suspected, a LP is *not* attempted because a quick reduction in the pressure in the spinal column can cause a herniation of the brainstem into the foramen magnum. This downward shift of the brain can put lethal pressure on the vital centers in the medulla (Bongard and Sue, 1994).

▼ PRETEST NURSING IMPLICATIONS RELATED TO LUMBAR PUNCTURE

Note the general nursing diagnoses for all invasive testing (e.g., consent forms and other policies). See the earlier discussion of EMLA as a local anesthetic. A doll and pictures may be used to demonstrate LP to a child and thus reduce anxiety and perceptions of pain (Mansson et al., 1993). The client does not need to maintain nothing-by-mouth status for LP. Sedation is usually not used but may be necessary for children or confused adults. A blood glucose sample must be drawn about 1/2–1 hr before the test to be used as a comparison with CSF glucose level. A serum chloride level may be used for comparison, but this is not routine.

▼ POSTTEST NURSING DIAGNOSES RELATED TO LUMBAR PUNCTURE

Risk for Altered Sensory Perceptions

See the general guidelines about vital signs and assessing for pain. Special attention should be paid to any change in the level of consciousness, particularly if increased intracranial pressure is suspected. The client may have a temporary problem voiding caused by the effect on nerves to the bladder. Damage to nerves may affect the legs.

Risk for Altered Comfort Related to Development of Spinal Headache

The exact reason for a spinal headache is not known, but it is assumed to be related to the loss of CSF. The use of a large needle or other trauma during the procedure may cause more loss of spinal fluid, and thus, there is less fluid to bathe the meninges of the brain. If a headache does begin, the client maintains bed rest and uses an ice cap and mild analgesics as ordered. The spinal headache usually is relieved in 24 hr, but it may persist longer, sometimes for weeks. Depending on the circumstances, the client may be instructed to stay flat in bed for several hours to prevent spinal headaches. If the LP is performed on an outpatient basis, the client may be allowed to go home without being prone for a period.

Altered Fluid Requirements

After a LP, the client can eat and drink as soon as he or she desires. Unless otherwise contraindicated, drinking plenty of fluids should be encouraged because this helps the body replace any lost CSF, and this may decrease risk for headache.

REFERENCE VALUES FOR CSF

Bilirubin	Negative
Cell count	0–5 mononuclear cells—infants and young children up to 20
Chloride	120–130 mEq/L—compare with serum, should be 10–20 mEq higher
Glucose	50–75 mg/dL—compare with serum glucose, should be about 60% of serum level; newborns have higher levels
Protein	15–45 mg/dL—Higher in newborns
Albumin	29.5 mg/dL
IgG	4.3 mg/dL
Oligoclonal bands	Absent
Pressure	70–180 mm H_2O infants and young children, 50–100 mm H_2O
Lactate	3 mmol/L—higher in newborns
Lactic dehydrogenase	About 10% of serum level

General Significance of Abnormal Findings in CSF

Blood in the Fluid. Normal fluid is clear. Bleeding from the tap itself usually does not make all the tubes bloody. The collection of samples should be marked #1, #2, and #3, so it is possible to see if the blood is less in the last tube than in the first tube. Grossly bloody CSF is a sign of hemorrhage somewhere in the CNS. It may not be possible to perform any other tests on the CSF when a great deal of blood is present.

Bilirubin. Bilirubin (the indirect portion) can cross the blood–brain barrier in infants. Bilirubin in the spinal fluid of a newborn (kernicterus) can cause brain damage (Chapter 11).

Cell Counts. Normally there are fewer than five cells per milliliter in CSF; all are lymphocytes. In bacterial infections there may be enough neutrophils to make the CSF cloudy. In tuberculosis and some viral diseases, lymphocytes may be increased. Tumor cells can also be identified with a Papanicolaou smear.

Chlorides. Chlorides are decreased in some bacterial infections, including tuberculosis. This test is not specific enough to be of much use and is not performed anymore unless specifically requested.

Glucose. The glucose level is lowered in bacterial infections because the bacteria use sugar. Viral infections do not cause a lowered CSF sugar. The blood glucose sample is needed for comparison. Ideally the blood glucose sample is drawn about 30 min before the LP because it takes glucose about 30 min to an hour to diffuse into the CSF.

Proteins. Degenerative diseases and brain tumors tend to cause increased protein in the CSF. Structural lesions that interrupt the blood–brain barrier cause increased total protein in the CSF because there is increased diffusion from the blood to the brain tissue. In general, an increase in the total protein of the CSF is a sign of a serious neurologic disorder. Because various diseases cause elevations in only some types of proteins, much research is directed toward identifying exactly what types of proteins are elevated in various diseases of the CNS. Demyelinating diseases of the CNS are those in which the myelin sheath covering the neurons is lost. During active demyelination a basic protein is present in the serum and the CSF. Immunoelectrophoresis can be performed on CSF. IgG and an abnormal type of protein band called oligoclonal bands are often present in multiple sclerosis (McBride and Distefano, 1988). IgG also increases in various CNS infections (Ravel, 1995).

Gram Stains and Cultures

Cultures are performed to identify any organisms found in the CSF. If a preliminary Gram stain identifies any organisms, the physician is notified immediately so treatment can begin at once (see Chapter 16 on culture and sensitivity tests).

Serologic Tests

The laboratory may perform various types of serologic tests to detect the presence of neurosyphilis. (See Chapter 14 for examples of serologic tests for syphilis.)

Lactate

Lactate levels are often more than twice normal in untreated bacterial meningitis and thus are useful in differentiating bacterial from viral meningitis (Latcha and Cunha, 1994). However, normal lactate levels are not always reliable in excluding bacterial meningitis, and other conditions can cause elevations (Ravel, 1995).

Lactic Dehydrogenase

An elevated LDH level is usually associated with inflammatory processes and bacterial meningitis. LDH isoenzymes (Chapter 12) give more detailed information on the origin of the LDH.

▼ BONE MARROW ASPIRATION OR BIOPSY

Description. Common sites used for bone marrow aspiration or biopsy in adults are posterior iliac crest, anterior iliac crest, and sternum. The tibia may be used in small children. If a biopsy, rather than aspiration alone, is planned, the iliac crest is used. The area is prepared, and a local anesthetic is administered. Hair may have to be shaved from the site. The physician or nurse-practitioner inserts the needle through the bone until the marrow is reached. For aspiration, the plunger of the syringe is pulled back to withdraw a small amount of marrow into the syringe. When the plunger is pulled back, the client often feels sharp pain. The client should be prepared for this momentary pain. Normal bone marrow is soft and semifluid, and thus, a sample can often be obtained by means of aspiration with a syringe. Otherwise, a bone marrow biopsy can be performed with a large needle that has a cutting blade. The specimen obtained must be carefully placed in the correct container. A smear may be microscopically examined immediately to make sure tiny bone particles, called *spicules*, are present. Six or more slides may be prepared. A culture tube may also be necessary. Usually only a small adhesive dressing is placed over the site because there is minimal bleeding or drainage. A small pressure dressing is used if a biopsy was performed.

Purposes. Bone marrow studies are performed when there are abnormal types of cells on a peripheral blood smear. They are used to confirm the presence of metastatic tumors or diseases such as leukemia or various types of anemia. Bone marrow studies may be performed periodically to evaluate the response to treatment.

▼ PRETEST NURSING DIAGNOSIS RELATED TO BONE MARROW ASPIRATION OR BIOPSY

Knowledge Deficit Related to Procedure Requirements

The client is usually not given sedation, but if sedation is deemed necessary, it does not interfere with the test. The client can eat and drink before the test. The procedure, including the momentary pain, should be explained to the client. The client is positioned with pillows under the thoracic spine if the sternum is used. When the iliac crest is used, the client is in a side-lying position or on his or her abdomen. The nurse helps the client get into as comfortable a position as possible, so the client can remain still during the procedure.

▼ POSTTEST NURSING IMPLICATIONS RELATED TO BONE MARROW ASPIRATION OR BIOPSY

Vital signs and other routines are performed as for other invasive tests, although the risk of bleeding is slight. The client may stay in bed for an hour or so to rest but then can resume normal daily activities. There may be a slight ache or pain, which requires the use of a mild analgesic. Chapter 2 discusses nursing diagnoses related to decreased red blood cell (RBC) counts and abnormal white blood cells (WBCs), which are often present when a bone marrow aspiration or biopsy is required.

▼ THORACENTESIS (PLEURAL TAP)

Description. The site usually used for a thoracentesis (pleural tap) is the seventh or eighth intercostal space. The clinician determines the exact site at which to insert the needle by studying the client's chest radiograph and by means of percussion and auscultation of the chest. To avoid large vessels, Doppler ultrasonography (Chapter 23) may be performed just before the tap (Bongard and Sue, 1994). The client is usually sitting so fluid pools at the base of the pleural space. If the client cannot sit, he or she may be turned toward the affected side and placed in a high Fowler position. The area is prepared and anesthetized. After the needle is positioned in the pleural space, fluid is withdrawn with a syringe and a three-way stopcock. The fluid for laboratory analysis, collected in a 50-mL syringe with 1 mL of heparin to assure accurate cell counts and pH reading, is then transferred to the appropriate containers (e.g., complete blood count (CBC) blood tube, chemistry blood tube, culture and sensitivity tube, and cytology jar). A catheter may be connected to the three-way stopcock to drain off a large amount of fluid. No more than 1,000–1,500 mL of fluid should be removed at one time. Vital signs should be monitored if large amounts of fluid are withdrawn. Atropine should always be immediately available for possible bradycardia due to a vasovagal effect (Qureshi et al., 1994). A pulse oximeter (Chapter 6) can be used to monitor for hypoxemia, and supplemental oxygen may be needed to relieve dyspnea. The client may feel some pain as the pleural space is entered, but the withdrawal of fluid is not uncomfortable. Once the fluid is withdrawn, a small bandage is placed over the site. Some clinicians may spray the site with a collodian seal. Thoracentesis is usually performed at the client's bedside or in the procedure room on the unit. Thoracentesis can also be performed in an office or clinic setting.

Purposes. A thoracentesis may be needed for aspiration of air, pleural fluid, or blood from the pleural cavity. A thoracentesis is often performed for therapy as well as for diagnosis. Inflammatory diseases of the lungs and neoplasms are common reasons for a large collection of pleural fluid. Blood in the pleural space (hemothorax) is usually from a traumatic injury.

Laboratory Examination of Pleural Fluid

For analysis of pleural fluid, the most cost-effective approach may be to first establish whether an exudate or transudate is present. Exudates have elevated LDH and protein levels, whereas transudates do not (Qureshi et al., 1994). Transudates occur when changes in hydrostatic or oncotic pressure allow fluid to leave the circulatory system. Examples of transudates are the pleural effusion that can occur with congestive heart failure, cirrhosis, and the nephrotic syndrome. Exudates are caused by inflammation, infections, malignant neoplasms, or other abnormalities that alter or injure the pleural surface and promote fluid collection. Further examination of exudates, besides protein and LDH, includes cell counts, pH, which becomes acidic with inflammation, and various chemistries such as glucose or amylase, if indicated. Tumor cells can be identified and organisms cultured.

▼ PRETEST NURSING IMPLICATIONS RELATED TO THORACENTESIS

The general pretest nursing diagnoses for bedside examinations are considered. An extra bedside table may be necessary to help position the client in a comfortable sitting position. The client can lean over the table with his or her feet on a chair for support. Chest radiographs are needed. The nurse should listen to the client's breath sounds to be used as a baseline for a posttest assessment. The nurse should also note any breathing difficulty and the color of the client's skin before the test is begun. Sedation, although not usually used, does not interfere with the procedure if needed. Food, fluids, and medicines need not be withheld.

▼ POSTTEST NURSING DIAGNOSES RELATED TO THORACENTESIS

Risk for Injury Related to Procedure

The client is usually turned on the *unaffected* side for 1 hr to allow the pleural puncture to seal. Vital signs are recorded as per routine. The amount of fluid withdrawn for diagnosis, if more than a few milliliters, should be recorded as part of the intake and output record, and the client should be assessed for hypovolemia. There is no restriction on food or fluids after the procedure. If the client has no respiratory or other problems within an hour after the test, all normal activity can be resumed.

Clients with pleural effusion caused by malignant tumors may have cytotoxic or antibiotic drugs injected into the pleural space after the fluid is withdrawn. The nurse must be aware of possible reactions to the drug injected into the pleural space.

Risk for Ineffective Breathing Patterns

Careful note should be made of the respiratory rate and the character of the respirations. The nurse should listen for any diminished breath sounds, which could be a sign of a pneumothorax. Any dyspnea or shortness of breath should be carefully compared with the respiratory status before the test. If a large amount of fluid is withdrawn as therapy, the client should be able to breathe with less effort. A chest radiograph is obtained to evaluate the amount of fluid removed and to check for any pneumothorax.

▼ PARACENTESIS (ABDOMINAL TAP)

Description. The word *paracentesis* actually means puncture of any cavity for the aspiration of fluid. An abdominal paracentesis is used for the removal of fluid from the peritoneal cavity. In general practice, abdominal paracentesis is usually simply called paracentesis because withdrawals of fluids from other cavities have specific names (i.e., thoracentesis, amniocentesis).

Paracentesis is performed at the client's bedside or in an outpatient setting. The client must sit with the feet supported. A bedside table may be used to support the arms in a comfortable position. The physician inserts a large-gauge needle or trocar through the abdominal wall. (It is essential that the bladder be empty so there is no accidental puncture of the bladder.) Doppler ultrasound (Chapter 23) can be used to avoid puncture of large abdominal collateral vessels (Bongard and Sue, 1994). Once the needle is in the peritoneal cavity, the fluid is withdrawn with a syringe if a small amount is needed for diagnosis. If the tap is also needed to relieve pressure from ascites, the needle may be connected to tubing, and a large collection bottle is used, which is much like the set-up used to withdraw blood. As much as 1,000 mL of fluid may be withdrawn at one time. Another technique is to perform slow, continuous drainage of ascites. The concern when a large amount of fluid is removed is that there may be a shift of fluid from the vascular space to the now-empty peritoneal cavity. Intravenous fluid or albumin may be used to prevent hypotension when large amounts of fluid are withdrawn. Once the needle or trocar is withdrawn, a small sterile dressing is placed over the site. If the client has a great deal of ascites and only a small amount of fluid is removed, the pressure of the remaining fluid may cause a continued leakage from the puncture site. The dressing may have to be changed frequently, and extra fluff gauze is used to absorb the leakage. The use of Montgomery straps eliminates the need to change the tape every time the dressing is changed.

Purposes. Paracentesis may be performed to assess for peritonitis. If the client has undergone peritoneal dialysis, the specimen may be aspirated from the peritoneal catheter. The nurse may collect this specimen by withdrawing a small amount of fluid with a syringe and using sterile technique.

An abnormal collection of fluid in the peritoneal cavity is called *ascites*. Ascites is most often seen in clients with advanced cirrhosis or widespread malignant disease in the abdomen. For these conditions, a paracentesis is performed for therapeutic rather than diagnostic reasons. The disadvantage of paracentesis for therapeutic reasons is that ascitic fluid contains a large amount of protein. Because paracentesis causes a loss of protein, other measures, such as diuretics, are used before paracentesis is performed for therapy.

In addition to diagnostic aids or therapeutic relief in cirrhosis and malignant disease, paracentesis is also performed as a diagnostic procedure for traumatic injuries to the abdomen. A peritoneal tap, or a peritoneal lavage with Ringer's lactate solution, is performed to see if there is any bleeding into the peritoneal cavity.

Laboratory Examinations of Peritoneal Fluid

Laboratory examination of the peritoneal fluid may include RBC count, WBC count, cultures, fecal content, bilirubin, and amylase (if pancreatitis is suspected). Normal peritoneal fluid is clear and yellowish. Blood in the fluid is abnormal. If the blood is intraperitoneal blood, it does not clot, but venous blood, which may be accidentally withdrawn from a vessel, clots. The amount of protein in the fluid helps differentiate a transudate from an exudate. Exudates, which usually result from inflammation, contain more protein and LDH than transudates, which are usually caused by pressure changes from mechanical factors.

▼ PRETEST NURSING IMPLICATIONS RELATED TO PARACENTESIS

In addition to the general nursing actions for invasive testing, the client should be weighed before and after the procedure to assess the fluid loss. (Recall that 1 L of fluid weighs 1 kg [2.2 lb].) The client *must have* an empty bladder so it is not pricked by the needle. If the client cannot void, a catheter may be necessary. The client needs to be in a comfortable sitting position with the feet supported on a bedside stool or chair.

▼ POSTTEST NURSING DIAGNOSES RELATED TO PARACENTESIS

Risk for Fluid Volume Deficit and Electrolyte Imbalance

When a large amount of fluid is being withdrawn, the client's blood pressure must be taken several times during the procedure. Equipment for an intravenous infusion should be readily available in case of hypotension from shifts of fluid out of the vascular space. Intravenous albumin is sometimes given immediately after the procedure. (See Chapter 10 on albumin levels.) Vital signs are checked after the paracentesis is completed and other routine aftercare for invasive procedures is carried out. The client's pre- and posttest weights should be compared. The amount, color, and character of the removed fluid should be recorded on the nurse's notes and as part of the intake and output (I&O) record. The client should record I&O for 24 hr. Depending on the causes of ascites, the client may follow a restricted fluid or sodium diet. Electrolytes must be closely monitored (Chapter 5).

Risk for Infection and Injury from Other Complications

If any excess fluid is left in the peritoneal cavity, there may be a problem with leakage from the site. The dressing may have to be changed frequently. Sterile technique must be used. The client's temperature should be taken every 4 hr for 24 hr. The nurse should carefully observe the client for other signs or symptoms of peritonitis, such as abdominal pain and tense, rigid abdominal muscles. For a client with cirrhosis, paracentesis may precipitate hepatic coma. (See Chapter 10 on ammonia levels.)

▼ GASTRIC ANALYSIS

Description. A gastric analysis is usually performed at the client's bedside, in a treatment room, or in an office or clinic. The nurse or physician may insert the tube, which should be well-lubricated with a water-soluble jelly. The client is seated upright. The nasogastric (NG) tube is passed into the stomach and left for the duration of the test. Either nostril may be used. The client may know that one side of his or her nose is more patent than the other side. The client's head should be hyperextended for the passage of the tube to the back of the throat. Once the tube reaches the posterior pharynx, the client can put his or her head back in a normal position or slightly forward. Sips of water, unless contraindicated, are given to help the tube go down the esophagus. A slight pulling back on the tube and a slight downward thrust are needed when the tube is felt to touch the posterior pharynx. Passing an NG tube is an unpleasant experience for the client. It may be necessary to stop for a moment to let the client relax. Once the tube is going down the esophagus easily, it should be passed rapidly so that the client does not gag. (It is possible to stimulate a vagal response by gagging and this can cause bradycardia, which can be dangerous to some clients.) If the NG tube is unintentionally put into the trachea of an alert client, this mistake is obvious because the client coughs violently and actively resists the tube, which suddenly blocks air passage. Once the tube is in the stomach, a fasting specimen is obtained by means of aspiration with a large syringe.

Use of Drugs in Gastric Analysis

Pentagastrin (Peptavlon), a synthetic form of an active peptide in natural gastrin, is given subcutaneously to stimulate gastric secretion. This drug has fewer adverse effects than the older histamine analogues that were once used as part of a gastric analysis. Pentagastrin begins stimulating gastric secretions within 10 min, has a peak effect in 20–30 min, and has a duration of 60–80 min. After the drug has been given to stimulate gastric secretion, secretions are collected at specified time intervals. The time collection of each specimen is marked on each collection tube, and all the specimens are sent to the laboratory for acidity analysis.

REFERENCE VALUES FOR GASTRIC ANALYSIS

Basal	
Men	3.0 ± 2.0 mEq/hr
Women	2.0 ± 1.8 mEq/hr

Maximal (after pharmacologic stimulation)	
Men	23 ± 5 mEq/hr
Women	16 ± 5 mEq/hr

Purposes. A gastric analysis is most commonly performed to measure the acidity of the gastric contents. The response of the gastric glands to drug stimulation with drugs such as pentagastrin is helpful in diagnosing peptic ulcer, gastric carcinoma, and pernicious anemia. Gastric acidity is usually increased with a peptic ulcer and decreased or absent (anacidity or achlorhydria) in pernicious anemia and gastric carcinoma. (See Chapter 22 on the Schilling test for pernicious anemia.) An analysis of gastric contents may also be performed to detect acid-fast bacillus in a client with undiagnosed tuberculosis. A client with tuberculosis usually swallows some sputum containing the organism that causes tuberculosis, which is acid-fast so it is not destroyed by the gastric juices. The gastric contents can also be examined for the presence of malignant cells by means of a Papanicolaou smear. Tests for occult blood may also be performed (Chapter 13).

Insulin may be given to test the gastric response to vagal stimulation. The vagus nerve causes increased production of hydrochloric acid by the stomach. Hypoglycemia, caused by the insulin, is a stimulus to the vagus nerve. The response of the stomach may be used to evaluate the effect of a vagotomy or to diagnose other problems of gastric acidity. The use of insulin with a gastric analysis is called the *Hollander test.*

▼ PRETEST NURSING IMPLICATIONS RELATED TO GASTRIC ANALYSIS

It is important that the client be asked about any history of allergic reactions. (See the general nursing diagnoses discussed at the beginning of this chapter.) The client must maintain nothing-by-mouth status for 6–8 hr before the test. The client should not smoke because it increases the secretion of gastric acid. Also, the client should not take anticholinergic drugs such as atropine or H2 blockers such as cimetidine because they markedly decrease gastric secretion.

▼ POSTTEST NURSING IMPLICATIONS RELATED TO GASTRIC ANALYSIS

Once all specimens are obtained, the NG tube can be removed. The client should be told that the tube will be removed quickly. The nurse can remove the tube by pinching it and quickly pulling it out. Paper towels should be handy to catch the tube, and the client needs tissues to blow his or her nose. The client may want to close his or her eyes or concentrate on something else while the tube is pulled out.

There are no restrictions on activity after a gastric analysis. Vital signs are necessary only to ensure the continued stable condition of the client. The client can eat as soon as he or she wishes. A sip of water or weak, warm tea may be offered first because the client may prefer to rest for a while.

▼ PAPANICOLAOU SMEARS OR EXFOLIATIVE CYTOLOGIC STUDIES

The Papanicolaou (Pap) smear usually refers to a test for malignant cells in the uterus, but the test can be performed on many body secretions. The Pap smear is named after Dr. George Papanicolaou, who in the 1940s developed a technique for identifying malignant cells in body secretions. Malignant cells slough off (exfoliate) more readily than do normal cells. The field that involves Pap smears is sometimes called *exfoliative cytology*. In addition to uterine or cervical secretions, exfoliative cytologic studies are conducted on sputum, pleural fluid, bronchial washings from a bronchoscope, gastric contents, bladder secretions, peritoneal fluid, and even secretions from the mammary glands. The collection of a sample for exfoliative cytologic examination is often part of an invasive study. The laboratory tells the nurse exactly how the specimen should be prepared. The results of a Pap smear used to be reported as

- Grade I: Normal-appearing cells
- Grade II: Atypical cytologic features but no evidence of malignancy
- Grade III: Suggestion of malignancy, but not conclusive
- Grade IV: Strongly suggestive of malignancy
- Grade V: Conclusive for malignancy

A newer system labels the grades as

- Normal
- Inflammatory
- Mild—cervical intraepithelial neoplasia (CIN)
- Severe CIN
- Cancer

Some clinicians use the term *dysplasia* rather than the term *intraepithelial neoplasia*. It must be remembered that all reports of exfoliative cytologic findings are used for screening, not for a final diagnosis. Thus, the presence of a malignant neoplasm is always confirmed with a biopsy.

Papanicolaou Smears of the Uterus

Description. A small amount of secretion is obtained from the cervix by means of swabbing the exterior of the cervix with an applicator. A jet washer may be used to obtain cells from the endometrium. Most sources suggest that two smears be taken to increase the chance of obtaining any atypical cells that may be present. The smears are placed on dry slides and immediately sprayed with a fixative. It is important that the cells not dry before they are fixed on the slide. Collection of Pap smears by nurse practitioners has been promoted for many years in the United States (Fisher et al., 1977). Research continues to support the ability of nurse practitioners to collect technically adequate specimens and arrange for appropriate follow-up care for women with abnormal findings (Mitchell, 1993).

Purposes. Cytologic examination of cells from the cervix can detect premalignant dysplasia that may be present 5–10 years before invasive carcinoma develops. The cause of dysplasia is not known, but it may be associated with some vaginal infections and condyloma (genital warts) caused by the human papilloma virus. Most authorities, such as the American Cancer Society, recommend that Pap smears be performed at least every 3 years, after three initial smears performed a year apart are normal. These guidelines apply to women 20 years of age and older, as well as to sexually active women younger than 20 years. Day (1990) noted that smears may be needed less often in women older than 65 years.

▼ PRETEST NURSING IMPLICATIONS RELATED TO PAP SMEARS

A Pap smear is usually performed 5–6 days after the menses. The client should not have intercourse or douche for 48 hr before the smear. If the client has used antibiotic vaginal creams, the examination should be delayed 1 month. The use of any medications, particularly oral contraceptives, should be recorded on the request slip. For some women, a pelvic examination is an unpleasant and embarrassing procedure, and the nurse must be sensitive to the need to respect the privacy of the client with actions like draping. There are do-it-yourself kits for Pap tests. If the woman is to collect the sample herself, she must be taught how deep in the vagina to collect the specimen and how to fix it in the proper preservative. As a guide, the woman can be told that the cervical os feels like the tip of the nose.

▼ POSTTEST NURSING IMPLICATIONS RELATED TO PAP SMEARS

There are no client restrictions after a Pap smear. If the cytology report shows atypical cells or cervical dysplasia, the client is followed up by means of colposcopy. Nursing research has investigated the affective and behavioral responses to unexpected, abnormal Pap results (Lauver et al., 1990). Some women may fear abnormal results of a Pap smear, whereas others may discount any risk because they have no symptoms. The news of an abnormal Pap smear and the need for colposcopy may be particularly anxiety producing for younger women and those with concurrent stressors (Nugent et al., 1993). Toole and Vigilante (1990) noted that public health nurses are often crucial in the successful follow-up care of women with dysplasia who do not return for follow-up appointments and treatment.

▼ CERVIGRAM

Description. Another way to screen for CIN is the use of photography to record an image of the cervix. After application of 5% acetic acid, photographs of the whole cervix are taken with a specially designed camera. The slide (cervigram) is then magnified 16 times to assess any changes in the cervix. Cervicography used as a complement to Pap smears is being investigated as one way to improve the rate of detection of cervical cancer. Whereas a Pap smear is used to detect cellular changes, cervicography helps detect disease at an enhanced macroscopic level and thus may help identify some malignant lesions missed on a Pap smear (Ferris et al., 1993).

▼ COLPOSCOPY, CERVICAL BIOPSY, AND ENDOMETRIAL BIOPSY

Description and Purposes. A colposcope, or colpomicroscope, is a binocular microscope with a magnifying glass and a high-intensity light source. It is used to examine the vagina and cervix and to collect a biopsy specimen if necessary. Nurses, as primary care practitioners, perform colposcopic examinations. The biopsy is planned for about 1 week after the client's menses because the cervix is more vascular before and after menses. The biopsy is performed after the menstrual period so there is no possibility of pregnancy. The client is prepared for a pelvic examination as described earlier. The client is not given any local anesthetic because the cervix is sensitive to pressure but not to burning or cutting, as is the skin. The momentary pressure is somewhat uncomfortable for some clients. The biopsy site may be sealed with a silver nitrate stick or cauterized. Packing will probably be put in the vagina.

With the colposcope, the clinician can identify areas of the cervix that appear atypical and thus perform direct punch biopsies. It takes about 10 min to view the cervical epithelium and note suspicious areas. Normally, the cervix is pink. During pregnancy, the cervix becomes dusky in color. After menopause the cervix is light pink. Any secretions should be odorless and clear. The stickiness of the secretions is related to ovulation time. If abnormal areas are seen in the cervix or if there are abnormal secretions, a cervical biopsy or an endocervical curettage should be performed. Endometrial biopsies may be performed as part of an infertility evaluation

(Chapter 28). An endometrial biopsy is performed with a special instrument inserted through the cervix. The pain is momentary, but sharp. This procedure is quite a bit more uncomfortable than a cervical biopsy. A local anesthetic may be used, or the client may be given medication such as ibuprofen 30 min before the procedure. Some bleeding may be expected, so a tampon or pad is needed.

▼ PRETEST NURSING IMPLICATIONS RELATED TO COLPOSCOPY

Women undergoing colposcopy for the first time may have many unanswered questions about the procedure as well as underlying concerns about cancer and the causes of CIN (Barsevick and Lauver, 1990). Preparatory information, including a review of female anatomy, the meaning of Pap results, and procedural and sensory information about colposcopy should be made available to women before the scheduled appointment (Nugent and Tamlyn-Leaman, 1992). Many institutions have written information, but the nurse should still be available to answer questions.

Preparation for colposcopy is similar to that for a Pap smear. The client should be told that the biopsy causes momentary discomfort. (If a cone biopsy is needed, the client needs anesthesia).

▼ POSTTEST NURSING IMPLICATIONS RELATED TO COLPOSCOPY

Vaginal packing or a tampon may be left in place for several hours. Any unusual bleeding or abdominal pain should be reported, but some spotting is expected for a few days. Intercourse can resume after 24 hours unless treatment was administered for the dysplasia. If cryotherapy or laser treatments were performed, the woman should abstain from intercourse for 2 weeks.

▼ BREAST BIOPSY AND NEEDLE ASPIRATION

Description and Purposes. A breast biopsy or needle aspiration as a diagnostic procedure for malignant tumors is usually performed in an outpatient setting. In the past, surgeons performed a breast biopsy with the client under general anesthesia so that a mastectomy could be performed immediately if the frozen section was positive for cancer. However, current practice is to wait and to perform the more extensive operation at a later date. Several reports demonstrated that a short delay between biopsy and mastectomy did not adversely affect survival. This delay gives the client and family more time to adjust to the idea of surgical intervention or to the other treatment options now available (Knobj & Gossage, 1990). For a breast biopsy, the skin is prepared and anesthetized in the usual manner. A small amount of tissue is incised. Either a biopsy or needle aspiration takes only a few minutes to complete. A probe may be placed when a mammogram is obtained (Chapter 20) to identify the exact site for the biopsy. If it is difficult to perform a biopsy on the mass, the client may need general anesthesia.

▼ PRETEST NURSING IMPLICATIONS RELATED TO BREAST BIOPSY

The setup for the procedure is similar to that for any other local biopsy—sterile drapes and local anesthetic. The physical discomfort is minimal, but the anxiety level of the client is likely to be high. Although most breast lumps are *not* malignant, there is always the possibility that this one may be. Roughly 80% of breast lumps are benign. Hall (1986) noted that the increase in mammograms may increase the number of unneeded biopsies.

▼ POSTTEST NURSING DIAGNOSIS RELATED TO BREAST BIOPSY

Knowledge Deficit Related to Health Maintenance

An ice bag may be used on the site. If a biopsy is performed, there may be a few stitches, which must be removed. The woman should wear a supportive bra 24 hr a day until healing is complete. The nipple may be numb for 1–2 months, which can interfere with sexual arousal (Wiley, 1981).

The nurse can also make sure that the client does know how to perform self-examinations of the breast. (See Chapter 20 for information on mammograms as screening devices for women at high risk.) The American Cancer Society has excellent material for client teaching on breast cancer. The Department of Health and Human Services also publishes a pamphlet on breast self-examination, which can be obtained free for client teaching.

Breast self-examination is an important self-care technique that nurses should teach all female patients. Only 25–35% of women in the United States regularly perform this detection procedure (Sternberger, 1994).

▼ LIVER BIOPSY

Description. A liver biopsy can be performed at the client's bedside or in a special treatment room. The skin is prepared and anesthetized. Before the biopsy needle is inserted into the liver, the client is asked to take a deep breath and then hold the breath after an expiration. Not breathing keeps the diaphragm motionless. Also, holding the breath after expiration leaves the diaphragm farther up in the thoracic cavity than after inspiration. (For a renal biopsy, the client is asked to hold his or her breath after inspiration, which is easier to do.) For children or confused adults, the nose can be momentarily blocked at the end of an expiration. At the end of a cry, a child has maximal expiration. It is much more desirable to have a quiet, cooperative client because jerking or thrashing about can tear the liver. An uncooperative client usually makes the procedure unsafe. The actual insertion of the needle and a collection of tissue takes only 1–2 min. The entire procedure can be performed in 10–15 min. When the needle is withdrawn, a pressure dressing is applied to the area.

Purposes. A liver biopsy may be useful in determining the exact nature of pathologic conditions in the liver, such as tumors, cysts, or cirrhosis. A sonogram (Chapter 23) or a liver scan (Chapter 22) gives the physician valuable information about the exact area to biopsy. Liver biopsies are also used to evaluate for rejection of a transplanted liver (Whiteman et al., 1990).

▼ PRETEST NURSING IMPLICATIONS RELATED TO LIVER BIOPSY

The client must undergo coagulation tests (prothrombin time [PT], partial thromboplastin time [PTT], and platelet counts) before the liver biopsy. A hct also is measured as a baseline assessment. For a liver biopsy, the rule is that PT activity should be more than 50% and not more than 3 sec over the control time. The platelets should be greater than 100,000/mm^3. Because a diseased liver may be unable to manufacture prothrombin in normal amounts, vitamin K may be ordered in an attempt to raise the PT percentage and decrease the time in seconds. (See Chapter 13 for a discussion of laboratory tests for prothrombin and the relation between prothrombin and liver disease and vitamin K.)

The client usually takes nothing by mouth for about 6 hr before the test. Fasting makes the liver less congested and the biliary ducts less turgid. Fasting also prevents any vomiting if complications occur. The client is usually not given any sedation, but some sedation may be needed by selected patients. Baseline vital signs are taken, and the client is given a chance to practice holding the breath after an expiration.

▼ POSTTEST NURSING DIAGNOSES RELATED TO LIVER BIOPSY

Risk for Injury Related to Internal Bleeding

The client is turned on his or her right side for 1–4 hr. Ambulatory clients may go home within 6 hr if there are no complications. It is important to check the dressing for any bleeding, but a pressure dressing should *not* be removed to look for bleeding. Usually serious bleeding is internal, and thus, it is not detected at visual inspection. Clients can bleed to death after a liver biopsy; therefore, vital signs are checked frequently, as with any invasive procedure. Food may be withheld until it is certain that the client is not having any immediate complications. For clients in the hospital, an 8-hr posttest hct may be performed to assess for any blood loss. Even a slight drop in hct should be called to the physician's attention immediately.

Risk for Injury from Other Complications

In addition to hemorrhage and shock, other complications that can occur from a liver biopsy include bile peritonitis, pneumothorax, or perforation of an abdominal organ (e.g., the colon). Any pain in the abdomen or any dyspnea calls for a thorough physical assessment of the thorax and abdomen. Slight pain at the biopsy sight and right shoulder pain can be expected as the local anesthetic wears off. The client may be instructed to maintain bed rest for an entire 24 hr or longer if there are any complications. The client should be cautioned not to cough or strain because this can increase intra-abdominal pressure. The day after the biopsy, the client can resume most activities but should not attempt strenuous activities or heavy lifting for a week or two.

▼ RENAL BIOPSY

Description. A renal biopsy is usually performed in a treatment room close to the ultrasound or radiology department because the insertion of the needle is monitored by means of fluoroscopy or scanning. Renal biopsies can also be performed with a cystoscope, through which a brush is inserted up into the ureter to obtain a fragment of renal tissue. The brush technique with a cystoscope requires general anesthesia and therefore is carried out in the operating room, as is an open biopsy when a wedge of renal tissue is obtained. A renal biopsy, under local anesthesia, is rendered through a skin puncture or through a small skin incision. The skin is prepared and anesthetized as usual. The client is usually not given any sedation, but the use of drugs does not interfere with the procedure. The client is asked to take a breath and hold it while the needle is being inserted to obtain the biopsy specimen. Only a very small piece of tissue is obtained. When the needle is withdrawn, a pressure dressing is applied to the area, and the client is transported back to the nursing unit.

Purposes. Renal biopsies are most helpful in the diagnosis of diseases that alter the structure of the glomeruli. Biopsies are performed only on the cortex, not the medulla. In acute renal failure a biopsy may be performed if inflammatory nephritis is suspected (Bongard and Sue, 1994). Renal biopsies may also help determine the exact nature of a mass, which could be a tumor, clot, or stone. Renal biopsies may be performed periodically to evaluate and monitor the course of chronic renal disease, such as the nephrotic syndrome.

▼ PRETEST NURSING IMPLICATIONS RELATED TO RENAL BIOPSY

Preparation is similar to that for a liver biopsy in that coagulation studies (PT, PTT, and platelet count) must be conducted, vital signs taken for a baseline, and blood drawn for a hct. In addition, the client should undergo urinalysis and an intravenous pyelogram (IVP) performed (Chapter 20) to determine that there are two functioning kidneys. Food and fluids are withheld before the procedure. Sedation does not affect the test and might be needed if the client is anxious even after optimal preparation. The client should be told approximately how long he or she will be in the radiology or ultrasound department and what the aftercare will be.

▼ POSTTEST NURSING DIAGNOSES RELATED TO RENAL BIOPSY

Risk for Injury Related to Bleeding

The client is usually instructed to remain motionless for 4 hr. Bed rest may be continued for 24 hr. If a piece of artery is discovered in the biopsy tissue, the bed rest may be prolonged. Vital signs are obtained and dressing-check routines are followed. A hct is usually ordered 8 hr after the procedure. During the first 24 hr, urine is collected in separate cups and left in the bathroom so hematuria can be monitored. The time at which each specimen is produced should be marked on the cup. Some urine may also be sent to the laboratory for microscopic examination. Microscopic hematuria occurs in about half of clients and a few clients have gross hematuria. There are dipsticks for detecting occult hematuria, but these are not as sensitive as a microscopic examination. (See Chapter 13 on guaiac tests and Chapter 2 on urinalysis.) Any severe jolt to the retroperitoneal area can cause bleeding, even several days after the biopsy. The client should be instructed to avoid strenuous activities or heavy lifting for several days. The client should also be told to report any flank pain, gross hematuria, or signs of dizziness or weakness.

Altered Urinary Pattern

Clients should have a large intake of fluids if permissible. Infection can occur after a biopsy so the client's temperature should be routinely checked for a few days after the biopsy. The client should report any burning on urination or frequency.

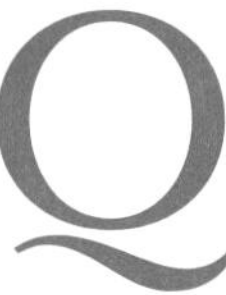

1. Which of the following nursing interventions is usually the *least useful* in alleviating the client's anxiety before a painful diagnostic procedure?

   a. Emphasizing the technical details of the procedure
   b. Preparing the client on ways to cope with painful sensations
   c. Explaining the purpose of any pretest preparations
   d. Providing privacy to maintain self-esteem

2. Epinephrine may be added to a local anesthetic, such as lidocaine (Xylocaine), to

   a. Increase the duration of local anesthesia and decrease bleeding
   b. Decrease the allergic effects of the anesthetic agent
   c. Maintain the blood pressure
   d. Cause vasodilation and better blood flow

3. Timmy, 7 years of age, must undergo bone marrow aspiration. Which of the following actions by the nurse would probably be *least* helpful in preparing Timmy for this invasive procedure?

   a. Letting Timmy play with replicas of some of the equipment
   b. Telling Timmy how he can help during the procedure
   c. Explaining the reason for the procedure
   d. Telling briefly about how the procedure will feel (i.e., some pain)

4. Mr. Fox has just undergone a lumbar puncture. Which of these factors seems to be the *most* important in preventing a spinal headache?

   a. Asking Mr. Fox to stay flat in bed for 24 hr after the procedure
   b. Maintaining nothing-by-mouth status for 2–3 hr before and after the procedure
   c. Encouraging fluids after the lumbar puncture
   d. Using prophylactic analgesics after the procedure

5. Which of the following nursing actions is *least* appropriate for Mrs. Sangria, who just underwent thoracentesis? Four hundred milliliters of clear fluid was obtained from the right pleural space.

   a. Encouraging extra fluids to rehydrate Mrs. Sangria
   b. Assessing the thorax for diminished breath sounds
   c. Positioning Mrs. Sangria on her left side for 1 hr after the thoracentesis
   d. Reporting any symptoms of blood in the sputum (hemoptysis) or shortness of breath (dyspnea)

6. Mr. Heppy is to undergo abdominal paracentesis this morning. Which of the following nursing actions is *not* routine for this diagnostic procedure?

   a. Making sure that the client's bladder is empty
   b. Using sterile equipment for the procedure
   c. Helping the client assume a comfortable side-lying position for the procedure
   d. Letting the client eat as tolerated

7. Procedures performed for a gastric analysis would *not* include

   a. Administration of atropine to dry up secretions before the test
   b. Insertion of nasogastric tube that stays in the stomach for the duration of the test
   c. Administration of a drug to stimulate gastric secretions
   d. Collection of several samples for determination of gastric acidity

8. The usual recommendation on the frequency of Papanicolaou smears for women aged 20–40 is that after three yearly Papanicolaou smears are normal the Papanicolaou smear should be performed at least

   a. Annually b. Every 2 years
   c. Every 3 years d. Every 4 years

9. Mr. Cronkite is to undergo a liver biopsy today. Which of the following nursing actions is appropriate in preparing Mr. Cronkite for the liver biopsy?

   a. Have him practice holding his breath after inspiration
   b. Encourage fluids to keep him well-hydrated
   c. Explain that a local anesthetic will be used to eliminate the pain
   d. Explain that he can resume normal activities as soon as the biopsy is finished and his vital signs are stable

10. Mr. Ralph has just returned from the radiology department, where he underwent a closed renal biopsy with local anesthesia. Which of the nursing actions is most appropriate?

    a. Have Mr. Ralph stay as motionless as possible in bed for 30 min to 1 hr
    b. Save all urine in one container for a 24-hr urine sample
    c. Administer the ordered analgesic for pain at the biopsy site
    d. Restrict fluid intake to no more than 1,000 mL per day

▼ REFERENCES

Barsevick, A., and Lauver, D. (1990). Women's informational needs about colposcopy. *Image, 22* (1), 23–26.

Beckemeyer, P., and Bahr, J. (1980). Helping toddlers and preschoolers cope while suturing their minor lacerations. *MCN: American Journal of Maternal Child Nursing, 5,* 326–330.

Bongard, F.S., and Sue, D.Y. (1994). *Current critical care diagnosis & treatment.* Norwalk, CT: Appleton & Lange.

Corbett, J.V. (1995). EMLA cream for local anesthetic. *MCN: American Journal of Maternal Child Nursing, 20* (3), 178.

Day, S. (1990). Cancer screening in the elderly. *Hospital Practice, 25* (9A), 13–25.

Ferris, D.G., Payne, P., Frisch, L.E., et al. (1993). Cervicography: Adjunctive cervical cancer screening by primary care clinicians. *Journal of Family Practice, 37* (2), 158–164.

Fisher, D., et al. (1977). Nurse-run Pap smear as hospital screening. *Connecticut Medicine, 41,* 143–145.

Gajraj, N.M., Pennant, J.H., and Watcha, M.F. (1994). Eutectic mixture of local anesthetics (EMLA) cream. *Anesthesia and Analgesia, 78,* 574–583.

Guarriello, D. (1984). When doctor's orders are not the best medicine. *RN, 47,* 19–20.

Hall, F. (1986). Screening mammography. Potential problems on the horizon. *New England Journal of Medicine 314* (1), 5335.

Hogue, E. (1986). Informed consent. *Nursing 86, 16* (6), 47–48.

Johnson, J., and Rice, V. (1974). Sensory and distress components of pain: Implications for study of clinical pain. *Nursing Research, 23,* 203–209.

Katzung, B. (1995). *Basic & clinical pharmacology* (6th ed.). Norwalk, CT: Appleton & Lange.

Knobj, M., and Gossage, J. (1990). Early-stage breast cancer: The options. *American Journal of Nursing, 90* (11), 28–30.

Latcha, S., and Cunha, B.A. (1994). *Listeria monocytogenes* meningoencephalitis: The diagnostic importance of the CSF lactic acid. *Heart & Lung, 23* (2), 177–179.

Lauver, D., Barsevick, A., and Rubin, M. (1990). Spontaneous causal searching and adjustment to abnormal Papanicolaou results. *Nursing Research, 39* (5), 305–308.

Mansson, M.E., Bjorkhem, G., and Wiebe, T. (1993). The effect of preparation for lumbar puncture on children undergoing chemotherapy. *Oncology Nursing Forum, 20* (1), 39–45.

McBride, E., and Distefano, K. (1988). Explaining diagnostic tests for M.S. *Nursing 88, 18* (2), 68–72.

Mitchell, H. (1993). Pap smears collected by nurse practitioners: A comparison with smears collected by medical practitioners. *Oncology Nursing Forum, 20* (5), 807–810.

Nugent, L.S., and Tamlyn-Leaman, K. (1992). The colposcopy experience: What do women know? *Journal of Advanced Nursing, 17,* 514–520.

Nugent, L.S., Tamlyn-Leaman, K., Isa, N., et al. (1993). Anxiety and the colposcopy experience. *Clinical Nursing Research, 2* (3), 267–277.

Pidgeon, V. (1985). Children's concepts of illness: Implications for health teaching. *Maternal Child Nursing Journal, 14* (1), 23–33.

Qureshi, N., Momin, Z.A., and Brandstetter, R.D. (1994). Thoracentesis in clinical practice. *Heart & Lung, 23* (5), 376–383.

Ravel, R. (1995). *Clinical laboratory medicine: Clinical application of laboratory data.* (6th ed.). St. Louis: Mosby–Year Book.

Sternberger, C. (1994). Breast self-examination: How nurses can influence performance. *MEDSURG Nursing, 3* (5), 367–371.

Suderman, J. (1990). Pain relief during routine procedures for children with leukemia. *MCN: American Journal of Maternal Child Nursing, 15* (3), 163–166.

Toole, K., and Vigilante, P. (1990). Cervical dysplasia and condyloma as risks for carcinoma. Two case studies. *MCN: American Journal of Maternal Child Nursing, 15* (3), 170–175.

Vessey, J.A., Carlson, K.L., and McGill, J. (1994). Use of distraction with children during an acute pain experience. *Nursing Research, 43* (6), 369–372.

Waidley, E. (1985). Preparing children for invasive procedures. *American Journal of Nursing, 85* (7), 811–812.

Whiteman, K., Nachtmann, L., Biondo, M., et al. (1990). Liver transplantation. *American Journal of Nursing, 90* (6), 68–72.

Wiley, K. (1981). Post-biopsy care. *American Journal of Nursing, 81* (9), 1553–1662.

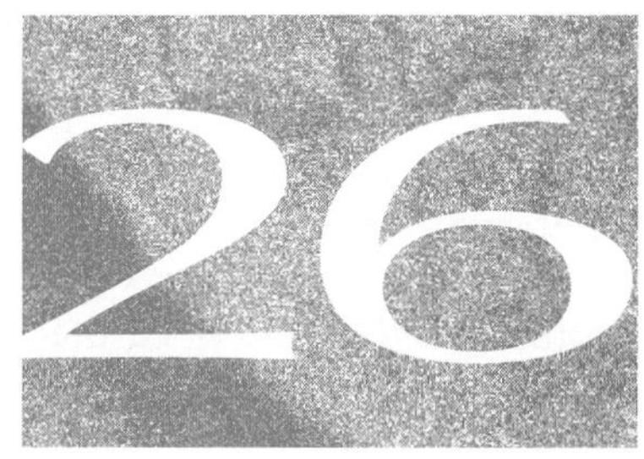

STRESS TESTS, CARDIAC CATHETERIZATIONS, AND ELECTROPHYSIOLOGIC STUDIES

- Stress Tests: ECG Treadmill Test and Exercise Tolerance Test
- Cardiac Catheterization
- Electrophysiologic Studies

OBJECTIVES

1. Describe the general purposes of stress testing (exercise treadmill electrocardiograms [ECGs]) for healthy people and for those with heart disease.
2. Explain what nurses should teach clients about stress testing.
3. Describe appropriate nursing interventions before and after stress tests.
4. Explain how stress test results are used to plan activity levels.
5. Compare the purposes and procedures of right-sided and left-sided cardiac catheterizations and electrophysiologic studies (EPS).
6. Describe appropriate nursing interventions before and after cardiac catheterization and EPS.
7. Identify expected effects of medications used before and during the cardiac tests discussed in this chapter.

Chapters 24 and 25 give basic information about noninvasive and invasive testing. This chapter discusses stress testing, a noninvasive test, which, unlike other noninvasive tests, is not risk-free. Although stress testing is fairly common, it is not always well understood by nurses or the general community. Even if nurses are not involved in stress-testing procedures, they should be able to explain the test and the needed precautions to clients and their families. Stress tests can be very dangerous if not conducted properly. Nurses help prepare clients for the tests, sometimes help administer the test, and more often are involved in follow-up programs for cardiac rehabilitation.

The other tests discussed in this chapter, cardiac catheterization and EPS, are sophisticated, invasive cardiac procedures.

The cardiac catheterization laboratory or the EPS laboratory not only requires elaborate equipment but also requires a team of highly skilled clinicians. A cardiologist trained to perform cardiac catheterization heads a team of technicians who are highly skilled in using the laboratory's monitoring equipment. In addition to being an assistant during the procedure, the nurse may also help prepare the client for the procedure and conduct follow-up assessment.

▼ STRESS TESTS: ECG TREADMILL TEST AND EXERCISE TOLERANCE TEST

Description. The forerunner of the modern heart stress test was the Master's two-step test, which involved stepping up and down on a 20-cm platform 30 times a minute while an ECG recorded the effect of the stress on the heart. The modern stress test is performed in a cardiology laboratory, which is set up to monitor blood pressure, ECG—and sometimes oxygen consumption—while the client exercises by walking on a treadmill. The treadmill is accelerated at intervals and the pitch is changed to determine the exercise tolerance of the person. The test is continued until a predetermined end-point has been obtained or the client shows signs of undue fatigue. A stationary exercise bicycle called a bicycle ergometer, which is portable and less expensive than a treadmill can be used. However, it is not as easy to standardize the results because many clients develop thigh muscle fatigue before they reach their maximum heart rate. The bicycle ergometer is more common Europe.

When exercise tolerance is assessed in clients with cardiac disease, a physician must be present so the test can be stopped if symptoms or dangerous arrhythmias develop. For a healthy client undergoing exercise tolerance testing, a physician or qualified delegate can observe the client's response while the client is using the treadmill. A certification examination for stress exercise testing is given by the American College of Sports Medicine. Nurses must realize that stress testing can be dangerous if not conducted properly. Only qualified personnel should conduct the tests. The American Heart Association has excellent information on quality control for operation of an exercise tolerance laboratory.

Before beginning the test, the client must be told exactly what to expect and that he or she can stop the test at any time, but the test is of greater value if the exercise is continued until a predetermined level is obtained. The predetermined levels are based on the client's age and expected response to a certain level of exercise. The target heart rate to be achieved is 75% or more of the maximal heart rate for a certain age (Table 26–1).

The client is connected to the apparatus necessary to monitor ECG and blood pressure. If oxygen consumption is measured, a mouthpiece is used. Baseline measurements are taken in advance, and the physician performs a brief physical examination to clear the client for the test.

TABLE 26–1. DETERMINING TARGET HEART RATE

Formula	Subtract current age from 220 and multiply results by 60–75%.
Example	220 − 56 = 164 164 × 60% = 98 164 × 75% = 123
Target Rate	This client, who is 56 years of age, needs to sustain a heart rate of 98–123 beats per minute for 20 minutes of an aerobic workout. He is asked to exercise at least at 123 beats per minute in a stress test.

The characteristic sign of myocardial ischemia is a depressed ST segment. However, some clients have a drop in the ST segment when hyperventilating, so before the treadmill is started an ECG is obtained while the patient is standing still and hyperventilating. After the client has a chance to practice walking on the treadmill, the test is begun with the increases in grade and miles per hour shown in Table 26–2. The ECG, blood pressure, and pulse are constantly monitored and fed into a computer for analysis. The development of a computer-aided method of analyzing treadmill exercise tests may eliminate some of the false-positives that were common before computers were used (Hollenberg et al., 1985). In addition to the concern for false-positive results, false-negative results also occur. Drugs such as dipyridamole, a vasodilator, may be given before a stress test to improve the detection of coronary artery disease (Picano et al., 1988).

During the test, clinicians assess for symptoms, such as vertigo, extreme dyspnea, pallor, or signs of exhaustion. Depending on the ECG reading and other circumstances, the client may be allowed to continue with mild or moderate angina, but severe angina necessitates an abrupt end of the test. Leg fatigue or severe pain in the calves (claudication) may also necessitate cessation of the test.

Other reasons to stop the test are

1. Decrease in systolic blood pressure of 22 mm Hg
2. Marked ST segment depression
3. Ventricular tachycardia (VT)
4. Heart block, second or third degree
5. Atrial fibrillation (AF)
6. Paroxysmal atrial tachycardia (PAT)

TABLE 26–2. EXAMPLE OF STAGES FOR EXERCISE TREADMILL TESTING

Stage	mph	km/hr	Grade (%)
1	1.7	2.7	10
2	2.5	4.0	12
3	3.4	5.4	14
4	4.2	6.7	16
5	5.0	8.0	18
6	5.5	8.8	20
7	6.0	9.6	22

The grade and miles per hour (mph) are increased every 8 min until the target rate is achieved as discussed in the text.

Some clients do have occasional ectopic beats with exercise, so a few premature atrial contractions (PACs) or even premature ventricular contractions (PVCs) are not indications to stop the test if there is no clinical evidence of a change in cardiac output. (See Chapter 24 for a detailed discussion on common types of arrhythmias and clinical assessment for changes in cardiac output.)

Nuclear Cardiology Stress Tests

A nuclear cardiology stress test uses radionuclides, also called radioisotopes, to assess the perfusion of the myocardium. The radionuclide may be injected before, during, or after the exercise. Thallium is injected during the peak of exercise, and scans are obtained for about 30 min. After this initial imaging, resting images are taken after 2–4 hr (Hochrein and Sohl, 1992). Technetium sestamibi (Cardiolite) is usually given when the client is at rest, images are obtained 1 hr after administration of the radionuclide, and then more of the radionuclide is injected at the height of exercise (Keeys, 1994).

If a client needs a stress test but has problems that prevent running or walking, a pharmacologic stress test can be conducted. Dipyridamole (Persantine), dobutamine, and adenosine may be used with radionuclides. (See Chapter 22 for more information about cardiac tests with radionuclides.)

Assessing Exercise Tolerance

In the planning of exercise programs, stress tests are administered to evaluate the exercise tolerance of the client. The information from a stress test is useful in planning a graduated exercise program. The exercise tolerance of clients with known heart disease also is evaluated. For example, a client with an uncomplicated myocardial infarction most likely undergoes an exercise test before discharge from the hospital. A long-term follow-up study of clients who underwent exercise screening tests after a myocardial infarction demonstrated that three findings were strong, independent predictors of cardiovascular mortality. These three predictors, after control for clinical variables, were (1) a hypotensive blood pressure response, (2) ST-segment depression, and (3) ST-segment elevation. Clients who have these findings on a stress test may benefit from close surveillance in the years after an infarction (Froelicher, 1994).

▼ PRETEST NURSING IMPLICATIONS RELATED TO STRESS TESTS

Obtaining Informed Consent. Although a stress test can yield valuable information, it is not risk-free, even when clients have been carefully screened. The exercise, which is equal in stress to walking briskly or running up a steep hill, can cause severe arrhythmias, a myocardial infarction, or a stroke in susceptible clients. Most authorities quote a mortality of about 0.01%, or one death in every 10,000 clients who undergo the test. Because of the morbidity and mortality, the client must sign an informed consent after the physician explains the benefits in relation to the risks. The nurse can reassure the client that trained personnel and emergency equipment are available in the laboratory to deal with any complications that may occur.

Clients need written information about stress tests, including the risks and benefits of the test. Clients should be given *time* to digest verbal and written information and then make an informed decision. (See Chapter 25 for more about the role of the nurse as the advocate for the client who is undergoing invasive tests or tests that can cause complications.)

Limiting Food and Fluid Intake. The client should eat a light meal 2 hr before the test. Some clinicians prefer that the client have no beverages containing caffeine, whereas others allow 1 cup of coffee or tea before the test. Milk or other foods, which may cause nausea during exercise, should be avoided. The client should be adequately hydrated before the test. Some procedures, particularly those with radionuclides, require the client to take nothing by mouth for 4 hours before the test.

Administering Medications. If the client is taking diuretics, assessment of the serum potassium level is completed before the exercise test. Hypokalemia, often a side effect of diuretics, predisposes the client to arrhythmias. Nitroglycerin or other vasodilators are not given before the test, unless the test is being given to evaluate the efficiency of the medications. The nurse must confer with the physician to see what medications are permissible before the test. For example, beta blockers may be withheld because they decrease the response to exercise. Clients need clear instructions on which routine medications are to be continued and which are to be withheld.

Clothing Needs. Comfortable *walking* shoes are a must for the test. Bedroom slippers, sandals, or high-heeled shoes are unsatisfactory. Rubber-soled shoes provide the best grip on the treadmill.

Men wear no clothes on the upper body so electrodes can be applied to the chest. Women can wear a bra and a hospital gown or blouse that opens in the front. A bra may interfere with imaging if a nuclear stress test is performed. Breast markers may be needed to avoid breast artifacts (Wackers, 1992). Pants, skirts, or trousers should be loose and comfortable because electrodes are placed on the extremities. Constricting clothing and nylon fabrics are to be avoided. Hair should be arranged off the face, and any bothersome jewelry should be removed.

(*continued*)

▼ PRETEST NURSING IMPLICATIONS RELATED TO STRESS TESTS (*continued*)

Resting Before the Test. A good night's sleep before the test is essential so that undue fatigue is not a factor in the results. Relaxation exercises before the test may be beneficial. The client performs warming-up exercises and cooling-down exercises in the laboratory.

▼ POSTTEST NURSING IMPLICATIONS RELATED TO STRESS TESTS

Assessing Vital Signs. The client remains in the cardiology laboratory until vital signs are normal. To ensure that levels have returned to baseline, ECG tracings are taken at various intervals. Rarely, the client may need to be monitored for several hours because of an arrhythmia or other complication.

Resuming Activities after Radionuclide Testing. If nuclear scanning has been performed as part of the stress test, more testing is done in 2–4 hours. Clients may be allowed a light meal, but this should be verified with the nuclear medicine department. (See Chapter 22 for precautions about urine after radionuclide testing.)

Follow-up Plans. An individualized exercise program is planned on the basis of the results of the stress test. An ideal exercise plan is one that helps the client achieve target heart rate for 20 min three times a week. Target heart rates are usually 60–75% of the client's maximum heart rate. Table 26–1 provides the formula for determining target heart rate. The American Heart Association has detailed guidelines for exercise prescriptions. Whatever the length and type of exercise prescribed by the physician, it is important that the client also understand the importance of warm-up and cool-down exercises.

If the stress test is given to evaluate angina and coronary ischemia, more diagnostic tests may be ordered by the physician. For example, the client may need instructions about cardiac catheterizations.

▼ CARDIAC CATHETERIZATION

Description. A cardiac catheterization is performed under local anesthesia because the client needs to cooperate by performing deep breathing and coughing maneuvers. (Coughing helps clear the dye from the coronary arteries.) The client may also be asked to perform bicycle-type leg exercises to see the effect of stress on cardiac function and coronary blood flow. (Small children undergo catheterization under general anesthesia.) Depending on the information needed, a catheter may be inserted into a vein for a study of the right side of the heart or into an artery (usually the femoral artery) for a study of the left side of the heart. The catheter for cardiac catheterization is a flexible, hollow tube 100 cm (40 inches), long. For a left-sided catheterization, an artery is punctured with a short stubby needle and a guide wire is inserted. The catheter slides over the guide wire into the artery. The guide wire makes it possible to guide the catheter through the left atrium into the left ventricle. Fluoroscopy is used to view the catheter; the room must be darkened. (See Chapter 20 for a discussion on fluoroscopy.) For a right-sided catheterization, a vein is used, and the catheter is threaded through the vena cava into the right atrium and right ventricle.

A transseptal technique uses a small needle inserted in the right side of the heart. The needle is gently maneuvered through the septum to obtain pressure readings and blood samples from the left side of the heart. In some cases of aortic stenosis, the heart valve cannot be crossed in the usual manner, and a transseptal technique is needed.

After the pressures and readings and blood samples are obtained, a catheter is threaded into the coronary artery, and a radiopaque dye is inserted to outline the coronary arteries. This dye contains iodine. (See Chapter 20 for the precautions when dye with iodine is used for a diagnostic procedure.) During the passage of the dye, the room is darkened so that the motion can be observed on the fluoroscope screen. Movies (cineography) may also be taken of the flow of the dye. The table is tilted to help with dye flow. Ultrasound may also be used (Chapter 23).

The entire procedure of a left-sided and right-sided cardiac catheterization takes about 1–2 hr, depending on the findings. However, clients may not need all the different aspects performed. For example, an adolescent with a valve defect may not undergo studies of the coronary arteries.

Because cardiac catheterization is an elaborate procedure that requires a specialized laboratory setup, it is not performed in small hospitals or clinics.

Purposes. As mentioned earlier in this chapter, a stress test may be a preliminary test before cardiac catheterization. Cardiac catheterization is used when noninvasive forms of cardiac diagnostic tests—such as ECGs (Chapter 24), cine computed tomography (CT) or cine magnetic resonance imaging (MRI) (Chapter 21) and radionuclide scans (Chapter 22)—have not provided enough diagnostic information. As with any invasive procedure, there is some risk to the client. If less complicated, less risky, and less costly procedures will suffice, they are preferred.

Cardiac catheterization is often needed to confirm the need for heart surgery. For example, the need for a coronary bypass procedure is assessed with cardiac catheterization, which demonstrates the lack of coronary perfusion. Cardiac catheterization also defines the nature of other cardiac problems, especially congenital heart defects (Hay et al., 1995). Cardiac catheterization can also help determine the severity of heart disease and evaluate the progress of the client after medical or surgical intervention.

Conventional cardiac catheterization measures the pressures and calculates the flows in the various chambers of the heart and great vessels. Blood samples are obtained to measure dilutions of dye and oxygen and carbon dioxide values. Radiopaque dye is used in radiography and fluoroscopy of the heart and vessels.

▼ PRETEST NURSING IMPLICATIONS RELATED TO CARDIAC CATHETERIZATION

Checking the Chart. The client's chart should contain the results of other diagnostic tests, such as coagulation studies and hematocrit (hct). In addition, vital signs and other baseline data are charted as for other invasive procedures (Chapter 25). The precatheterization physical stability of the client must be assessed and documented. For example, strokes do occur as a complication of cardiac catheterization, so a careful neurologic evaluation before the procedure makes evaluation afterward more reliable (Bongard and Sue, 1994).

Although the risks of serious complications, such as a myocardial infarction or cerebrovascular accident, are slight, they sometimes occur with a catheterization. Thus, the client must sign a consent form that lists the possible complications, including such things as the possibility of a loss of a limb or cardiac arrest. The client's physician must explain the possibility of such risks in relation to the potential greater benefits of the procedure.

Physical Preparation of Client. The client usually consumes nothing by mouth after midnight for a morning procedure. If the test is not scheduled until the afternoon, a clear liquid breakfast may be given. Peripheral pulses should be assessed and the skin over the pulse points marked with ink to assist with posttest assessment. The client's groin, used for the femoral puncture, should be shaved. Shaving may be performed on the unit or in the laboratory. The client should void and empty his or her bowels, if possible, because the procedure is a long one. The client is transported to the laboratory on a gurney. A hospital gown is worn. Glasses can be worn, as can a watch, because the client is awake. Dentures are left in place because they may be needed if the client is to perform any breathing exercises with a mouthpiece. Hearing aids should be worn if needed. The client's chart should document the presence of a hearing difficulty or any communication problems.

Use of Medications Before and During the Procedure. Routine medications are usually not withheld, but this should be checked with the cardiologist. Some drugs, such as long-term anticoagulants, are usually contraindicated before the procedure because of the risk of bleeding. Thus, if a client has been taking warfarin (Coumadin), this must be evaluated by the physician. The premedications differ from institution to institution. Some cardiologists prefer no sedation for clients. Others routinely order a sedative. Antihistamines or a cortisone preparation may be ordered for clients who are allergy-prone. Some institutions have a policy to give cortisone or antihistamine drugs 1–2 days before cardiac catheterization. Test doses of the contrast medium also may be given. During the procedure, the client may be given vasodilators, such as nitroglycerin, to promote arterial dilation or ergonovine to constrict the arteries. Pain medications, other than a local anesthetic, are not routine before or during the procedure. More than one intravenous infusion may be started in the laboratory. Protamine is given at the end of the procedure to neutralize the effect of heparin. Clients who take NPH insulin may have antibodies to protamine and thus have an allergic reaction (Stewart et al., 1984). Emergency drugs should be readily available. Manipulation of the catheter can stimulate the vagus nerve and cause bradycardia, so atropine should be one of the emergency drugs. In the past, when catheters were larger, atropine was used routinely before catheterization.

▼ PRETEST NURSING DIAGNOSES RELATED TO CARDIAC CATHETERIZATION

Anxiety Related to Lack of Knowledge About Procedure

A nurse from the cardiac catheterization laboratory or from the general unit should reinforce the explanation of the cardiac catheterization procedure. Most cardiac catheterization laboratories have client information booklets that describe the procedure and answer common questions that clients may have about the preparation for the test. For example, Kaiser Permanente Medical Centers in northern California have a booklet that explains not only the catheterization procedure but also why the client must go to the San Francisco facility. The booklet contains a map of the medical center to help the referred client find the hospital and parking lot. The client arrives the day of the procedure. Some institutions use audiovisual material to explain the cardiac catheterization procedure. This can be accomplished the morning of the examination. Past studies have not shown whether it is more or less effective to have clients visit the cardiac laboratory before the procedure (Edwards and Payton, 1976). Without adequate preparation, viewing the "cath lab" may be anxiety-producing. Teasley (1982) suggested a checklist for teaching the client about the procedure, followed by viewing the laboratory, if feasible. Ventura (1984) suggested describing the environment.

(*continued*)

▼ PRETEST NURSING DIAGNOSES RELATED TO CARDIAC CATHETERIZATION (*continued*)

Rice et al. (1986), in a pilot study, found relaxation training did not significantly decrease anxiety before cardiac catheterization but suggested the effects need to be explored with a larger sample. A 1994 study suggested that videotaped procedural-sensory modeling information may be more useful to clients than written information alone (Davis et al., 1994a,b).

Risk for Pain and Discomfort from Cardiac Catheterization

Some clients experience much discomfort during a cardiac catheterization, whereas others do not. The anxiety level of the client seems to be an important factor. Certainly, the idea of a catheter entering one's heart is a frightening idea. The nurse should explain to the client that he or she may experience a small amount of discomfort so that he or she does not imagine the worst. Because the positioning of the catheter may cause a rapid or irregular pulse, the client may feel his or her heart "flip-flop" or race. Therefore, it may be comforting for the client to know that arrhythmias are common during the threading of the catheter and usually disappear without treatment. The client should be told that there will be constant monitoring for serious arrhythmias and that emergency equipment and drugs are present for immediate use. Clients should also be aware that a vigorous cough may suddenly be needed if they have an arrhythmia. This cough cardiopulmonary resuscitation (CPR) can help convert a potentially lethal ventricular arrhythmia to a normal sinus rhythm. The cough closes the epiglottis and increases intrathoracic pressure, which increases blood flow through the heart, hence coronary ischemia may be decreased.

Another discomfort is a venous or, even more so, an arterial puncture. A local anesthetic is used before an arterial puncture, but there is usually some pain associated with the procedure. Needles in general are very unpleasant for some clients. (See Chapter 25 on ways nurses can help prepare clients for momentary pain.) The injection of the dye may be a source of pain or discomfort for some clients, because of a metallic taste, a warm feeling, or a more intense rush from the dye. (The symptoms of an allergic reaction can occur, but this is not common; see Chapter 20.) Another discomfort may be the length of time the client must lie relatively still on the table—this may be very taxing for some clients. Nevertheless, the discomforts should be explained to the client.

▼ POSTTEST NURSING DIAGNOSES RELATED TO CARDIAC CATHETERIZATION

Risk for Altered Cardiac Output

Vital signs are checked the same as for other invasive procedures. Arrhythmias usually occur during the procedure, not afterward, but an *apical* pulse should be part of the assessment each time the client's vital signs are taken. If there is any arrhythmia, the client may need to be monitored for a time. (See Chapter 24 on monitoring.) An intravenous line is kept open (k/o rate) if arrhythmias have persisted. (See Chapter 20 on anaphylactic reactions from contrast medium, which could also cause altered cardiac output.)

Risk for Altered Tissue Perfusion

Because more than one entry site may be used, the nurse needs to check for more than one bandaged area after catheterization. Occasionally, a surgical cutdown may be performed to find the vessel for the catheter. If so, the client has skin sutures at the cutdown site.

The outside of the pressure dressing should be checked for any bleeding or hematoma formation. The pulse distal to the arterial puncture site should be checked and compared with the uninvolved site for a thrombus in the artery. Spasms of the artery can also cause diminished arterial flow. The venous site is less likely to have any serious complications. Phlebitis (inflammation of the vein) can develop later and may be relieved with warm compresses.

The length of bed rest depends on whether the procedure was left-sided, right-sided, or both. Bed rest for an arterial entry may be 4–6 hr depending on the size of the catheter used. Institutions used to require strict bed rest until the day after a catheterization (Teasley, 1982). The client can turn from side to side during bed rest, but the extremity used for the arterial puncture should not be moved for several hours.

Altered Fluid Requirement

The client can eat and drink as soon as he or she desires. An adequate intake of fluids is needed to help excretion of the dye. The dye, a hypertonic solution, can produce a fluid volume deficit. Clients can have delayed allergic reactions to the iodine dye, so the nurse must keep this in mind when assessing any pain or discomfort. (See Chapter 20 on radiopaque dyes.)

Altered Comfort

Back pain from the positioning is common, and a backrub may be helpful. Mild analgesics may be needed for pain at the puncture site. Pain distal to the puncture site is not expected and could mean an embolus to the extremity.

Clients undergoing catheterization usually exhibit some of the following symptoms: fatigue, dyspnea on exertion, edema, paroxysmal nocturnal dyspnea (PND), or angina. Nurses need to know what symptoms were present before catheterization so new symptoms can be identified and called to the physician's attention. New symptoms should not be masked by pain medication.

(continued)

▼ POSTTEST NURSING DIAGNOSES RELATED TO CARDIAC CATHETERIZATION (*continued*)

Risk for Injury Related to Cardiac Tamponade and Other Complications

In addition to arrhythmias, emboli, and infarctions, cardiac tamponade can occur after cardiac catheterization. Bleeding into the pericardial sac causes reduced cardiac output, because the heart is compressed in the pericardial sac. Symptoms of cardiac tamponade include anxiety, tachypnea, distended neck veins (when the client sits forward), muffled heart sounds, narrowing pulse pressure, and a paradoxical pulse. To detect a paradoxical pulse, the nurse must take the systolic blood pressure during inspiration and expiration, noting if the systolic pressure is less during inspiration. A difference of more than 10 mm Hg in the two is evidence of a paradoxical pulse. One easy way to detect a paradoxical pulse is to ask the client to hold his or her breath after the first systolic reading (Kinnebrew, 1981). Any questionable symptoms or marked change in vital signs should be immediately called to the attention of the physician. Although cardiac tamponade and other complications are unlikely after cardiac catheterization, they can occur, and a prudent nurse is always alert for adverse reactions after all invasive tests.

Knowledge Deficit Related to Home Care

In the past clients were admitted to the hospital for cardiac catheterization. Now many clients go home within 6–8 hr after the procedure. Institutions provide written discharge instructions that include the information discussed earlier and specific guidelines for activities and care of the insertion site. For example, no bending or squatting or unnecessary activity should be performed the evening after the catheterization. If the client feels or notices any bleeding, direct hand pressure should be applied to the site and the physician called for instructions.

The next day the client can gradually resume some activity with no heavy lifting or exercise. The dressing can be removed during a bath or shower and replaced with a small dry dressing, which is then changed daily until healing occurs. If stitches were used, they should be removed in about 1 week. The physician should also state when the client can return to work and how much exercise is allowed the first week.

▼ ELECTROPHYSIOLOGIC STUDIES

EPSs are performed under laboratory conditions similar to those for cardiac catheterization. Electrodes that can both pace and stimulate the rhythm of the heart are connected to catheters that are inserted through the femoral, brachial, or basilic vein to the right side of the heart. Arterial catheters are used if there is a need to stimulate the left ventricle. A typical study may require three to six of these intracardiac pacing catheters. The intracardiac ECG is recorded simultaneously with the regular or surface ECG (Chapter 24). This very sophisticated monitoring can give a detailed evaluation of the entire conduction system with mapping of both normal and abnormal (aberrant) pathways. EPSs are also useful to evaluate if dangerous arrhythmias can be induced. An arrhythmia may be artificially induced in a drug-free state to try to assess what has caused syncope or a previous cardiac arrest. Induction of an arrhythmia is also attempted after the client has reached a steady state with an antiarrhythmic drug to see if the drug does prevent the arrhythmia. If the drug fails the test (i.e., the arrhythmia can be elicited with an EPS), another antiarrhythmic drug is tried, and the EPS is performed again when the drug produces a steady state. Mason (1993) compared EPSs with Holter monitoring (Chapter 25) and noted that both can be effective in monitoring the efficacy of drugs, so other factors to consider are the cost of testing, the safety of the procedure, and the experience of physicians and staff members with the two methods.

▼ PRETEST NURSING IMPLICATIONS RELATED TO ELECTROPHYSIOLOGIC STUDIES

Although the physical and psychological preparation for an EPS is similar to that for a cardiac catheterization, the risk for anxiety may be even greater. During an EPS, arrhythmias are purposely induced, and the client may experience a life-threatening arrhythmia that requires emergency drug therapy or defibrillation. Also, some clients have to undergo several EPSs to find and evaluate an effective drug for their particular type of arrhythmia. EPSs are performed in large medical centers where specialists in cardiovascular nursing are usually available to help clients understand the purpose of repeated EPSs and to deal with the fear that an EPS can generate (Rogers, 1986; Mercer, 1987).

▼ POSTTEST NURSING IMPLICATIONS RELATED TO ELECTROPHYSIOLOGIC STUDIES

The nursing implications for care after cardiac catheterization also apply to an EPS. Sometimes a catheter may be left in place because of the need to repeat a study. The client may stay flat for 4 hr and then be propped up with pillows. The leg should be kept straight with no bending at the groin. A small bedpan creates less need to bend the leg than does a conventional bedpan. The client should be turned toward the side of the puncture. If using a bedpan seems to put strain on the groin site, the client may need to have a Foley catheter inserted. Lines left in place for repeat EPSs require specific orders for the care and flushing of the catheter.

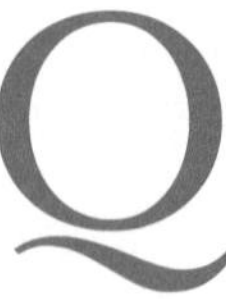

1. Mr. Bodansky asks the nurse why the physician has ordered a nuclear cardiology stress test rather than a conventional stress test. The nurse should base an answer on the fact that radionuclides are used with an exercise stress test for
   a. Assessing the location of partially obstructed coronary arteries
   b. Evaluating exercise tolerance after a myocardial infarction
   c. Evaluating myocardial perfusion during exercise
   d. Assessing the relation between arrhythmias and stress level

2. Mrs. Dunbar, 48 years of age, is scheduled for a stress test tomorrow because she has had some heart palpitations while exercising. She asks the clinic nurse about the procedure. The nurse would be correct in informing Mrs. Dunbar that
   a. Blood pressure cuff and electrocardiogram leads are used during the test
   b. A treadmill is adjusted to decreasing and increasing speeds during the test
   c. If Mrs. Dunbar has any angina, the test will be stopped
   d. Clients must be admitted to the hospital in preparation for the test

3. Mr. Faber has been scheduled for a stress test in the cardiology laboratory tomorrow morning. He had an uncomplicated myocardial infarction a week ago. Which of the following nursing interventions is most appropriate in preparing Mr. Faber for the test?
   a. Reassuring him that there are no risks from the test
   b. Instructing him to consume nothing by mouth for 12 hours before the test
   c. Giving him nitroglycerin tablets, if needed before the test
   d. Asking his family to bring him walking shoes for the test

4. Regina, 16 years of age, is to undergo cardiac catheterization, right-sided and left-sided, this morning. She takes digitalis and consumes a no-added-salt (NAS) diet. Which of the following is *not* an appropriate nursing action in preparing Regina for the cardiac catheterization?
   a. Checking to see if all ordered laboratory reports are on the chart, such as PT, PTT, and hct
   b. Allowing liquids but withholding all oral medicines
   c. Explaining that Regina will be awake and that she will be asked to do such maneuvers as coughing and deep breathing during the procedure
   d. Allowing Regina to wear her glasses and a watch to the cardiac catheterization laboratory

5. Regina was given atropine sulfate during the cardiac catheterization procedure. The desired effect of atropine in relation to cardiac catheterization is to

   a. Promote sedation
   b. Decrease respiratory secretions
   c. Prevent bradycardia
   d. Eliminate gastrointestinal spasms

6. Regina has just returned from the cardiac catheterization laboratory. She underwent a right-sided and left-sided (left femoral artery was used) catheterization with no complications, except a minor arrhythmia during the procedure. Her vital signs are stable. Which nursing action is *unnecessary* for the first hour that Regina is back on the unit?

   a. Keeping the left leg immobilized
   b. Offering her something to drink and telling her fluids help eliminate the dye
   c. Checking the pulses distal to the left femoral artery and comparing these with the pulses in the right foot
   d. Taking her temperature every 15 min for three times

7. In comparing electrophysiologic studies (EPSs) and cardiac catheterization, the nurse should know that these two procedures are similar in that

   a. Catheters may be left in place for repeated tests
   b. The client's anxiety tends to be minimal
   c. Catheters may be threaded into the left and right sides of the heart
   d. The client must maintain bed rest for 24 hr

▼ REFERENCES

Bongard, F.S., and Sue, D.Y. (1994). *Current critical care diagnosis & treatment.* Norwalk, CT: Appleton & Lange.

Davis, T., Maguire, T.O., Haraphongse, M., et al. (1994a). Preparing adult patients for cardiac catheterization: Informational treatment and coping style interactions. *Heart & Lung, 23* (2), 130–139.

Davis, T., Maguire, T.O., Haraphongse, M., et al. (1994b). Undergoing cardiac catheterization: The effects of informational preparation and coping style on patient anxiety during the procedure. *Heart & Lung, 23* (2), 140–150.

Edwards, M., and Payton, V. (1976). Cardiac catheterization: technique and teaching. *Nursing Clinics of North America, 11,* 271–281.

Froelicher, E.S. (1994). Usefulness of exercise testing shortly after acute myocardial infarction for predicting 10 year mortality. *American Journal of Cardiology, 74,* 318–323.

Hay, W.W., Groothuis, J.R., Hayward, A.R., and Levin, M.J. (1995). *Current pediatric diagnosis & treatment.* (12th ed.). Norwalk, CT: Appleton & Lange.

Hochrein, M.A., and Sohl, L. (1992). Heart smart: A guide to cardiac tests. *American Journal of Nursing, 92* (12), 22–25.

Hollenberg, M., Zoltick, J.M., Go, M., et al. (1985). Comparison of a quantitative treadmill exercise score with standard electrocardiographic criteria in screening asymptomatic young men for coronary artery disease. *New England Journal of Medicine, 313* (10), 600–606.

Keeys, M.U. (1994). Nuclear cardiology stress testing. *Nursing 94, 24,* 63–64.

Kinnebrew, M. (1981). Add paradoxical pulse to your assessment routine. *RN, 44* (11), 32–33.

Mason, J.W. (1993). A comparison of electrophysiologic testing with Holter monitoring to predict antiarrhythmic-drug efficacy for ventricular tachyarrhythmias. *New England Journal of Medicine, 329* (7), 445–451.

Mercer, M. (1987). The electrophysiology study: A nursing concern. *Critical Care Nurse, 7* (2), 58–67.

Picano, E., Lattanzi, F., Masisni, M., et al. (1988). Usefulness of the dipyridamole-exercise echocardiography test for diagnosis of coronary artery disease. *American Journal of Cardiology, 62,* 67–70.

Rice, V., Caldwell, M., Butler, S., et al. (1986). Relaxation training and response to cardiac catheterization: A pilot study. *Nursing Research, 35* (1), 39–43.

Rogers, R. (1986). Your patient is scheduled for EPS. *American Journal of Nursing, 86* (5), 573–575.

Stewart, W., et al. (1984). Increased risk of severe protamine reactions in NPH insulin-dependent diabetics undergoing cardiac catheterization. *Circulation, 70* (5), 788.

Teasley, D. (1982). Don't let cardiac catheterization strike fear in your patient's heart. *Nursing 82, 12* (3), 52–56.

Ventura, B. (1984). What you need to know about cardiac catheterization. *RN, 47* (9), 24–30.

Wackers, F.J. (1992). Diagnostic pitfalls of myocardial perfusion imaging in women. *Journal of Myocardial Ischemia, 4* (10), 23–37.

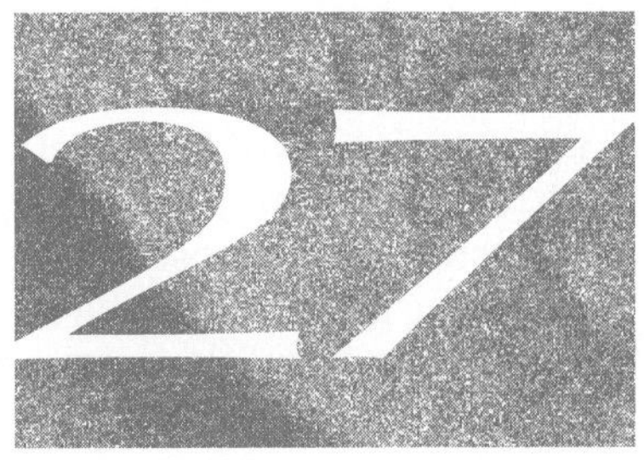

ENDOSCOPIC PROCEDURES

- Bronchoscopy
- Gastroscopy
- Esophagogastroduodenoscopy
- Endoscopic Retrograde Cholangiopancreatography
- Sigmoidoscopy or Proctoscopy (Proctosigmoidoscopy)
- Colonoscopy and Enteroscopy
- Cystoscopy and Ureteroscopy
- Laparoscopy
- Arthroscopy

OBJECTIVES

1. Describe nursing assessments for seven possible complications that may occur after endoscopic procedures.
2. Identify at least five general nursing diagnoses for clients undergoing endoscopic procedures.
3. Compare and contrast the nursing interventions before and after bronchoscopy, gastroscopy, or other endoscopic procedures involving the upper airway.
4. Identify areas for client teaching about sigmoidoscopy and other endoscopic procedures of the lower gastrointestinal (GI) tract.
5. Identify endoscopic procedures that may require conscious sedation.
6. Describe nursing interventions for a client who has undergone cystoscopy under local anesthesia.

Endoscopes are used for direct visualization of hollow organs or body cavities. Specifically designed endoscopes are named for the cavity that is being viewed, such as a gastroscope, bronchoscope, or sigmoidoscope. Table 27–1 presents examples of endoscopic procedures. The scopes contain lights so that the interior or cavity of the organ can be seen. The scopes are hollow instruments with suction tips, biopsy forceps, and other accessories for obtaining tissue samples. Electrodes for cauterization may also be an accessory. Photocoagulation can be used to control GI bleeding, and gallstones can be removed with a special adaptor. Endoscopes are also used with lasers to vaporize small tumors and cysts and to cut more precisely than a scalpel (Freeman, 1986). Cameras can be used to record the findings for later reference.

Earlier scopes were all rigid instruments, but newer models are flexible nylon tubes, which can more easily be advanced into a body cavity, such as the intestinal tract. Fiberscopes or fiber-optic scopes are made of strands of glass fibers that reflect light and actually make it possible to see around corners. A flexible fiberscope can be threaded from the mouth into the duodenum (duodenoscopy) or from the rectum through the ileocecal valve into the small intestine (enteroscopy). The first fiberscopes were used in the early 1960s. Industry also uses fiber-optic instruments to peer into cavities, such as automobile engines, so that the engine does not have to be dismantled (Hirschowitz, 1979).

POSSIBLE COMPLICATIONS OF ENDOSCOPIC PROCEDURES

Although endoscopic procedures cause some pain and discomfort, topical anesthetics or conscious sedation make the procedure tolerable for a cooperative client. An endoscopic procedure may save the client the risk and expense of a surgical

TABLE 27–1. AREAS VISUALIZED WITH ENDOSCOPIC PROCEDURES

Name of Procedure	Area Visualized[a]
Arthroscopy	Knee or other joints
Bronchoscopy	Bronchial tree
Colposcopy	Vagina and cervix (Chapter 25)
Culdoscopy	Female pelvic organs
Cystoscopy	Urinary bladder
Endoscopic retrograde cholangiopancreatography (ERCP or ECPG)	Common bile duct and pancreatic duct
Enteroscopy	Upper colon and small intestine
Esophagoscopy	Esophagus
Esophagogastroduodenoscopy (EGD)	Esophagus to small intestine
Fetoscopy	In amniotic sac to view fetus (Chapter 28)
Gastroscopy	Stomach
Laparoscopy	Abdominal cavity
Proctoscopy	Anus and rectum
Sigmoidoscopy	Sigmoid colon
Ureteroscopy	Ureters

[a]Preparation discussed in this chapter unless noted.

procedure under general anesthesia. Specific complications for the different types of endoscopic procedures are discussed later, but there are at least seven possible risks of any type of endoscopic procedure. These risks are

1. The possibility of perforation of the organ or cavity being examined.
2. Aspiration of saliva or gastric contents when the upper airway or esophagus is being examined.
3. Untoward reactions to the drugs used, which include topical anesthetics and medications such as meperidine (Demerol) and the benzodiazepines, diazepam (Valium), and midazolam (Versed). Although other drugs may be used for conscious sedation, meperidine may be better than the other opioids with regard to client comfort and amnesia (Chokhavatia et al., 1994). The worst unwanted effects of these drugs are respiratory depression and hypotension. Naloxone (Narcan), a specific antagonist for the opioids, and other emergency drugs should be available. As mentioned later, other drugs may be used during some endoscopy procedures and these, too, may cause unwanted effects.

   Flumazenil (Mazicon), a specific benzodiazepine antagonist, may be used to reverse the effects of a benzodiazepine used during an endoscopic procedure. The drug eliminates sedation rapidly, so at the end of the procedure the client is awake, oriented to the surroundings, and cooperative. The client may have little recall of the endoscopic procedure. However, clients still need assessment for respiratory depression because the drug may not reverse hypoventilation. Also, resedation may occur, so a second dose of the antagonist may be needed (Deglin and Vallerand, 1995).
4. Cardiovascular problems, such as arrhythmias and even myocardial infarction, due to the psychological and physical stress of the procedure. A vasovagal effect can be stimulated. The vagus can cause bradycardia because the effect of the vagus nerve is to slow the heart. Atropine should be available to treat the bradycardia.
5. Hemorrhage, particularly if a biopsy has been performed as part of the diagnostic procedure.
6. Infections and transient bacteremia. The danger of bacteremia is explored in the section on cystoscopy.
7. Hypersensitivity to contrast medium. In a survey of 10,000 endoscopic procedures in which iodinated contrast medium was locally instilled, the incidence of hypersensitivity was 0.3% compared with 10% for intravenous delivery (Sable et al., 1983). Because locally instilled dye reaches peak serum levels after endoscopy is completed, clients should be monitored for delayed reactions. (See Chapter 20 on contrast media.)

The risks of these complications are low, and the exact rates of occurrence depend on the skill of the clinician performing the procedure, the physical status of the client, and the type of instrumentation used. Because of the possible risks mentioned, the physician has the client sign a special consent form. (See Chapter

25 on consent forms.) This form should be in the client's chart before any sedative medications are given. Baseline studies, hematocrit (hct), and urinalysis are routine in most clinic and inpatient settings. Coagulation studies (i.e., partial thromboplastin time [PTT] and platelet studies) are needed if bleeding is a potential problem. If the client has undergone any other diagnostic tests before endoscopy, those results should be available on the chart.

▼ GENERAL PRETEST NURSING DIAGNOSES RELATED TO ENDOSCOPY

Anxiety Related to Unknowns About Procedure

Because the client usually is awake during the procedure, he or she should understand the general procedure. As emphasized in Chapter 25, most clients particularly want to know how the procedure feels (Johnson and Rice, 1974). Some clients may want a detailed explanation of the technical aspects; others do not. Clients should also be told what causes the sensations—if they know what to expect they are less likely to misinterpret the experience. Physical sensations should be described but not evaluated by the nurse because this may cause more anxiety (McHugh et al., 1982).

Because endoscopy is performed in a specialized procedure room or operating room, the nurse is usually not present during the procedure. Thus, the nurse performs his or her anxiety-relieving function well before the client goes for the examination. As with other diagnostic tests, the nurse can reinforce the information given by the physician and try to find out answers to those questions that continue to bother the client about the test. Nurses who work in the procedure rooms have specific functions during the test but can also focus on helping clients deal with anxious feelings.

Knowledge Deficit Related to Physical Preparation

With the exception of sigmoidoscopy, all the endoscopic procedures discussed in this chapter require that the client maintain nothing-by-mouth status. Vital signs must be taken for baseline data, and a notation should be made of the client's general physical status before the examination (e.g., a client may have abdominal cramps before the examination or shortness of breath). Any signs and symptoms present before the procedure should be documented. The client should void before the procedure so he or she does not have to urinate during the procedure. If general anesthesia is planned, the client should be instructed on deep breathing and coughing exercises and other postoperative care. The nurse must protect the client from injury by instructing the client to stay in bed, with side rails up, after any premedications are given. The client should be informed that the drugs used before or during the procedure may cause drowsiness, euphoria, or a feeling of "not self," and that monitoring may include pulse oximetry (Chapter 6) and other devices for monitoring vital signs.

▼ GENERAL POSTTEST NURSING DIAGNOSES RELATED TO ENDOSCOPY

Risk for Injury Related to Adverse Reactions or Complications

The frequency with which to record the client's vital signs is determined by the routine practices discussed for other invasive procedures in Chapter 25. The client may want to rest, because the procedures are somewhat of an ordeal. The nurse should check for specific complications each time vital signs are taken. The nurse should particularly assess for bleeding if a biopsy was part of the procedure. The nurse needs to know what medicines were used both before and during the test so that untoward reactions can be identified. (See the earlier discussion of seven possible complications.)

Risk for Pain Related to Procedure

Mild analgesics may be needed when local anesthesia wears off. Because severe pain can be caused by a perforation, any severe or persistent pain should be carefully assessed. The risk of perforation increases if laser therapy was part of an endoscopic procedure (Zettel, 1986).

Risk for Ineffective Airway Clearance Related to Use of Local Anesthesia

When a scope is inserted via the throat, the gag reflex can be abolished by administration of a topical anesthetic. The nurse must check to see if a local anesthetic was used. Even though the client can swallow, he or she may still not have a gag reflex. The return of the gag reflex can be checked by gently touching a tongue blade to the back of the throat. Once the gag reflex returns, the client is allowed to resume whatever diet is tolerated.

Knowledge Deficit Related to Home Care

Any specific instructions for follow-up care, such as sitz baths or warm gargles, should be explained to the client. If the client is going home after the diagnostic procedure, he or she needs explicit instructions on symptoms that should be reported immediately to the physician or clinic. The client should

(continued)

▼ GENERAL POSTTEST NURSING DIAGNOSES RELATED TO ENDOSCOPY (*continued*)

be accompanied to the procedure by a friend or family member who, in addition to driving the client home, can also be taught what to look for because the drugs used during procedure can produce some amnesia in the client.

▼ BRONCHOSCOPY

Description and Purposes. For bronchoscopy, a lighted bronchoscope is passed into the bronchial tree. A local anesthetic may be sprayed or swabbed on the throat. The client lies on his or her back with the head hyperextended. The bronchoscope is inserted via the nose or mouth into the trachea and main stem bronchi. The client must breathe around the tube. This can cause a fear of suffocation. It is important that the client be relaxed and not fight the tube. Oxygen may be administered to maintain Po_2. Visualization of the mucosa of the bronchi shows the surgeon the area on which to perform a biopsy when cancer is suspected. Bronchial washings or brush biopsy specimens can be obtained for culturing fungi, acid-fast bacilli, *Pneumocystis carinii*, and *Legionella pneumophila*. (Immune-deficient clients are prone to parasitic infections as with *P. carinii*, and simple sputum cultures do not identify the organism.) Bronchoscopy is also used therapeutically to remove foreign objects or for deep suctioning. For suctioning, the bronchoscopy may be performed at the client's bedside but is usually performed in the operating room or a specially equipped room. Bronchoscopy is usually performed with topical anesthesia or with some conscious sedation. Sometimes general anesthesia is used.

▼ PRETEST NURSING IMPLICATIONS RELATED TO BRONCHOSCOPY

Completing Routine Preoperative Care. Most institutions have a routine preoperative checklist that is completed before bronchoscopy. The consent form must be signed. Hct and urinalysis must be performed. The client consumes nothing by mouth for about 6–8 hr before the procedure. Good mouth care is important before the procedure so that less bacteria are present in the mouth. Dentures must be removed, and the physician must be warned about any loose teeth.

Patient Teaching. During the procedure, the client breathes through the nose with the mouth open. The client may need time to practice. The client is not able to talk while the bronchoscope is in his or her throat; therefore, the nurse should explain that the client must communicate with hand signals.

Administering Medications. The pretest medications given parenterally usually include atropine (to dry up respiratory secretions); a narcotic, usually meperidine (Demerol), and a sedative such as diazepam (Valium). Diazepam is also a muscle relaxant, which helps with passage of the tube. As noted in the general nursing diagnoses, respiratory depression can occur.

▼ POSTTEST NURSING DIAGNOSES RELATED TO BRONCHOSCOPY

Risk for Ineffective Airway Clearance Related to Increased Secretions

The client is kept in a semi-Fowler position but may be turned to either side. The client should not smoke. Tissues and a paper bag are needed for expectorations. An emesis basin, lined with tissue, may be useful for copious secretions. (Lining the basin makes it easier to empty.) Once the gag reflex has returned, encouraging fluids to keep the client well-hydrated makes secretions less viscous and easier to expectorate. Vigorous coughing after a biopsy can loosen a clot. A suction machine should be available. Some institutions have routine orders for oxygen for 4 hr after bronchoscopy. Pulse oximeters (Chapter 6) may be used to assess persistent hypoxemia. Because severe respiratory embarrassment can occur, a tracheostomy set should be nearby. An absence of breath sounds may indicate pneumothorax. Subcutaneous emphysema (a collection of air in tissues) can occur if there is a leak in the pleural space. (See the discussion on thoracentesis or pleural taps in Chapter 25.) Some pink-tinged mucus or small amounts of blood in the sputum are not unusual after bronchoscopy, but hemoptysis can signal hemorrhage from a biopsy site.

Altered Comfort Related to Procedure

The client should not do much talking. A pad and pencil can be used for communication. Fluids, particularly warm fluids that are soothing, are encouraged once the gag reflex has returned. A gargle with warm saline solution may help relieve throat discomfort. Throat lozenges may be used. A soft diet may be better tolerated if swallowing is painful. The client may be very anxious to hear the results of the biopsy, because this test is often the determinant of whether a malignant tumor of the lung is operable.

▼ GASTROSCOPY

Description and Purposes. Gastroscopy may include viewing the esophagus (esophagoscopy) as well as the interior of the stomach. The presence of ulcers can be verified and a biopsy taken. If a client has GI bleeding, it may be possible to control the bleeding with photocoagulation, so early endoscopic treatment may be advisable. With a gastroscopy, a percutaneous endoscopic gastrostomy (PEG) tube can be easily inserted or removed at the bedside or in an outpatient setting (Thompson, 1995). The next section discusses upper GI endoscopy in general and the associated nursing implications.

▼ ESOPHAGOGASTRODUODENOSCOPY

Description and Purposes. All endoscopic procedures on the upper GI tract are performed with the client in the left lateral recumbent position. Appropriate intravenous medications and local anesthetics are given to make the procedure tolerable. In addition to drugs for sedation, the client may receive atropine or glucagon to slow peristalsis. A plastic mouthpiece is used to help relax the jaw and protect the endoscope. The client may be asked to swallow once or twice while the scope is advanced down the esophagus. After that the client should not swallow—secretions can drain from the side of the mouth or be suctioned out. The client may feel a sensation of pressure as air is instilled to help with visualization of the GI tract. This is more uncomfortable with duodenoscopy. Most of the air is removed at the end of the procedure. Burping is common. With active esophageal bleeding, endotracheal intubation may be necessary to prevent aspiration both during and after the procedure.

Esophagogastroscopy may include viewing the esophagus to detect lesions or varices. Gastric and duodenal ulcers can also be viewed and biopsies performed. Color instant photographs of the ulcerations may be placed in the client's chart. Diagnosis of a gastric infection with *Helicobacter pylori*, a gram-negative bacterium, is usually made by means of biopsy of gastric mucosal samples, although noninvasive testing for the bacteria may include serologic testing or the urea breath test (Moulton-Barrett et al., 1993).

If the client has GI bleeding it may be possible to pinpoint and cauterize the bleeding site. The use of a cautery is not painful for the client, but if monopolar cautery is used he or she feels the cold, sticky grounding pad applied to the thigh. The pad is not necessary with bipolar cautery (Renkes, 1993). Thermal coagulation is usually used rather than laser coagulation because of the risk for tissue injury during laser coagulation, the cost of the laser instrument, and the inferior success rate of laser therapy compared with use of contact devices (Bongard and Sue, 1994).

▼ PRETEST NURSING IMPLICATIONS RELATED TO UPPER GI ENDOSCOPY

A general preoperative preparation is completed, including consent forms and laboratory work. As with bronchoscopy, it is important that dentures be removed and the client checked for any loose teeth. The client consumes nothing by mouth for 8–12 hr before the procedure.

▼ POSTTEST NURSING IMPLICATIONS RELATED TO UPPER GI ENDOSCOPY

The client may be kept in a semi-Fowler position or turned to the side to help expectorate any fluids. The standard vital sign routine is followed, as is careful evaluation for any signs of gastric bleeding. If a local anesthetic is used, no liquids are allowed until the gag reflex returns (see bronchoscopy care). Warm saline gargles may be used to relieve a sore throat, or throat lozenges can be used. As with other procedures, the use of drugs may cause specific posttest reactions.

▼ ENDOSCOPIC RETROGRADE CHOLANGIOPANCREATOGRAPHY

Description and Purposes. Endoscopic retrograde cholangiopancreatography (ERCP or ECPG) involves the passage of a flexible fiberscope through the mouth, stomach, and into the duodenum, as for esophagogastroduodenoscopy (EGD), discussed in the previous section. As in EGD, the procedure starts with the client placed on the left side. However, after the scope is in the mouth, the client is turned to a supine position with the head turned to the right. When the endoscope reaches the ampulla of Vater, dye is injected to outline the common bile duct and the pancreatic ducts. Radiographs are taken of the biliary tree (cholangiogram). ERCP is an important diagnostic tool for clients with cholestatic jaundice. The usual precautions before and after esophagoscopy or gastroscopy are applicable to ERCP. The additional concerns related to the injection of dye into the biliary system are discussed in the section on cholangiograms (Chapter 20). Possible complications of ERCP are acute pancreatitis, cholangitis, pancreatic abscess, drug reactions, and instrument injury. Serum amylase and lipase levels are useful in assessing for pancreatitis (Chapter 12). ERCP can be combined with a surgical procedure (sphincterotomy) to remove a gallstone from the common bile duct. Transient pancreatitis after sphincterotomy is considered normal, and the client has an elevated amylase level for a few days (Peternel, 1985). Other types of therapeutic procedures also may be performed with ERCP, including insertion of stents or catheters (Renkes, 1993). After complicated procedures, such as removal of stones or insertion of stents, the client may consume nothing by mouth or only clear liquids until the next morning. Assessment of pain, abdominal distention, and bowel sounds is important, and the findings should be documented.

Another type of endoscopy, laparoscopy, has revolutionized the treatment of gallstones (Gholson et al., 1994). General anesthesia is needed for this approach, as discussed in the section on laparoscopy.

▼ SIGMOIDOSCOPY OR PROCTOSCOPY (PROCTOSIGMOIDOSCOPY)

Description and Purposes. Sigmoidoscopes are used to view the lower, or sigmoid, colon, and proctoscopes are used to view the anus and rectum. When the scope is put through the rectal sphincter, the client has a strong sensation of a need to defecate. This is only a sensation because the client undergoes intestinal preparation before the examination. The flexible scope is advanced about 40 cm into the colon. Air, inserted to help with visualization of the colon, may cause an uncomfortable sensation of pressure and cramps. The procedure lasts 5–10 min and is well tolerated by most clients. However, for some clients the procedure may cause considerable discomfort, and the scope cannot be advanced as far as needed to produce the best view. Having the client relax and take deep breaths may help, as may removing some air. Newer scopes are equipped with monitors that may be viewed by the client as the scope is advanced. This may or may not be an appropriate diversion for the client.

Endoscopy of the lower colon is used to detect and perform biopsies on polyps and tumors. The clinician can sometimes see the site of bleeding or the extent of an inflammatory process. Because most cancer of the large intestine occurs in the lower colon, sigmoidoscopy is a useful detection tool for cancer.

The American Cancer Society, the National Cancer Institute, and the American College of Physicians all recommend that all adults older than 50 years undergo sigmoidoscopy as a screen for cancer of the colon, a leading cause of death in this age group. The screening may be performed every 3–5 years according to the advice of the physician. After 75 years of age, the guidelines may differ (Day, 1990). In addition, a test for occult blood in the stool should be performed once a year after 50 years of age. (See Chapter 13 on occult blood testing.) However, some authorities do not support routine sigmoidoscopy or stool screening tests unless the client has a personal or family history that suggests higher-than-average risk (Goldbloom et al., 1993). Maule (1994) found that specially trained nurses can perform screening flexible sigmoidoscopy as accurately and as safely as physicians. Thus widespread screening may become less expensive and more readily available as preventive health care than it is now.

▼ PRETEST NURSING IMPLICATIONS RELATED TO SIGMOIDOSCOPY

Clients should continue to take all their routine medications except iron pills, bismuth subsalicylate (Pepto-Bismol), or bulk-forming laxatives, all of which should be discontinued for 3 days. Regular meals may be taken until 2 hours before the examination. Two sodium phosphate/biphosphate (Fleet) enemas are given 2 hours before the exam-ination. Because this procedure is usually performed on an outpatient basis, the client needs to be clear on how to obtain and administer the ready-to-use enema sets. No sedation is used, so the clients needs to be prepared on how to relax during the procedure.

▼ POSTTEST NURSING IMPLICATIONS RELATED TO SIGMOIDOSCOPY

Clients may drive home after this procedure. The client may have some mild abdominal cramping because of the air instilled for the test, and air may continue to be expelled for several hours.

▼ COLONOSCOPY AND ENTEROSCOPY

Description and Purposes. These procedures use flexible fiberscopes to view the upper colon and small intestine. Some enteroscopes are 9 feet (270 cm) long and are passed nasally (Lewis and Waye, 1988). See the discussion of oral insertions. For colonoscopy, a scope inserted through the rectum provides access to the lower GI tract. Colonoscopy may last from 20 min to more than 1 hr depending on the tortuosity of the intestine and the procedures performed. The client lies on the left side as the scope is inserted in the rectum, but later may need to lie prone with the right knee flexed. Introduction of air into the colon, to help distend the intestine and aid visualization, causes some pressure and cramping. The discomfort tends to be more intense as the coloscope is maneuvered through the curves in the colon. Conscious sedation makes the procedure tolerable. Atropine or glucagon may be given to decrease peristalsis. Atropine may also be used for the bradycardia that may occur from the vagal effect of stimulating the colon.

Colonoscopy is useful for diagnosing inflammatory bowel disease without a complex abdominal operation. Also, polyps can be removed and biopsies performed. If electrocautery is used, the client needs to be prepared for the cold, sticky ground pad used with the monopolar cautery (Renkes, 1993).

▼ PRETEST NURSING IMPLICATIONS RELATED TO COLONOSCOPY

In addition to the general nursing implications for endoscopic procedures, attention must be given to ensuring a thorough cleansing of the intestine so

(*continued*)

▼ PRETEST NURSING IMPLICATIONS RELATED TO COLONOSCOPY (*continued*)

that fecal matter does not obscure viewing. In the past, intestinal preparation included 2 days of clear liquids, in combination with cathartics and enemas. Now intestinal preparation is usually completed with a balanced electrolyte solution in a polyethylene glycol base. Because electrolyte lavage is expensive and some clients may not comply with taking the large volumes needed, oral sodium phosphate may be better tolerated and more effective (Kolts et al., 1993). Whatever the type of intestinal preparation the nurse needs to make sure the client understands the importance of a thorough intestinal cleaning. (See Chapter 20 for more detailed discussion of intestinal preparation and the procedure for GI irrigation.)

▼ POSTTEST NURSING DIAGNOSIS RELATED TO COLONOSCOPY

Altered Comfort Related to Flatus

The client has abdominal cramps after the procedure because of the air injected during the examination. A rectal tube may be used, depending on the site of treatment (Zettel, 1986). Changing positions or walking, if permissible, can also relieve gas pains. (See the beginning of this chapter for other concerns such as bleeding or perforation.)

▼ CYSTOSCOPY AND URETEROSCOPY

Description and Purposes. A cystoscope is passed through the urethra into the bladder so the interior of the bladder can be examined for inflammation, tumors, stones, or structural abnormalities. For some diagnostic studies, such as for interstitial cystitis, it is necessary that the bladder be distended during examination to assess for changes in the mucosal lining of the bladder. Small stones may be removed with the scope. Ureteral catheters may be passed into each ureter to obtain samples of urine from the pelvis of each kidney. A radiopaque dye (Chapter 20) may be injected for a retrograde pyelogram. Cystoscopy can be performed with topical anesthesia, but more extensive procedures require the use of general or spinal anesthesia. The topical anesthetic is in jelly form and is put into the urethra. Ureteroscopy may be used in conjunction with ultrasound (Chapter 23) to remove stones (Stone, 1988).

▼ PRETEST NURSING IMPLICATIONS RELATED TO CYSTOSCOPY

Routine preparations are performed in relation to procedures such as consent forms, vital sign checks, and laboratory work. If the client is to undergo general anesthesia, he or she should be instructed on routine deep breathing and other routines for recovery from general anesthesia. The client is allowed a full liquid diet if the procedure is to be performed with local anesthesia. Administration of prophylactic antibacterial agents may be started.

▼ POSTTEST NURSING DIAGNOSES RELATED TO CYSTOSCOPY

Risk for Bleeding

The standard vital sign routine is followed. Some hematuria is not uncommon, but the client should be carefully watched for hemorrhage if a biopsy was performed. The client may maintain bed rest for up to 4 hr. If the procedure was performed in a urology clinic, the client and the client's family should be instructed on these routine assessments and other pertinent aftercare.

Risk for Urinary Retention

The client's intake and output should be monitored for at least 24 hr. Adult clients should have an intake of 2,500–3,000 mL, unless contraindicated. If the client does not have a Foley catheter, the nurse must check for the possibility of urinary retention with overflow. Small amounts of urine, 50–100 mL frequently, may be a sign of urinary retention with overflow. Cholinergic drugs, such as bethanechol chloride (Urecholine), may be needed to stimulate bladder contraction. If the client has a Foley catheter, the catheter must be kept connected to a sterile drainage system.

The client may have a ureteral catheter. These catheters are very tiny and are usually fastened on a splint. It is important that there not be any tension on the catheter or any kinking. Nurses do not routinely irrigate ureteral catheters. If the catheter is to be irrigated, only a few cubic centimeters of sterile normal saline solution are used because the renal pelvis holds only about 5 mL of urine. Because the renal pelvis does not have room for much collection of urine, it is important that the physician be notified if a ureteral catheter is not draining properly.

(*continued*)

▼ POSTTEST NURSING DIAGNOSES RELATED TO CYSTOSCOPY (*continued*)

Risk for Infection

Clients are sometimes given antibacterial agents after cystoscopy because of the high risk for urinary tract infections from the instrumentation. Any break in the tissue of the bladder may let bacteria into the bloodstream; consequently, the client may have chills and fever from transient bacteremia. This transient bacteremia may be dangerous for clients with mitral valve disease because bacterial endocarditis can occur. The client should be instructed about the signs of urinary tract infection, such as burning on urination or cloudy, foul-smelling urine. Some burning after urination is expected the first day after instrumentation. A urinalysis is usually performed as a posttest procedure. (See Chapter 3 for interpretation of routine urinalysis and Chapter 16 for culture and sensitivity tests.)

Altered Comfort Related to Bladder Spasms

The client may have some pain when urinating (dysuria) and bladder spasms. Sometimes antispasmodic drugs, such as oxybutynin (Ditropan) are given for bladder spasms. Mild analgesics may also be needed, such as phenazopyridine (Pyridium). If permitted, warm tub baths may be soothing. Clients with interstitial cystitis may need instructions on foods and drugs that irritate the bladder wall.

▼ LAPAROSCOPY

Description and Purposes. An instrument can be used to inspect the pelvic viscera. If the instrument is inserted into the abdomen through a small incision in the lower abdominal wall, the procedure is called *laparoscopy*. Carbon dioxide is instilled into the peritoneal cavity to distend the abdomen so that visualization is easier. A laparoscopic examination is sometimes performed to help diagnose infertility (Chapter 28). Operations performed with a laparoscope are sometimes called "Band-Aid" operations, because the incision, only 1–2 cm long, requires only a small dressing.

Most laparoscopic procedures are performed with the aid of general anesthesia, but some procedures on selected clients can be performed with local anesthesia combined with intravenous conscious sedation. When local anesthesia is used the client may be discharged 1 hr after the procedure (DeCherney and Pernoll, 1994). Even complex operations such as removal of the gallbladder are performed with a laparoscope. This has revolutionized the postoperative care of clients with cholelithiasis (Gholson et al., 1994). Clients have a shorter hospital stay than when a laparotomy is performed.

▼ NURSING IMPLICATIONS RELATED TO LAPAROSCOPY

If a laparoscopy is performed under light, general anesthesia, the client needs routine preoperative preparation. A Foley catheter is inserted to keep the bladder deflated. Aftercare is the standard care discussed at the beginning of this chapter.

Gas injected into the abdominal cavity during laparoscopy can irritate the diaphragm and cause referred pain in the shoulder area. Clients can be assured the pain disappears in 1–2 days. Mild analgesics may be needed.

▼ ARTHROSCOPY

Description and Purposes. An arthroscope is a fiberoptic endoscope used to examine the interior of joints. Although other joints can be visualized, the most common arthroscopic procedure involves the knee joint. Arthroscopy of the interior of the knee joint can reveal injuries to the meniscus as well as other abnormalities. Normal saline solution is used to flush the knee and to remove loose objects and allow easier scope management. Simple surgical repairs can be performed with the use of an arthroscope. General anesthesia is used if surgical repair is anticipated or if the client has a great deal of pain. Arthroscopy is another "Band-Aid" operation made possible with fiber-optic endoscopes and microscopic surgical instruments.

▼ NURSING IMPLICATIONS RELATED TO ARTHROSCOPY

Pre- and postprocedure care depends on whether the client undergoes local or general anesthesia. Nursing diagnoses discussed at the beginning of this chapter are pertinent. In addition, the nurse should assess for any possible infection, which can be serious in a joint. The risk for infection may be increased by the use of intraoperative intraarticular corticosteroids (Armstrong and Bolding, 1994). Some clients may be given prophylactic antibiotics when joints are entered to prevent osteomyelitis. Ice bags may be used to reduce postprocedure swelling. Any limitations on weight bearing are related to the procedure performed. (See Chapter 20 on arthrograms, which may be obtained with an arthroscope.)

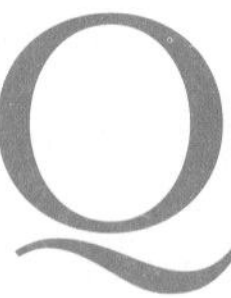

1. Which of the following is *not* a potential complication for clients undergoing endoscopic procedures?

   a. Shock caused by perforation of a body organ
   b. Hemorrhage caused by bleeding from a biopsy site
   c. Oversedation related to the use of sedatives before or during the procedure
   d. Burns from the light on the end of the instrument

2. Which of the following nursing actions is more important in preparing a client for bronchoscopy than for other types of endoscopic procedures?

   a. Obtaining informed consent
   b. Emphasizing oral hygiene
   c. Preparing the client for discomfort and the effects of conscious sedation
   d. Demonstrating the use of a nose clip to ensure mouth breathing

3. When a client has had an anesthetic sprayed on the throat, the assessment that determines the client can have fluids is

   a. Ability to swallow without discomfort
   b. Presence of gag reflex when a tongue blade touches the back of throat
   c. Absence of nausea or abdominal distention
   d. Presence of active bowel sounds

4. Clients should be taught that the usual recommendation for routine sigmoidoscopies for adults without symptoms is

   a. Annually for all people older than 40 years
   b. Annually for all people older than 50 years
   c. Every 3–5 years after 40 years of age
   d. Every 3–5 years after 50 years of age

5. Standard nursing care after general anesthesia is most often necessary for a client undergoing

   a. Laparoscopy b. Enteroscopy
   c. Gastroscopy d. Sigmoidoscopy

6. An *inappropriate* nursing intervention after a client has undergone cystoscopy under local anesthesia is

   a. Recording input and output for at least 24 hr
   b. Checking for urinary retention with overflow

c. Keeping the client on nothing-by-mouth status for 4–6 hr after the procedure
d. Assessing for bladder spasms and giving ordered analgesics as needed

▼ REFERENCES

Armstrong, R.W., and Bolding, F. (1994). Septic arthritis after arthroscopy: The contributing roles of intraarticular steroids and environmental factors. *American Journal of Infection Control, 22,* 16–18.

Bongard, F.S., and Sue, D.Y. (1994). *Current critical care diagnosis & treatment.* Norwalk, CT: Appleton & Lange.

Chokhavatia, S., Nguyen, L., Williams, R., et al. (1993). Sedation and analgesia for gastrointestinal endoscopy. *American Journal of Gastroenterology, 88* (3), 393–396.

Day, S. (1990). Cancer screening in the elderly. *Hospital Practice, 25* (9A), 13–25.

DeCherney, A.H., and Pernoll, M.L. (1994). *Current obstetric & gynecologic diagnosis & treatment* (8th ed.). Norwalk, CT: Appleton & Lange.

Deglin, J.H., and Vallerand, A.H. (1995). *Davis's drug guide for nurses* (4th ed.). Philadelphia: FA Davis.

Freeman, D. (1986). Lasers in the OR. *American Journal of Nursing, 86* (3), 278–282.

Gholson, C.F., Sittig, K., and McDonald, J.C. (1994). Recent advances in the management of gallstones. *American Journal of Medical Science, 307* (4), 293–304.

Goldbloom, R., Oboler, S., and Sox, H.C. (1993). Periodic health evaluation. *Patient Care, 27*(4), 14–28.

Hirschowitz, B. (1979). A personal history of the fiberscope. *Gastroenterology, 76,* 864–869.

Johnson, J., and Rice, V. (1974). Sensory and distress components of pain: Implications for study of clinical pain. *Nursing Research, 23,* 203–209.

Kolts, B.E., Lyles, W.E., Achem, S.R., et al. (1993). A comparison of the effectiveness and patient tolerance of oral sodium phosphate, castor oil, and standard electrolyte lavage for colonoscopy or sigmoidoscopy preparation. *American Journal of Gastroenterology, 88* (8), 1218–1223.

Lewis, B., and Waye, J. (1988). Chronic gastrointestinal bleeding of obscure origin: Role of small bowel enteroscopy. *Gastroenterology, 94,* 1117–1120.

Maule, W.F. (1994). Screening for colorectal cancer by nurse endoscopists. *New England Journal of Medicine, 330* (3), 183–187.

McHugh, N., Christman, N.J., and Johnson, J.E. (1982). Preparatory information: What helps and why. *American Journal of Nursing, 82* (5), 780–782.

Moulton-Barrett, R., Triadafilopoulos, G., Michener, R., et al. (1993). Serum C-bicarbonate in the assessment of gastric *Helicobacter pylori* urease activity. *American Journal of Gastroenterology, 88* (3), 369–374.

Peternel, E. (1985). A high-tech approach to a GI problem. *RN, 48* (6), 44–47.

Renkes, J. (1993). GI endoscopy: Managing the full scope of care. *Nursing 93, 23* (6), 50–55.

Sable, R., Rosenthal, W.S., and Siegel, W. (1983). Absorption of contrast medium during ERCP. *Digestive Diseases and Science, 28,* 801–806.

Stone, L. (1988). Ureteroscopy: Treatment for distal ureteral stone. *Ethicon: Point of View, 25* (3), 16–17.

Thompson, L. (1995). Percutaneous endoscopic gastrostomy. *Nursing 95, 25* (4), 62–63.

Zettel, E. (1986). Beaming in on the G.I. tract. *American Journal of Nursing, 86* (3), 280–282.

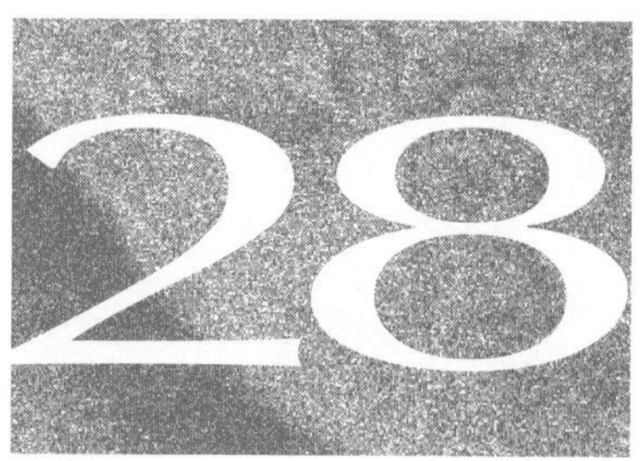

DIAGNOSTIC PROCEDURES RELATED TO CHILDBEARING YEARS

- Basal Body Temperature
- Ovulation Tests
- Semen Analysis
- Postcoital Examination: Sims–Huhner Test (Huhner Test)
- Tubal Patency Tests, Hysterosalpingogram, and Tubal Insufflation (Rubin's Test)
- Amniocentesis: Amniocentesis for Prenatal Diagnosis of Genetic Defects: Three Assessments, Amniocentesis in Isoimmune Disease (Rh Factor), and Amniocentesis for Assessing Fetal Maturity
- Chorionic Villus Sampling
- Percutaneous Umbilical Blood Sampling and Fetal Biopsy
- Fetal Monitoring Nonstress Test
- Contraction Challenge Test

OBJECTIVES

1. Identify appropriate nursing diagnoses for clients undergoing tests related to reproduction.
2. Explain client instruction needed for each of the five basic fertility tests.
3. Describe basic facts about amniocentesis and chorionic villus sampling (CVS) biopsy that are helpful in planning nursing care for a couple in which the woman is to undergo a procedure for prenatal genetic diagnosis.

4. Name some common genetic diseases that are detected with three types of tests of amniotic fluid or CVS.
5. Explain the therapeutic value of amniocentesis in assessment of isoimmune disease (Rh factor).
6. Explain the clinical significance of determining lecithin-to-sphingomyelin ratio (L/S ratio) and creatinine levels in amniotic fluid.
7. Describe the routine preparation, including client teaching, for a client who is to undergo amniocentesis in the last trimester.
8. Compare and contrast the contraction stress test (CST) and the nonstress test for antepartum monitoring.

Even a nurse who is not a specialist in maternal–child health nursing may at times be called on to assist with diagnostic procedures commonly performed during the childbearing years. The intent of this chapter is to give the reader an overview of the diagnostic procedures used to assess the ability to conceive or to carry a fetus to term. The chapter begins with the basic tests of fertility because the inability to become pregnant is a common problem. The technique of CVS for prenatal diagnosis is discussed and compared with early amniocentesis. Amniocentesis is discussed in regard to tests for chromosome defects, inborn errors of metabolism, and neural tube defects. Two other uses of amniocentesis, evaluation of the severity of hemolysis from the Rh factor and assessment of fetal maturity, are explained. Basic information about fetal monitoring is presented at the end of the chapter.

▼ GENERAL NURSING DIAGNOSES RELATED TO FERTILITY AND PRENATAL TESTING

Family Coping: Potential for Growth

During the childbearing years, many couples suffer disappointments because of the inability to have the longed-for "perfect" child. For many years, nurses have become involved in helping families deal with unexpected or crisis situations. Leavitt (1982) described the impact of nurses who provide primary preventive care to families who are at high risk. Nurses who contract with couples for follow-up visits after a family crisis can help strengthen the adaptive capability of a family. The key point is for the nurse to focus on the family as a unit. Whether it is the crisis of infertility, an unhappy report from amniocentesis, or the stress of fetal monitoring, a professional nurse can be instrumental in helping the family cope and even grow from the experience.

Anxiety Related to Test Procedures and Effect on Self-concept

The nurse's sensitivity to the needs of clients undergoing diagnostic tests is important for short-term care as well as for follow-up care. For example, when clients are connected to monitors or undergoing technical procedures, they may begin to feel depersonalized. However, in one study of 50 mothers who had been monitored during labor, none found the monitor depersonalizing. The investigators found that the nurses did not walk in the room and look at the monitor first—a tendency when machines are being used. Rather, the nurse first spoke with the woman and asked her how she was doing. After the personal interaction and after feeling the woman's contractions, the nurse correlated the clinical findings with the readouts from the monitors (McDonough et al., 1981). Sandelowski (1993) presented a preliminary conceptual framework for nursing research on technology dependency and warned that nurses must counter the magnetic quality of monitors that tends to draw attention to the machines and away from clients. As more and more diagnostic procedures are used to assess the natural events of childbearing, the nurse can continue to supply the essential human element of caring. (See Chapter 25 for discussion of relieving anxiety about diagnostic procedures.)

FERTILITY TESTING

A growing number of couples in the United States seek medical help for **infertility**. Three possible reasons for an increased focus on infertility tests are (1) the diminished number of children available for adoption because of legalized abortion; (2) a rising incidence of sexually transmitted diseases, which can cause pelvic inflammatory disease (PID) and sterility; and (3) the fact that more women are opting to delay pregnancy until after 30 years of age, when reproduction may not be easy.

Infertility is defined as the inability of a couple to achieve pregnancy after 1 year of unprotected intercourse. Estimates suggest that as many as one in five or six couples may seek help for infertility (Blackwell, 1989; Beastall, 1993). For some couples, such circumstances as past PID, suspected hormone imbalances, or other physical problems indicate sterility may be a problem. If there are no obvious reasons why a couple should not be able to conceive, fertility tests are not advocated until after a year of unprotected intercourse. For women older than 35 years, tests may be conducted sooner than a year. A nurse can reassure a couple who seems healthy that not becoming pregnant after only a few months is not an indication to seek medical help too quickly.

For couples who have tried for much longer than 1 year to conceive, the decision to begin fertility testing may be difficult. The tests may be expensive. They are an invasion into an area that is usually very private. And beginning the tests is, in a way, an acknowledgment of failure to do something that is thought of as being natural. Clients may discuss with nurses the frustration in not being able to become pregnant. The nurse can assess if the couple needs a referral for fertility testing. The nurse can emphasize that infertility may be caused by a problem with the man, woman, or both; therefore, both people need to be tested once the couple have decided they need help. Some basic tests for fertility are summarized in Table 28–1.

TABLE 28–1. EXAMPLES OF BASIC TESTS FOR INFERTILITY

Test	Purpose
Basal body temperature recordings and LH ovulation test kits	Presumptive evidence of ovulation
Semen analysis	Assessment of number and characteristics of sperm in one ejaculation
Hormone analysis	Assessment of hormonal imbalances, which may be primary or secondary hypofunction (Chap. 15). Some physicians use endometrial biopsy (Chap. 25)
Postcoital examination (Sims–Huhner)	Assessment of mobility and number of sperm in cervical mucus after intercourse and of characteristics of mucus at time of ovulation
Hysterosalpingogram	Assessment of tubal patency and any structural defects in uterus or tubes (Rubin's test tests only tubal patency). (See Chap. 20 on hysterosalpingogram).

See text for explanation of these and other tests and client teaching.
LH, luteinizing hormone.

▼ BASAL BODY TEMPERATURE

The term *basal* refers to the lowest possible level of a physiologic measurement (i.e., baseline). The basal body temperature (BBT) is taken early in the morning before the woman gets out of bed. Because this test requires only a thermometer and a graphic chart, women may perform this test before they seek medical advice. There are special BBT or ovulation thermometers that are measured in tenths of degrees rather than the two-tenths on conventional thermometers. An electronic thermometer linked to a microcomputer also can be purchased. If the woman can determine her ovulatory pattern, the couple can plan intercourse to take advantage of her fertile period. (Using a temperature chart to avoid conception is not always reliable because the change in temperature occurs with ovulation, not before.)

In women who have a normal menstrual cycle, BBT is usually less than 98°F (36.7°C) in the preovulatory phase. Before ovulation occurs, an increasing production of estrogen may cause a slight downward trend in BBT. Then with ovulation, progesterone is secreted by the corpus luteum. Progesterone affects the hypothalamus, so there is up to a 1°F (0.37°C) rise in BBT. The increase in temperature at ovulation usually makes the woman's basal temperature greater than 98°F (36.7°C). If the woman keeps an accurate graphic recording for a few months, a physician can interpret the charts and determine if there is presumptive evidence that ovulation is occurring. The client needs to record on the chart any colds or infections, which would disrupt the normal temperature pattern.

Preparation of Client for BBT Recordings

The client should be instructed on exactly when to take the temperatures and how to record them on the graph. (Nurses seem to forget that shaking down a thermometer, reading the results in tenths, and plotting the number on a graph are skills that may need to be learned.) The woman should be given the chance to practice any of the necessary skills of which she is unsure. Each morning as soon as she awakens, the client should take and record her temperature. The woman should be instructed to take the temperature before she goes to the bathroom or performs any physical activity, including sex. Oral temperatures are usually sufficient. The client is given a special chart to record the temperatures, which is brought back to the physician's office or infertility clinic for analysis. The newer electronic thermometers keep a daily record.

▼ OVULATION TESTS

In the past few years, simple home ovulation test kits have been available for over-the-counter purchase. These self-test kits measure the surge of luteinizing hormone (LH) that appears in the urine 12–36 hr *before* ovulation. The ovulation tests are useful as a beginning assessment for infertility in women. (See Chapter 15 on LH levels.) For a woman who wishes to avoid pregnancy, Fehring (1990) noted that self-observation of cervical mucous after teaching by a qualified natural family planner may be as helpful and less expensive than the commercial kits. However, the kits can be used to avoid intercourse during the time of ovulation or to plan intercourse to enhance fertility. These tests, based on monoclonal technology, are quite specific and sensitive.

Preparation of Client and Collection of Sample

The various commercial test kits for LH in the urine contain written information on how to conduct the test and all the needed equipment. Some tests require droppers or vials, and some require only a stick that can be held in the stream of urine. Toll-free numbers are included with most of the test kits if the client needs more information.

Clients can begin a daily test a few days after the end of the menses. Some kits contain enough supplies to test the urine for up to 10 days each month. The first voided urine specimen in the morning is ideal because the urine is concentrated. When the surge of LH appears in the urine, a positive test results in a sharp color change.

Urine samples may be brought to a clinical laboratory for measurement of pregnanediol, a urinary metabolite of progesterone (Chapter 15). Sonograms may be obtained daily to validate ovulation (Chapter 23). A substantial number of women do not demonstrate sonographic evidence of ovulation until the second morning after detection of the urine LH surge (Pearlstone and Surrey, 1994).

▼ SEMEN ANALYSIS

An investigation of semen is the most important initial diagnostic study for infertility in men. If the analysis seems normal, more intensive investigation of the woman's fertility is in order. In the laboratory, a sperm count is performed, as is an examination of the form of the sperm, its mobility, and the amount and characteristics of the semen. If any abnormalities are detected, or if the count is low, a second specimen is examined because there are variations with each ejaculation. Semen analysis is performed after a vasectomy to determine that the operation has been successful.

Preparation of Client and Collection of Sample

The client needs specific instructions on how to collect the specimen. Semen is collected after 2 or more days of sexual abstinence. The client may be given privacy in a bathroom to collect the specimen in a jar by means of masturbation. This is a highly intimate matter and may cause tension and anxiety in the man. Some men, for psychological or religious reasons, prefer to collect semen at home by using a condom during intercourse. The condom should not contain lubricants or substances that may interfere with the analysis. The client may be given a plastic sheath to use as the condom. (Religious practices may necessitate a small puncture in the sheath.) All the semen is put into a clean jar and kept at room temperature. It must be sent to the laboratory within 1–2 hr after ejaculation.

REFERENCE VALUES FOR SEMEN ANALYSIS

Color	Grayish white
pH	7.3–7.8
Volume	2.0–5.0 mL
Sperm count	20–250 million/mL
Motility	>60%
Normal sperm	>60%
Viscosity	Can be poured from pipette in droplets rather than a thick strand

Reference for semen analysis is from Ravel (1995). Note that sperm penetration assay (hamster test) is performed in vitro to assess if sperm are able to penetrate ova from hamsters (DeCherney and Pernoll, 1994).

▼ POSTCOITAL EXAMINATION: SIMS–HUHNER TEST (HUHNER TEST)

The Sims–Huhner test is an examination of the number and motility of the sperm found in the cervical mucous of a woman after intercourse. The test is performed 1–2 days before expected ovulation because an increased secretion of estrogen causes characteristic changes in the mucous. Estrogen increases the elasticity and sodium content of the cervical mucous. The elasticity of the mucous is called *spinnbarkeit.* Normally, these mucous changes enhance sperm survival. (Learning the mucous changes for ovulation is the basis for a form of contraception [Fehring, 1990].) *Ferning* refers to the pattern produced when cervical mucous dries under the influence of estrogen. Postcoital examination of the mucous and the sperm can help determine if an immunologic or hormonal problem is contributing to the infertility. Some authorities do not use postcoital testing as part of the basic evaluation but may use it to evaluate the effect of clomiphene, a fertility drug, on the cervical mucous (Blackwell, 1989).

Preparation of Client and Collection of Sample

The test is planned for 1–2 days before the woman's expected time of ovulation. The couple has intercourse, and the woman then goes to the clinic or office for a pelvic examination. The woman may be told to stay in bed for about half an hour after intercourse. The sample of cervical mucous must be obtained 2–4 hr after intercourse. The couple should not use any lubricants, and the woman should not douche. These instructions may seem obvious, but the health professional must make sure that the client understands the test.

REFERENCE VALUES FOR SIMS–HUHNER TEST

The microscopic examination shows the quality of the mucous, including the pattern it makes on a slide. Patterns such as ferning are considered normal. The number and motility of the sperm are observed. Ten or more sperm per high-power field is considered a normal count.

▼ TUBAL PATENCY TESTS, HYSTEROSALPINGOGRAM, AND TUBAL INSUFFLATION (RUBIN'S TEST)

The tubes can be insufflated with carbon dioxide (Rubin's test) or radiopaque dye (hysterosalpingogram) to see if the tubes are patent. Instillation of carbon dioxide can be performed in the physician's office, but it does not give the detailed information a study with dye does. A hysterosalpingogram is useful for identifying any structural defects in the uterus or tubes. A hysterosalpingogram is obtained in the radiology department. (See Chapter 20 for the discussion of nursing implications related to a hysterosalpingogram.)

A hysterosalpingogram or Rubin's test may have a therapeutic effect because it breaks up adhesions in a tube or removes debris that may have been blocking the tube.

MEASUREMENT OF HORMONES

The levels of follicle-stimulating hormone (FSH) and LH, as well as testosterone, progesterone, and estrogen, may be assessed with laboratory tests to determine normal hormonal balance in both the man and the woman. (See Chapter 15 for detailed information.) Some physicians prefer an endometrial biopsy to determine the quantity of progesterone rather than serum levels of the hormone. Others consider an endometrial biopsy part of a second phase. An endometrial biopsy can be performed as part of a cervical examination (Chapter 25).

OTHER FERTILITY TESTS AND TREATMENT OPTIONS

Laboratory tests may or may not be sufficient to identify the cause of infertility. Depending on the results of the basic tests, the physician may order other procedures, such as laparoscopy, to examine the female reproductive organs in more detail (Chapter 27). Surgical reconstruction may be needed. For women who are not ovulating, medications may be prescribed by the physician. The nurse's role depends on the particular treatments tried.

Since the first "test-tube" baby in 1978, many other options have become possible, including implantation of ova from other women into women who are postmenopausal (Sauer et al., 1990). A survey of client's perceptions of infertility treatment indicated that although technologic advances have allowed for more definitive diagnoses and increased changes in conception, the rigorous and sometimes experimental treatment, the long duration and expense of treatment, and the need to make complex decisions about termination of treatment are all stressful. Professional competency, sensitivity, and environmental comfort can mediate the stress (Blenner, 1992).

▼ NURSING DIAGNOSES RELATED TO FERTILITY TESTS

Risk for Ineffective Coping Related to Inability to Conceive

Although treatment can help many infertile clients, the success rate for all infertility clients, irrespective of the cause of infertility, is approximately 50% at most centers. The final pronouncement that it is highly unlikely that a couple can have a child by the usual biologic means is difficult for many couples to accept. Adoption may or may not be the answer for a couple. Couples may benefit from talking to other couples who have been unable to conceive. There are various support groups for infertile couples. The nurse can find out if there is a support group in an area. Resolve, Inc., is a nationwide organization that serves the needs of the infertile population. A person who has an infertility problem may feel guilt over the perceived inadequacy. If the couple does not remain a couple, the person may have problems explaining the infertility to a new partner.

Anticipatory Grieving Related to Loss of a Desired Goal

The loss of a child, either real or desired, does cause a period of grieving. Wong (1980) wrote about the empty-mother syndrome. Although Wong's work was with mothers who lost children after a long illness, the four interventions she used to help resolve grief may be applied to several situations discussed in this chapter, including infertility, the birth of a child with a defect, or the termination of a pregnancy. Interventions to help relieve grief can include (1) preparing the couple for anticipating *normal* feelings of emptiness, loneliness, and failure; (2) helping the couple reevaluate their roles in a childless family (or in a family that does not have the perfect or longed-for child); (3) encouraging the couple to explore fulfilling activities that use their special talents and abilities; and (4) supporting the couple by helping them communicate with each other and with other family members who have been affected by the loss of a child (Wong, 1980). For example, potential grandparents can feel hurt by the lack of a grandchild, so they need help to express their feelings of loss. The meaning of the loss is individualized and varies from situation to situation. Devore and Baldwin (1986) gave excellent guidelines for counseling clients who have lost a fetus because of an ectopic pregnancy, and Sherrod (1988) and Blenner (1990) gave examples of the role of nurses in helping couples deal with infertility.

SCREENING TESTS PERFORMED DURING PREGNANCY

The introduction of oral contraceptives gave women more control over the decision of when or whether to have a child. Also, as women's roles change, more women are opting to have children at a later age—for example, after a career is established. Many years ago, in *McCall's* magazine, the question, "How old is too old to have a baby?" was answered with a quotation from a physician who said, "When you quit menstruating" (Pines, 1980). With the advent of ova donations to postmenopausal women, Angell (1990) noted the determination of how old is too old to have a baby may be related to stamina (labor and 2 AM feedings) rather than reproductive function. The use of amniocentesis and CVS has increased the probability of healthy normal babies for what used to be called elderly (older than 35 years) primigravidas. These two screening techniques have made it possible for couples who may be at high risk for genetic defects to undergo a pregnancy knowing that some defects can be detected with laboratory testing. Nurses need to be aware of some of the basic tests genetic counseling can offer prospective parents because people often ask nurses for referrals and information on new trends in health care. Genetic counseling is recommended (1) for women older than 35 years of age, (2) for couples who already have one child with a genetic defect, (3) for couples with a family history of genetic defects, (4) as a positive serum-marker test for neural tube defects and for Down syndrome (see Chapter 18 for AFP, serum estriol and HCG maternal blood tests), and (5) for women taking anticonvulsant medication (Chapter 17). To avoid arbitrariness and discrimination on the basis of maternal age, some clinicians explain the risks and benefits of amniocentesis to pregnant women of all ages (Pauker and Pauker, 1994).

▼ AMNIOCENTESIS

Purposes. Amniocentesis is the removal of some amniotic fluid for diagnostic purposes. The three most important reasons for amniocentesis for diagnostic purposes include (1) prenatal detection of genetic disorders, (2) follow-up and possible treatment of isoimmune disease due to the Rh factor, and (3) assessment of fetal maturity. Table 28–2 provides a summary of the different purposes of amniocentesis.

Amniocentesis for Prenatal Diagnosis of Genetic Defects: Three Assessments

Karyotyping for Chromosome Study

A variety of diseases can be detected through a study of the cells and chemicals in the amniotic fluid. Identification of the chromosomes is called *karyotyping*. Karyotyping of chromosomes is a pattern of the 22 pairs of autosomal chromosomes and

TABLE 28–2. THREE PURPOSES OF AMNIOCENTESIS

Purposes	Timing	Results	Usual Follow-Up
1. Assessment of genetic defects a. Karyotyping of chromosomes	15th–18th week of gestation (Some centers may perform test earlier)[a]	Can identify Down syndrome and other chromosomal abnormalities	Takes 10–14 days to obtain all results Couple may opt for abortion if serious genetic defect found
b. Biochemical defects		>60 defects can be identified	
c. α-Fetoprotein levels		May indicate improper closure of neural tube	
2. Assessment of isoimmune disease (Rh factor)	After 24–25 weeks of gestation	Level of bilirubin in amniotic fluid indicates severity of hemolysis	Increasing levels of bilirubin may indicate need for intrauterine transfusions or induced labor
3. Assessment of fetal maturity a. Lecithin-to-sphingomyelin ratio	Near end of gestation	Ratio of 2:1 is usually evidence of lung maturity	Labor may be induced if tests indicate mature fetus
b. Creatinine levels		Level of 2 mg/dL is evidence of maturity of kidneys	
c. Staining of fat cells		Evaluate fetal maturity with fat cells	

See text for discussion on CVS, which is also performed to assess for genetic defects but does not detect neural tube defects.
[a]See text on advantages of early (before 15 weeks) amniocentesis.

one pair of sex chromosomes: XX of the woman or the XY of the man. All the severe chromosomal abnormalities can be detected with fetal karyotyping. Trisomy of chromosome 21 (Down syndrome) is the most common abnormality found and the most common genetic birth defect.

If there is a possibility of a sex-linked defect such as hemophilia, the sex of the fetus may be important. Some diseases, such as hemophilia, are linked to the X chromosome; therefore, if the fetus is a girl, there is little if any possibility of the disease. The hemophilia trait is transmitted by women and occurs in males. A woman must have two defective X chromosomes, which is a rare possibility. Although the sex of the fetus is always identified with a chromosomal study, the parents may prefer to not know the results unless there is a possibility of a sex-linked disease. Centers inform the prospective parents that they can learn the sex if they so desire.

Biochemical Defects

Numerous enzymes or biochemical abnormalities can be detected with amniocentesis as research finds more and more gene markers for diseases such as Huntington's chorea and muscular dystrophy. Some of the metabolic diseases tested for are galactosemia, maple syrup urine disease, Gaucher's disease, and Tay–Sachs disease. Some of these diseases are tested for only if it is known that both parents are carriers. For example, Tay–Sachs disease can be detected in the carrier state in parents, and because the disease is caused by a recessive gene, both parents must be carriers for the fetus to be at risk. (See Chapter 18 for laboratory tests of carrier states for biochemical defects and the impact of mass screening.)

α-Fetoprotein Levels to Detect Neural Tube Defects

α-Fetoprotein (AFP) is manufactured by the fetal liver. Normally, there is a low level of this protein in the amniotic fluid, but if the neural tube does not close properly, large amounts of AFP leak into the amniotic fluid. If the neural tube does not close at the top, a normal brain does not develop (anencephaly). If the defect in the neural tube is lower, the fetus has spina bifida. A meningocele or myelomeningocele may be associated with spina bifida. The more involvement of the spinal cord, the more severe is the handicap. The child may be paralyzed from the waist down and lack bowel and bladder control, or the damage may be slight and amenable to therapy. Severe omphalocele (protrusion of intestines) or congenital nephrosis can also cause increased levels of AFP. If the amniotic fluid is contaminated with fetal blood, the AFP level may be falsely high because the protein level is normally high in the blood. Thus a test of fetal hemoglobin (hgb) can be performed to rule out this artifact.

High levels of AFP in pregnant women do not always indicate a problem with neural tube defects because there may be an incorrect estimation of fetal age, twins, or other reasons for an increase, which are not well understood. Still, even with these disadvantages, AFP blood screening must by law be offered to pregnant women in some states in the United States (Chapter 18). If the AFP blood-screening level is elevated, a repeat test is performed. If the test is positive on a second blood sample, the woman undergoes ultrasonography (Chapter 23) and amniocentesis. (See Chapter 2 for the role of folic acid in decreasing the risk of neural tube defects. See Chapter 18 for a discussion of the use of serum AFP with other tests for screening for Down syndrome.)

Counseling Before Amniocentesis for Prenatal Diagnosis. Although the technical preparation of the client for amniocentesis is simple, the psychological care of the client may be complex. If amniocentesis is being performed for genetic counseling, the ultimate question is "what action will be taken if an abnormality is found?" Counseling is initiated before amniocentesis to help the couple fully understand the ramifications of the test so they can make an informed decision.

Although amniocentesis is considered to have little risk for the mother and less than 1% risk for the fetus, the couple must be aware of the possibility of damage to or death of the fetus. The physician in a particular center or a genetic counselor, who may be a nurse or other health professional, can explain the statistics of a particular center.

Although a couple may not want to terminate a pregnancy if the results show a defect, they may desire the amniocentesis to better plan for the birth of a child with a defect. The nurse who works in a setting where amniocentesis is performed must be aware of the difficult decisions couples must make about whether the findings from an amniocentesis are reason for an abortion. Pressures from family and friends, and society in general, may make it difficult for the couple to choose what is right for them.

A genetic counselor can be invaluable in supplying the couple with correct data to help them make their decision. Several bioethical issues are raised when prenatal diagnosis is conducted, and nurses have been involved in helping clients work through the highly charged emotions surrounding prenatal diagnosis (Neidhardt, 1986; Green and Malin, 1988). Nurses need to stay involved in the ethical concerns of prenatal testing as technology advances (Sandelowski, 1993).

Timing of Early and Conventional Amniocentesis. Since the late 1960s, the standard time for amniocentesis to ensure adequacy of the amniotic fluid analysis has been between 15–20 weeks gestation. Testing takes 10 days to more than 2 weeks, so results are not available until well into the second trimester, when abortions are complicated. In the early 1980s, CVS became available as a first trimester test. (CVS is discussed later in this chapter.) In the late 1980s, early amniocentesis was introduced. In some studies in which early amniocentesis was compared with CVS, both tests were performed at 10–13 weeks gestation (Nicolaides et al., 1994). Early amniocentesis, before 15 weeks, and conventional amniocentesis, after 15 weeks, also have been compared (Crandall et al., 1994). At present, all three tests are useful in certain situations. Conventional amniocentesis is still needed for definite diagnosis of neural tube defects and as a follow-up examination for ambiguous results with the earlier tests. In general, CVS results are available between 12 and 14 weeks gestation, early amniocentesis results between 13 and 16 weeks, and conventional amniocentesis results between 17 and 22 weeks. Crandall et al. (1994) reported the risk of spontaneous abortion to be 3% or less with CVS, 2% or less with early amniocentesis, and 1% or less with conventional amniocentesis. However the success and complications of the three methods may differ depending on the competence of individual clinicians conducting the tests.

▼ NURSING DIAGNOSIS RELATED TO AMNIOCENTESIS

Anxiety Related to Waiting for Results After Conventional Amniocentesis

The waiting period after amniocentesis is a time of extreme anxiety for most couples. The woman may be trying to conceal the pregnancy until she knows the fetus is all right. (A pregnancy of 17 or more weeks may be difficult to conceal.) The couple tends to have ambivalent feelings about the fetus because it is possible that it may be aborted. Crying and indecision about the pregnancy are common. If the results indicate a serious defect and the decision is made to abort the fetus, the abortion must be carried out by induction because the client is in the second trimester. Fortunately, the most common result of amniocentesis is a *prediction* of normality. It is important that couples understand not all possible defects can be detected with amniocentesis, and there is always a possibility of error. It is emphasized that no test can *guarantee* a healthy baby. But for a couple with reason to fear one of the defects that can be identified with amniocentesis, a report of no defect is joyous news. A woman who does not have the support of the father of the child may have an even more difficult time awaiting the report of the amniocentesis than a woman who has emotional support.

Amniocentesis in Isoimmune Disease (Rh Factor)

If the mother has a rising titer of Rh antibodies, amniocentesis may be performed several times during the pregnancy to monitor the welfare of the fetus. (A rising bilirubin level in the amniotic fluid indicates hemolysis of fetal red blood cells.) Usually the first amniocentesis is performed as early as 18 weeks if the mother has a high antibody titer and a history of previously affected fetuses. It is performed as late as 24 weeks if there is a low fixed antibody titer and no history of an affected fetus (Perry et al., 1986; DeCherney and Pernoll, 1994). Elevated or rising Rh antibody titers in the mother indicate that the fetus may have hemolytic disease of the newborn (HDN). This disease, formerly called *erythroblastosis fetalis,* was even more common before the introduction of immunoglobulins of Rh antibodies (RhoGam), which can be given to prevent an Rh negative mother from making antibodies against the Rh factor of the fetal cells. Other isoimmune factors, such as ABO incompatibility, can cause some hemolytic reactions, but it is the Rh factor that causes the severe increase in bilirubin due to massive hemolysis of the red blood cells of the fetus. (See Chapter 14 for a discussion on Rh testing.)

REFERENCE VALUES FOR BILIRUBIN IN AMNIOTIC FLUID

The amount of bilirubin in the amniotic fluid is measured by how it changes patterns of light at a certain wave length (spectrophotometry). Charts are available to compare the concentration of bile pigments at different gestational ages.

Clinical Significance. If there is an abnormal amount of bilirubin for the gestational age, the obstetrician must decide whether to perform intrauterine transfusions of the fetus or to induce labor. One of the considerations for inducing labor is the maturity of the fetus. (See the L/S test discussed next.) Perry et al. (1986) discussed the role of the nurse in helping with exchange transfusions for the fetus.

Amniocentesis for Assessing Fetal Maturity

Lecithin-to-Sphingomyelin Ratio

The lecithin/sphingomyelin ratio (L/S ratio) is a test for fetal lung maturity. Lecithin and sphingomyelin are two phospholipids found in amniotic fluid and serum. Sphingomyelin, which is associated with nervous tissue, remains at about the same level in the amniotic fluid throughout the pregnancy. Lecithin is a component of alveolar surfactant. If there is sufficient surfactant to lubricate the alveolar surfaces, the lungs can inflate normally at birth. Without sufficient surfactant, the newborn infant is prone to hyaline membrane disease or respiratory distress syndrome (RDS). Lecithin begins to rise in the amniotic fluid at about 35 weeks gestation. This rise parallels the development of lung maturity. When the lecithin level is about double the sphingomyelin level in the amniotic fluid, the lungs are usually mature. However, the predictive value of the L/S ratio may differ among races. Black infants seem to fare better with lower ratios than do white infants (Richardson and Torday, 1994).

REFERENCE VALUES FOR LECITHIN-TO-SPHINGOMYELIN RATIO

A ratio of 2:1 is strong evidence that the fetus has mature lungs.

Shake Test for L/S Ratio. A quick way to check if sufficient lecithin is present is to mix equal parts of alcohol and saline solution with a sample of amniotic fluid and shake the test tube for 15 sec. If bubbles persist in the sample for 15 min, it is presumed that adequate lecithin is present. Factors such as dirty glassware may interfere with this test, so a quantitative measurement of L/S ratio is much more accurate.

Other Tests on Amniotic Fluid for Fetal Maturity

The L/S ratio is the most heavily used indicator of fetal maturity because if there is evidence of mature lung function the risk of RDS is much decreased. The laboratory can also stain fetal fat cells to assess the maturity of the fetus. Phosphatidylglycerol, a small component of lung surfactant is almost completely synthesized by mature lung alveolar cells and may be used to assess lung maturity in complicated pregnancies (Ravel, 1995). Creatinine levels are an indication of maturity of the kidneys. The creatinine level usually begins to rise at about 34 weeks of gestation. By 37 weeks gestation the level is 2 mg/dL or greater. The interpretation of all the data from amniocentesis requires the skilled judgment of the obstetrician because no one test can be viewed in isolation of the overall clinical condition of the mother and the fetus.

▼ PRETEST NURSING DIAGNOSES RELATED TO AMNIOCENTESIS

Anxiety Related to Unknowns About Procedure

The physical preparation of the client for amniocentesis is the same whether the collection of fluid is for prenatal diagnosis of a genetic defect, to assess isoimmune disease, or to determine if the fetus is mature enough for induced labor. As noted earlier, detailed counseling is important if amniocentesis is being performed because of possible genetic defects. Even at the time of the procedure, a couple may need last-minute reassurance. Sammons (1985) found that clients undergoing prenatal amniocentesis identified as helpful (1) ongoing physician explanation, (2) use of Lamaze relaxation techniques, and (3) presence of a trusted support person, be it husband, mother, or nurse. If the amniocentesis is being performed to determine if transfusions are needed or if labor should be induced, the client needs immediate reassurance about the purpose of the test and how the physician uses the results to make a decision about care. The client needs to sign a special consent form that indicates that she understands the purposes of the procedure and the complications that can occur. (See Chapter 25 on consent for invasive tests.)

Risk for Injury to Fetus

The nurse should take baseline vital signs. If amniocentesis is being performed in late pregnancy, the fetal heart rate should be monitored for a baseline reading. No premedication is given. Depending on the timing of the procedure, the

(*continued*)

▼ PRETEST NURSING DIAGNOSES RELATED TO AMNIOCENTESIS (*continued*)

client may or may not need a full bladder for visualization with ultrasound. (See Chapter 23 for a detailed explanation of the use of ultrasound in pregnancy.) Ultrasound is used to visualize the placenta and the position of the fetus to avoid injury.

Procedure. The client lies in a recumbent position throughout the sonogram and withdrawal of the fluid. The skin of the abdomen is prepared with an iodine solution (Betadine or Iodophor). Because only one needle puncture is used to remove the fluid, the physician does not usually use a local anesthetic. (Chapter 25 describes the medications that are used for local anesthesia.) The physician inserts a long needle through the abdominal wall into the amniotic sac and withdraws amniotic fluid. The client feels the stick, but the aspiration is not painful. The fluid sample is placed in clearly marked test tubes. If the specimen is to be tested for bilirubin, the fluid should be collected in a dark tube and protected from the light because light changes the composition of indirect bilirubin. (Light is actually used as therapy, phototherapy, for high indirect bilirubin in the newborn.) After the needle is withdrawn, a small adhesive bandage is placed over the puncture site on the abdomen.

▼ POSTTEST NURSING DIAGNOSIS RELATED TO AMNIOCENTESIS

Knowledge Deficit Related to Follow-up Care

If amniocentesis is performed in early pregnancy for prenatal diagnosis, the client can go home after the test. The woman may be told to avoid strenuous exercise, douching, or sexual activity for at least 24 hours. The client is told she may have some mild cramps for a short time and is given instructions to notify the physician or clinic if severe cramps develop or if bleeding occurs. Nursing research (Stringer and Librizzi, 1994) documented that minor complications within 24 hours after amniocentesis included soreness (44%), cramping (31.8%), fluid leak (9.5%), and vaginal spotting (2%). The genetic counselor has already impressed on the couple that the results of the test are not available for 10–14 days, but the couple should be reminded again that they will be called as soon as the results are known. (See the earlier discussion of the anxiety of waiting for results.) Amniocentesis carries a risk of about 11% for sensitizing susceptible Rh-negative pregnant women, so an injection of Rh IgG antibodies may be ordered for these women (DeCherney and Pernoll, 1994). (See Chapter 14 for a discussion on the importance of prenatal Rh testing and the use of immunoglobulins.)

If the amniocentesis is done in late pregnancy to assess the status of the fetus, the client may or may not be hospitalized. The fetal heart rate is monitored for 30 min after the test to assess for any difficulty. The pregnant woman's vital signs also are assessed.

▼ CHORIONIC VILLUS SAMPLING

This test of a chorionic sample is a test of cells similar to those of the fetus. The physician inserts a small catheter through the vagina and cervix into the uterus. Suction is applied to obtain some cells. As an alternative method, CVS may be performed with needle insertion through the abdominal wall. As with amniocentesis, ultrasound is used to guide the needle. The preparation of the client is similar to that for amniocentesis. The great advantage of CVS over amniocentesis is that it can be performed earlier in pregnancy. (See the discussion of the timing of CVS in the section on amniocentesis.) CVS cannot be used to detect neural tube defects. A multicenter study (Rhoades et al., 1989) demonstrated that CVS is slightly more risky, 0.8% higher fetal loss rate, than amniocentesis. The study also revealed that amniocentesis has an accuracy rate of 99.4% compared with 97.8% for CVS. Ambiguous results of CVS may necessitate amniocentesis at a later date, and inability to obtain a sample at CVS may also necessitate amniocentesis. In addition to the higher rate of spontaneous abortion after CVS, which may be as high as 3.4%, reports also suggest that there may be a higher risk of limb and facial abnormalities after CVS (Crandall et al., 1994).

▼ PRE- AND POSTTEST NURSING IMPLICATIONS RELATED TO CVS

See the pre- and posttest implications for amniocentesis. Nursing research (Stringer and Librizzi, 1994) noted the incidence of minor complications within 24 hours after CVS were cramping (31.9%), spotting (27.7%), soreness (14.9%), and fluid leak (6.4%).

▼ PERCUTANEOUS UMBILICAL BLOOD SAMPLING AND FETAL BIOPSY

The use of ultrasound has made it possible to obtain fetal blood and to conduct fetal tissue sampling. Access to the fetal circulation and other tissues makes it possible to perform many types of tests to confirm genetic disease and infections. Because these procedures carry greater risks than amniocentesis or CVS, they are reserved for situations in which diagnostic information cannot be obtained by safer means (D'Alton and DeCherney, 1993).

▼ FETAL MONITORING NONSTRESS TEST

Fetal monitoring, a noninvasive technique to evaluate the status of the fetus, is called the nonstress test to differentiate it from the contraction stress test, which does put stress on the fetus. The client is attached to a fetal monitor and the fetal heart rate (FHR) is recorded. The specific patterns of FHR acceleration may be termed reactive, nonreactive, or equivocal. A nonstress test is considered reactive when two or more FHR accelerations occur in a 20-min period. These accelerations must be at least 15 beats per minute above the baseline and must last at least 15 sec. If only one acceleration occurs or if the accelerations do not meet the foregoing criteria, the test results may be called *equivocal.* If no accelerations occur the test is *nonreactive.* A second 20-min period may be recorded.

▼ NURSING IMPLICATIONS RELATED TO NONSTRESS TESTS

A nonstress test may be performed in a clinic, office, or in a quiet room in an obstetric unit. The client is put in a recliner chair or a comfortable bed. A semi-sitting position with a slight left tilt helps avoid supine hypotension from pressure on the vena cava. The client should void before the procedure to remain comfortable. It is also advisable for the client to eat before the test because the active bowel sounds of an empty stomach may interfere with the test. Also, the fetus is more active after a meal. The nurse should take a baseline blood pressure measurement. The monitors are applied per hospital routine. The sleep–awake pattern of the fetus is observed for about 40 min because a rest—activity pattern of the fetus is usually in a 20–40 min pattern. Some women may have to be monitored longer to obtain a reactive pattern. If the client is taking sedative drugs, the fetus may be less active. One way to shorten the time required to obtain a reactive nonstress test is to use vibroacoustic stimulation of the fetus by the use of an artificial larynx placed on the pregnant woman's abdomen. Sleutel (1990) found that FHR tracings after stimulation had more acceleration and were of greater amplitude and duration than those in the control group. The length of time required to obtain a reactive nonstress test was almost 15 min shorter than in controls.

Experienced obstetric nurses may perform the entire monitoring procedure, including interpretation of the findings. Research by Chez et al. (1990) supported the position that obstetric nurses can demonstrate the same skills as physicians in interpreting a nonstress test. Consultation and follow-up readings of the strip may require the services of a physician or nurse expert. The use of the auscultated acceleration test (AAT), which is performed with a fetoscope but no fetal monitors to auscultate a change in FHR after manual stimulation, has been investigated by nurse researchers and may prove useful after further investigation (Paine et al., 1992).

Although the nonstress method of antepartum monitoring does not cause any pain or physical discomfort for the woman, most women are highly anxious about the results. Fetal monitoring is performed when there is a probability of fetal jeopardy, as when a client has diabetes or hypertension or other risk factors. The nurse should allow the woman to express her concerns and anxieties. The nurse can get answers for any questions the woman may have about her prenatal care or the process of labor and delivery. The nurse can also help the client use some of the relaxation techniques she may be learning in childbirth classes. A study of maternal reactions to fetal monitoring revealed that the women wanted the nurse with them much or most of the time. The women in the study wanted "someone to hold onto, someone who cares" (Shields, 1978).

▼ CONTRACTION CHALLENGE TEST

In the contraction challenge test, also called the contraction stress test (CST), to determine the ability of the fetus to withstand the contractions of labor, contractions once were stimulated with oxytocin. Now the test is often performed by means of intermittent nipple stimulation. With either oxytocin or nipple stimulation, the test often requires 1–2 hr to complete (DeCherney and Pernoll, 1994). Because contractions produce a transient decrease in the uteroplacental blood flow, some fetuses may be stressed during labor. The CST may indicate if a fetus would be in less jeopardy if a cesarean delivery were initiated. Because there is some risk of inducing labor with this test, the test must be conducted close to a delivery suite. CST is definitely contraindicated with rupture of membranes or a previous classic cesarean delivery and usually contraindicated with multiple pregnancies, previous premature labor, placenta previa, hydramnios, and previous low transverse cesarean incision. Because a CST does have some risks, qualified personnel are needed to administer the test. A CST takes longer and is more expensive than a nonstress test in antepartum monitoring.

REFERENCE VALUES FOR CONTRACTION STRESS TEST

The specific patterns must be carefully evaluated by the physician in conjunction with other clinical data. A negative CST shows no late deceleration in fetal heart rate after a contraction. In essence, a negative test is evidence that the fetus is not in jeopardy and the pregnancy may be allowed to progress normally because the fetus can withstand the stress of labor contractions.

▼ PRETEST NURSING IMPLICATIONS RELATED TO CONTRACTION STRESS TEST

A CST is given near a delivery suite. The general preparation of the client is the same as for a nonstress test, except the client is asked to sign a special consent form, which explains the possible risks of the procedure. (See Chapter 25 on informed consent.) If nipple stimulation is not effective, the usual procedure is to give oxytocin intravenously at a dilution ordered by the physician. The drip rate is increased until the client is having three contractions in 10 min. The fetus is monitored for at least 30 min. The nurse must carefully monitor the client during the test. The client can be helped to more easily tolerate the contractions by using the techniques she is learning in her childbirth class.

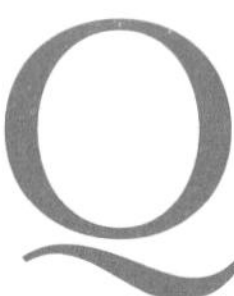

1. John and Mary Menendez, both 27 years of age, have been married a little more than 2 years. Although they have used no form of birth control for the past 16 months, pregnancy has not occurred. The couple desire a child, so they have asked a nurse in a clinic about fertility testing. Which statement contains appropriate information?
   - **a.** Infertility is most likely not a problem because they have only been having unprotected intercourse for a little more than a year
   - **b.** Infertility is usually due to female problems so Mary needs to be tested first
   - **c.** Most infertility problems can be treated with drugs such as clomiphene (Clomid) or a simple surgical procedure
   - **d.** Basic infertility tests include semen analysis, ovulation tests, and tubal patency tests such as a hysterosalpingogram

2. As part of an infertility evaluation, Mary is to keep a record of her basal body temperature on a daily basis. The nurse is assessing to see if Mary can accurately read the thermometer. In addition, the nurse should emphasize
   - **a.** The temperature should be taken before Mary gets out of bed in the morning
   - **b.** An increase in temperature is expected before ovulation occurs
   - **c.** Rectal temperatures are the only way to obtain a basal reading
   - **d.** A 1-month graph of temperatures is usually sufficient

3. Which of the following statements about amniocentesis is important when planning care for a client who is to undergo amniocentesis for prenatal diagnosis of genetic defects?

   a. The amniocentesis must be performed as early as possible, usually before the eighth week of gestation
   b. The test is a guarantee of a healthy baby
   c. The results take 10–14 days, so this is a period of great anxiety for a couple who may decide to terminate the pregnancy
   d. There is a risk of 5–10% for the fetus

4. Mrs. Sanders is a 39-year-old primigravida who has elected to undergo chorionic villi sampling for prenatal diagnosis. The advantage of CVS over amniocentesis is that CVS is

   a. Less hazardous to the fetus
   b. Less expensive
   c. Able to detect neural tube defects
   d. Performed earlier in pregnancy

5. One of the tests performed on amniotic fluid is a test for α-fetoprotein because an elevation of this protein is suggestive of

   a. Fetal lung immaturity
   b. Immunologic deficiencies
   c. Neural tube defects
   d. Phenylketonuria

6. Mrs. Ragella is 34 weeks pregnant. An amniocentesis revealed an increased bilirubin level as compared with levels performed a week ago. This rising bilirubin level is indicative of

   a. Possible fetal jeopardy caused by hemolytic disease
   b. Normal liver functioning
   c. Renal immaturity
   d. Fetal distress caused by hypoxia

7. The physician is concerned because a too early cesarean delivery may predispose Mrs. Ragella's infant to respiratory distress syndrome (RDS). Which of these tests of amniotic fluid is used to assess lung maturity in the fetus?

   a. Lecithin-to-sphingomyelin ratio
   b. Creatinine levels
   c. Karyotyping of chromosomes
   d. Spectrophotometric analysis of bilirubin levels

8. Mrs. Foster has diabetes and is near term with her second pregnancy. Her other pregnancy was a stillbirth. She has been admitted to the obstetric unit for a possible early delivery. She is scheduled for amniocentesis this afternoon to assess fetal matu-

rity. Mrs. Foster asks the nurse about the procedure. The nurse should explain to Mrs. Foster that

a. Premedication will be used to relax her
b. Local anesthesia must be used to eliminate pain
c. Ultrasound will be performed to visualize the placenta and fetus
d. Radiography of the abdomen is routine after the procedure is completed

9. Mrs. Foster is scheduled for more tests. She asks the nurse if a contraction stress test is the same as the routine fetal monitoring she had with her last pregnancy. The nurse should explain that the CST *differs* from the nonstress technique of antepartum monitoring in that the CST

a. Requires that fetal heart rate be assessed with internal fetal monitors to detect any abnormal patterns
b. Uses a drug or nipple stimulation to cause contractions
c. Is used for women who have high-risk pregnancies
d. Cause anxiety whereas the nonstress test is anxiety-free for the client

▼ REFERENCES

Angell, M. (1990). New ways to get pregnant. *New England Journal of Medicine, 323* (17), 1200–1202.

Beastall, G.H. (1993). Role of endocrine biochemistry laboratories in the investigation of infertility. *Journal of Clinical Pathology, 46,* 790–794.

Blackwell, R. (1989). The infertility workup and diagnosis. *Journal of Reproductive Medicine, 34* (suppl 1), 81–84.

Blenner, J.L. (1990). Passage through infertility treatment: A stage theory. *Image, 22* (3), 153–158.

Blenner, J.L. (1992). Stress and mediators: Patients' perceptions of infertility treatment. *Nursing Research, 41* (2), 92–97.

Chez, B., Skuurnick, J., Chez, R., et al. (1990). Interpretations on nonstress tests by obstetric nurses. *JOGN Nursing, 19* (3), 227–232.

Crandall, B.F., Kulch, P., and Tabsh, K. (1994). Risk assessment of amniocentesis between 11 and 15 weeks: Comparison to later amniocentesis controls. *Prenatal Diagnosis, 14,* 913–919.

D'Alton, M.E., and DeCherney, A.H. (1993). Prenatal diagnosis. *New England Journal of Medicine, 328* (2), 114–120.

DeCherney, A.H., and Pernoll, M.L. (1994). *Current obstetric & gynecologic diagnosis & treatment* (8th ed.). Norwalk, CT: Appleton & Lange.

Devore, N., and Baldwin, N. (1986). Ectopic pregnancy on the rise. *American Journal of Nursing, 86* (6), 674–678.

Fehring, R. (1990). Methods used to self-predict ovulation: A comparative study. *JOGN Nursing, 19* (3), 233–237.

Green, D., and Malin, J. (1988). Prenatal diagnosis: When reality shatters parents' dreams. *Nursing 88, 18* (2), 61–64.

Leavitt, M. (1982). Families at risk: Primary prevention in nursing practice. Boston: Little, Brown.

McDonough, M., et al. (1981). Parents' response to fetal monitoring. *MCN: American Journal of Maternal Child Nursing, 6,* 32–34.

Neidhardt, A. (1986). Why me? Second trimester abortion. *American Journal of Nursing, 86* (10), 1133–1135.

Nicolaides, K., Brizot, M., Patel, F., et al. (1994). Comparison of chorionic villus sampling and amniocentesis for fetal karyotyping at 10–13 weeks gestation. *Lancet, 344,* 435–439.

Paine, O., Benedict, M.I., Strobino, S.M., et al. (1992). A comparison of the auscultated acceleration test and the nonstress test as predictors of perinatal outcomes. *Nursing Research, 41* (2), 87–91.

Pauker, S.P., and Pauker, S.G. (1994). Prenatal diagnosis: Why is 35 a magic number? (Editorial) *New England Journal of Medicine, 330* (16), 1151–1152.

Pearlstone, A.C., and Surrey, E.S. (1994). The temporal relation between the urine LH surge and sonographic evidence of ovulation determinants and clinical significance. *Obstetrics & Gynecology, 83* (2), 184–188.

Perry, S., Parer, J., and Inturrisi, M. (1986). Intrauterine transfusion for severe isoimmunization. *MCN: American Journal of Maternal Child Nursing, 11* (3), 182–189.

Pines, M. (1980). How old is too old to have a baby? *McCall's, 107* (June issue).

Ravel, R. (1995). *Clinical laboratory medicine: Clinical application of laboratory data* (6th ed.). St. Louis: Mosby–Year Book.

Rhoades, G.G., Jackson, L.G., Schlesselman, S.E., et al. (1989). The safety and efficacy of chorionic villus sampling for early prenatal diagnosis of cytogenetic abnormalities. *New England Journal of Medicine, 320* (10), 609–617.

Richardson, D.K., and Torday, J.S. (1994). Racial differences in predictive values of the lecithin/sphingomyelin ratio. *American Journal of Obstetrics and Gynecology, 170* (5), 1273–1278.

Sammons, L. (1985). Effects of preparation for amniocentesis on anxiety (Abstract). *California Nurse, 81* (10), 8.

Sandelowski, M. (1993). Toward a theory of technology dependency. *Nursing Outlook, 41* (1), 36–42.

Sauer, M.V., Paulson, R.J., and Lovo, R.A. (1990). A preliminary report on oocyte donation for extending reproductive potential in women over 40. *New England Journal of Medicine, 323* (17), 1157–1160.

Sherrod, R. (1988). Coping with infertility: A personal perspective turned professional. *MCN: American Journal of Maternal Child Nursing, 13* (3), 191–194.

Shields, D. (1978). Maternal reactions to fetal monitoring. *American Journal of Nursing, 78* (12), 2110–2112.

Sleutel, M. (1990). Vibroacoustic stimulation and fetal heart rate in nonstress tests. *JOGN Nursing, 19* (3), 199–204.

Stringer, M., and Librizzi, R. (1994). Complications following prenatal genetic procedures. *Nursing Research, 43* (2), 184–186.

Wong, D. (1980). Bereavement: The empty-mother syndrome. *MCN: American Journal of Maternal Child Nursing, 5,* 385–389.

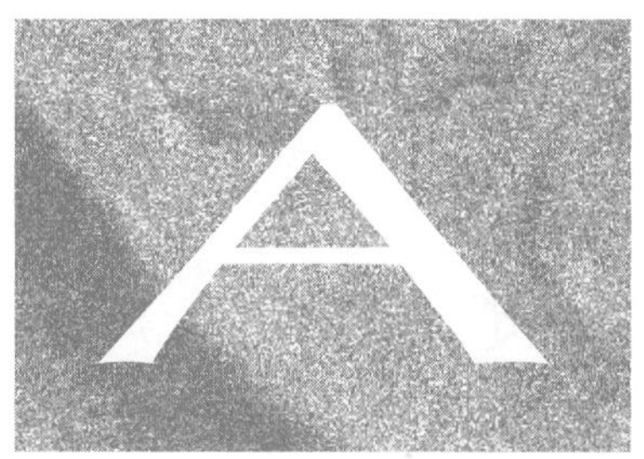

APPENDICES

REFERENCE VALUES AND OTHER INFORMATION

As emphasized in Chapter 1, laboratory books such as this one cannot provide a table of *normal* values for laboratory tests because each laboratory must provide its own normal range for the particular technique that it uses and for the population it serves. Values listed in a book are only *reference* values, and they must be adapted to a particular setting. The primary source for reference values used in this text are those printed periodically in the *New England Journal of Medicine,* with whose permission the four tables in Appendix A are reprinted. Reprints and updates of the normal reference values are available by ordering from:

Normal Reference Values
New England Journal of Medicine
P.O. Box 9125
Waltham, MA 02254-9125

In addition to the reference values listed in Appendix A, Appendix B contains a summary of changes in newborns and in children. Appendix C presents the changes in the elderly, and Appendix D, those in pregnancy. Documentations of the changes in various populations are included with the tables and throughout the text.

The collection of blood is most often performed with a Vacutainer or other commercial system, which has different-colored tops on the collection tubes to indicate the additive present. Table 1–3 in Chapter 1 lists the meaning of the color-coded tops. Most serum blood samples require no additives, so blood is collected in a red-topped tube.

The tables of reference values also contain the values in SI units, which are explained in Chapter 1. Because reference tables contain many abbreviations and measurement terms, lists of common abbreviations are presented in Appendix E and Appendix F. Measurements to help the reader decipher laboratory reports are provided in Appendix G. Answers to the self-test questions are contained in Appendix H and Appendix I.

APPENDIX A. NORMAL REFERENCE LABORATORY VALUES

TABLE A–1. GENERAL CHEMISTRY VALUES

Analyte	Fluid	MGH Units	SI Units	Method or Instrument	Factor for Conversion to SI Units
Acid phosphatase, prostatic	S	0–0.8 U/liter	0.0–13.0 nkat/liter	Kinetic method	16.67
Alanine aminotransferase (ALT, SGPT)	S			Kinetic method	0.01667
Female		7–30 U/liter	0.12–0.50 µkat/liter		
Male		10–55 U/liter	0.17–0.91 µkat/liter		
Albumin	S	3.1–4.3 g/dl	31–43 g/liter	Colorimetry (bromocresol purple)	10
Aldolase	S	0–7 U/liter	0–117 nkat/liter	Kinetic method	16.67
Alkaline phosphatase	S			Kinetic method	0.01667
Female		30–100 U/liter	0.5–1.67 µkat/liter		
Male		45–115 U/liter	0.75–1.92 µkat/liter		
Alkaline phosphatase, leukocyte	WB			Histochemistry	
Female (not taking oral contraceptives)		30–160	None		None
Male		33–188	None		None
$Alpha_1$-antitrypsin	S	85–213 mg/dl	0.85–2.13 g/liter	Nephelometry	0.01
Alpha-fetoprotein (nonmaternal)	S	<10 IU/ml	<7.75 µg/liter	Immunoassay	0.775
Ammonia	P	12–55 µmol/liter	12–55 µmol/liter	Enzymatic analysis	1
Amylase	S	53–123 U/liter	0.88–2.05 nkat/liter	Kinetic method	0.01667
	U	0–375 U/liter	0–6.25 µkat/liter	Kinetic method	
Angiotensin-converting enzyme (ACE)	S	10–50 U/liter	167–834 nkat/liter	Kinetic method	16.67
Aspartate aminotransferase (AST, SGOT)	S			Kinetic method	0.01667
Female		9–25 U/liter	0.15–0.42 µkat/liter		
Male		10–40 U/liter	0.17–0.67 µkat/liter		

Bicarbonate (HCO_3^-)	WB, S	22–26 meq/liter	22–26 mmol/liter	Calculation	1
Bilirubin, direct	S	0.0–0.4 mg/dl	0–7 μmol/liter	Colorimetry	17.1
Bilirubin, total	S	0.0–1.0 mg/dl	0–17 μmol/liter	Colorimetry	17.1
CA-19-9	S	<37.0 U/ml	<37.0 kU/liter	Immunoassay	1
CA-125	S	<20.0 U/ml	<20.0 kU/liter	Immunoassay	1
Calcium	S	8.5–10.5 mg/dl	2.1–2.6 mmol/liter	Colorimetry	0.25
	U	0.0–300 mg/day	0.0–7.5 mmol/day	Atomic absorption	0.025
Calcium, ionized	P	1.14–1.30 mmol/liter	1.14–1.30 mmol/liter	Ion-selective electrode	1
Carbon dioxide content, total	S	24.0–30.9 mmol/liter	24.0–30.9 mmol/liter	Carbon dioxide electrode	1
Carbon dioxide, partial pressure, arterial (Pa_{CO_2})	WB	35–45 mm Hg	4.7–6.0 kPa	Carbon dioxide electrode	0.1333
Carboxyhemoglobin	WB	<5% of total hemoglobin	<0.05 fraction of total hemoglobin saturation	Multiwavelength spectrophotometry	0.01
Carcinoembryonic antigen (CEA)	P, S	0.0–3.0 ng/ml	0.0–3.0 μg/liter	Immunoassay	1
Cerebrospinal fluid (adult)	CSF				
Albumin		11–48 mg/dl	0.11–0.48 g/liter	Nephelometry	0.01
Cell count		0–5 mononuclear cells/μl	0–5 × 10^6 cells/liter	Manual count	1 × 10^6
Chloride		120–130 mmol/liter	120–130 mmol/liter	Coulometry	1
Glucose		50–75 mg/dl	2.8–4.2 mmol/liter	Enzymatic analysis	0.05551
IgG		8.0–8.6 mg/dl	0.08–0.086 g/liter	Nephelometry	0.01
Pressure		70–180 mm of water	70–180 arbitrary units	Manual measurement	1
Protein		15–45 mg/dl	0.15–0.45 g/liter	Turbidometry	0.01
Ceruloplasmin	S	23–43 mg/dl	230–430 mg/liter	Oxidase activity	10
Chloride	P, S	100–108 mmol/liter	100–108 mmol/liter	Coulometry	1
	U	10–200 mmol/liter	10–200 mmol/liter	Coulometry	1
Cholesterol	S			Colorimetry	0.02586
Desirable		<200 mg/dl	<5.18 mmol/liter		
Borderline high		200–239 mg/dl	5.18–6.19 mmol/liter		
High		≥240 mg/dl	≥6.20 mmol/liter		
Copper	P	70–155 μg/dl	11.0–24.4 μmol/liter	Atomic absorption	0.1574
	U	0–60 μg/dl/day	0.0–0.94 μmol/day	Atomic absorption	0.01574
Creatine kinase (CK)	S			Kinetic method	0.01667
Female		40–150 U/liter	0.67–2.50 μkat/liter		
Male		60–400 U/liter	1.00–6.67 μkat/liter		

(continued)

TABLE A–1. GENERAL CHEMISTRY VALUES (*Continued*)

Analyte	Fluid	MGH Units	SI Units	Method or Instrument	Factor for Conversion to SI Units
Creatine kinase isoenzymes, MB fraction	S	0–7.5 ng/ml	0–7.5 µg/liter	Immunoassay	1
Creatine kinase isoenzyme index	S	0.0–3.0% relative index	None	$\frac{\text{ng/ml}}{\text{total CK (U/liter)}} \times 100$	None
Creatinine	S	0.6–1.5 mg/dl	53–133 µmol/liter	Colorimetry	88.4
	U	15–25 mg/kg/day	0.13–0.22 mmol/kg/day		0.0088
Fecal fat (as stearic acid)		1–7 g/day	3.5–25 mmol/day	Gravimetry	3.515
Gamma-glutamyl transpeptidase (GGT)	S	1.0–60.0 U/liter	0.02–1.00 µkat/liter	Kinetic method	0.01667
Globulin	S	2.6–4.1 g/dl	26–41 g/liter	Calculation: total protein − albumin	10
Glucose, fasting	P	70–110 mg/dl	3.9–6.1 mmol/liter	Enzymatic analysis	0.05551
High-density lipoprotein, cholesterol, as major risk factor	S	<35 mg/dl	<0.91 mmol/liter	Colorimetry	0.02586
Ketones	S, U	Negative	Negative	Colorimetry (nitroprusside)	
Lactic dehydrogenase (LDH)	S	110–210 U/liter	1.83–3.50 µkat/liter	Kinetic method	0.01667
Lactic dehydrogenase isoenzymes	S			Electrophoresis	0.01
LD_1		17–27%	0.17–0.27		
LD_2		28–38%	0.28–0.38		
LD_3		18–28%	0.18–0.28		
LD_4		5–15%	0.05–0.15		
LD_5		5–15%	0.05–0.15		
Total LDH (when isoenzymes determined)		110–250 U/liter	1.83–4.23 µkat/liter		
Lactic acid	P	0.5–2.2 mmol/liter	0.5–2.2 mmol/liter	Enzymatic analysis	1
Lipase	S	4–24 U/dl	0.67–4.00 µkat/liter	Kinetic method	0.1667
Low-density lipoprotein cholesterol	S			Calculation	0.02586
Desirable		<130 mg/dl	<3.36 mmol/liter		
Borderline high risk		130–159 mg/dl	3.36–4.11 mmol/liter		
High risk		≥160 mg/dl	≥4.13 mmol/liter		

Magnesium	S	1.5–2.0 meq/liter	0.8–1.0 mmol/liter	Colorimetry	0.5
5′-Nucleotidase	S	1–11 U/liter	0.02–0.18 μkat/liter	Kinetic method	0.01667
Osmolality	S	280–296 mOsm/kg of water	280–296 mmol/kg	Freezing-point depression	1
Oxygen, partial pressure, arterial (PaO_2); room air, age dependent	WB	75–100 mm Hg	10.0–13.3 kPa	Oxygen electrode	0.1333
Oxygen saturation, arterial	WB	96–100%	0.96–1.00	Pulse oximetry	0.01
pH, arterial	WB	7.35–7.45 pH units	7.35–7.45 pH units	pH electrode	1
Phosphorus, inorganic	S	2.6–4.5 mg/dl	0.84–1.45 mmol/liter	Spectrophotometry	0.3229
	U	average, 1 g/day	average, 32 mmol/day		32.29
Potassium	S	3.5–5.0 mmol/liter	3.5–5.0 mmol/liter	Ion-selective electrode	1
	U	Diet dependent	Diet dependent	Ion-selective electrode	1
Prostate-specific antigen	S			Immunoassay	1
Female		0.0–0.5 μg/liter	0.0–0.5 μg/liter		
Male <40 yr old		0.0–2.0 μg/liter	0.0–2.0 μg/liter		
Male ≥40 yr old		0.0–4.0 μg/liter	0.0–4.0 μg/liter		
Protein, total	S	6.0–8.0 g/dl	60–80 g/liter	Colorimetry	10
	U	<165 mg/day	<0.165 g/day	Turbidometry	0.001
Sodium	S	135–145 mmol/liter	135–145 mmol/liter	Ion-selective electrode	1
	U	Diet dependent	Diet dependent	Ion-selective electrode	1
Triglycerides (fasting)	S	40–150 mg/dl	0.45–1.69 mmol/liter	Spectrophotometry	0.01129
Urea nitrogen (BUN)	S	8–25 mg/dl	2.9–8.9 mmol/liter	Conductivity	0.357
Uric acid	S			Colorimetry	59.48
Female		2.3–6.6 mg/dl	137–393 μmol/liter		
Male		3.6–8.5 mg/dl	214–506 μmol/liter		

MGH, Massachusetts General Hospital; S, denotes serum; WB, whole blood; P, plasma, U, urine; CSF, cerebrospinal fluid.

Reprinted with permission from the New England Journal of Medicine *327:718–724 (September 3), 1992*

TABLE A–2. ENDOCRINE CHEMISTRY VALUES

Analyte	Fluid	MGH Units	SI Units	Method or Instrument	Factor for Conversion to SI Units
Aldosterone					
Standing (normal-salt diet)	S, P	4–31 ng/dl	111–860 pmol/liter	Immunoassay	27.74
Recumbent (normal-salt diet)	S, P	<16 ng/dl	<444 pmol/liter	Immunoassay	27.74
Normal-salt diet (100–180 meq of sodium)	U	6–25 μg/day	17–69 nmol/day	Immunoassay	2.774
Low-salt diet (10 meq of sodium)	U	17–44 μg/day	47–122 nmol/day	Immunoassay	2.774
High-salt diet	U	0–6 μg/day	0–17 nmol/day	Immunoassay	2.774
Androstenedione	S	60–260 ng/dl	2.1–9.1 nmol/liter	Immunoassay	0.0349
Antidiuretic hormone (arginine vasopressin)	P	1.0–13.3 pg/ml	1.0–13.3 ng/liter	Immunoassay	1
Calcitonin	S			Immunoassay	1
Female		0–20 pg/ml	0–20 ng/liter		
Male		0–28 pg/ml	0–28 ng/liter		
Catecholamines					
Dopamine	U	65–400 μg/day	424–2612 nmol/day	Liquid chromatography	6.53
	P	0–30 pg/ml	0–196 nmol/liter	Liquid chromatography	6.53
Epinephrine	U	1.7–22.4 μg/day	9.3–122 nmol/day	Liquid chromatography	5.458
Supine	P	0–110 pg/ml	0–600 pmol/liter	Liquid chromatography	5.458
Standing	P	0–140 pg/ml	0–764 pmol/liter	Liquid chromatography	5.458
Norepinephrine	U	12.1–85.5 μg/day	72–505 nmol/day	Liquid chromatography	5.911
Supine	P	70–750 pg/ml	0.41–4.43 nmol/liter	Liquid chromatography	0.005911
Standing	P	200–1700 pg/ml	1.18–10.0	Liquid chromatography	0.005911
Chorionic gonadotropin (hCG) (nonpregnant)	S	<10 mIU/ml	<10 IU/liter	Immunoassay	1
Corticotropin (ACTH)	P	6.0–76.0 pg/ml	1.3–16.7 pmol/liter	Immunoassay	0.2202
Cortisol	P			Immunoassay	27.59
Fasting, 8 a.m.–12 noon		5.0–25.0 μg/dl	138–690 nmol/liter		
12 noon–8 p.m.		5.0–15.0 μg/dl	138–410 nmol/liter		
8 p.m.–8 a.m.		0.0–10.0 μg/dl	0–276 nmol/liter		
Cortisol, free	U	20–70 μg/day	55–193 nmol/day	Immunoassay	2.759
C peptide	S	0.30–3.70 μg/liter	0.10–1.22 nmol/liter	Immunoassay	0.33

11-Deoxycortisol (after metyrapone)	P	>7.5 μg/dl	>216 nmol/liter	Immunoassay	28.86
1,25-Dihydroxyvitamin D	S	16–42 pg/ml	38–101 pmol/liter	Immunoassay	2.4
Erythropoietin	S	<19 mU/ml	≤19 U/liter	Immunoassay	1
Estradiol	S,P			Immunoassay	3.671
Female					
Premenopausal adult		23–361 pg/ml	84–1325 pmol/liter		
Postmenopausal		<30 pg/ml	<110 pmol/liter		
Prepubertal		<20 pg/ml	<73 pmol/liter		
Male		<50 pg/ml	<184 pmol/liter		
Gastrin	P	0–200 pg/ml	0–200 ng/liter	Immunoassay	1
Growth hormone	P	2.0–6.0 ng/ml	2.0–6.0 μg/liter	Immunoassay	1
Hemoglobin A_{1c}	P	3.8–6.4%	0.038–0.064	Liquid chromatography	0.01
Homovanillic acid	U	0.0–15.0 mg/day	0–82 μmol/day	Liquid chromatography	5.489
17-Hydroxycorticosteroids	U			Colorimetry	2.759
Female		2.0–6.0 mg/day	5.5–17 μmol/day		
Male		3.0–10.0 mg/day	8–28 μmol/day		
5-Hydroxyindoleacetic acid (lower in women than in men)	U	2–9 mg/day	10–47 μmol/day	Colorimetry	5.23
17-Hydroxyprogesterone	S			Immunoassay	3.026
Female					
Prepubertal		0.20–0.54 μg/liter	0.61–1.63 nmol/liter		
Follicular		0.02–0.80 μg/liter	0.61–2.42 nmol/liter		
Luteal		0.90–3.04 μg/liter	2.72–9.20 nmol/liter		
Postmenopausal		<0.45 μg/liter	<1.36 nmol/liter		
Male					
Prepubertal		0.12–0.30 μg/liter	0.36–0.91 nmol/liter		
Adult		0.20–1.80 μg/liter	0.61–5.45 nmol/liter		
25-Hydroxyvitamin D	S	8–55 ng/ml	20–137 nmol/liter	Immunoassay	2.496
Insulin	S	0–29 μU/ml	0–208 pmol/liter	Immunoassay	7.175
17-Ketogenic steroids	U			Colorimetry	3.467
Female		3.0–15.0 mg/day	10–52 μmol/day		
Male		5.0–23.0 mg/day	17–80 μmol/day		
17-Ketosteroids	U			Colorimetry	3.467
Female and male ≤10 yr old		0.1–3.0 mg/day	0.4–10.4 μmol/day		
Female and male 11–14 yr old		2.0–7.0 mg/day	6.9–24.2 μmol/day		

(continued)

TABLE A–2. ENDOCRINE CHEMISTRY VALUES (*Continued*)

Analyte	Fluid	MGH Units	SI Units	Method or Instrument	Factor for Conversion to SI Units
Female ≥15 yr old		5.0–15.0 mg/day	17.3–52.0 μmol/day		
Male ≥15 yr old		9.0–22.0 mg/day	31.2–76.3 μmol/day		
Metanephrines, total	U	0.0–0.90 mg/day	0.0–4.9 μmol/day	Spectrophotometry	5.458
Parathyroid hormone	P	10–60 pg/ml	10–60 ng/liter	Immunoassay	1
Parathyroid-related protein	P	<1.5 pmol/liter	<1.5 pmol/liter	Immunoassay	1
Pregnanediol	U			Gas chromatography	3.12
Female		0.2–6.0 mg/day	0.6–18.7 μmol/day		
Follicular phase		0.1–1.3 mg/day	0.3–5.3 μmol/day		
Luteal phase		1.2–9.5 mg/day	3.7–29.6 μmol/day		
Pregnancy		Gestation-period dependent	Gestation-period dependent		
Male		0.2–1.2 mg/day	0.6–3.7 μmol/day		
Pregnanetriol	U	0.5–2.0 mg/day	1.5–6.0 μmol/day	Gas chromatography	2.972
Prolactin	S			Immunoassay	1
Female		0–15 ng/ml	0–15 μg/liter		
Male		0–10 ng/ml	0–10 μg/liter		
Renin activity	P			Immunoassay	0.2778
Normal salt intake					
Recumbent 6 hr		0.5–1.6 ng/ml/hr	0.14–0.44 ng/(liter · sec)		
Upright 4 hr		1.9–3.6 ng/ml/hr	0.53–1.00 ng/(liter · sec)		
Low salt intake					
Recumbent 6 h		2.2–4.4 ng/ml/hr	0.61–1.22 ng/(liter · sec)		
Upright 4 hr		4.0–8.1 ng/ml/hr	1.11–2.25 ng/(liter · sec)		
Upright 4 hr, with diuretic		6.8–15.0 ng/ml/hr	1.89–4.17 ng/(liter · sec)		
Somatomedin C	P			Immunoassay	1
Female					
Preadolescent		60.8–724.5 ng/ml	60.8–724.5 μg/liter		
Adolescent		112.5–450.0 ng/ml	112.5–450.0 μg/liter		
Adult		141.8–389.3 ng/ml	141.8–389.3 μg/liter		
Male					
Preadolescent		65.5–841.5 ng/ml	65.5–841.5 μg/liter		

Adolescent		83.3–378.0 ng/ml	83.3–378.0 μg/liter		
Adult		54.0–328.5 ng/ml	54.0–328.5 μg/liter		
Testosterone, total, morning sample	P			Immunoassay	0.03467
Female		20–90 ng/dl	0.7–3.1 nmol/liter		
Male, adult		300–1100 ng/dl	10.4–38.1 nmol/liter		
Testosterone, unbound, morning sample	P			Equilibrium dialysis	34.67
Female, adult		0.09–1.29 ng/dl	3–45 pmol/liter		
Male, adult		3.06–24.0 ng/dl	106–832 pmol/liter		
Thyroglobulin	S	0–60 ng/ml	0–60 μg/liter	Immunoassay	1
Thyroid-hormone–binding index		0.83–1.17	0.83–1.17	Charcoal resin	1
Thyroid-stimulating hormone	S	0.5–5.0 μU/ml	0.5–5.0 mU/liter	Immunoassay	1
Thyroxine, free	S	0.8–2.7 ng/dl	10–35 pmol/liter	Direct equilibrium dialysis	12.87
Thyroxine-binding globulin	S	Age and sex dependent	Age and sex dependent	Immunoassay	
Thyroxine, free, index		4.6–11.2	4.6–11.2	Calculation	1
Thyroxine, total (T_4)	S	4–12 μg/dl	51–154 nmol/liter	Immunoassay	12.87
Triiodothyronine, total (T_3)	S	75–195 ng/dl	1.2–3.0 nmol/liter	Immunoassay	0.01536
Vanillylmandelic acid (VMA)	U	1.4–6.5 mg/day	7.1–32.7 μmol/day	Liquid chromatography	5.046

MGH, Massachusetts General Hospital; S, serum; P, plasma; U, urine.

TABLE A–3. IMMUNOLOGY VALUES

Analyte	Fluid	MGH Units	SI Units	Method or Instrument	Factor for Conversion to SI Units
Autoantibodies					
Adrenal gland	S	Negative at 1:10 dilution	Not applicable	Indirect immunofluorescence	
Anticentromere antibodies	S	Negative at 1:40 dilution	Not applicable	Indirect immunofluorescence	
Anti–native DNA antibodies	S	Negative at 1:10 dilution	Not applicable	Indirect immunofluorescence	
Antineutrophil antibodies, direct	WB	Negative	Not applicable	Autologous immunologic assay	
Antineutrophil antibodies, indirect	S	Negative	Not applicable	Staphylococcal conjugated immunologic assay	
Antinuclear antibodies	S	Negative at 1:8 dilution	Not applicable	Indirect immunofluorescence	
La	S	None detected	Not applicable	Indirect immunofluorescence	
Mitochondrial	S	Negative at 1:20 dilution	Not applicable	Indirect immunofluorescence	
RNP	S	None detected	Not applicable	Indirect immunofluorescence	
Ro	S	None detected	Not applicable	Indirect immunofluorescence	
Sm	S	None detected	Not applicable	Indirect immunofluorescence	
Smooth muscle	S	Negative at 1:20 dilution	Not applicable	Indirect immunofluorescence	
Thyroid colloid and microsomal antigens	S	Negative at 1:10 dilution	Not applicable	Indirect immunofluorescence or hemagglutination	
C1-esterase-inhibitor protein	S	12.6–24.6 mg/dl	0.13–0.25 g/liter	Nephelometry	0.01
Complement					
C3	S	83–177 mg/dl	0.83–1.77 g/liter	Nephelometry	0.01
C4	S	15–45 mg/dl	0.15–0.45 g/liter	Nephelometry	0.01
Total hemolytic (CH_{50})	S	150–250 U/ml	150–250 U/liter	Sheep red-cell hemolysis	1
Factor B	S	17–42 mg/dl	0.17–0.42 g/liter	Nephelometry	0.01
Immunoglobulin, quantitation	S			Nephelometry	
IgA		70–312 mg/dl	0.7–3.12 g/liter		0.01
IgG		639–1349 mg/dl	6.39–13.49 g/liter		0.01
IgM		56–352 mg/dl	0.56–3.52 g/liter		0.01
IgE		<103 IU/ml	<247 μg/liter		2.4
Rheumatoid factor (fasting sample)	S	<30 IU/ml	<30 kIU/liter	Nephelometry	1
Viscosity	S	1.4–1.8 relative viscosity units, as compared with water	1.4–1.8 relative viscosity units, as compared with water	Ostwald viscometry	1

MGH, Massachusetts General Hospital; S, serum; WB, whole blood.

Reprinted with permission from the New England Journal of Medicine *327:718–724 (September 3), 1992*

TABLE A–4. HEMATOLOGY AND COAGULATION VALUES

Analyte	Fluid	MGH Units	SI Units	Method or Instrument	Factor for Conversion to SI Units
Alpha$_2$-antiplasmin, functional	P	80–130%	0.80–1.30	Chromogenic assay	0.01
Anti–factor VIIIC titer	P	0 Bethesda units	0 Bethesda units	Automated clotting assay	1
Antiplatelet antibodies	P	Negative	Negative	Serotonin release	1
Antithrombin III	P				
Immunologic		22–39 mg/dl	220–390 mg/liter	Immunoassay	10
Functional		80–120%	0.80–1.20	Chromogenic assay	0.01
Bleeding time		2–9.5 min	2–9.5 min	Surgicutt	1
Clot retraction	P	50–100%/2 hr	0.50–1.00/2 hr	Manual	0.01
D-Dimer screen	P	<0.5 μg/ml	<0.5 mg/liter	Latex agglutination	1
Differential blood count	WB			Automated cell counter	0.01
Neutrophils		45–74%	0.45–0.74		
Bands		0–4%	0.00–0.04		
Lymphocytes		16–45%	0.16–0.45		
Monocytes		4–10%	0.04–0.10		
Eosinophils		0–7%	0.00–0.07		
Basophils		0–2%	0.00–0.02		
Erythrocyte count	WB	4.15–4.90 × 10^6/mm^3	4.15–4.90 × 10^{12}/liter	Automated cell counter	1
Erythrocyte sedimentation rate	WB			Manual (modified Westergren method)	1
Female		1–30 mm/hr	1–30 mm/hr		
Male		1–13 mm/hr	1–13 mm/hr		
Factor I, fibrinogen	P	0.15–0.35 g/dl	4.0–10.0 μmol/liter	Automated clotting assay	29.41
Factor II, prothrombin	P	60–140%	0.60–1.40	Automated clotting assay	0.01
Factor V	P	60–140%	0.60–1.40	Automated clotting assay	0.01
Factor VII	P	60–140%	0.60–1.40	Automated clotting assay	0.01
Factor VIII	P	50–200%	0.50–2.00	Automated clotting assay	0.01
Factor IX	P	60–140%	0.60–1.40	Automated clotting assay	0.01
Factor X	P	60–140%	0.60–1.40	Automated clotting assay	0.01
Factor XI	P	60–140%	0.60–1.40	Automated clotting assay	0.01

(continued)

TABLE A–4. HEMATOLOGY AND COAGULATION VALUES *(Continued)*

Analyte	Fluid	MGH Units	SI Units	Method or Instrument	Factor for Conversion to SI Units
Factor XII	P	60–140%	0.60–1.40	Automated clotting assay	0.01
Factor XIII screen	P	Negative	Negative	Urea clot dissolution	1
Ferritin	S			Immunoassay	1
Normal		>20 ng/ml	>20 µg/liter		
Borderline deficient		13–20 ng/ml	13–20 µg/liter		
Deficient		0–12 ng/ml	0–12 µg/liter		
Excessive		>400 ng/ml	>400 µg/liter		
Fibrin(ogen) degradation products	S	<10 µg/ml	<100 mg/liter	Latex agglutination	10
Fletcher factor screen	P	Negative	Negative	Automated clotting assay	1
Folate (folic acid)	S			Immunoassay	2.266
Normal		≥3.3 ng/ml	>7.3 nmol/liter		
Borderline deficient		2.5–3.2 ng/ml	5.7–7.3 nmol/liter		
Deficient		<2.5 ng/ml	<5.7 nmol/liter		
Glucose-6-phosphate dehydrogenase (erythrocyte)	WB	5–15 U/g of hemoglobin	5–15 U/g of hemoglobin	Colorimetry	1
Haptoglobin	S	13–163 mg/dl	0.13–1.63 g/liter	Nephelometry	0.01
Hematocrit	WB			Automated cell counter	0.01
Female		37–48%	0.37–0.48		
Male		42–52%	0.42–0.52		
Hemoglobin	WB			Automated cell counter	0.6206
Female		12–16 g/dl	7.4–9.9 mmol/liter		
Male		13–18 g/dl	8.1–11.2 mmol/liter		
Iron	S	50–150 µg/dl	9.0–26.9 µmol/liter	Colorimetry	0.1791
Iron-binding capacity	S	250–410 µg/dl	45–73 µmol/liter	Colorimetry	0.1791
Leukocyte count	WB	$4.3–10.8 \times 10^3/mm^3$	$4.3–10.8 \times 10^9$/liter	Automated cell counter	1
Lupus inhibitor tests				Automated clotting assay	1
Tissue-thromboplastin-inhibition test	P	Negative	Negative		
Dilute Russell's viper venom test	P	Negative	Negative		
Platelet neutralization procedure	P	Negative	Negative		

Anticardiolipin antibody	S			Immunoassay	1
IgG		0–23 Anti-IgG units	0–23 arbitrary units		
IgM		0–11 Anti-IgM units	0–11 arbitrary units		
Mean corpuscular hemoglobin (MCH)	WB	28–33 pg/cell	28–33 pg/cell	Automated cell counter	1
Mean corpuscular hemoglobin concentration (MCHC)	WB	32–36 g/dl	320–360 g/liter	Automated cell counter	10
Mean corpuscular volume (MCV)	WB	86–98 μm^3	86–98 fl	Automated cell counter	1
50:50 Mixing studies	P	Correction = factor deficiency		Automated clotting assay	1
Osmotic fragility of erythrocytes	WB	Increased if hemolysis occurs at >0.5% sodium chloride		Spectrophotometry	1
Partial-thromboplastin time, activated	P	24–37 sec	24–37 sec	Automated clotting assay	1
Peroxide hemolysis	WB	<10%	<0.10	Manual	0.01
Plasminogen, functional	P	80–130%	0.80–1.30	Chromogenic assay	0.01
Platelet aggregation	PRP	>65% aggregation in response to adenosine diphosphate, epinephrine, collagen, ristocetin, and arachidonic acid		Platelet aggregometry	Not applicable
Platelet count	WB	150–350 × $10^3/mm^3$	150–350 × 10^9/liter	Automated cell counter	1
Platelet, mean volume	WB	6.6–11.0 μm^3	6.6–11.0 fl	Automated cell counter	1
Protein C					0.01
Immunologic		70–140%	0.70–1.40	Immunoassay	
Functional		70–140%	0.70–1.40	Automated clotting assay	
Protein S	P				0.01
Total antigen		70–140%	0.70–1.40	Immunoassay	
Functional		70–140%	0.70–1.40	Automated clotting assay	
Prothrombin time	P	8.8–11.6 sec	8.8–11.6 sec	Automated clotting assay	1
Red-cell distribution width	WB	11.5–14.5%	0.115–0.145	Automated clotting assay	0.01
Reptilase time	P	Within 5 sec of control	Within 5 sec of control	Automated clotting assay	1
Reticulocyte count	WB	0.5–2.5% red cells	0.005–0.025 red cells	Manual	0.01
Ristocetin cofactor (functional von Willebrand factor)	P	50–150%	0.50–1.50	Platelet agglutination	0.01
Thrombin time	P	Within 5 sec of control	Within 5 sec of control	Automated clotting assay	1

(continued)

TABLE A–4. HEMATOLOGY AND COAGULATION VALUES (*Continued*)

Analyte	Fluid	MGH Units	SI Units	Method or Instrument	Factor for Conversion to SI Units
Vitamin B_{12}	S			Immunoassay	0.7378
Normal		205–876 pg/ml	151–646 pmol/liter		
Borderline		140–204 pg/ml	103–150 pmol/liter		
Deficient		<140 pg/ml	<103 pmol/liter		
von Willebrand factor (vWF) antigen (factor VIII:R antigen)	P	50–150%	0.50–1.50	Immunoassay	0.01
von Willebrand factor multimers	P	Normal distribution	Normal distribution	Western blotting	1

MGH, Massachusetts General Hospital; P, plasma; WB, whole blood; S, serum; PRP, platelet-rich plasma.
Reprinted with permission from the New England Journal of Medicine *327:718–724 (September 3), 1992*

APPENDIX B. REFERENCE VALUES FOR NEWBORNS AND CHILDREN COMPARED WITH ADULT VALUES

Name of Test	Change in Value	Explanation for Change Found In
Acid phosphatase	Higher in newborns and children	Chap. 12
Aldolase	Higher in newborns and children	Chap. 12
Alkaline phosphatase	Higher until puberty	Chap. 12
ALT (SGPT)	Higher in newborns	Chap. 12
Ammonia	Higher in newborns, particularly premature infants. Also higher in children	Chap. 10
Amylase	Low or absent in newborns	Chap. 12
AST (SGOT)	Higher in newborns and children	Chap. 12
Bicarbonate	Lower in newborns and slightly lower in children	Chaps. 5, 6
Bilirubin	Higher until 1 month of age	Chap. 11
BUN	Slightly lower in newborns and infants	Chap. 4
C3, C4	Lower at birth	Chap. 14
Calcium	Lower in newborns first few days. Slightly higher in children	Chap. 7
Carbon dioxide content	Lower in infants and children	Chaps. 5, 6
Cholesterol	Lower in children	Chap. 9
Creatinine	Lower in children. Increases with age. Higher in males after puberty	Chap. 4
Creatine kinase	Higher in newborns	Chap. 12
Fibrinogen	Lower in newborns	Chap. 13
GGTP	5 times higher in newborns	Chap. 12
Gonadotropins (FSH and LH)	Lower in children	Chap. 15
Glucose	Lower in newborns and slightly lower in children	Chap. 8
Growth hormone (GH)	Higher in newborns and children	Chap. 15
Hgb, hct, and RBC	High in newborns, lower by 1 year of age, and adult levels by 8–13 years. Infants have some fetal hgb	Chap. 2
Immunoglobulins—IgG, IgA, etc.	Newborns contain some from mother, varies with age	Chap. 10
17-Ketogenic steroids	Low in newborns and increases with age	Chap. 15
LDH	Very high in newborns, child 1–2 times adult	Chap. 12
Magnesium	Slightly lower?	Chap. 7
Metanephrines (urine)	Higher in infants	Chap. 15
pH	Lower in newborns	Chap. 6

(*continued*)

APPENDIX B. REFERENCE VALUES FOR NEWBORNS AND CHILDREN COMPARED WITH ADULT VALUES (*Continued*)

Name of Test	Change in Value	Explanation for Change Found In
Po_2	Lower in newborns	Chap. 6
Phosphorus	Highest in newborns, levels decline by puberty	Chap. 7
Potassium	Slightly higher in newborns	Chap. 5
Pregnanediol	Lower in children	Chap. 15
Pregnantriol	Lower in children	Chap. 15
PT (prothrombin time)	Higher in newborns	Chap. 13
PTT (partial thromboplastin time)	Higher in newborns	Chap. 13
Platelets	Slightly lower in newborns	Chap. 13
Reticulocytes	Higher in newborns	Chap. 2
Sedimentation rate	Slower in newborns and children	Chap. 2
Specific gravity	Lower until 2 years of age	Chap. 3
Testosterone	Much lower in children	Chap. 15
Total protein	Slightly lower in children	Chap. 10
Triglycerides	Lower in children	Chap. 9
T_4	Higher in children and especially newborns	Chap. 15
Uric acid	Lower values until puberty	Chap. 4
Urine osmolality	Lower in newborns	Chap. 4
WBC	Extremely high in newborns, differential also different in children	Chap. 2

Also see other references for specific tests in each chapter. Note that the values for premature infants are not the same as for newborns at term. Consult a specialty text for high-risk neonate care.

References for Appendix B

Cherian, G., and Hill, G. (1978). Percentile estimates of 14 chemical constituents in sera of children and adolescents. *American Journal of Clinical Pathology, 69*, 24–31.

DeCherney, A.H., and Pernoll, M.L. (1994). *Current obstetric & gynecologic diagnosis & treatment* (8th ed.). Norwalk, CT: Appleton & Lange.

Gottfried, E.L. (1994). *Clinical laboratory manual.* San Francisco: San Francisco General Hospital.

Hay, W.W., Groothuis, J.R., Hayward, A.R., and Levin, M.J. (1995). *Current pediatric diagnosis & treatment* (12th ed.). Norwalk, CT: Appleton & Lange.

Kaplan, A., Jack, R., Opheim, K.E., et al. (1995). *Clinical chemistry interpretation and techniques* (4th ed.). Baltimore: Williams & Wilkins.

Meites, S. (1977). *Pediatric clinical chemistry: A survey of normals, methods and instrumentation with commentary.* Washington, DC: American Association for Clinical Chemistry.

Ravel, R. (1995). *Clinical laboratory medicine: Clinical application of laboratory data* (6th ed.). St. Louis: Mosby–Year Book.

APPENDIX C. POSSIBLE ALTERATIONS IN REFERENCE VALUES FOR THE AGED[a]

Name of Test	Possible Change in Value	Explanation for Change Found In
Albumin	Slight decrease	Chap. 10
Alkaline phosphatase	Increase	Chap. 12
Amylase	Increase	Chap. 12
Antinuclear antibodies (ANA)	May be present	Chap. 14
AST	Increase	Chap. 12
Bilirubin	Slight increase	Chap. 11
Blood sugar, fasting and 2-hr pc	Increase	Chap. 8
BUN	Increase	Chap. 4
C3, C4	Increase	Chap. 14
Calcium	May decrease, but still in normal range	Chap. 7
Cholesterol	Increase until older than 70 years	Chap. 9
Cold agglutinins	Increase	Chap. 14
Creatinine clearance	Decrease	Chap. 4
Glucose tolerance test (GTT)	Change in curve	Chap. 8
Gonadotropins (LH, FSH)	Eventual decrease, but increase postmenopausal	Chap. 15
Immunoglobulins	Decreases and alterations	Chap. 10
Lymphocytes	May decrease	Chap. 2
17-Ketosteroids	Decrease	Chap. 15
Magnesium	Slight decrease	Chap. 7
Po_2	Decrease	Chap. 6
Phosphorus	May decrease with age	Chap. 7
Pregnanediol	Decrease in woman	Chap. 15
Rheumatic factor (RF)	May be present	Chap. 14
Sedimentation rate (ESR)	Increase	Chap. 2
T_3 RIA	Decrease?	Chap. 15
Triglycerides	Increase except in very elderly	Chap. 9
Transaminases (SGOT, SGPT)	Slight increase	Chap. 12
Uric acid	Slight increase	Chap. 4
VDRL	May become reactive?	Chap. 14
Vitamin B_{12}	Slight decrease	Chap. 2
WBC	Decrease	Chap. 2

Also see the reference values for specific tests in each chapter. Note that the effect of age on many tests is not known. The figures used for normal may sometimes be more reflective of the common underlying chronic diseases of the elderly rather than of a normal healthy stage. For example, hypertension affects many elderly clients, and it can cause some renal changes that can change the values of various laboratory tests.

[a]References for Appendix C appear on page 764.

References for Appendix C

Cavalieri, T.A., Chopra, A., and Bryman, P.N. (1992). When outside the norm is normal: Interpreting lab data in the aged. *Geriatrics, 47* (5), 66–70.

Cooley, E. (1989). Laboratory tests in the elderly: What is abnormal? *Postgraduate Medicine, 85*, 336–337.

Fülöp, T., Worum, I., Varga, P., et al. (1989). Blood laboratory parameters of carefully selected healthy elderly people. *Archives of Gerontology and Geriatrics, 8*, 151–163.

Gerbodes, K., et al. (1979). Is the elderly patient accurately diagnosed? *Geriatrics, 34*, 91–96.

Gottfried, E.L. (1994). *Clinical laboratory manual.* San Francisco: San Francisco General Hospital.

Harnes, J. (1980). Normal values with increasing age. *Journal of Chronic Disease, 33*, 593–594.

Kaplan, A., Jack, R., Opheim, K.E., et al. (1995). *Clinical chemistry interpretation and techniques* (4th ed.). Baltimore: Williams & Wilkins.

Melillo, K.D. (1993). Interpretation of laboratory values in older adults. *Nurse Practitioner, 18*(7), 59–67.

Ravel, R. (1995). *Clinical laboratory medicine: Clinical application of laboratory data* (6th ed.). St. Louis: Mosby–Year Book.

APPENDIX D. ALTERED REFERENCE VALUES FOR COMMON LABORATORY TESTS IN NORMAL PREGNANCIES

Name of Test	Change in Value	Explanation for Change Found In
ACTH	Decrease	Chap. 15
Aldosterone	Increase	Chap. 15
Alkaline phosphatase	Marked increase	Chap. 12
Albumin	Decrease	Chap. 10
Bilirubin	Occasional increase	Chap. 11
Bicarbonate	Decrease	Chap. 6
Blood glucose	Variations in trimesters	Chap. 8
BUN	Decrease	Chap. 4
C-reactive protein	Increase	Chap. 14
Calcium	Decreases with albumin levels	Chap. 7
P_{CO_2}	Decrease	Chap. 6
Cholesterol	Increase	Chap. 9
Cortisol	Increase	Chap. 15
Creatinine clearance	Increase	Chap. 4
Creatinine (serum)	Decrease	Chap. 4
Fibrinogen levels	Increase	Chap. 13
Folic acid levels	Decrease	Chap. 2
GGTP	Increase	Chap. 12
Hemoglobin, hematocrit	Decrease (dilutional)	Chap. 2
Iron	Decrease	Chap. 2
Magnesium	May decrease	Chap. 7
5′ Nucleotidase	Increase	Chap. 12
Phosphorus	May decrease	Chap. 7
Protein electrophoresis	Change in pattern	Chap. 10
PT	May decrease or same	Chap. 13
PTT	May decrease	Chap. 13
Platelets	Increase	Chap. 13
Retic	Increase	Chap. 2
Sed rate	Increase	Chap. 2
T_3-T_4 and thyroid-binding globulin	Altered values	Chap. 15
Triglycerides	Increase	Chap. 9
Uric acid	Decrease in early pregnancy	Chap. 4
Vitamin B_{12}	Decrease	Chap. 2
WBC	Increase in total and in neutrophils	Chap. 2

Increases or decreases are in relation to the woman's prepregnancy values.
Also see references for specific tests discussed in each chapter.
References for Appendix D appear on page 766.

References for Appendix D

DeCherney, A.H., and Pernoll, M.L. (1994). *Current obstetric & gynecologic diagnosis & treatment* (8th ed.). Norwalk, CT: Appleton & Lange.

Hytten, F., and Lind, T. (1975). Diagnostic indices in pregnancy. Summit, NJ: Ciba-Geigy.

Kaplan, A., Jack, R., Opheim, K.E., et al. (1995). *Clinical chemistry interpretation and techniques* (4th ed.). Baltimore: Williams & Wilkins.

Milne, J.A. (ed.). (1979). Physiological response to pregnancy in health and disease. *Post Graduate Medical Journal, 55,* 293–367.

Ravel, R. (1995). *Clinical laboratory medicine: Clinical application of laboratory data* (6th ed.). St. Louis: Mosby–Year Book.

APPENDIX E. COMMON ABBREVIATIONS FOR LABORATORY TESTS

ABG	Arterial blood gases
ABO	Blood types
ACD	Acid citrate dextrose (anticoagulant)
ACT	Activated coagulation time
ACTH	Adrenocorticotropic hormone
ADH	Antidiuretic hormone
AFB	Acid-fast bacillus
AFP	α-Fetoprotein
AHG	Antihemophilia globulin
A/G ratio	Albumin-to-globulin ratio (outdated)
ALA	(δ) aminolevulinic acid
ALT	Alanine aminotransferase (new term for SGPT)
APPT	Activated partial thromboplastin time (also PTT)
ANA	Antinuclear antibodies
ASO	Antistreptolysin O titer
AST	Asparate aminotransferase (new name for SGOT)
BC	Blood culture
BCP	Biochemical profile; also, birth control pills
BMR	Basal metabolic rate
Br	Bromide
BS	Blood sugar
BSP	Bromsulphalein (dye for liver function test)
BUN	Blood urea nitrogen
C3, C4	Complement factors
C&S	Culture and sensitivity
Ca^{2+}	Calcium
CBC	Complete blood count
CEA	Carcinoembryonic antigen
CF	Complement fixation
CL^-	Chloride
CO_2	Carbon dioxide (P_{CO_2} = partial pressure)
CPK or CK	Creatine phosphokinase
Cr	Chromium
CRP	C-reactive protein
Crit	Hematocrit
CSF	Cerebrospinal fluid
Cu	Copper

(continued)

CUA	Clean urinalysis
Diff	Differential (white blood cell count)
EDTA	Ethylenediaminotetracetate (anticoagulant for blood samples)
ESR	Erythrocyte sedimentation rate
Fe	Iron
FBS	Fasting blood sugar
FEP	Free erythrocyte porphyrins
FSH	Follicle-stimulating hormone
FTA	Fluorescent treponemal antibodies
GC	Gonococcus
GFR	Glomerular filtration rate
GGTP	γ-Glutamyl transferase
GH	Growth hormone
GHB	Glycosylated hemoglobin (A_{1c})
G-6-PD	Glucose-6-phosphatase dehydrogenase
GTT	Glucose tolerance test
HAA	Hepatitis-associated antigen
HAT	Heterophile antibody titer
Hgb	Hemoglobin
HBD	Hydroxybutyric dehydrogenase
HBsAg	Hepatitis B surface antigen
HCG	Human chorionic gonadotropin
Hct	Hematocrit
Hg	Mercury
5HIAA	5-Hydroxyindoleacetic acid
ICSH	Interstitial cell-stimulating hormone (LH in women)
IFA	Immunofluorescence antibody test (may be direct or indirect)
Ig	Immunoglobulin (IgA, IgM, etc.)
IEP	Immunoelectrophoresis
K^{2+}	Potassium
17-KGS	17-Ketogenic steroids
17-KS	17-Ketosteroids
LAP	Leucine aminopeptidase
LDH	Lactic dehydrogenase
LDL	Low-density lipoprotein
LE Prep	Lupus erythematosus test
LE (urine)	Leukocyte esterase
LEP	Lipoprotein electrophoresis
LFT	Liver function tests
LH	Luteinizing hormone (ICSH in men)
Li	Lithium
lytes	Electrolytes (Na, K, Cl, bicarbonate)
MCH	Mean corpuscular hemoglobin (erythrocyte indices)
MCHC	Mean corpuscular hemoglobin concentration (erythrocyte indices)
MCV	Mean corpuscular volume (erythrocyte indices)

MHA	Microhemagglutination test
Mg	Magnesium
MIC	Minimal inhibitory concentration
N	Nitrogen
Na^{2+}	Sodium
NC	Normal color
NL	Normal
NPN	nonprotein nitrogen
O_2	Oxygen (Po_2 = partial pressure)
O&P	Ova and parasites
17-OH	17-Hydroxysteroids
OTC	Over-the-counter (drugs)
P	Phosphorus
Pb	Lead
PBI	Protein-bound iodine (outdated)
PCV	Packed cell volume (hematocrit)
pH	Hydrogen-ion concentration
PKU	Phenylketonuria
Pl.ct.	Platelet count
PMN	Polymorphonuclear (type of WBC)
PMV	Platelet mean volume
PSP	Phenolsulfonphthalein (dye for renal excretion test)
PPLO	Pleuropneumonia-like organism (has characteristics between virus and bacteria)
PT	Prothrombin time
PTH	Parathyroid hormone or parathormone
PTT	Partial thromboplastin time (*see also* APTT)
PP or PC	Postprandial (or after meals)
QNS	Quantity not sufficient
RAST	Radioallergosorbent test
RAI	Radioactive iodine
RBC	Red blood cell count
RDW	Red cell distribution width
Retic	Reticulocyte count
RF	Rheumatoid factor (also called RA factor)
Rh	Rhesus; Rh factor in blood
RIA	Radioimmunoassay
R/O	Rule out
RPR	Rapid plasma reagin
segs	Segmented neutrophils of WBC
S&A	Sugar and acetone
SG	Specific gravity
SGOT	Serum glutamic-oxaloacetic transaminase (newer name is AST)
SGPT	Serum glutamic-pyruvic transaminase (newer name is ALT)
SMA	Sequential multiple analyzer (SMA-6 does 6 tests; SMA-12, 12 tests)
SPEP	Serum protein electrophoresis
Stat	Immediately

(*continued*)

APPENDIX E. COMMON ABBREVIATIONS FOR LABORATORY TESTS (*Continued*)

STS	Serologic test for syphilis
T-C	Type and cross match
T&S	Type and screen
T_3	Triiodothyronine
T_4	Thyroxine
TPI	Treponema pallidum immobilization
TBG	Thyroid-binding globulin
TIBC	Total iron-binding capacity
TP	Total protein
TRH	Thyroid-releasing hormone
TSH	Thyroid-stimulating hormone (thyrotropin)
TSP	Total serum proteins
UA	Urinalysis
UC	Urine culture
UrAc	Uric acid
VDRL	Venereal Disease Research Laboratories (test for syphilis)
VLDL	Very low-density lipoprotein
VMA	Vanillylmandelic acid
WBC	White blood cell count
WNL	Within normal limits
WNR	Within normal range
X match	Cross match (of blood)
X	Female chromosome
Y	Male chromosome

Compiled from various sources. Some abbreviations are common in Canada. See Watson, E.M. (1974). Clinical Laboratory Procedures. *Canadian Nurse, 70,* 25–44.

APPENDIX F. COMMON ABBREVIATIONS FOR DIAGNOSTIC PROCEDURES

ABG	Arterial blood gases
AFP	α-Fetoprotein
BE	Barium enema
BMR	Basal metabolic rate
CT scan	Computed tomography (*also* CAT)
CSF	Cerebrospinal fluid
CVS	Chorionic villus sampling
ECG	Electrocardiogram
ECHO	Echocardiogram
EEG	Electroencephalogram
EGD	Esophagogastroduodenoscopy
EMG	Electromyelogram
ERCP	Endoscopic retrograde cholangiopancreatography (*also* ECPG)
FEF	Forced expiratory flow
FEV_1	Forced expiratory volume in 1 sec
FVC	Forced vital capacity
GA	Gastric analysis
GB series	Gallbladder series
GFR	Glomerular filtration rate
GI series	Gastrointestinal series
I-131, I-123, etc.	Radioactive iodine
IVC	Intravenous cholangiogram
IVP	Intravenous pyelogram
KUB	Kidneys, ureters, bladder (flat plate of abdomen)
LP	Lumbar puncture
L/S ratio	Lecithin-to-sphingomyelin ratio
MBC	Maximal breathing capacity (*also* MVV)
MRI	Magnetic resonance imaging (*see* NMR)
MVV	Maximum voluntary ventilation (*also* MBC)
NMR	Nuclear magnetic resonance (*see* MRI)
NSR	Normal sinus rhythm
NST	Nonstress test (for fetus)
OCG	Oral cholecystogram
OCT	Oxytocin challenge test
PEG	Pneumoencephalogram
PET	Positron emission tomography
PFT	Pulmonary function tests
RAI	Radioactive iodine
RIHSA	Radio-iodinated human serum albumin (for blood volume)
Tc-99	Technetium (radionuclide)
TV	Tidal volume
UGI	Upper gastrointestinal
VC	Vital capacity
VE	Volume exhaled per minute at rest

APPENDIX G. UNITS OF MEASURE

cc	cubic centimeter (same as mL, 1/1,000 liter, which is the preferred term)
cm	centimeter
dL	deciliter (1/10 of a liter)
g	gram (1/1,000 of a kilogram, 15 grains)
hpf	high-power field (microscope)
G%	grams in 100 milliliters
IU	international unit
kg	kilogram (1,000 grams, or 2.2 pounds)
L	liter (1,000 milliliters or 1,000 cubic centimeters)
lpf	low-power field (microscope)
μg	micrograms (1/1,000 milligram)
mCi	millicurie
mEq	milliequivalent (*see* Chapter 5 for formula)
mg	milligram (1/1,000 gram)
mg%	milligrams in 100 milliliters (same as dL)
mIU	milliinternational unit (1/1,000 IU)
mL	milliliter (1/1,000 liter, same as cc)
mm	millimeter (1/10 centimeter)
mm^3	cubic millimeter (*see* RBC, Chap. 2)
mm Hg	millimeters of mercury (*see* blood gases, Chap. 6)
mmol	millimoles (*see* Chap. 1 on SI units)
mOsm	milliosmoles (*see* Chap. 4)
ng	nanogram (1/1,000 microgram, *see* Chap. 15)
pg	picogram (1/1,000 nanogram, *see* Chap. 15)
QNS	quantity not sufficient
SI	international system (*see* Chap. 1)
u	international enzyme unit
μ	micro
μg	microgram (1/1,000 milligram)
w/v	weight/volume
μCi	microcurie (1/1,000 of a millicurie)
WNL	within normal limits
WNR	within normal range
$<$	less than
$>$	greater than

APPENDIX H. ANSWERS TO QUESTIONS FOR PART I (LABORATORY TESTS)

CHAPTER 1

1. c
2. d
3. b
4. c
5. d
6. b
7. c
8. b
9. d

CHAPTER 2

1. d
2. c
3. b
4. a
5. c
6. c
7. d
8. a
9. d
10. c
11. a
12. c
13. a
14. d
15. a

CHAPTER 3

1. c
2. d
3. d
4. a
5. d
6. c
7. d
8. b
9. d
10. c
11. b

CHAPTER 4

1. c
2. a
3. b
4. d
5. c
6. b
7. b
8. c
9. a
10. b
11. a

CHAPTER 5

1. b
2. a
3. b
4. b
5. b
6. c
7. a
8. b
9. a
10. c
11. c
12. a
13. b
14. b
15. c
16. b
17. d

CHAPTER 6

1. b
2. a
3. a
4. d
5. d
6. d
7. b
8. b
9. a
10. b
11. d
12. b
13. b
14. c
15. a
16. a
17. b
18. d
19. d
20. b
21. c

CHAPTER 7

1. a
2. c
3. d
4. c
5. d
6. b
7. c
8. c
9. d
10. a
11. a
12. d
13. c
14. b

CHAPTER 8

1. c
2. d
3. b
4. c
5. d
6. a
7. a
8. c
9. b
10. c
11. c
12. a
13. a
14. d

(continued)

CHAPTER 9

1. a
2. c
3. a
4. d
5. b
6. b
7. d
8. a

CHAPTER 10

1. d
2. c
3. d
4. b
5. b
6. b
7. a
8. b
9. c
10. a
11. c
12. c
13. d

CHAPTER 11

1. d
2. d
3. c
4. c
5. b
6. a
7. d
8. d
9. c
10. a
11. c
12. b

CHAPTER 12

1. a
2. a
3. a
4. d
5. a
6. a
7. a
8. c
9. d
10. a
11. b

CHAPTER 13

1. d
2. a
3. a
4. b
5. d
6. d
7. d
8. b
9. d
10. d
11. c
12. d
13. b
14. b
15. b
16. a
17. b

CHAPTER 14

1. d
2. b
3. a
4. b
5. a
6. c
7. d
8. d
9. d
10. a
11. d
12. c
13. d
14. b

CHAPTER 15

1. c
2. a
3. c
4. b
5. c
6. b
7. d
8. c
9. d
10. c
11. a
12. b

CHAPTER 16

1. c
2. d
3. b
4. a
5. c
6. a
7. b
8. d
9. a
10. b
11. c
12. b
13. b
14. a

CHAPTER 17

1. c
2. c
3. d
4. b
5. a
6. b
7. c
8. b
9. c
10. c
11. d
12. c

CHAPTER 18

1. b
2. a
3. b
4. c
5. a
6. a
7. c
8. d
9. c

APPENDIX I. ANSWERS TO QUESTIONS FOR PART III (DIAGNOSTIC PROCEDURES)

CHAPTER 20

1. a
2. c
3. d
4. b
5. d
6. d
7. a
8. d
9. a
10. d
11. a
12. a
13. c

CHAPTER 21

1. c
2. b
3. a
4. d
5. b
6. b
7. b

CHAPTER 22

1. b
2. c
3. d
4. b
5. c
6. a
7. a
8. d
9. a

CHAPTER 23

1. b
2. c
3. c
4. a
5. d
6. b
7. d
8. d
9. b

CHAPTER 24

1. c
2. d
3. c
4. c
5. d
6. c
7. a
8. a
9. d
10. d
11. d
12. b

CHAPTER 25

1. a
2. a
3. c
4. c
5. a
6. c
7. a
8. c
9. c
10. c

CHAPTER 26

1. c
2. a
3. d
4. b
5. c
6. d
7. c

CHAPTER 27

1. d
2. b
3. b
4. d
5. a
6. c

CHAPTER 28

1. d
2. a
3. c
4. d
5. c
6. a
7. a
8. c
9. b

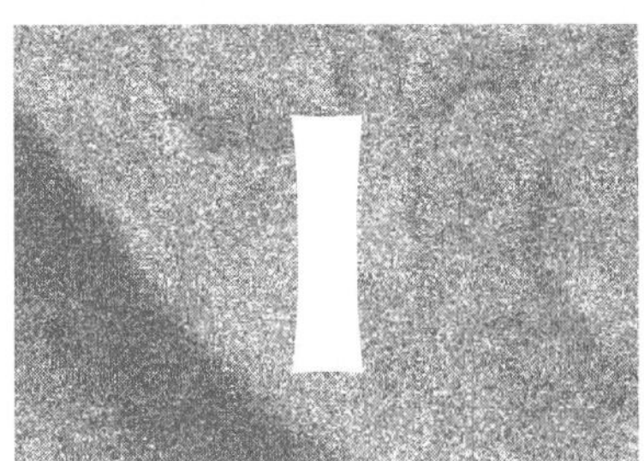

INDEX

A

Entries followed by *t* or *f* refer to tables or figures, respectively.

Entries followed by *t* or *f* refer to tables or figures, respectively.

B

Entries followed by *t* or *f* refer to tables or figures, respectively.

C

Entries followed by *t* or *f* refer to tables or figures, respectively.

D

Entries followed by *t* or *f* refer to tables or figures, respectively.

E

Entries followed by *t* or *f* refer to tables or figures, respectively.

Entries followed by *t* or *f* refer to tables or figures, respectively.

H

Entries followed by *t* or *f* refer to tables or figures, respectively.

I

Entries followed by *t* or *f* refer to tables or figures, respectively.

J

K

L

M

Entries followed by *t* or *f* refer to tables or figures, respectively.

N

Entries followed by *t* or *f* refer to tables or figures, respectively.

O

P

Entries followed by *t* or *f* refer to tables or figures, respectively.

Q

R

S

Entries followed by *t* or *f* refer to tables or figures, respectively.

T

U

Entries followed by *t* or *f* refer to tables or figures, respectively.

V

W

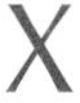

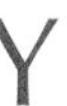

Z

SI Conversion Factors for Values in Clinical Chemistry *(continued from first page)*

Component	Present Reference Intervals (Examples)	Present Unit	Conversion Factor	SI Reference Intervals	SI Unit Symbol	Suggested Minimum Increment
imipramine (P)						
therapeutic	50–200	ng/mL	3.566	180–710	nmol/L	10 nmol/L
insulin (P, S)	5–20	μU/mL	7.175	35–145	pmol/L	5 pmol/L
iron (S)						
male	80–180	μg/dL	0.1791	14–32	μmol/L	1 μmol/L
female	60–160	μg/dL	0.1791	11–29	μmol/L	1 μmol/L
iron binding capacity (S)	250–460	μg/dL	0.1791	45–82	μmol/L	1 μmol/L
lactate (P) (as lactic acid)	0.5–2.0	mEq/L	1.00	0.5–2.0	mmol/L	0.1 mmol/L
	5–20	mg/dL	0.1110	0.5–2.0	mmol/L	0.1 mmol/L
lactate dehydrogenase (S)	50–150	U/L	0.01667	0.82–2.66	μkat/L	0.02 μklat/L
lead (B)-toxic	>60	μg/dL	0.04826	>2.90	μmol/L	0.05 μmol/L
		mg/dL	48.26		μmol/L	0.05 μmol/L
lipase (S)	0–160	U/L	0.01667	0–2.66	μkat/L	0.02 μkat/L
lipoproteins (P)						
low density (LDL) as cholesterol	50–190	mg/dL	0.02586	1.30–4.90	mmol/L	0.05 mmol/L
lithium ion (S)						
therapeutic	0.50–1.50	mEq/L	1.00	0.50–1.50	mmol/L	0.05 mmol/L
luteinizing hormone (S)						
male	3–25	mIU/L	1.00	3–25	IU/L	1 IU/L
female	2–20	mIU/L	1.00	2–20	IU/L	1 IU/L
metanephrines (U) (as normetanephrine	0–2.0	mg/24 h	5.458	0–11.0	μmol/d	0.5 μmol/d
osmolality (P)	280–300	mOsm/kg	1.00	280–300	mmol/kg	1 mmol/kg
osmolality (U)	50–1200	mOsm/kg	1.00	50–1200	mmol/kg	1 mmol/kg
phenobarbital (P)						
therapeutic	2–5	mg/dL	43.06	85–215	μmol/L	5 μmol/L
phenytoin (P)						
therapeutic	10–20	mg/L	3.964	40–80	μmol/L	5 μmol/L
phosphate (S) (as phosphorus, inorganic)	2.5–5.0	mg/dL	0.3229	0.80–1.60	mmol/L	0.05 mmol/L
potassium ion (S)	3.5–5.0	mEq/L	1.00	3.5–5.0	mmol/L	0.1 mmol/L
		mg/dL	0.2558		mmol/L	0.1 mmol/L
potassium ion (U) (diet dependent)	25–100	mEq/24 h	1.00	25–100	mmol/d	1 mmol/d
pregnanediol (U)						
normal	1.0–6.0	mg/24 h	3.120	3.0–18.5	μmol/d	0.5 μmol/d
pregnancy	depends on gestation					

(see reverse side)

SI Conversion Factors for Values in Clinical Chemistry

Component	Present Reference Intervals (Examples)	Present Unit	Conversion Factor	SI Reference Intervals	SI Unit Symbol	Suggested Minimum Increment
pregnanetriol (U)	0.5–2.0	mg/24 h	2.972	1.5–6.0	μmol/d	0.5 μmol/d
procainamide (P)						
therapeutic	4.0–8.0	mg/L	4.249	17–34	μmol/L	1 μmol/L
toxic	>12.0	mg/L	4.249	>50	μmol/L	1 μmol/L
N-acetylprocainamide (P)						
therapeutic	4.0–8.0	mg/L	3.606	14–29	μmol/L	1 μmol/L
progesterone (P)						
follicular phase	<2	ng/mL	3.180	<6	nmol/L	2 nmol/L
luteal phase	2–20	ng/mL	3.180	6–64	nmol/L	2 nmol/L
prolactin	<20	ng/mL	1.00	<20	μg/L	1 μg/L
protein, total (S)	6.0–8.0	g/dL	10.0	60–80	g/L	1 g/L
quinidine (P)						
therapeutic	1.5–3.0	mg/L	3.082	4.6–9.2	μmol/L	0.1 μmol/L
toxic	>6.0	mg/L	3.082	>18.5	μmol/L	0.1 μmol/L
salicylate (S) (salicylic acid)						
toxic	>20	mg/dL	0.07240	>1.45	mmol/L	0.05 mmol/L
sodium ion (S)	135–147	mEq/L	1.00	135–147	mmol/L	1 mmol/L
sodium ion (U)	diet dependent	mEq/24 h	1.00	diet dependent	mmol/d	1 mmol/d
testosterone (P)						
female	0.6	ng/mL	3.467	2.0	nmol/L	0.5 nmol/L
male	4.6–8.0	ng/mL	3.467	14.0–28.0	nmol/L	0.5 nmol/L
theophylline (P)						
therapeutic	10.0–20.0	mg/L	5.550	55–110	μmol/L	1 μmol/L
thyroid tests:						
thyroid stimulating hormone (TSH) (S)	2–11	μU/mL	1.00	2–11	mU/L	1 mU/L
thyroxine (T_4) (S)	4.0–11.0	μg/dL	12.87	51–142	nmol/L	1 nmol/L
thyroxine binding globulin (TBG) (S) (as thyroxine)	12.0–28.0	μg/dL	12.87	150–360	nmol/L	1 nmol/L
thyroxine, free (S)	0.8–2.8	ng/dL	12.87	10–36	pmol/L	1 pmol/L
triiodothyronine (T_3) (S)	75–220	ng/dL	0.01536	1.2–3.4	nmol/L	0.1 nmol/L
T_3 uptake (S)	25–35	%	0.01	0.25–0.35	1	0.01
transferrin (S)	170–370	mg/dL	0.01	1.70–3.70	g/L	0.01 g/L
triglycerides (P) (as triolein)	<160	mg/dL	0.01129	<180	mmol/L	0.02 mmol/L
urea nitrogen (S)	8–18	mg/dL	0.3570	3.0–6.5	mmol/L UREA	0.5 mmol/L
urea nitrogen (U)	2.0–20.0	g/24 h	35.700	450–700	mmol/d	10 msmol/d
urobilinogen (U)	0.0–4.0	mg/24 h	1.693	0.0–6.8	μmol/d	0.1 μmol/d